PLEASE

THE

A

The PRIMARY PREVENTION *of* RHEUMATIC DISEASES

This book is published in collaboration with the

International League Against Rheumatism

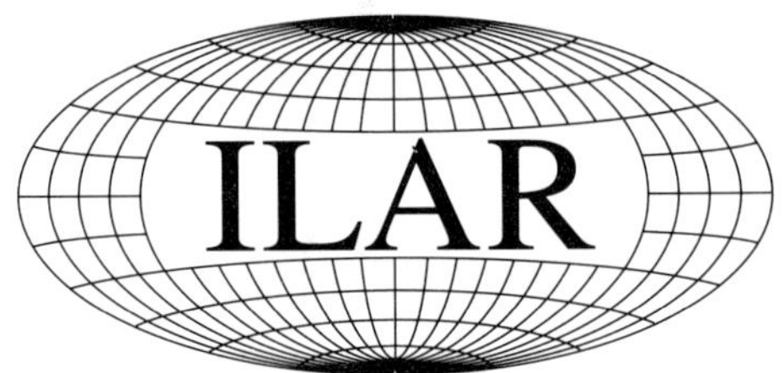

The
PRIMARY
PREVENTION
of
RHEUMATIC
DISEASES

EDITED BY R. D. WIGLEY

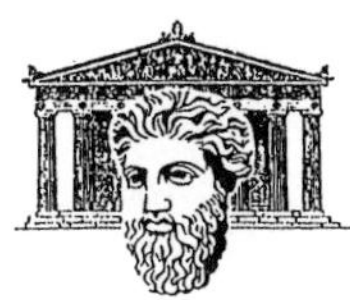

The Parthenon Publishing Group

International Publishers in Medicine, Science & Technology

Casterton Hall, Carnforth,
Lancs LA6 2LA, UK

One Blue Hill Plaza, Pearl River
New York 10965, USA

Published in the UK and Europe by
The Parthenon Publishing Group Limited
Casterton Hall, Carnforth
Lancs, LA6 2LA, England

Published in the USA by
The Parthenon Publishing Group Inc.
One Blue Hill Plaza
PO Box 1564, Pearl River
New York 10965, USA

British Library Cataloguing in Publication Data
Primary Prevention of Rheumatic Diseases
  I. Wigley, R.D.
  616.7

ISBN 1-85070-366-3

Library of Congress Cataloging-in-Publication Data
Primary prevention of rheumatic diseases / edited by R.D. Wigley.
        p.   cm.
    Includes bibliographical references and index.
    ISBN 1-85070-366-3 : $65.00
    1. Rheumatism—Prevention.   2. Musculoskeletal system—Diseases—
Prevention.   I. Wigley, R. D. (Richard Drummond), 1921–
    [DNLM: 1. Rheumatic Diseases—prevention & control.   WE 544 P952]
RC927.P668   1992
616.7′2305—dc20
DNLM/DLC
for Library of Congress   92–49960
                                                                          CIP

First published 1994

Lasertypesetting by Martin Lister Publishing Services, Bolton-le-Sands, Carnforth, Lancs

Printed in Great Britain by Butler & Tanner Limited, Frome and London

CONTENTS

LIST OF CONTRIBUTORS

Professor Erik Allander
Department of Social Medicine
Karolinska Institute, Huddinge Hospital
Huddinge, Sweden

Professor John A.D. Anderson
Faculty of Medicine and Health Sciences
United Arab Emirates University
UAE

Dr David Barraclough
Department of Rheumatology
Royal Melbourne Hospital
Parkville, Melbourne
Victoria 3050, Australia

Professor Lydia I. Benevolenskaya
Institute of Rheumatology
USSR Academy of Medical Sciences
Moscow, Russia

Professor Anders Bjelle
Department of Medicine
University of Gothenburg
Sahlgren Hospital
Gothenburg, Sweden

Dr Angelina Blaauw
Department of Rheumatology
University of Limburg
Maastricht, The Netherlands

Professor W. Watson Buchanan
Department of Medicine
McMaster University
Hamilton, Ontario, Canada

Dr John Darmawan
President, APLAR
Seroja Arthritis Center
Jalan Seroja Dalam 7
Semarang 50241, Indonesia

Professor Peter Disler
Director, Medical Rehabilitation Unit
Palmerston North Hospital and Massey
    University
Palmerston North, New Zealand

Dr Clifford Eastmond
Department of Rheumatology
City Hospital
Aberdeen AB9 8AU, Scotland, UK

Professor Bryan Emmerson
Department of Medicine
Princess Alexandra Hospital
University of Queensland
Brisbane, Queensland 4102, Australia

Professor William R. Felts
Department of Medicine
George Washington School of Medicine
Washington, DC, USA

Professor Robert Fraser
Department of Medicine
Royal Melbourne Hospital
Parkville, Melbourne
Victoria 3050, Australia

Dr Anthony Gear
Department of Rheumatology
Palmerston North Hospital
Palmerston North, New Zealand

Professor James Gear
South African Institute for Medical Research
    and National Institute for Virology
Private Bag X4
Sandringham 2131, South Africa

Professor Nortin M. Hadler
Department of Medicine
University of North Carolina
Chapel Hill, NC 27599-7280, USA

Dr Marc C. Hochberg
Department of Rheumatology
Welch Center for Prevention, Epidemiology
    and Clinical Research
University of Maryland
Baltimore, MD 21205, USA

Dr Nikolai Khaltaev
Department of Non-Communicable Diseases
World Health Organization
CH-1211 Geneva 27, Switzerland

Dr Muhammad Asim Khan
Director, Division of Rheumatology
Case Western Reserve University
Metro Health Medical Center
3395 Scranton Road, Cleveland, Ohio, USA

Dr Peter Lee
Department of Rheumatology
The Wellesley Hospital
160 Wellesley Street
Toronto, M4Y 1J3, Canada

Professor Kenneth D. Muirden
Department of Medicine
Royal Melbourne Hospital
Parkville, Melbourne
Victoria 3050, Australia

Professor Patrick J. Rooney
Department of Medicine
McMaster University
Hamilton, Ontario, Canada

Dr Alan J. Silman
Director, ARC Epidemiology Unit
Medical School, Manchester University
Manchester, UK

Dr Richard Talbot
Department of Cardiology
Waikato Hospital, Hamilton, New Zealand

Professor Sjef van der Linden
Department of Internal Medicine, Division of
    Rheumatology
University of Limburg
Maastricht, The Netherlands

Dr Richard Wigley
Director, WHO Collaborating Centre for
    Epidemiology of Rheumatic Diseases
Palmerston North Hospital
Palmerston North
New Zealand

Dr Ann Williamson
Principal Research Scientist
National Institute of Occupational Health and
    Safety
Sydney, NSW 2001, Australia

FOREWORD

Disease prevention depends firstly on a clear understanding of causation and secondly, on practical methods for controlling major etiological factors. What has to be acknowledged is that virtually all diseases are caused by multiple factors and frequently are due to the summation of complex genetic, hormonal, viral and psychosocial influences. Thus, infection depends not only on the virulence of the microorganism but on host resistance mechanisms. The remarkable decline in infant mortality and the extension in human life-span, involving both developing and developed countries alike, has been influenced by social and economic developments and public health-orientated measures (such as clean water and sewerage) rather more than by developments in medical research. However, the identification of important disease risk factors for a number of common conditions such as smoking, solar exposure, dietary fat and alcohol has led to further reductions in disease prevalence and mortality in some countries at least.

The very success of strategies to reduce the mortality from circulatory, nutritional and diseases due to infection has had the predictable result of leaving communities more exposed to the chronic non-communicable diseases, especially those affecting the elderly. It is possible that the burden of pain and disability as well as from an economic point of view could be substantial if effective preventative strategies are not identified and implemented. An important World Health Organization (WHO) memorandum of as long ago as 1976 puts this as follows:

... so far much effort has been directed at killing diseases whereas crippling diseases are relatively neglected – yet the social and economic burden which the latter imposes is probably greater.

Arthritic and musculoskeletal diseases (sometimes categorized erroneously as 'diseases of affluence') may not dominate mortality statistics. However, they figure in the top three causes of acute illness, chronic illness and disability using Australian Health Survey figures. They account for 9% of acute hospital bed days and 9% of general practitioner consultations.

The message must be that to redress this problem of enormous proportions, preventive strategies must be identified and urgently acted upon. However, as Richard Wigley has so clearly articulated, rheumatologists seem blinded by their frustration at not being able to control the progress of some major rheumatic diseases such as rheumatoid arthritis and osteoarthritis and are inclined to forget that the causes of many rheumatic complaints are understood to the extent that control measures are feasible. Some of the dramatic public health measures applicable to other fields, such as compulsory motor vehicle seat belt usage, limitation of tobacco and alcohol advertising require legislative action backed by a sizeable positive public attitude. Others, however, require the action of individual doctors with the motivation and necessary skill to offer preventative care. Preventative care may be seen by health departments as equated with cost savings or minimization of the impact of the elderly on health budgets. In fact, resources may not always be saved by preventive strategies because many people may need to be subjected to interventions to prevent a small group of people developing a problem. For example, the cost benefit of hormone replacement therapy to prevent postmenopausal osteoporosis still needs to be clarified more fully.

This publication, sponsored by WHO and the International League Against Rheumatism (ILAR) sets out to review what is known about preventing arthritis and the musculoskeletal disorders. Like other biomedical sciences, preventive medicine is now based on firm scientific foundations and the application of knowledge, much of it recently compiled, is essential to provide optimal benefits in the pursuit of world health and the promotion of well-being.

Kenneth D. Muirden
President, The International League
Against Rheumatism

1. NATIONAL AND INTERNATIONAL STATISTICS

William R. Felts

INTRODUCTION

Most forms of arthritis have etiologies which are as yet unspecified and pose a significant impediment to primary prevention activities. The secondary prevention applied to rheumatic disease focuses upon efforts to diminish the complications of illnesses, or to reduce the disability from arthritis that has already developed. National and international statistical data are helpful in the development of initiatives directed toward prevention, and in addressing other problems associated with these diseases confronting society and the afflicted individuals. Data gathered from focused and general studies are important in the study of specific conditions and in aggregates of rheumatic diseases. Epidemiological analysis seeks to ascertain prevalence, incidence, mortality and etiology, and has been expanded to encompass such concerns as costs, outcome assessment and optimal allocation of resources. Dependable statisticians are essential for these studies.

IMPACT OF RHEUMATIC DISEASES

The burdens imposed by rheumatic and musculoskeletal diseases upon society, families and individuals must be examined when one seeks to predict the potential impact of prevention activities. Although arthritis produces a broad array of 'peripheral' effects on society, including the needs for health care facilities, manufacture of drugs, assistive and prosthetic devices, construction of buildings with barrier-free entrances,

establishment of a transfer of payments system for income loss, and other effects, the most profound effect is the loss of productivity through unemployment[1].

In the United States, the aggregated economic impact of rheumatic diseases was projected to equal nearly 1% of the gross national product. Ten percent of lost wages in the entire population are attributed to rheumatic co-morbidity, and account for as much as a third of such costs in the non-institutionalized population. These diseases affect 7% of the population and account for 14% of all physician office visits, 9% of all physician in-patient visits, almost 20% of hospital utilization, 10% of all hospital procedures, and 5% of all hospital discharges. These conditions also account for 32% of all persons in the US who claim to be unable to perform major life activities (activities of daily living, ADL), for over 40% of those claiming other limitations in ADL, 32% of all those limited in the amount or kind of major activities, 29% of all those limited in outside activities, and 31% of those experiencing any form of activity limitations. They are directly responsible either as a main or secondary cause for over 2 million persons being unable to perform major activity at all, and for over 5 million having activity limitation in other ways. They are responsible either as a main or secondary cause for limitations in ADL for nearly 1 million Americans and may be directly responsible for the ADL limitations of a million more. They account for

1

close to 800 million restricted activity days (of which over 400 million are for the musculoskeletal condition itself), and over 300 million bed days (of which over 150 million are for this condition) in the last data-year studied. It is noteworthy that between one quarter and one half of labor force participants leave work within a decade of the onset of rheumatic disease[2]. When all age groups are combined, musculoskeletal diseases are the leading cause of limitation of mobility and the second most common cause of activity limitation in the US[3]. The impact of these conditions on society is likely to increase as the US population ages, since the prevalence and severity of rheumatic diseases are greater in the elderly[2].

Measuring the impact of illness, although an imperfect exercise, is important as it directs attention to significant related or secondary problems. As an example, efforts to improve functionality in persons with musculoskeletal conditions may serve to corroborate studies that conclude that the greatest costs incurred by these illnesses are indirect in the form of lost productivity, rather than direct medical expenditures. Effective secondary prevention efforts are needed to reverse these trends.

Changing and varied demographics and economies alter the impact of disease. Musculoskeletal morbidity, although great in any era, is relative to time and place[4]. For public policy to respond to the needs of individuals with musculoskeletal disorders, and to assess their health care 'consumption', the data analyzed should be current and dynamic, an objective that is rarely achievable.

Although these findings may not be directly comparable with those from other developed nations, and may be even less so in developing nations, they serve to underscore the magnitude of the burden imposed by these conditions on one large western nation, and should stimulate others to perform similar assessments with a goal of initiating primary and secondary prevention activities whenever feasible.

ADDITIONAL APPLICATIONS AND DATA GAPS

Health statistics are used by institutions, governments and policy-makers as guides to disease mortality, prevalence, and incidence allowing these sectors to prioritize a population's health care needs. (Note: it is currently easier to derive prevalence than incidence of specific conditions within a population; longitudinal cohort studies are best suited to establish incidence). The existence of large databases and computers allows manipulation of large blocks of data, providing opportunities to fill many gaps in knowledge. Because data analysis is a dynamic science, and accurate quantification of the effects on society and individuals of various disease states is necessary, newer methods for outcome (intervention effectiveness) assessments are needed. One such technique, meta-analysis, is already showing its strength in interpreting the results of multiple small studies, which suffer from the lack of statistical 'power' because of the limited size of the cohort. Conclusions drawn from statistical studies are also affected by the quality of the data, which depends on the accuracy from the original point of data origin through all pathways into the final database. As applications of data to outcome assessments increase, and the need to modify resource allocation priorities expands, there is an increasing demand for more precise information and enhanced analytical techniques[5]. Standardization of major data elements, from diagnoses to outcome measures, is evolving slowly. The achievement of global standardization in data collection would enable more confident international comparisons, but requires much more work, as it is currently hampered by differences among nations in definitions, classifications and taxonomical structures.

2

MUSCULOSKELETAL DISEASE LIMITATIONS

Many unique challenges and obstacles to statisticians are provided by rheumatic and musculoskeletal diseases. Dr Sidney Cobb observed:

The full extent of the rheumatism problem is not demonstrated by reports of diagnosable rheumatic disease. As every practitioner knows, a large proportion of persons seeking treatment for rheumatic diseases have conditions that are not assignable with any confidence to one or another of the diagnostic categories [6].

Although numerous new diagnostic labels have been coined subsequent to Dr Cobb's statement, his observation typifies the experience of clinicians. Most retrospective studies based upon diagnostic data underestimate the prevalence of musculoskeletal diseases, a problem that is further exacerbated by cross-sectional studies in which patients experiencing partial disease remission are statistical 'blind spots'.

Other limitations must be acknowledged. For example, hospital-based statistics regarding rheumatic disease are of limited usefulness when they are applied to a patient population with a group of diseases largely present in ambulatory settings. The data are further complicated by the fact that many patients with these conditions do not seek medical care and are statistically invisible. Furthermore, there are very few tests that establish a definitive diagnosis of rheumatic diseases, which are often identified by applying lists of criteria. Conflicts therefore exist between the epidemiological and clinical diagnoses of rheumatoid arthritis in population samples[7], as, in general, rheumatic diseases lack uniformly accepted diagnostic criteria, and some of the clinical findings are too rare to be reported in currently available surveys. Data from national surveys in the USA are available for osteoarthritis, rheumatoid arthritis, bursitis and gout. Estimates for juvenile arthritis, alkylosing spondylitis, systemic lupus erythematosus, scleroderma and osteoporosis have been projected and are based upon limited regional surveys[8].

Case identification is also problematic, as in many regions the only existent data have been coded and entered in the databases by laymen with limited skills. In addition, the lay individual, general practitioner, epidemiologist and specialist may define and report cases differently. Linguistic and semantic barriers between and among countries may adversely affect the ability to compare data. These limitations illustrate the magnitude of the challenges for researchers in epidemiological applications, impact surveillance, and intervention outcome assessments.

CLASSIFICATION SYSTEMS

Classifications by which observations are catalogued, stored, retrieved and manipulated serve to expedite most studies. Some components of these systems include diagnoses, symptoms and reasons for encounters with the health care system, as well as services and procedures provided, diagnostic criteria, glossaries, the consequences of disease, including impairments, disabilities and handicaps, outcome measurements and functional assessments. Classifications often introduce unique problems, as they may have been formulated for a specific application, but have been subsequently adapted to new tasks with additional, differing objectives. Such goals vary greatly among countries and among researchers.

The International Classification of Diseases[9] is the most prominent example of such a taxonomical system, and provides an excellent example of an approach toward international consensus. It originated as the International List of Causes of Death (ICD) and was first published in 1893 to assist in standardizing and promulgating mortality statistics. With time, the creation and maintenance of the ICD became the responsibility of the World Health Organization (WHO). The ICD is determined by a WHO voting structure representing participating member countries and is influenced by the politics inherent in such an arrangement. Traditionally, member countries are represented by statisticians and epidemiologists, whose epidemiological bias often prevails over the interests of clinicians. This trend changed somewhat during the revision process for ICD-10, as clinicians in several nations became more actively involved in formulating the ICD.

Since the ICD taxonomic classification axes are based primarily upon etiology, it is frequently difficult to perceive a clinical relationship for some of the tabulation sequences of the rheumatic and musculoskeletal disorders. Other than infectious and overuse disorders, most rheumatic diseases are of unknown etiology. The ICD accommodates some clinical entities of undemonstrated causation through the inclusion of syndromes (clusters of symptoms/findings occurring repetitively). 'Rheumatoid arthritis' and 'osteoarthritis' represent syndromes which may ultimately be proven to have multifactorial etiologies and require changes in definitions. Diagnostic criteria for these syndromes change periodically, thereby contributing to distortions of trend analyses. Such effects are inevitable in the absence of known etiologies, and exemplify the inherent limitations of classification systems for epidemiological and other studies.

An overview of the problems of musculoskeletal disease classifications is contained in the ICD for Rheumatology and Orthopedics (ICD-R and O)[11] promulgated by the International League Against Rheumatism (ILAR), in which the principles of classification are reviewed, along with applications to musculoskeletal diseases. Also presented in the ICD-R and O is a tabular listing from ICD-9 of the diagnostic terms and codes most commonly used by rheumatologists and orthopedists. A separate section entitled the 'International Classification of Musculoskeletal Diseases' (ICMSD) provides an alternative sequencing of the diagnoses and codes in a format selected by rheumatologists. It categorizes various arthritic illnesses by clinical patterns rather than by anatomical systems. A section on 'standardization' reviews selected international initiatives that seek to stimulate and promote commonality of data in the quest to improve comparisons among multiple studies. Among such initiatives are the International Classification for Health Problems in Primary Care (ICHPPC-2)[12], the International Classification of Procedures in Medicine[13], the Current Procedural Terminology (CPT-4)[14], the International Classification of Impairments, Disabilities, and Handicaps[15], and other selected examples illustrating the changing dynamics of classification and taxonomies. The coding and descriptive systems, and the processes through which they are derived are important tools in the generation of statistics. They are also worthy of emulation as a framework for progressive international efforts. A second edition based upon ICD-10 is scheduled for publication in 1993.

APPLICATION OF DATA TO DISEASE PREVENTION

An analytical vehicle is required for measuring the results of prevention activities focused on specific conditions. Changes in incidence and prevalence can be effective gauges of primary prevention, and recognition of changes in the incidence or degree of disability can assist in evaluating the outcome of secondary prevention efforts. Rehabilitative interventions can be adjusted accordingly.

Large databases have become major resources for investigators. Compilations of health-related data are increasingly available for public access as a result of enhanced computer technology, its expanding capacities for storage and retrieval,

4

and the development of linkages or networks. Hospitals and other institutions, state and regional health services, national aggregates of mortality statistics, focused surveys, health-care claims data, and relevant information pools contribute to increasingly large and sophisticated databases. However, much work remains in applying analytical techniques for research purposes. Since the quality of the information contained in the databases is highly variable, the diagnostic criteria of these diseases are not standardized, and measurements of impairment and functional capacity are often lacking in uniformity, only gross conclusions are warranted. Continued efforts are required to ensure that sequential generations of these databases will achieve better standardization and enhance their effectiveness for problem evaluation and formulation of public policies by which to address them.

Disability is often considered as a loss or diminishment of work capability. It also has been defined as a functional limitation of greater than 6–12 months on the kind or amount of work an individual would normally do resulting from an acute or chronic health health condition or impairment[16]. Functional limitation and socioeconomical factors are stronger indicators of the likelihood of disability than is the medical diagnosis. Older individuals are more likely to be severely disabled than younger persons with the same condition, and are more prone to co-morbid conditions that exacerbate the severity of the disability. US Social Security Administration data demonstrate that disability rates are more clearly associated with prevalence of conditions in the population than with variations in the specific medical condition causing a disability. In the USA, the National Arthritis Data Group utilized multiple data resources in evaluating disability and identified four diagnostic conditions wherein preventive intervention is recommended to reduce the prevalence and morbidity of musculoskeletal diseases[1]:

(1) *Osteoporosis* Proven effective measures in people over 50 years of age are cyclic administration of estrogens to women whose ovaries have been removed prior to age 50; a calcium intake of 1–1.5 g/day; regular weight-bearing exercises; and measures to reduce the likelihood of falls. Trade-offs associated with estrogen therapy include slightly increased risks of genital and breast malignancies. Low doses of vitamin D may be helpful. Additional medications are under investigation. Weight control lessens the likelihood of developing severe osteoarthritis of weight-bearing joints.

(2) *Rheumatoid arthritis* Improved working conditions for people with rheumatoid disease could substantially reduce their functional limitations. Major elements would include increased job autonomy, improved transportation, redesign of working ergonomics, vocational training of selected individuals and developing home-based job opportunities.

Yelin and colleagues[17] noted that demographic factors, such as social and work-related interactions, are more important than disease status in determining employment outcome. Marital status is the most important single variable in American society, with the unmarried more likely to continue working. Job autonomy is also very important, as a self-employed person or an employee with the latitude to adjust his own hours and working conditions is more likely to remain employed than an assembly-line worker who is bound to a fixed schedule. Surprisingly, working activities and environmental elements such as the requirement for lifting, stooping, climbing, and exposure to high humidity, do not play a significant role in employment status, although these factors are emphasized in determining a patient's functional status in government programs.

In a Canadian study, Robinson and Walters[18] noted that educational level, a relative long employment history in the same position, a non-physically demanding job, marital stability, and enjoyment of the job itself were the prevailing characteristics of patients with rheumatoid arthritis remaining employed despite disability. Morning stiffness and impediments in public transportation were the most difficult obstacles to overcome.

(3) *Back pain* A reduction in 'occupational' back pain would be achieved by a program emphasizing job screening based on a proper ratio of individual muscular strength to job demand, the use of a profile of employee characteristics (height, weight, spinal curvature, etc.) and appropriate job motivational techniques.

(4) *Scoliosis* The amount of psychological stress, back pain and cardiorespiratory impairment resulting from the long-term effects of scoliosis, as well as the expense of corrective surgery, could be reduced by expanded scoliosis screening programs for teenagers and a close follow-up of all identified abnormalities.

(5) *Traumatic morbidity and mortality* The causal relationship between injuries and post-traumatic forms of arthritis and musculoskeletal pain is well known. An example of the usefulness of such data in identifying injuries, analyzing their epidemiology, and maximizing the use of limited resources in initiating preventive measures is epitomized by the following report[19].

The Indian Health Service is responsible for the health care delivery to native Indian Americans. Indian Service Hospitals have been required to report injuries utilizing ICD-9 'E' codes for over 20 years. Aggregate data studies disclosed types of accidents to vary among geographical regions with drowning the most common cause of death in Alaska and burns in the upper continental US. High school injuries were more common on a reservation in Montana. Focused efforts are under way to develop effective prevention interventions concentrating upon the needs of the specific region.

Two geographical areas of high mortality and morbidity from vehicular accidents also were identified on reservations in the states of Arizona and North Carolina. Focused analysis of available data from the former indicated the high incidence locale to be limited to a 1 mile stretch of highway where all the accidents occurred at night. Eight to ten deaths per year and even greater morbidity occurred consistently. A modest expenditure of US$ 39 000 made available jointly by the tribal Council and the county to install adequate lighting on this segment of roadway resulted in accident elimination.

Similar studies in the second state also noted a short segment of highway where pedestrian accidents had been numerous over time with injuries and deaths. Construction of a short, lighted, pedestrian pathway was undertaken. Measurable improvements thereafter were the elimination of mortality and near-total elimination of injuries. The prevention of delayed traumatic arthropathy and rheumatism is apparent but impossible to quantify.

The International Classification of Diseases contains a supplementary classification section devoted to 'External Causes of Injury and Poisoning', in common usage referred to as 'E' codes. Utilization of the section permits classification of environmental events, circumstances, and conditions as the cause of injury, poisoning and other adverse affects. In most countries, including the USA, use of this section is elective and not mandated. However, it is of note that when recording of the ICD 'E' codes was implemented by a limited group of hospitals, problem identification resulted and led to the development of effective prevention strategies[20].

Occupational exposure with injury represents another area where prevention opportunities abound. In 1986, the category 'accidents and adverse effects' ranked first as the cause of death for every age group from 1 year to 45 years of age in the United States[21]. The absence of mandatory 'E' code reporting for most of the American population leaves injury epidemiology in a deplorable state with numerous potential prevention activities unidentified.

HEALTH DATA RESOURCES

Availability of health data from various types of epidemiological and statistical studies varies considerably between developed and developing countries. One information source by which various national resources can be identified is the International Health Data Reference Guide, 1990[22] compiled by the US National Center for Health Statistics (NCHS), which lists the agencies and principal individuals to be contacted for detailed information by nation. This guide contains data about birth, marriage and divorce rates, mortality, hospital statistics including outpatient visits, discharge statistics, and health manpower statistics identified by individual countries. For each country, major population-based surveys, if available, are listed, as are the data contained in each.

An example of the usefulness of multisource data was provided by the National Arthritis Advisory Work Group, which in 1989 generated estimates of the prevalence of selected arthritic and musculoskeletal diseases in the US from available national data and numerous related, but more focused studies[8]. Special epidemiological problems for uncommon diseases can be illustrated by the example of juvenile rheumatoid arthritis[23].

The major databases from which these assessments were made included the National Health Examination Survey which later evolved into the National Health and Nutrition and Examination Surveys (NHANES), and the National Health Interview Survey (NHIS). Both surveys are based on probability samples of the US civilian, non-institutionalized population. The NHIS series obtains information from household questionnaires, and yields a probability sample of circa 111 000 individuals annually. Data are obtained by interview, so the derived statistics measure health status and experience rather than precisely-defined disease-specific prevalence. Oversampling techniques are applied to selected ethnic groups to assure adequate representation. The 1960–62 NHIS and the 1971–75 NHANES focused on data obtained by extensive medical histories, direct examination, clinical and laboratory tests, and radiographs. The latter was based upon a probability sample of 20 749 non-institutionalized civilians, aged 1 to 74 years. A 'detailed' subsample of 6910 adults was administered additional survey elements with radiographs of the knees and hips (excluding women under age 50 years). The 1976–79 NHANES II included osteoarthritis and disc degeneration as target conditions, and radiological examinations from lumbar and cervical spine radiographs became available for public use data tapes.

An example of a large database dedicated to rheumatic diseases in the US is ARAMIS (American Rheumatism Association Medical Information System), which is based primarily at Stanford University. Verified and standardized patient data are collected longitudinally and stored with the participation of numerous regional centers. The ARAMIS has been used to investigate many of the problems of standardization identified in this review, including the dimensions of health outcomes[24]. Other centers have also developed measurement tools for outcome studies in rheumatic disease[25].

Although these surveys illustrate the usefulness of multiple national data-gathering activities, they also underscore the limitations imposed when such data are amassed using multiple methodologies. Caution must be exercised when attempting to compare data among countries, regions and from different studies.

CONCLUSION

It is apparent that the ability to compare health statistics internationally is increasing. National and international collaborations may eventually allow facile epidemiological comparisons and universal interpretation of data. It is recognized (and understandable) that most efforts to standardize the 'tools' of epidemiological research have to date occurred at national levels. The International Classification of Disease has been the most notable international success as a taxonomical system. In spite of the many language and social barriers, professional communication and efforts to expand consensus activities beyond national boundaries are becoming increasingly apparent. The International League Against Rheumatism (ILAR), and its joint efforts with the World Health Organization has become an important organ for furthering efforts focused on the rheumatic diseases. ILAR's epidemiology projects performed jointly by representatives from different countries is also stimulating standardization of these evaluation tools. The US National Institute of Arthritis, Musculoskeletal and Skin Diseases (NIAMS), with the assistance of ILAR is exploring the feasibility of an international clearinghouse of epidemiological study instruments which have met validation criteria. This is viewed as another major step toward standardizing rheumatic disease epidemiological research.

Through continued efforts such as these, the ability for international acquisition and comparison of data will be enhanced. Undoubtedly, the identification of enhanced opportunities for preventive intervention will be a welcome result.

REFERENCES

1. McDuffie FC, Felts WR, Hochberg MC, Lawrence RC *et al*. Arthritis and musculoskeletal diseases, 'Closing the Gap: The Burden of Unnecessary Illness', The Carter Presidential Center, Inc., supplement to Am J Prevent Med. 1987; 5:19–29
2. Felts W, Yelin E. The economic impact of the rheumatic diseases in the United States. J Rheumatol. 1989; 16:867–84
3. Kelsey J. Epidemiology of Musculoskeletal Disorders. New York, Oxford University Press, 1982
4. Yelin EH, Felts WR. A summary of the impact of musculoskeletal conditions in the United States. Arthritis Rheum. 1990; 33:750–755
5. Felts WR Taxonomies for application in rheumatic diseases: quests for uniformity. J Rheumatol. 1983; Suppl. 10:74–77
6. Cobb S The Frequency of the Rheumatic Diseases. Cambridge, Harvard University Press, 1971
7. Allander, E. Conflict between epidemiological and clinical diagnosis of rheumatoid arthritis in a population sample. Scand J Rheumatol. 1973; 1:109–112
8. Lawrence RC, Hochberg MC, Kelsey JL, McDuffie FC, Medsger TA *et al*. Estimates of the prevalence of selected arthritis and musculoskeletal diseases in the United States. J Rheumatol. 1989; 16:427–441
9. International Classification of Diseases, Ninth Revision. Geneva, World Health Organization, 1977
10. International Classification of Diseases, 9th edn, Clinical Modification (ICD-9-CM), Ann Arbor, Michigan, Commission on Professional and Hospital Activities, 1978
11. ICD R and O (International Classification of Diseases to Rheumatology and Orthopedics), International League Against Rheumatism (ILAR), Academy Professional Information Services, 116 West 32nd St., New York, NY 10001, USA, 1985
12. ICHPPC International Classification of Health Problems in Primary Care, 3rd edn (ICHPPC-2-Defined). WONCA, London, Oxford University Press, 1983
13. ICPM International Classification of Procedures in Medicine, 2 vols. Geneva, World Health Organization, 1978

14. Current Procedural Terminology, 4th edn (CPT-4), Monroe, Wisconsin, American Medical Association, 1992

15. International Classification of Impairments, Disabilities and Handicaps. Geneva, World Health Organization, 1980

16. Haber L. Disabling efforts of chronic disease and impairment. J Chronic Dis. 1971; 24:469–489

17. Yelin EH, Meenan R, Nevitt M, Epstein, WV. Work Disability in rheumatoid arthritis: effects of disease, social and work factors. Ann Intern Med. 1980; 93:551

18. Robinson HS, Walters K. Patterns of work – rheumatoid arthritis. Int Rehabil Med. 1978; 1:121

19. Smith R: Presentation to the National Committee on Vital and Health Statistics Subcommittee on Ambulatory and Hospital Care Statistics. Washington, DC, Jan. 16, 1991

20. Felts WR, Ashley JT, Cannon NL, Ertel PY, Jones JM, Steinwald B, Van Amburg GH. Report of the National Committee on Vital and Health Statistics on the Need to Collect External Cause-of-Injury Codes in Hospital Discharge Data. NCHS Working Paper Series #38, 70 pp, June 1991

21. Health United States and Prevention Profile 1989. USA Dept. of Health and Human Services. DHHS Pub. #(PHS) 90-1232, 53-57, Hyattsville, Md, 1990

22. International Health Data Reference Guide, 1990, US Department of Health and Human Services, Office of Planning and Extramural Programs, National Center for Health Statistics, 6525 Belcrest Road, Hyattsville, Md 20782, USA

23. Hochberg MD. The epidemiology of juvenile rheumatoid arthritis; review of current status and approaches for future research. In Lawrence RC, Shulman LE, eds., Epidemiology of Rheumatic Disease. New York, Gower Medical, 1984, pp. 220–230

24. Fries JF, Spitz, PW, Young DY. The dimensions of health outcomes: the health assessment questionnaire, disability and pain scales. J Rheumatol. 1982; 9:789–793

25. Meenan RF, Gertman PM, Mason, JH, Dunaif R. The arthritis impact measurement scales: further investigations of a health status measure. Arthritis Rheum. 1982; 25:1048–1053

2. PREVALENCE OF MAJOR CHRONIC RHEUMATIC DISEASES IN THE USSR[*]

Nikolai Khaltaev[†] and Lydia I. Benevolenskaya[‡]

INTRODUCTION

Chronic rheumatic disease and other disorders of the musculoskeletal system, which include more than 180 distinct nosologies[1], are among the most frequently reported causes of impairment in the adult population in the USSR[2], and are a major cause of work-related disability. Rheumatic diseases are responsible for 15.6% of all first-time disabilities in the recorded year[3]. The records from the Institute of Rheumatology, USSR Academy of Medical Sciences[4] reveal that 75% of all rheumatic diseases that required hospitalization and accompanied by prolonged disability, first occurred under 40 years of age; one-third of them became disabled within the first 3 years of disease onset; 36% remained invalids for more than 11 years.

Epidemiology of chronic rheumatic disease

Often the most prevalent diseases in an adult population are not the most well studied, given the great diversity of these conditions, the lack of unified diagnostic criteria, and the high cost of screening. For the development of effective preventive strategies, knowledge of the true prevalence of these diseases and their risk factors in different populations is critical. In this paper, data on four chronic rheumatic diseases are presented from representative epidemiological surveys of different cities and regions in the USSR. The study methods and diagnostic criteria for these four conditions (rheumatoid arthritis, osteoarthritis, ankylosing spondylitis and gout) are detailed in recent work by Benevolenskaya[5] and Brzhezovsky[6].

RHEUMATOID ARTHRITIS

Rheumatoid arthritis is a chronic systemic disorder of unknown etiology, which is characterized by debilitating musculoskeletal deformities secondary to the destruction of articular tissues and bone erosion resulting in mechanical joint abnormalities. Current understanding of rheumatoid arthritis suggests that it is pathogenically linked to both humoral and cellular immune defects, which may be affected by host immune status and genetics. The reported prevalence of rheumatoid arthritis ranges from 1 to 5%, making it one of the most common inflammatory joint diseases[7,8]. The earliest epidemiological surveys of rheumatoid arthritis in the USSR were conducted from 1962 to 1973 by the Institute of Rheumatology of

---

*The data were collected in different republics of the USSR before its collapse; [†]from the Division of Non-Communicable Disease and Health Technology, World Health Organization, Geneva, Switzerland; [‡]from the Institute of Rheumatology, USSR Academy of Medical Sciences, Moscow

Table 1 Prevalence of rheumatoid arthritis (RA) (%) in different cities of the USSR (> age 15 years)

City	Population screened	*Definite RA* Patient number $M \pm m$		*Probable RA* Patient number $M \pm m$		*Definite & probable RA* Patient number $M \pm m$	
Vilnius[1]	5 640	7	0.12 ± 0.04	0	—	7	0.12 ± 0.04
Novosibirsk[2]	5 404	7	0.13 ± 0.04	1	0.02 ± 0.02	8	0.15 ± 0.05
Krasnovodsk[3]	5 531	16	0.29 ± 0.06	11	0.20 ± 0.05	27	0.49 ± 0.09
Irkutsk[4]	5 811	18	0.31 ± 0.07	7	0.12 ± 0.04	25	0.43 ± 0.08
Yaroslavl[5]	5 967	21	0.35 ± 0.07	13	0.22 ± 0.06	34	0.57 ± 0.09
Odessa[6]	6 592	15	0.23 ± 0.05	31	0.47 ± 0.08	46	0.70 ± 0.10
Total	34 945	84	0.24 ± 0.06	63	0.18 ± 0.05	147	0.42 ± 0.07

	1–4	1–3 $p < 0.05$	1–3
	1–5 $p < 0.05$	1–4	1–4
	2–5	1–5 $p < 0.01$	1–5
		1–6	1–6 $p < 0.01$
		2–3	2–3
		2–5	2–4
		2–6 $p < 0.001$	2–5
			2–6

the USSR Academy of Medical Sciences, in which different cultural and geographical regions with a population of circa 80 000 were investigated, using the Rome criteria (1961) for the diagnosis of rheumatoid arthritis. As shown in Figure 1 the prevalence of definite and probable rheumatoid arthritis in population samples ranged from 0.24 to 1.44%, averaging 0.8%, including 0.2–1.03% prevalence of definite rheumatoid arthritis, average 0.57%, and 0.04–0.89% of probable rheumatoid arthritis, average 0.2%. The prevalence of rheumatoid arthritis as well as definite rheumatoid arthritis was highest in the Baltic Republics of Lithuania and Estonia (Tartu) and lowest in the middle Asian Republics of Uzbekistan (Tashkent) and Tadzhikistan (Dushanbe). A low prevalence of definite rheumatoid arthritis was observed in the far east region (Vladivostok). The prevalence of rheumatoid arthritis is lowest in the middle Asian and far eastern regions of the USSR, and highest in the western part of the country (with the exception of Arkhangelsk, located on the northern coast of the White Sea, which also has a low prevalence). These data also included a category of 'probable' rheumatoid arthritis, which is likely to have included in addition to early and non-typical variants of rheumatoid arthritis, other arthropathies with similar clinical presentations. Thus, the category of 'definite' rheumatoid arthritis provides more accurate information on the prevalence of rheumatoid arthritis. Our data find the typical patient to be a female between 45–64 years of age. One-third of these followed a relatively benign course which did not impair the patient's work capacity.

In Table 1, the results of the latest studies undertaken in six cities are presented. Much attention was paid in these studies to the unification of the diagnostic criteria and standardization. Of 34 945 people aged 15 years and older who were screened, 147 patients with rheumatoid arthritis were identified. According to the more strict and widely used New York criteria (1966) (*see* Chapter 20), the prevalence of definite rheumatoid arthritis was 0.24%; probable rheumatoid arthritis occurred in an additional 0.18%, yielding a total prevalence of rheumatoid arthritis of 0.42%.

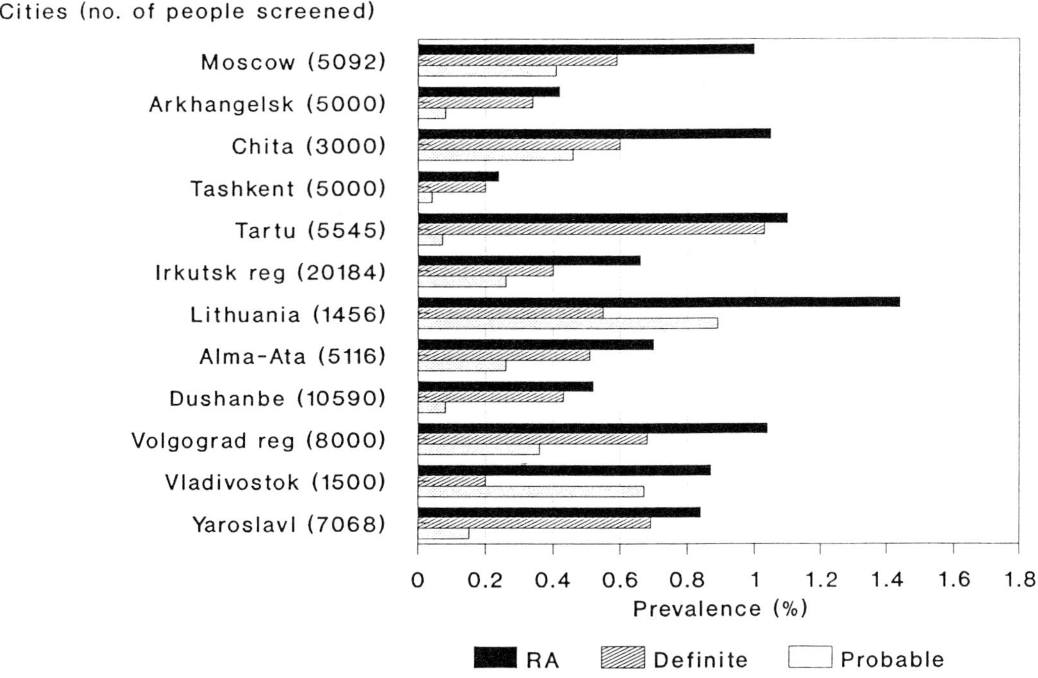

Figure 1 Results of surveys made in 1962–72, illustrating the prevalence of rheumatoid arthritis (RA) in different regions of the USSR. (Reproduced with kind permission from reference 3)

Standardization of the data by sex and age slightly reduced these figures to 0.23% for definite rheumatoid arthritis, 0.17% for probable rheumatoid arthritis, thus totalling 0.40% (Table 2). A low prevalence of rheumatoid arthritis is reported in Vilnius (Lithuania) and Novosibirsk (west Siberian part of the USSR), while in Krasnovodsk (Turkmenistan), Irkutsk (east Siberian part of the USSR), Yaroslavl (central part of USSR) and Odessa (Ukraine) rheumatoid arthritis is two to four times more common. The results of the survey show no obvious influence of climate or geographical location on the prevalence of rheumatoid arthritis. There was a statistically significant difference in rheumatoid arthritis prevalence among males and females in the analysis of the whole data. As elsewhere in the world, in the USSR, rheumatoid arthritis is a 'female' disease, and in our statistics was two to eight times more common in women, affecting 0.34% of females and 0.12% of males, respectively. Rheumatoid arthritis is most prevalent in women 55–64 years of age. In males, there is a similar trend of increased prevalence of rheumatoid arthritis with age. In four out of six cities, the highest prevalence was in those over the 65 years of age, although two-thirds of all patients at the time of screening were in the working age group.

This study shows a prevalence of rheumatoid arthritis in different USSR populations of 0.42±0.07% (definite rheumatoid arthritis in 0.24±0.06%), which is lower than in earlier studies. This finding can be explained by the use of the stricter New York diagnostic criteria (1966), rather than the Rome criteria (1961), which exclude those diseases, e.g. Bekhterew's disease, systemic lupus erythematosus and

Table 2 Age and sex standardized prevalence of rheumatoid arthritis (RA) in different cities of the USSR (standardized by Irkutsk; population of 15 years and older)

City	Definite RA			Probable RA			Total RA		
	Male $M \pm m$	Female $M \pm m$	Both $M \pm m$	Male $M \pm m$	Female $M \pm m$	Both $M \pm m$	Male $M \pm m$	Female $M \pm m$	Both $M \pm m$
Vilnius[1]	0	0.19±0.08	0.11±0.04	0	0	0	0	0.19±0.08	0.11±0.04
Novosibirsk[2]	0.18±0.08	0.17±0.08	0.19±0.06	0	0.03±0.03	0.02±0.02	0.18±0.08	0.20±0.08	0.21±0.06
Krasnovodsk[3]	0.17±0.08	0.53±0.13	0.35±0.08	0.11±0.07	0.26±0.09	0.21±0.06	0.18±0.08	0.79±0.16	0.56±0.10
Irkutsk[4]	0.16±0.08	0.42±0.11	0.31±0.07	0.08±0.06	0.15±0.07	0.12±0.04	0.24±0.10	0.56±0.13	0.43±0.08
Yaroslavl[5]	0.21±0.09	0.33±0.10	0.27±0.07	0.14±0.07	0.23±0.09	0.19±0.06	0.36±0.11	0.57±0.13	0.47±0.09
Odessa[6]	0.04±0.04	0.29±0.09	0.16±0.05	0.17±0.08	0.48±0.12	0.31±0.07	0.21±0.08	0.76±0.15	0.47±0.08
M±m standardized			0.23±0.06			0.17±0.05			0.38±0.06
M±m non-standardized			0.24±0.06			0.18±0.05			0.42±0.07
			$1-3\,p<0.05$ $1-4$	$1-3\,p<0.01$ $1-4\,p<0.05$ $1-5\,p<0.01$ $1-6\,p<0.001$		$2-3\,p<0.01$ $2-5\,p<0.05$ $2-6\,p<0.001$	$1-3,4,5,6\,p<0.001$		$2-3\,p<0.01$ $2-5,6\,p<0.05$

scleroderma, Sjögren syndrome, and psoriatic arthropathy, which may have features in common with rheumatoid arthritis. Nevertheless, a real decrease in the prevalence of rheumatoid arthritis should be also considered (*see* Chapter 20).

OSTEOARTHRITIS

Osteoarthritis, also known as osteoarthrosis or degenerative joint disease, is characterized by degeneration of articular cartilage with proliferation and remodelling of subchondral bone. An estimation of the prevalence of osteoarthritis is difficult for several reasons. First, radiological examination of all joints of the body is required for a definitive diagnosis, which is unjustified both ethically and economically in mass population surveys. Second, standardized diagnostic criteria have not been available. Most estimates of the prevalence of osteoarthritis are based on clinical evaluation, with a limited number of joints involved in the radiographical examination. The prevalence of osteoarthritis for the US population of 25–74 years of age, diagnosed by history and examination is 12.1%, i.e., an estimated 15.8 million persons have osteoarthritis in the USA[9]. In other populations, osteoarthritis of the knee is rare before the age of 35, but 20–40% of those over 70 have significant radiographical changes of the knee; 30% of those with radiographical abnormalities are symptomatic, with a smaller proportion being severely disabled. Hip osteoarthritis is less common, but a higher proportion of cases are symptomatic and/or are associated with severe disability. Women are more often affected than men, at a ratio of around 2 : 1 in most surveys, which is an inequity that decreases with increasing age[10].

In Table 3 the latest data on the prevalence of osteoarthritis in different regions of the country are shown. A sample of 41 348 people (45.7% males; 54.3% females) aged 15 years and older, from seven cities in different regions of the USSR were screened. The diagnostic criteria included complaints of pain in at least one joint, appearing in the evening or at night, after mechanical load, with joint deformity due to bone proliferation, e.g. Heberden's nodes, accompanied by radiographical changes such as the narrowing of the joint space, osteosclerosis of the joint surface and presence of osteophytes. Primary selection of the patients was directed to all those with the complaints of pain in the joints of the hands, feet, knees, hips and spine with a detailed examination, followed by radiological examination of the joints. A total of 2659 patients with osteoarthritis (33.2% males and 66.8% females) were detected, representing 6.43% of those surveyed. The prevalence of definite osteoarthritis was 5.11%, and of probable osteoarthritis was 1.33%. As can be seen from Tables 3 and 4, there was no geographical tendency in the prevalence of osteoarthritis, but as expected, the prevalence of osteoarthritis was on average, two-fold greater in females than in males in all the cities (Table 5). The knee was involved in 76.8% of males, 68% of females; the hand joints were involved in 50.3% of females, 27% of males; the spine was involved in 47.7% of males, 41.6% of females; the hip was involved in 12.8% of females, 7.7% of males. The onset of osteoarthritis in women was 5–10 years earlier than in men, and was most prevalent in females ages 55 to 64 and in males 65 years and older. Most cases identified in this survey were mild with slow progression. Only 20% of patients with osteoarthritis took medical advice for treatment, and thus from this vantage point, an epidemiological approach to osteoarthritis, the early detection of the disease and timely measures for the treatment and prevention are difficult to over-estimate.

ANKYLOSING SPONDYLITIS

This systemic chronic inflammatory disorder of the spinal joints commonly begins in the sacroiliac joints and gradually ascends the spine, sometimes causing fusion of the costovertebral, intervertebral, and apophyseal joints, and in some

Table 3 Prevalence of osteoarthritis (OA) (%) in different cities of the USSR (population 15 years of age and older)

City	Number screened	Definite OA Abs no.	Definite OA M±m	Probable OA Abs no.	Probable OA M±m	Total Abs no.	Total M±m
Irkutsk[1]	5 781	395	6.83±0.33	27	0.47±0.09	422	7.30±0.34
Vilnius[2]	5 640	366	6.49±0.33	22	0.39±0.08	388	6.88±0.34
Krausnovodsk[3]	5 531	331	5.98±0.32	41	0.74±0.12	372	6.73±0.34
Yaroslavl[4]	5 967	325	5.45±0.29	59	0.99±0.13	384	6.43±0.32
Vladivostok[5]	6 433	298	4.63±0.26	161	2.50±0.19	459	7.14±0.32
Odessa[6]	6 592	225	3.41±0.22	170	2.58±0.20	395	5.99±0.29
Novosibirsk[7]	5 404	171	3.16±0.24	68	1.26±0.15	239	4.42±0.28
Total	41 348	2111	5.11±0.11	548	1.33±0.06	2 659	6.43±0.12

2–4,3–5,4–5 $p<0.05$	2–3 $p<0.05$	2–6 $p<0.05$
1–4 $p<0.01$	1–7,3–7 $p<0.01$	3–5,6 $p<0.01$
1–5,6,7; $p<0.001$	1–4,5,6; 2–4,5,6 $p<0.001$	1–4; 2–4; 3–4;4–5,6,7
2–5,6,7;	2–7,3–5,6; 4–5,6; 5–7, $p<0.001$	
3–6,7; 4–6,7; 5–6,7	6–7 $p<0.001$	

Table 4 Standardized prevalence (Std Prev) by age and sex, and non-standardized prevalence (non-Std Prev) of definite osteoarthritis (OA) in different cities of the USSR (population 15 years and older, standardized by Yaroslavl)

City	Males (M±m) Std Prev	Males (M±m) non-Std Prev	Females (M±m) Std Prev	Females (M±m) non-Std Prev	Both (M±m) Std Prev	Both (M±m) non-Std Prev
Krasnovodsk[1]	5.31±0.42*	4.02±0.39	9.67±0.53*	7.72±0.49	7.60±0.34	5.98±0.32
Irkutsk[2]	5.27±0.42	5.11±0.44	9.77±0.53*	8.09±0.47	7.63±0.34	6.83±0.33
Vilnius[3]	4.52±0.39	5.28±0.45	8.61±0.50	7.47±0.47	6.67±0.32	6.49±0.33
Vladivostok[4]	3.68±0.35	3.15±0.32	6.78±0.45	5.82±0.40	5.31±0.29	4.63±0.26
Yaroslavl[5]	2.86±0.31	2.86±0.31	7.77±0.48	7.77±0.48	5.45±0.29	5.45±0.29
Novosibirsk[6]	2.71±0.31*	1.66±0.25	6.33±0.43*	4.62±0.40	4.61±0.27*	3.16±0.24
Odessa[7]	1.91±0.26	2.34±0.27	4.50±0.37	4.33±0.34	3.27±0.23	3.41±0.22
Mean	3.42±0.13	3.42±0.13	7.91±0.16	6.53±0.16	5.78±0.11	5.11±0.11

3–4,4–5 $p<0.05$	6–5 $p<0.05$	3–4,5 $p<0.01$
1–4,2–4,4–6,5–7	2–5,3–4 $p<0.01$	1–4,5,6,7)
6–7 $p<0.01$	1–4,5,6,7)	2–4,5,6,7)
1–5,6,7)	2–4,2–6,2–7) $p<0.001$	3–6,7; 4–7) $p<0.001$
2–5,6,7) $p<0.001$	3–6,3–7)	5–6,7)
3–5,6,7)	4–7,5–7,6–7)	6–7)
4–7))		

*Statistically significant difference between standardized and non-standardized parameters ($p<0.05$)

Table 5 Prevalence of definite osteoarthritis (OA) (%) in different cities of the USSR (males and females 15 years of age and older)

| City | Males | | | Females | | | Male/female ratio |
| | Number screened | Patients with OA | | Number screened | Patients with OA | | |
		Abs no.	$M \pm m$		Abs no.	$M \pm m$	
Krasnovodsk	2 589	104	4.02 ± 0.39	2 942	227	7.72 ± 0.49	1.9
Irkustk	2 445	125	5.11 ± 0.44	3 336	270	8.09 ± 0.47	1.6
Vilnius	2 519	133	5.28 ± 0.45	3 121	233	7.47 ± 0.47	1.4
Vladivostok	2 857	90	3.15 ± 0.32	3 576	208	5.82 ± 0.40	1.9
Yaroslavl	2 828	81	2.86 ± 0.31	3 139	244	7.77 ± 0.48	2.7
Novosibirsk	2 656	44	1.66 ± 0.25	2 748	127	4.62 ± 0.40	2.9
Odessa	3 036	71	2.34 ± 0.27	3 556	154	4.33 ± 0.34	1.9
Total	18 930	648	3.42 ± 0.13	22 418	1 463	6.53 ± 0.16	1.9

cases, may involve the peripheral joints, especially the hips and shoulders. Ankylosing spondylitis (AS) has been inadequately studied in epidemiological surveys. In Rochester, Minnesota, AS occurs in $197/10^5$ males, and in $73/10^5$ females. The diagnosis of AS requires the presence of back pain plus grade II-IV radiological changes[11]. The use of radiological criteria alone for the diagnosis of sacro-iliitis in three English surveys[12] of male populations yielded an average prevalence of $2933/10^5$. A strong association of sacro-iliitis with HLA-B27 has been shown in most studies[13,14].

In Table 6 the prevalence is shown for ankylosing spondylitis in different USSR populations. Of 47 787 people screened, 24 cases of ankylosing spondylitis were found. According to the New York criteria, the prevalence of AS was 0.05%, or 0.50 per 1000 of population (0.31 definite AS and 0.19 probable AS). There were no statistically significant differences in its prevalence among different cities. Males are affected 6.5 times more often than females. In males, definite AS had a prevalence of 0.91/1000 and probable AS had a prevalence of

0.59/1000, and 0.15 and 0.08, respectively in females. The maximal prevalence of ankylosing spondylitis was observed in the 40–49 age group at 1.5 per thousand; very rare cases of ankylosing spondylitis occur in older women.

There is an obvious genetic component in the development and prevalence of AS. Investigation of 50 probands with this condition (43 men and 7 women) and 109 first-degree relatives (52 men and 57 women) has shown a strong hereditary influence of AS within families. In all cases the disease presented between 8 and 40 years of age, with a mean age of onset at 32.1 years and an average duration of disease of 11.7 years. All patients fit both the Rome (1961) and New York (1966) criteria. Of the 50 patients, 10 had a central form of disease (7 male and 3 female), 39 had a peripheral (35 male and 4 female) form and one had a visceral form. The disease was active in 29 first-degree and 21 second-degree cases. Bilateral sacro-iliitis was found in 31 second-degree and 19 third- and fourth-degree relatives. Clinical and radiological investigation of the first-degree relatives revealed secondary AS in two families, and in the relatives of two of 52 males

Table 6 Prevalence (*n*) of ankylosing spondylitis (AS) in different cities of the USSR (per 1000, population 15 years and older)

City	Screened (*n*)	Definite AS		Probable AS		Total AS	
		n	*M±m*	*n*	*M±m*	*n*	*M±m*
Vilnius	5 640	1	0.17±0.17	1	0.17±0.17	2	0.35±0.25
Irkutsk	5 781	4	0.69±0.34	1	0.17±0.17	5	0.86±0.38
Krasnovodsk	5 531	2	0.36±0.26	1	0.18±0.18	3	0.54±0.31
Odessa	6 592	1	0.15±0.15	1	0.15±0.15	2	0.30±0.21
Yaroslavl	5 967	0	—	1	0.17±0.17	1	0.17±0.17
Novosibirsk	5 404	2	0.37±0.26	1	0.19±0.19	3	0.56±0.32
Vladivostok	6 433	0	—	2	0.31±0.22	2	0.31±0.22
Dushanbe	6 439	5	0.78±0.35	1	0.16±0.16	6	0.94±0.38
Total	47 787	15	0.31±0.08	9	0.19±0.06	24	0.50±0.10

(3.8%). When one considers that the prevalence of AS in the male population is 0.06%, a 63-fold increase among relatives of AS patients is very impressive; no AS was found among relatives of the women.

GOUT

The prevalence of gout, a metabolic disease characterized by recurrent attacks of acute arthritis, an increase in serum urate concentration and deposits of serum urate monohydrate crystals in and around the joints of the extremities has been inadequately documented in the USSR, as most reports have been based on medical records or postmortem examinations, and the criteria used to establish the diagnosis of gout are over-simplistic. In the USA, the prevalence of gout determined by questionnaire for males is $1360/10^5$ and for females, $640/10^5$, increases with age, and most frequently occurs in those aged 65 years and older[15]. In South Africa, gout which was formerly a disease exclusive to Whites, is increasing among urban Blacks, who have higher concentrations of serum urate than their kinsfolk in rural communities[16]. The latest data on the prevalence of gout in different cities of the USSR are presented in Table 7. These were based on stand-

ardized diagnostic criteria[3] used in all centers participating in the study. The rarity of gout in the very young justified the choice of age group, i.e. older than 15 years for this study.

Of 41 384 persons screened, 40 cases of gout were found (0.10%). In 25 cases, 'definite gout' was diagnosed (0.06%) and in 15 cases (0.04%), 'probable gout'. The male/female ratio among patients was 5.5 : 1, thus representing a male bias that is typical of gout in other populations. Most of the gout patients were 35–64 years of age, with the highest prevalence in the 55–64 year age group (0.30%, where 'definite gout' was 0.19%). There was not one case of gout in those under 25 years old. The highest prevalence of gout was found in Odessa (0.26%) and the lowest in Irkutsk (0.02%). Of all cases of gout in women, 69.2% were from Odessa. A higher prevalence of gout was seen among males in Dushanbe (0.26% of 'definite gout'). These figures correlate well with the concentration of uric acid in the populations screened. In Table 8 the mean levels of uric acid measured in random samples from the screen populations are presented. Uric acid concentration of more than 0.413 mmol/l (US: 7 mg/dl) for males and more than 0.407 mmol/l (US: 6.9 mg/dl) for fe-

Table 7 Prevalence of gout in different cities of the USSR (population 15 years and older), probable (Prob), definite (Def), absolute number (*n*)

City	Number	Males	*Prob + Def*		*Def*		*Def males*	
			n	*%*	*n*	*%*	*n*	*%*
Vilnius	5 640	3 519	3	0.05	2	0.04	2	0.08
Dushanbe	6 439	3 050	8	0.12	8	0.12	8	0.26
Irkutsk	5 811	2 445	1	0.02	1	0.02	1	0.04
Krasnovodsk	5 531	2 589	3	0.05	2	0.04	2	0.08
Novosibirsk	5 404	2 656	3	0.06	2	0.04	1	0.04
Odessa	6 592	3 036	17	0.26	8	0.12	4	0.26
Yaroslavl	5 967	2 828	5	0.05	2	0.03	0	0
Total	41 384	19 123	40	0.10	25	0.06	18	0.09

Table 8 Mean serum level of uric acid in random samples from the screened populations in eight cities of the USSR

City	*Number screened*			*Mean level of uric acid* (mg/l)		
	Males	*Females*	*Total*	*Males*	*Females*	*Total*
Vilnius	102	252	354	53	49	50
Vladivostok	39	99	138	41	43	43
Dushanbe	257	639	896	63	55	58
Irkutsk	160	398	558	36	31	34
Krasnovodsk	244	454	698	47	36	40
Novosibirsk	19	25	44	32	33	33
Odessa	181	443	624	71	63	66
Yaroslavl	73	182	255	36	43	40
Total	1075	2492	3567	54	47	50

males was considered as hyperuricemic[17]. From Table 8 the highest mean level of uric acid was in Odessa, 0.389 mmol/l (US: 6.6 mg/dl) and Dushanbe, 0.342 mmol/l (US: 5.8 mg/dl); the lowest was in Novosibirsk, 0.195 mmol/l (US: 3.3 mg/dl) and Irkutsk, 0.201 mmol/l (US: 3.4 mg/dl). The mean level of uric acid is higher in the average male, 0.319 mmol/l (US: 5.4 mg/dl), than in the average female, 0.277 mmol/l (US: 4.7 mg/dl). The prevalence of 'hyperuricemia' was highest in Odessa (26.7%) and lowest in Irkutsk (1.1%), and was present in 78% of patients with 'definite gout' and 90% of patients with 'probable gout'. Thus, the association between uric acid concentration and prevalence of gout opens perspectives for the primary prevention of this disease in contrast to other chronic rheumatic disease where the perspectives for primary prevention are still unclear. More comprehensive epidemiological studies are clearly needed.

REFERENCES

1. Decker J and The Glossary Subcommittee of the ARA Committee on Rheumatologic Practice. American Rheumatism Association: Nomenclature and classification of arthritis and rheumatism. Arthritis Rheum. 1983; 26:1029–1032

2. Nasonova VA, Benevolenskaya LI, Zborovski AB. Epidemiology of rheumatic disease in socialist countries. Proceedings of the ILAR 1989 Congress, Rio de Janeiro, Brazil, 17th–23rd September 1989, pp. 585–589

3. Benevolenskaya LI, Brzhezovsky MM. Epidemiology of Rheumatic Disease, Moscow, Meditsina, 1988 (In Russian)

4. Maksakova EN, Bolotina A Yu, Troffimova TM *et al*. The problems of invalidation of patients with rheumatic diseases. Vopr Rheum. 1980; 1:51–54 (In Russian)

5. Benevolenskaya LI. The strategy of the risk factor study in rheumatic diseases. Proceedings of the International Symposium on 'Risk Factors in Rheumatic Diseases', Pitsunda, November 19–22, 1986. Moscow, 1986, p. 93

6. Brzhezovsky MM. On certain methodological principles in the study of risk factors. Proceedings of the International Symposium on 'Risk Factors in Rheumatic Diseases', Pitsunda, November 19–22, 1986. Moscow 1986, p. 98

7. Lawrence JS. Rheumatism in Population. London, Heinemann Medical Books, 1977, p. 156

8. Lawrence RC, Hochberg MC, Kelsey JL *et al*. Estimates of the prevalence of selected arthritic and musculoskeletal diseases in the United States. J Rheumatol. 1989; 16:427–441

9. Cunningham LS, Kelsey JL. Epidemiology of musculoskeletal impairments and associated disability. Am J Public Health. 1984; 74:574–579

10. Felson DT. Epidemiology of hip and knee osteoarthritis. Epidemiol Rev. 1988; 10:1–28

11. Carter ET, McKenna CH, Brian DD *et al*. Epidemiology of ankylosing spondylitis in Rochester, Minnesota, 1935–1973. Arthritis Rheum. 1979; 22:365–370

12. Gofton JP, Lawrence JS, Bennett PH *et al*. Sacroiliitis in eight populations. Ann Rheum Dis. 1966; 25:528–533

13. Calin A, Elswood J. Relative role of genetic and environmental factors in disease expression sib–pair analysis in ankylosing spondylitis. Arthritis Rheum. 1989; 32:77–81

14. Cohen LM, Mittal KK, Schmid FR *et al*. Increased risk for spondylitis stigmata in apparently healthy HLA-B27-positive men. Ann Intern Med. 1976; 84:1–7

15. Collins JG. Prevalence of selected chronic conditions, United States 1983–85, Advance data from Vital and Health Statistics of the National Center for Health Statistics, No. 155, USDHHS, 1988

16. Scott, JT. In Copeman's Textbook of the Rheumatic Diseases, Churchill Livingstone, 1986

17. Khaltaev NG, Zakharbekov RR, Khaltaeva ED, Akhmeteli MA. Hyperuricaemia, coronary heart disease risk factors and diet. Cardiology. 1982; 8:56–59 (In Russian)

3.   RHEUMATIC PROBLEMS IN THE ASIA PACIFIC REGION

Richard Wigley

INTRODUCTION

The World Health Organization (WHO) appropriately in the 1950–70 period concentrated on the control of communicable diseases which affected vast numbers in rural areas of developing countries, where the majority of the world population resided. As these complaints came under control, attention was directed to those non-communicable diseases for which control measures existed, i.e. diabetes, hypertension, coronary disease and rheumatic fever. The latter, though primarily a rheumatic disorder and secondarily a heart disorder, was the only rheumatic disease included and that, rather inappropriately, under heart disease, which is a complication of some cases only. WHO control programs were in place for the other non-communicable disease groups.

To fill the gap in international initiatives against rheumatic diseases, a joint meeting of the International League against Rheumatism (ILAR) and the WHO was held in Geneva in 1981, where plans were initiated for a global program for the control of rheumatic diseases. This collaboration was named the Community Oriented Program for the Control of Rheumatic Disease (COPCORD). The following year, a Kroc conference was convened to further identify specific needs for both developing and developed countries[1]. Through the work of Lawrence[2], Valkenburg (personal communication), Bennett[3], Duff[4], Shichikawa[5] and their many co-workers, the prevalence of

rheumatic diseases was established for the developed countries. However, little progress could be made in the control of rheumatic disease in the developing countries until the prevalence of rheumatic complaints was known. Determining the nature of local problems in the rural areas of these countries was given priority. The surveys were to be followed by educational programs appropriate to the profile of disorders found in each region, and to control risk factors where feasible. Questionnaires were developed from experience gained by earlier surveys in Tokelau Islanders and migrants to New Zealand[6,7] and in Quemoy[3].

The first study was organized in the Philippines by Manahan in San Antonio, Luzon, sixty miles south of Manila[8]. Volunteer primary health care workers administered a simple questionnaire, the district nurse further questioned the positive responders, and as a final step, those with significant rheumatic complaints were called to the health center for medical examination. A 2-year delay in completion of the second questionnaire, and therefore the medical examination of the severely affected patients was caused by a combination of uncontrolled activities of the New People's Army, a guerrilla faction, difficulty in patient access, and a severe bout of malaria in the district nurse. These factors resulted in a high drop-out rate in examinees, so the prevalences were probably underestimated at the examination phase[9].

Table 1 Prevalence of rheumatic complaints in South East Asia COPCORD

	Philippines[9]	Indonesia[10]		Malaysia[13]			Australia[12]
	Phase II	Rural	Urban	Malay	Chinese	Indian	
Urban and rural	950	4 683	1 071	1 267	474	853	1 437
Rheumatism ever	33	24[†]	32[†]				
Last 2 weeks	28			23	13	24	
Joint symptoms		18	28	9	4.9	11	32[§]
Neck pain	7.1	5	12	3.6	1.0	6.2	17
Dorsal pain	93	5	9	7	1.9	6.7	6.2
Lumbar pain	11	15	23	7	4.4	10	22
Knee pain	6.1	12.2	14.8	11	3.6	11	15
Shoulder pain	1.8	11		4	1.9	6	10
Elbow pain	1.7	10		2.7	1.7	6	6.3
Rheumatoid arthritis*	0.2	0.2	0.3	0.3	0	0	0.7
Ankylosing spondylitis	nil			0	0.1	0.2	0.2
Osteoarthritis	4.0	5.1		3.2	1.0	1.3	8.2
Heberden's nodes	1.8	2.9		0.7	0.2	0.5	
Gout	0.5	1.7	4.8	0.1	0.1	0.2	1.5
Fibromyalgia	—	15[‡]		0.5	0.2	1.5	5.8[‡]
Disability	—	3.0	1.0	2.8	1.9	3.8	4.4

[†]Past pain in limbs; [§]pain within the last week; [‡]any soft tissue rheumatism; *definite rheumatoid arthritis

Other initiatives in rheumatic disease epidemiology of the Asia Pacific region include studies by Darmawan[10,11], Muirden[12] and Veerapen[13]. Darmawan examined an urban and a rural population from central Java, using as controls, subjects without rheumatic complaints[10]. A similar study of urban and rural populations in a developed country was performed in Victoria Australia by Muirden[12].

A study recently completed by Veerapen[13] in Malaysia compared different ethnic groups (Malays, Chinese and Tamil Indians) living in a similar rural environment. Fibromyalgia was more common in Tamil Indians and Malays than in Chinese women, who also had a lower incidence of other rheumatic complaints. In this study, nurses and nurse aids with 18 months training carried out the initial screening. Soft tissue rheumatism was systematically sought, by routine counting of fibromyalgic 'tender' points, using the criteria delineated by the American College of Rheumatology[14] (*see* Chapter 6). There is a need to develop precise definitions of the many soft tissue rheumatism syndromes common in all populations to allow accurate accrual of statistics and to plan interventional strategies.

Extensive population studies in China sponsored by ILAR[15–18] were primarily intended to determine the prevalence of rheumatoid arthritis (RA), ankylosing spondylitis (AS) and systemic lupus erythematosus (SLE). ILAR's questionnaire included questions also used in the COPCORD studies, facilitating comparison with the COPCORD, Tokelau, and the Dutch Zoetemeer studies (Tables 1 and 2). Certain caveats are relevant, as these studies differ in methodologies.

Table 2 Non-COPCORD comparable studies

	China[20]		Tokelau[7]		Holland[2]
	Beijing	Shantou	Island	Migrant	Zoetemeer
Sample size	4 213	5 058	794	1 333	4 683
Rheumatism ever			28	66	
Rheumatism currently					33
Joint pain	33[‡]	7.6[‡]			
Neck pain	4.6[‡]	1.9[‡]	0.3[*]	0.1[*]	
Dorsal pain	1.5[‡]	1.9[‡]	0.8[*]	0.9[*]	
Lumbar pain	28	12.1[‡]	13[*]	12[*]	43
Shoulder pain	4.6	1.0	4.3[*]	2.5[*]	13
Elbow pain	4.0	1.0	0.4[*]	—	6.5
Knee pain	27	2.1	8.0[†*]	9.7[†*]	12
Rheum. arthritis[§]	0.3	0.2	0.1	0.2	0.9
Ankylosing spond.	0.2	0.4	0.1	0	
Osteoarthritis	—	—	29[†*]	31[†*]	
Heberden's nodes	0.01		11[*]	5.2[*]	5.6
Gout	0	0	0.7[*]	3.0[*]	
SLE	0.1	0.02	0	0.1	
Disability	1.1	0.5			

* Rates adjusted to Tokelauans resident in the islands; [‡]age standardized to the sum of the Beijing and Shantou populations; [†]clinical diagnosis of osteoarthritis and [§]definite rheumatoid arthritis; SLE, systemic lupus erythematosus

In the China and Tokelau studies, all subjects were examined by qualified physicians, while in the COPCORD studies, screening was by primary health care workers of differing levels of training and experience, and only the positive respondents were examined by rheumatologists. To minimize the ethnic and language-related differences, rheumatologists of the COPCORD and China study committees assisted with the examination phase of these studies (K.D. Muirden, H.A. Valkenburg, I. Duff, P.H. Bennett, Zhang Nai-Zheng and R.D. Wigley).

The spectrum of complaints seen in the developing nations differs from that of the older Dutch (personal communication) and Australian[12] populations (Table 1), in that spinal pain is less prevalent and knee pain is more prevalent in the north Chinese population[14–18]. Knee pain is a more important cause of pain in the east where squatting is an essential daily living activity. The inability to squat is a major handicap that would be relatively unimportant in the west. Morimoto[19] has described a particular pattern of osteoarthritis of the knees in Japanese who squat and kneel regularly for ceremonial and domestic purposes. Studies are in progress to develop a non-invasive method of detecting cartilage degeneration in the knees for population studies and to identify risk factors[20]. An association of genu varum (bow legs) and knee pain was shown in the Beijing rural study. There was no cohort effect to suggest a transitory fall in calcium intake which may be a factor as milk is little used in that part of China.

The lower rate of back pain in South East Asia than in Holland, Australia and north China may be partially explained by use of the carrying pole. This may be an optimal method for carrying large weights, as the load is raised and lowered with the knees, balanced to prevent lateral flexion, twisting is unnecessary and shock loading is absorbed by the flexibility of the pole. A potential disadvantage is the skin thickening across the shoulders, which may be painful[10].

There is a higher rate of all rheumatic symptoms, and in particular, knee pain in Han Chinese in the Beijing rural district than in the warmer coastal area of east Quantung (Chenghai), which suggests that there are differences in environmental risk factors. This finding requires further clarification, as some suggestions, e.g. that there is greater stoicism leading to a lower complaint rate in the south of China seems unlikely. The high fish intake and rice-based diet along the warmer and more moist southern coast may have a protective effect in contrast to the wheat based diet, supplemented with domestic animal proteins in the colder, drier north. Rheumatoid arthritis and ankylosing spondylitis were not significantly different in prevalence between the north and the south or from prevalence in Caucasians. Ergonomic differences between populations require detailed study to explain regional differences in soft tissue rheumatism and joint pain. A study is planned in a southern coastal fishing village to elucidate this difference and hopefully to disclose risk factors. Systemic lupus erythematosus (SLE) is too uncommon to disclose any difference in prevalence in China, although most SLE studies in Caucasians have been clinical, and thus would underestimate its actual prevalence in a population

EDUCATION

The educational phase of the COPCORD has been studied by Darmawan (*see* Chapter 30) in a rural village in Indonesia[21] using the traditional Wyang shadow play method to convey messages (as the population is largely illiterate), concerning the optimal way to carry out daily activities. One major success from the COPCORD projects has been recorded, that of eliminating 'natural' herbal remedies containing phenylbutazone and prednisone, which had disturbing consequences in Indonesia[22]. Implementation of these and other strategies presents great challenges; much work remains to be done.

REFERENCES

1. Conference on Epidemiology of Rheumatic Diseases. Specific needs of developing and developed countries. J Rheumatol, Special Issue, Vol 10, 1983
2. Lawrence JS. Rheumatism in Populations. London, Heinemann, 1977
3. Beasley RP, Bennett PH, Chien CL. Low prevalence of rheumatoid arthritis in Chinese. J Rheumatol, Special Issue, Vol 10, pp. 11–15, 1983
4. Mikkelsen WM, Dodge HJ, Duff IF *et al*. Estimates of the prevalence of rheumatic diseases in the population of Tecumseh, Michigan 1959–60. J Chronic Dis. 1967; 20:351–369
5. Shichikawa K, Mayeda A, Komatsubara *et al*. Rheumatic complaints in urban and rural populations in Osaka. Ann Rheum Dis. 1966; 25:25–31
6. Wigley RD, Prior IAM, Salmond C, Stanley D, Pinfold B. Rheumatic complaints in Tokelau I. Migrants resident in New Zealand. The Tokelau migrant study. Rheumatol Int. 1967; 7:53–59
7. Wigley RD, Prior IAM, Salmond C, Stanley D, Pinfold B. Rheumatic complaints in Tokelau II. A comparison of migrants in New Zealand and non-migrants. The Tokelau migrant study. Rheumatol Int. 1987; 7:61–65
8. Manahan L, Caragay R, Muirden KD, Allander E, Valkenburg HA, Wigley RD. Rheumatic pain in a Philippine village. A WHO COPCORD study. Int J Rheumatol. 1985; 5:149–153.11
9. Wigley RD, Manahan L, Muirden KD, Caragay R, Pinfold B, Couchman KG, Valkenburg HA. Rheumatic disease in a Phillipine village II. COPCORD study, phases II and III. Int J Rheumatol. 1991; 11:157–161

10. Darmawan JD. Rheumatic conditions in the northern part of central Java. An epidemiological survey. Doctoral thesis, Erasmus University, Rotterdam, Holland

11. Darmawan J, Valkenburg HA, Muirden KD, Wigley RD. Epidemiology of rheumatic diseases in rural and urban populations in Indonesia: a World Health Organization International League against Rheumatism COPCORD study, Stage I, Phase 2. Ann Rheum Dis. 1992; 51:525–528

12. Muirden KD, Valkenburg HA *et al*. The Australian COPCORD. In press

13. Veerapen K, Wigley RD, Couchman KG. *et al.*, The Malaysian COPCORD. In press

14. Wolfe F, Smythe H, Yunus MB, Bennett RM *et al*. The American College of Rheumatology 1990 criteria for the classification of fibromyalgia. Arthritis Rheum. 1990; 33:160–172

15. Wigley RD, Zhang NZ, Duff ID, Bennett PH. ILAR study of rheumatic disease in China. SEAPAL Bull. 1987; 5:34–39

16. Wigley RD, Zhang NZ, Duff ID, Bennett PH. ILAR study of rheumatic diseases in China II. SEAPAL Bull. 1988; 6:47–49

17. Wigley RD, Zhang NZ, Duff ID, Bennett PH. ILAR study of rheumatic disease in China III. APLAR Bull. 1990; 7:51–53

18. Wigley RD, Zhang NZ, Duff ID, Bennett PH. ILAR study of rheumatic disease in China. APLAR Bull. 1990; 7:72–75

19. Morimoto I. Attrition lesions of articular cartilage in Japanese knee joint due to formal sitting and squatting. J Anthropol Soc Nippon Suppl. 1989; 90:51–53

20. Wigley RD, Zhang NZ, Hu DW, Sheng SC, Couchman KG, Duff ID, Bennett PH. ILAR study of rheumatic disease in China IV. Knee pain in Shiao Hong Men village. APLAR Bull. 1990; 7:76–77

21. Darmawan JD, Muirden KD. Primary community arthritis education by means of the Wayang shadow play at a rural primary health centre in Bandungan, Central Java, Indonesia. SEAPAL Bull. 1986; 4:10

22. Darmawan JD, Wigley RD, Valkenburg HA. Disturbing findings in Indonesia. SEAPAL Bull. 1986; 4:6–7

4.   RHEUMATIC SYNDROMES CAUSED BY ACCIDENTS

Peter Disler and Ann Williamson

Accidents will occur in the best-regulated families...they may be expected with confidence, and must be borne with philosophy

Mr Micawber in 'David Copperfield

INTRODUCTION

Accidents are the cause of approximately 15% of severe disabilities in the world, which affect an estimated 80 million people. As Mr Micawber noted, accidents respect no social class, nor age or sex, and their effect on the health and economic well-being of their victims, and the society in which these affected individuals live, is considerable.

It is generally accepted that accidents involving the musculoskeletal system may result in the development of 'rheumatic conditions'; indeed rheumatoid arthritis, tuberculous arthritis, and gout have all, at one time or another, been said to be caused by trauma. Although other alternate etiological factors for these conditions have been identified, there is little doubt that a relationship may exist in some cases. It is well accepted, for example, that gout may be precipitated by acute injury, and there have been numerous case reports of classic seronegative spondyloarthropathy presenting for the first time after physical injury in HLA-B27-positive individuals[1], perhaps through release of antigens from injured joints[2].

Critical examination of the literature reveals little in the way of comprehensive studies specifically linking rheumatic disease and either particular types of injury, or the specific types of accidents that might cause them. This chapter will review some of the current evidence for these links and discuss some aspects of how rheumatic disease might be minimized by reducing accidents. In order to do so, we need to examine the circumstances under which accidents occur, and then determine whether rheumatic disease is more common under such circumstances. Similarly, in planning prevention we must in the first instance focus on how and where the accident took place, then use this knowledge for the primary prevention of injuries likely to lead to rheumatic disease.

EPIDEMIOLOGICAL INFORMATION

The first step in analyzing a postulated relation between accidents and 'rheumatic' conditions is the rational examination of epidemiological data. This is made difficult by the relative paucity of statistics linking accidents to rheumatic disease, in part, because 'rheumatic condition' and 'accident' are terms that are broadly and inconsistently defined. Rheumatic symptoms, for example are defined for this volume as *'any pain or discomfort that arises in the joints or other parts of the musculoskeletal system'*; an accident is defined by the Oxford English Dictionary as *'An unforeseen contingency'*. Another reason for the paucity of data is that accident-related mortality is more commonly recorded than accident-related morbidity, and people with rheumatic symptoms from accidents obviously fall into the latter category. It has been estimated that for one death from accidents there are 15 severe and 30 minor injuries[3], a ratio that will vary in accordance with the standards of medical management.

Relatively accurate data are available in certain countries, and in this chapter we will be drawing from New Zealand and Australian statistics. New Zealand is a particularly rich source of information as it has a single legislated 'no fault' compensation scheme for all victims of 'personal injury by accident' (the Accident Compensation Corporation or ACC). Direct extrapolation of these data to other countries may be difficult, as Australia and New Zealand have strong rural economies, relatively sparse populations and it is reasonable to expect accidents to rise with industrialization and urbanization. The ACC statistics are also biased by their focus on 'earning-related' compensation; members of the working population are far more likely to be registered than children, the elderly, the unemployed or women working without salary in their own homes. Home and sport injuries are covered in Chapter 5. Despite these caveats, the data base does provide a valuable vantage point.

In New Zealand's ACC data from 1/4/88 to 31/3/89 the age mode of both sexes was in the late teens and early twenties[4]; females have a lower overall injury rate for both work-related and non-work-related injuries until they reach the sixth and seventh decades, where female accidents are more common and consist largely of osteoporosis-related fractures. Seventy-eight percent of accidents occurred in wage earners, but more than 50% of the injuries were not work related. This is important in terms of the discussion of prevention that will follow.

ENVIRONMENTAL CIRCUMSTANCES OF AN ACCIDENT

If one is to plan prevention, then a useful starting place is to look at where the accidents occur, which may be divided into a number of broad categories.

Traffic accidents

In developed countries, these are the most common cause of accident-related mortality and morbidity, and the number of injured people is increasing faster than the number killed, a datum that is attributed to use of safety (seat) belts[5]. A specific area of interest is the effect of the extremes of age on the incidence of accidents. Accidents on the public highway are particularly common in persons over 65 years of age[6], possibly relating to failing vision and hearing loss, and not uncommonly result in multiple injuries. Children are also commonly involved in traffic accidents, as they discriminate poorly between right and left, misjudge vehicular speeds and traffic volume, and it has been said that 'on the practical level, a child is incapable of crossing a street alone without excessive risk before the age of 9 years and the use of bicycles outside protected zones is not safe before the age of 12'[6]. The age of the driver is also relevant; according to ACC statistics, 46% of all motor vehicle injuries involve persons between ages 15 and 24 in New Zealand, where the minimum legal driving age is 15. The type of vehicle is also important, as New Zealand's ACC statistics reveal that the annual accident rate of $6177/10^5$ licensed motorcycles is more than 10-fold greater than the rate $(603/10^5)$ reported for motorcars.

Household accidents

Every year 100 000 people are admitted to hospital with household accidents in Great Britain and about a million receive treatment from their general practitioner[6]. In a study of domestic accident victims treated at 20 hospitals in England and Wales, hospitalization was required in 6.6%, and was greater than 1 month in duration in 15%. Of the injuries suffered, 31.7% were due to fractures, dislocation, contusions and sprains, and would be expected to lead to rheumatic symp-

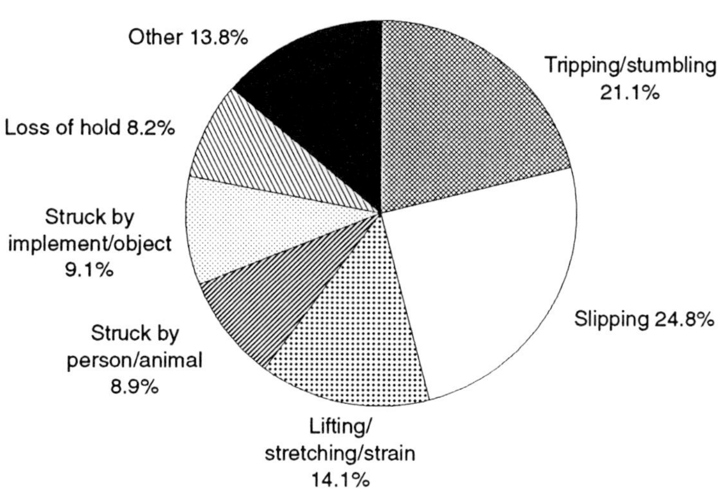

Figure 1 Causes of injuries in the home. These data are based on 24 534 claims. (Reproduced with kind permission from reference 4)

toms, at least acutely. The ACC statistics record the commonest causes of household accidents, and this is shown in Figure 1 (based on 24 534 claims).

Occupational accidents

An estimated 160 000 industrial accidents occur each day in the world[7], and in New Zealand comprise 36% of the accidents registered annually with New Zealand's ACC. The incidence of occupational accidents in developing ('third world') nations may be quite different, as more developed nations can afford the 'luxury' of occupational safety and hygiene and commonly maintain valid statistics. It is tragic to note that in their attempt to control costs, large industries may build factories in less developed parts of the world, precisely so they may lower their high (but cost-ineffective) standards of occupational safety.

New Zealand's ACC data not surprisingly reveal that the more 'physical' occupations are more accident-prone (Figure 2). Figure 3 correlates the injury rates to specific industries; again, it is not entirely unexpected that mining and quarrying

have the highest rate (99.7/1000, followed by factory work, construction and forestry.

Rural regions in general have poor 'track' records with more accidents than more industrial regions; even in those countries where great efforts are expended on protecting factory workers, scant attention is paid to simple accident-preventive measures within the farming community.

TYPE OF INJURY THAT MAY CAUSE RHEUMATIC DISEASE

Injuries which are likely to cause rheumatic complaints result from either direct trauma to joints, or from forced, inappropriate movement of a joint beyond its normal range of motion, which might, for example, be rotatary in the case of a non-rotatary joint such as the knee. The role of hemorrhage, secondary to minor trauma in people with bleeding disorders, and secondary infection, due to foreign body 'implantation' should not be disregarded as causing rheumatic complaints. An array of long-term indwelling foreign bodies have been described, including bullets[8], and the

29

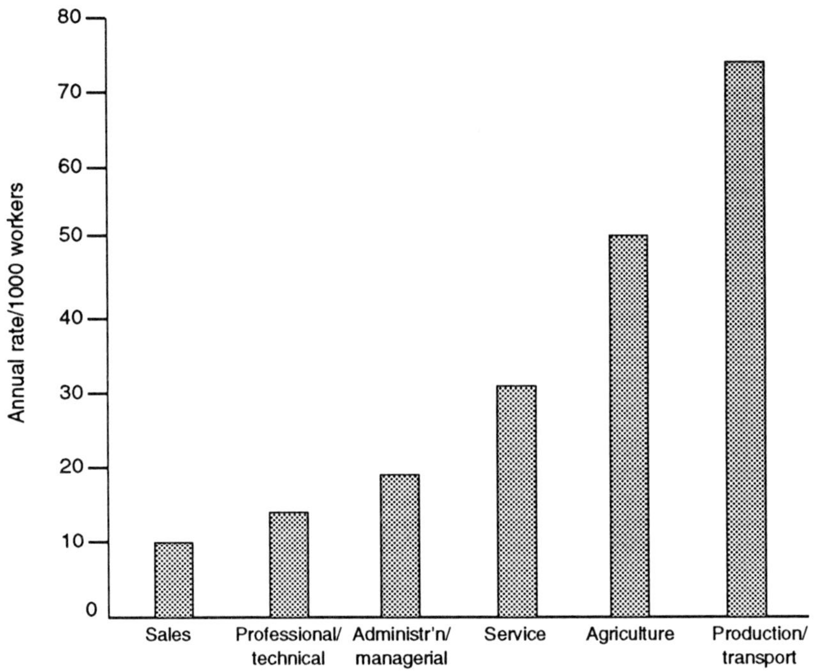

Figure 2 Distribution of work-related injuries on the basis of occupation of injured person. (Reproduced with kind permission from reference 4)

more exotic spines of sea urchins and other marine creatures[9].

Osteoarthritis (OA) is often divided into an idiopathic or primary form and a secondary form, which is classically induced by trauma and associated with joint injury. Both forms have similar pathological changes. The earliest event is degeneration of cartilage, a substance that provides mechanical support and congruous motion of joints, which can be damaged if the biomechanical capacities of the joint and surrounding muscle are exceeded, either acutely by a precipitous injury or chronically through repeated use. Cartilage is vulnerable to repeated impact loading, as shown in animal studies, to chemical and physical changes similar to human OA[10]. Radin and co-workers suggest that this explains the preferential involvement of the distal interphal-

angeal joints in OA of the hand in humans, as they bear the greatest stress in hand gripping[11].

Sports-related activities present a framework for examining the relationship between injury and OA in later life. As this will be discussed more fully in Chapter 5, it suffices to say here that the Framingham Study showed that if a man had suffered a knee injury requiring the use of crutches or sticks, the relative risk of future OA was 3.46[12]. As further corroboration, a history of knee injury is linked to OA of the same side, while obesity is associated with bilateral OA[13]. Finally, retired American football players have a high prevalence of OA of the hip and knee joints[14], although this article did not examine in detail specific sites of injury that occurred during the athletically active periods.

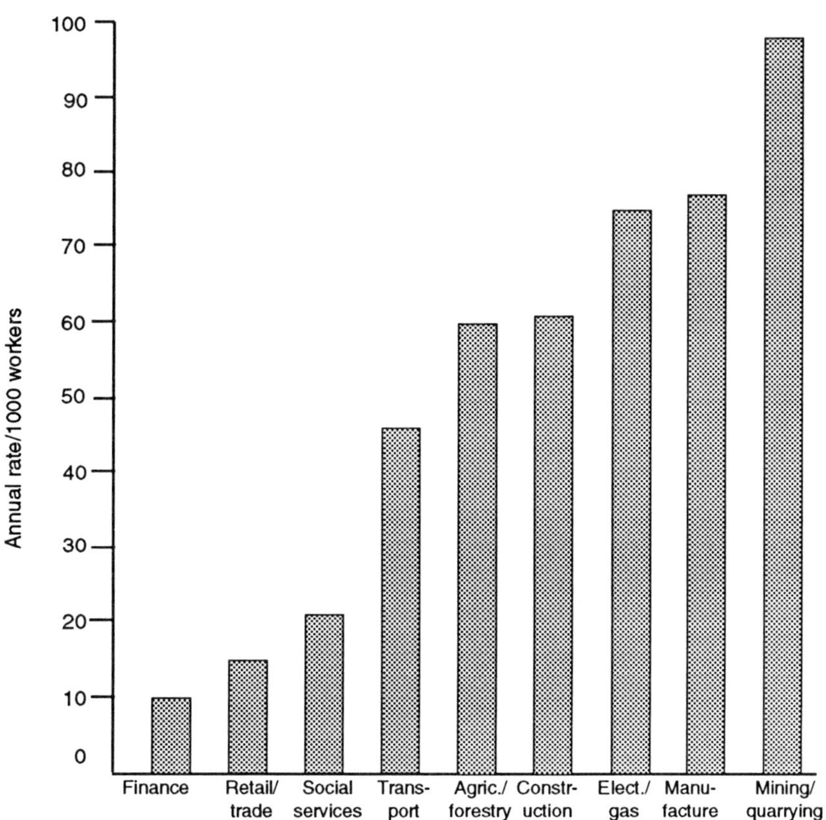

Figure 3 Distribution of work-related injuries on the basis of the industry in which the injured person works. (Reproduced with kind permission from reference 4)

Common sites of injury

While the ACC statistics (see above) do not indicate the incidence or prevalence of chronic rheumatic symptoms, they do record in detail the body site for which a claim was made. One can thus focus on those injury sites that might lead to such rheumatic symptoms. Figure 4 shows the distribution of claims on the basis of the site of injury. Although injuries of the head and face (29.4%), chest (1.7%) and abdomen (2.7%) are not primary sites of rheumatic symptoms, the remaining 66.2% of injuries may affect joints. If the analysis is restricted to work-related injuries, the anatomical distribution of injuries changes; facial injuries decrease and the balance shifts further towards injuries that might be expected to lead to rheumatic symptoms (Figure 5). The back and lower spine account for 25% of all work-related injuries, and both regions are common sites of chronic rheumatic symptoms.

Arthritis following on fractures

We found no record of prospective studies that link injuries to rheumatic symptoms; all such studies are retrospective in nature. However, a seminal report on this subject was presented recently by Wright[15] in response to four critical medicolegal questions raised by a retired Judge to the British Arthritis and Rheumatism Council, *viz:*

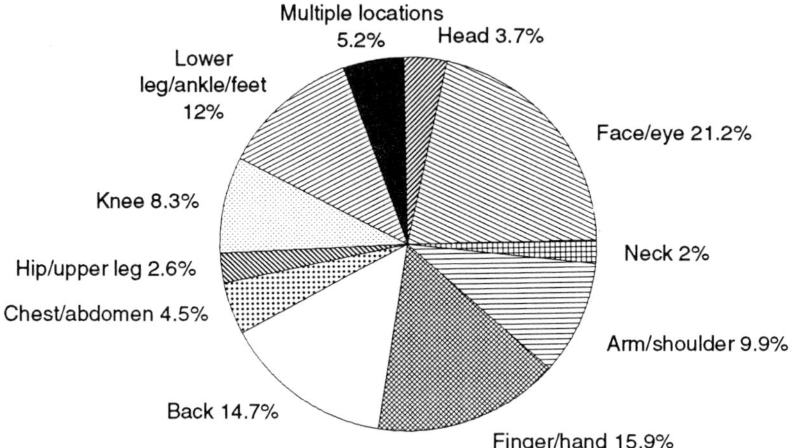

Figure 4 Anatomical sites of injury (all types). (Reproduced with kind permission from reference 4)

(1) What is the likelihood of arthritis following a fracture?

(2) Are some areas of the body more likely to develop arthritis following trauma?

(3) Does age affect the relationship of trauma to arthritis?

(4) How soon after a fracture is arthritis likely to occur?

Wright, prefacing his discussion with a comment on the 'scanty literature on the subject', presented a consensus opinion from 108 colleagues to whom these questions were then referred. Some of these will be summarized below.

Wright's colleagues differ widely regarding the frequency that arthritis follows a fracture through an articulation, suggesting that this ranges between 10% and 100%! There are nevertheless strong biomechanical arguments for the development of arthritis in this setting, which relates to a break in continuity of the bony articular surface, leading to 'peak loading during different phases of motion at the interface between the intact and missing surfaces', predisposing the joint surface to instability and shear forces. OA is thought to develop if a 2–3 mm 'step' or defect is present in the joint surface. It would follow that joints that are not directly load-bearing have lesser risks of chronic and/or progressive problems. This may also vary within a single joint, depending on the defective regions, e.g. with an acetabular fracture, the long-term functional status is better if the weight-bearing dome is intact than if it is disrupted. Early orthopedic surgeons recognized this in fractures of the knee and suggested that OA would occur unless precise and anatomical reduction was achieved.

Almost all of Wright's respondents felt that the lower limb was generally at greater risk than the upper limb for developing rheumatic diatheses. One study in parachutists suggests that ankle fractures are almost invariably followed by OA[16], and the amount of force involved in the injury appears to be critical in the development of OA[17]. It has been suggested that if fibrocartilage alone is damaged by a traumatic impact, then

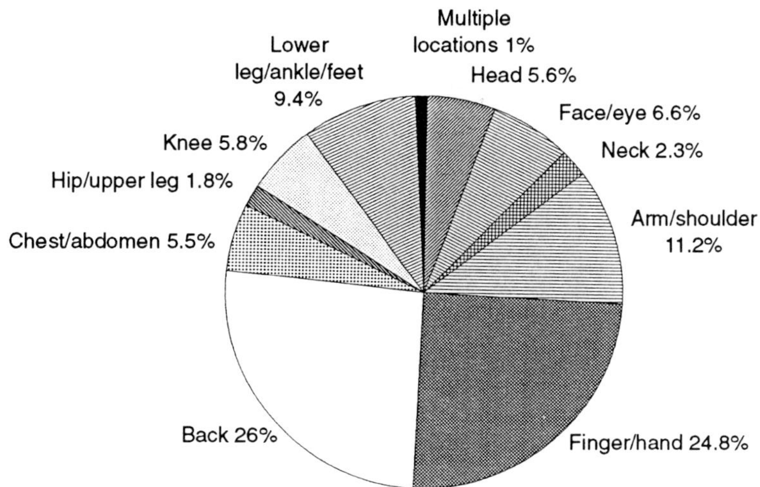

Figure 5 Anatomical sites of injury (work related). (Reproduced with kind permission from reference 4)

this can be repaired but if the force is sufficient to damage bone too, then repair does not occur without OA.

Analysis of individual joints reveals more information. Some fractures are more likely to lead to OA, possibly because the blood supply is more likely to be disrupted, for example, the neck of femur, scaphoid, talus and tibial condyle. The incidence of OA following fracture–dislocation of the hip is (38–40%), with a higher incidence of arthritis with posterior dislocations, and in patients who are fully ambulatory (and weight bearing) in the first 3 months after an accident.

With the knee, persuasive evidence for a relationship between intra-articular fracture and OA came from a large study by Rasmussen[18], in which OA developed in 21% of knees on the side that suffered tibial condylar fractures and only 2% on the other side. The development of post-traumatic OA depends in part on the joint's alignment, and is more common with varus deformity. The pathogenesis of OA of the knee secondary to meniscal injury has proven controversial, since although there is little doubt that meniscal tears

are associated with OA[19], it is uncertain whether open meniscectomy also predisposes to OA[20,21]. Most authors agree that it does, but it is unclear whether recent trends in arthroscopic management of joint diseases have altered the situation.

With respect to extra-articular fractures, one of Wright's respondents indicated that OA rarely (<5%) develops from long bone fractures if the limb's alignment is maintained, while OA is more common in misaligned joints (a critical angle of >10% for the knee and ankle joints). Wright also suggested that the risk of that in the malalignment in the axial or coronal planes was ten times the risk of that in the sagittal (flexion/extension) plane for an equivalent degree of deformity.

An example of how fractures can cause long-term rheumatic disease is seen in the scaphoid bone of the wrist, where over time, nearly 100% of non-union fractures ultimately evolve towards osteo-arthritis[22–24]. Bone displacement appears to play a critical role in this relationship, and Fisk[25] suggests that this displacement may be due either to damage to periscaphoid ligaments or to resorption at the fracture site. In another study of non-united scaphoid fractures, Vender and colleagues[26] showed that all articular surfaces are not equally susceptible to developing arthritis. In the scapho-capitate, arthritis developed in 24% at 1 year, 38% at 4 years and 60% at 9 years; luno-capitate arthritis was slower to develop, but occurred in 50% at 20 years; radio-scaphoid arthritis was most common and was present in 75% at 4 years.

With respect to the third question addressed by Wright, i.e. the effect of age on OA, he notes that postfracture OA is more common in the elderly. This may be because as a whole, those of advanced years suffer from a 'background substrate' of arthritis that is present, even before a fracture occurs, and because more years may have elapsed since a fracture's occurrence. Wright's final question is the time-span over which OA develops after fracture. It is said that radiological changes of OA occur within 2–5 years of a fracture accompanied by joint deformity. He noted an anecdotal case of secondary OA occurring in as little as 20 weeks after a subarticular fracture of the acetabulum. At the other extreme, the time lapse between fracture and OA was 15 years with supracondylar fractures, 20 years with broken femoral shafts and up to 44 years with tibial shaft fractures.

ARTHRITIS FOLLOWING DAMAGE TO PERIARTICULAR SOFT TISSUE

An important factor in development of OA following fracture is the joint's stability.[18] In addition to the induction of arthritis by trauma to, or fracture of the joint, arthritis may also follow damage to periarticular soft tissues, e.g. tendons, ligaments, bursae and muscles. Although it is widely accepted that interruption of structural integrity around the joint predisposes to OA[27], little has been written to systemically explain this relationship. The knee is possibly the most well-studied joint, perhaps because it is the most often involved in OA, and because ligamentous injury is one of the most frequent predisposing causes[28]. Funk noted that knees with OA requiring replacement by prosthetic devices have a high frequency of previous ligamentous injury[29]. Iseki and Fujikawa[30] described medial instability in 43% of 516 patients with OA of the knee, and anterior instability in another 27%. In a systematic study of people with medial collateral ligament insufficiency, Kannus and Jarvinen showed that OA was more common on the medial side and that the amount of pathological change was a function of the degree of the instability[28]. These authors constructed a model of post-traumatic OA of the knee joint in which they postulated that knee injury leads to immobilization and wasting of the quadriceps muscles, and this, together with ligamentous and meniscal damage leads to instability of the knee, a sure formula for OA. The obverse, however also applies, i.e. thinning of cartilage leads to laxity of the medial ligament and further instability.

ACCIDENTS THAT MAY CAUSE RHEUMATIC DISEASE

Information about the type of accident also helps to shed light on the link between accidents and rheumatic disease. In Australia, information on specific occupation-related accidents and injuries is provided by the Work Related Fatalities Study conducted at the Australian National Occupational Health and Safety Commission[31]. Data were collected from coroners' records of all work-related traumatic fatalities over a 3-year period (1982–84). It is noteworthy that only a few types of accidents lead to injuries that are likely precursors of rheumatic disease. For example, fractures, dislocations and contusions or crush injuries were most likely to be caused by being struck by a moving object. Other common, but far less frequent causes for 'rheumatic-type' injuries include falls from heights, being struck by a falling object or striking against an object (Figure 6). It seems possible, therefore, to target these

34

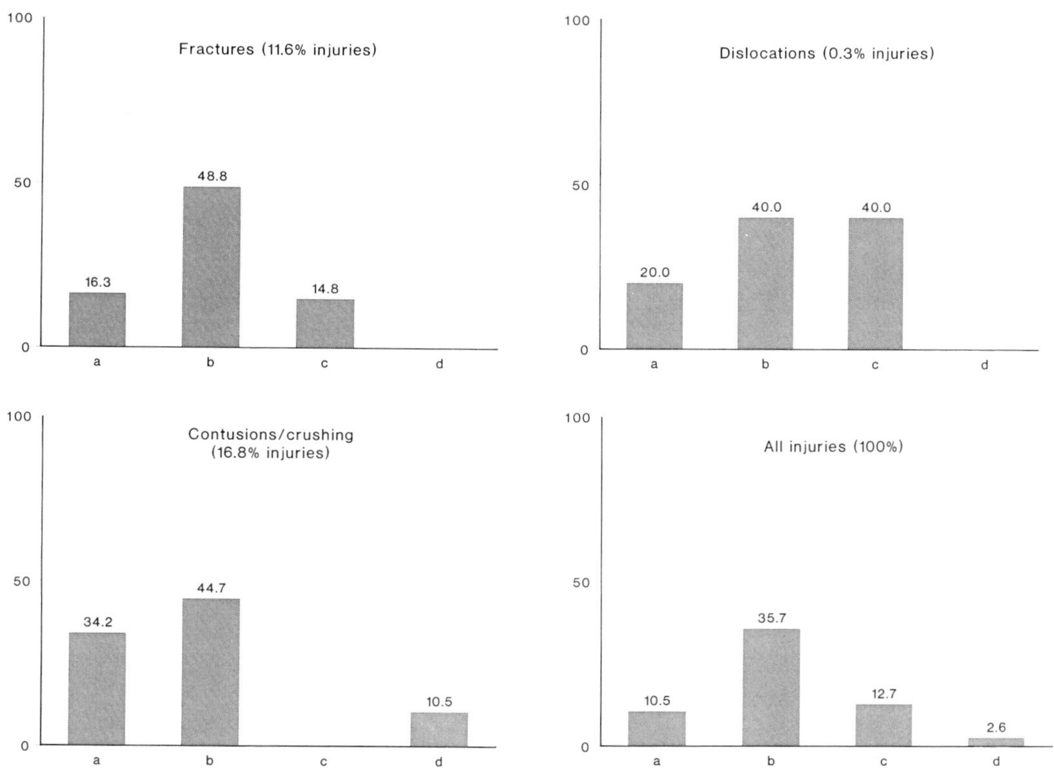

Figure 6 Specific injuries and the accidents that cause them. (Unpublished material from Worksafe Australia's Work-Related Fatalities Study[31]). Injury types: a, fall from other level; b, struck by moving object; c, struck by falling object; d, caught on, in, between

accidents to reduce trauma-related rheumatic disease.

It must be remembered, however, that these data were derived from fatal accidents and the same relationship may not apply to non-fatal accidents; obviously, rheumatic disease can only occur in non-fatal injuries! Nevertheless, similar types of injury should be represented in both fatal and non-fatal accidents, with the only difference being in the severity of the injuries[32,33] and the size, weight or speed of the impacting object. This heuristically logical contention is not supported, however, by the ACC data which deal with the 'mechanism' of work-related morbidity. These data bring into focus the important con-

tribution of 'lifting and stretching' (34%), which results in the well-known high incidence of back injuries (Figure 7). Further, in terms of the activity of the individual at the time of the accident, 'lifting and lowering' is highly significant, another common risk activity for back injury (Figure 8).

Establishing a link between the type and cause of injury, is only the first step in establishing why accidents occur. Much more must be known about the circumstances under which an activity becomes 'hazardous' before we can understand how to prevent its occurrence, factoring in such variables as the working environment (e.g. poor lighting, or loud noise) at the time of the accident,

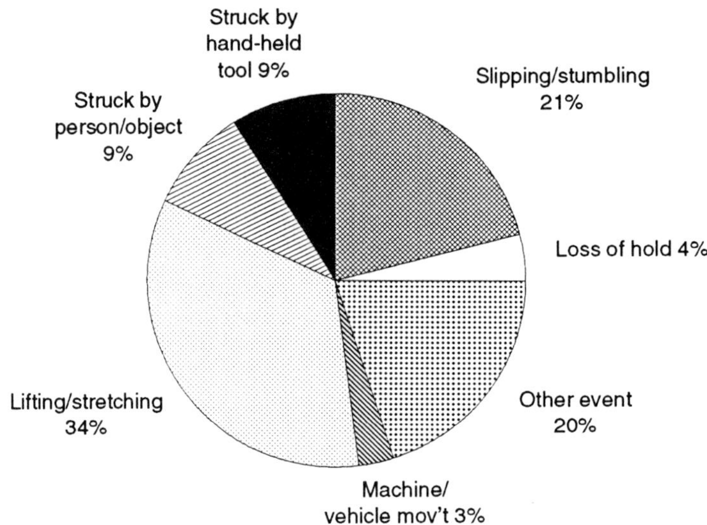

Figure 7 Mechanism of work-related injury. (Reproduced with kind permission from reference 4)

the equipment used, the work-related behavior of the person or others (e.g., habitually leaving objects on stairs or in walkways, poor supervision or training) or even the medical condition of the accident victim. If these factors are not considered, the effectiveness of preventive strategies may be diluted.

It must also be stressed that safety devices such as seat belts, pedestrian crossing signs, helmets and machine guards do not prevent the accident from occurring, but aim to prevent or limit injuries. Unfortunately, safety measures have a number of significant limitations. First, these devices must perform adequately under conditions imposed by the accident; for example, a harness or seat belt must have the strength to withstand the forces applied to it in an accident. In order for safety devices to effectively prevent injury, they must be available and fully operational where accidents are likely to occur. Second, a person must be sufficiently motivated to use such devices, which is often not the case. As an example, a recent study by the New South Wales Road Traffic Authority, found that 20% of children do not wear seat belts even though they are mandatory in that state, and there is considerable public awareness of their benefits[34]. Similarly, a common problem in industry is motivating workers to use personal protective equipment of all kinds[35].

Given these limitations, reliance solely on safety devices to prevent injuries in accidents is clearly an inadequate control measure. Additional methods need to be used to decrease the likelihood that injury will occur. This, coupled with the fact that these methods focus on injury-reduction rather than on prevention, leads one to examine the circumstances preceding accidents.

MODELS OF ACCIDENT CAUSATION

Various models have been proposed that attempt to describe how and why accidents occur. Laflamme[36] described four distinct models for examining how occupational accidents occur.

(1) Energy transfer models which describe accidents as occurring due to a chronological

36

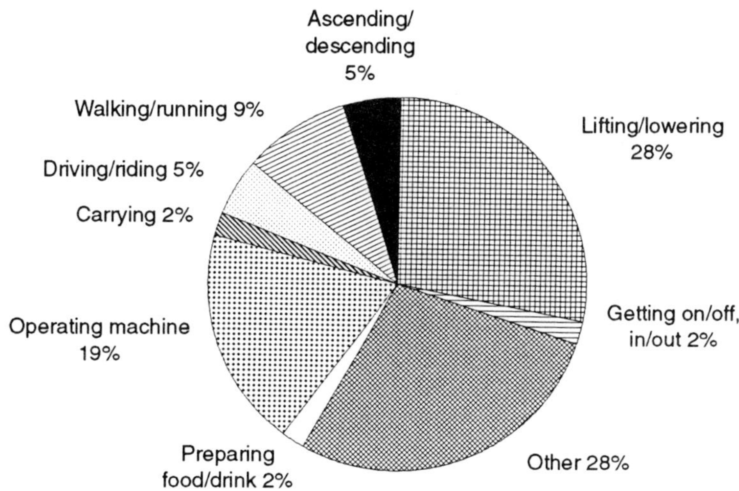

Figure 8 Activity of injured person at time of work-related accident. (Reproduced with kind permission from reference 4)

chain of events, usually involving unsafe actions of a person leading to the build up and release of unwanted energy in a situation[37,38];

(2) Sequential models which attempt to describe disturbances in normal performance of a task by putting together the sequences of events that led up to the accident occurring (e.g. the INRS method[39,40]);

(3) Decisional models which attempt to analyze how people make decisions in the sequence of events leading up to the accident and how the different aspects of the work situation interact to cause the accident[41,42]; and

(4) Organizational models which attempt to describe in detail the wider organizational factors that influence the occurrence of accidents[36].

Implicit in all models is the idea that investigating the sequences of causation will assist in determining what factors to target for prevention. Un-fortunately, many of them fall short of this goal for a range of reasons, often because they are not suitable for practical accident analysis applications or because they are far too abstract or too complex. The MORT procedure[40], for example, is a standardized check-list based on a logic tree that attempts to identify specific oversights, omissions, assumed risks and general management system weaknesses in nearly 300 problem areas. This is often considered to be too detailed and time-consuming for normal use, particularly if accident analysis is being used to investigate a large number of accidents. Many models include factors that cannot be assessed reliably following the accident. For example, decision-type models require that information about the individual's behavior and decision-making process be regarded as factors in analyzing an accident sequence. This information often cannot be determined by reviewing the sequence of events leading up to the accident, nor can it be obtained accurately from those persons involved in an accident, due to problems of recall, time delays or simply due to the effect of having been involved in the accident. Some models, in particular the energy transfer-based models, fail to consider all factors, particularly the highly-relevant psychological and organizational factors.

DEFINING TARGETS FOR ACCIDENT PREVENTION

Models of accident causation use different methods to determine appropriate targets for prevention. Probably the most common approach is to use information already gathered such as accident and incident reports or compensation statistics to identify preventive targets[43]. This approach has major limitations, since such reports generally only allow very superficial descriptions of the final events in the accident sequence. Other models acknowledge the need for more information, and develop their own information-gathering systems tailored to emphasize what they consider to be important aspects of accident causation[41], allowing for more in-depth analysis of circumstances and events preceding the accident. In practice, such analyses are hampered by an inverse relationship between the depth and details of information needed to explain the wider causes of accidents and the likelihood that such data are available. Thus, although there are a number of comprehensive models of how accidents occur, and these might provide very useful suggestions for preventive targets, they are poorly applicable to the 'art' of accident analysis in the real world. For example, the INRS system[39] was developed for the nuclear industry and has been effective in establishing targets for accident prevention in a high risk, low probability environment, but has limited application in analyzing the extent and nature of human involvement in accidents in other settings.

It has been argued that a major limitation of all models that require data on past accidents in order to develop preventive strategies, is that they are only useful when enough data has been collected[44], or 'enough fitters fall off ladders'[45].

Some models develop preventive strategies by predicting the probability of events occurring in a particular accident sequence, by either studying similar situations or via expert input and general experience, which is an approach most often used in risk assessment. The drawbacks of preventive strategy analysis are that it relies on definitions of normal circumstances in order to calculate the probability of abnormal situations occurring; such definitions may be very inaccurate.

It is thus clear that the use of accident causation models to develop targets for prevention is limited by the lack of sufficient detail to allow one to target specific 'at risk' situations and activities. These models should not, on the other hand, provide so much detail that reliable data cannot be reasonably collected, which is often the case when models attempt to include details of the role of human action in accident causation.

Attempts have been made to avoid some of these problems by reversing the reasoning of accident analysis[46,47]. Rather than developing a model of accident causation, and then collecting data to fit into it or exploring the likelihood of deviations therefrom, Williamson and Feyer[46] have developed a classification system for information relating to accidents and applied it to large data sets in order to establish a 'data-derived' model of accident causation. This data-driven approach to the question of why accidents occur circumvents many of the problems inherent in the more conventional models described above, and has been applied to the data collected as part of the Work-Related Fatalities Study[31]. The classification system codes the sequence of precursor events leading up to an accident and any other factors that contributed to unsafe circumstances. The nature of the precursor events were coded into one of four categories: environmental, equipment, medical or behavioral and the last category was subdivided in terms of whether it constituted an error, and if so its type. Contributing factors were classified in any number of eight possible categories; environmental, equipment, work practice, supervision, training, task error, medical, alcohol and drug use and other. Precursor events and contributing factors were ranked in terms of their significance for the occurrence of each fatality, allowing one to infer the root cause(s) of the accident itself, a critical consideration for accident prevention. A total of 1020 coded fatalities were analyzed and revealed that four patterns of event sequences accounted for two-thirds of all deaths. Environmental and behavioral influences were involved in approximately equal proportions immediately before the accident, but behavioral factors were reported as being much more influential in causing the accident. Further analysis of the type of behavior showed that errors during skill-based behavior were the most common. Of the contributing factors, poor work practices were by far the most common and the most influential in causing the accident, and where they occurred were most likely to be the root cause of the accident.

Examination of the types of accident patterns by industry showed that aside from a few specific industries, the same four patterns involving mainly behavioral and environmental influences impacted on accidents. The occupations with unique accident patterns were timber getters (lumberjacks), maritime workers, who are strongly influenced by environmental factors, and air transport workers, whose equipment plays a major role in accident causation.

These analyses provide important insights required to formulate preventive strategies. Since the root causes of most accidents are skill-based errors and/or unsafe work practices, this greatly narrows the areas that need to be targeted to those that should be most productive for preventing accidents. It also shows that commonly used preventive strategies such as more, or improved, training of workers are unlikely to be successful in circumstances where skill-based errors are the root cause of accidents because these types of errors can not be eliminated through training. Rather it would appear that environments need to be made more tolerant such that when skill-based errors occur, they do not lead to injury. This is one situation where safety devices built into the working environment could successfully prevent the injury, if not the accident. For most industrial accidents however, targeting unsafe work practices may be the most effective preventive goal. These analyses also show what not to target. Except for the air transportation industry, equipment failure and health problems are rarely implicated as contributing factors in the event sequence, and are even less involved as root cause(s) of the accident.

This project has demonstrated that data on the causes of accidents can be used to develop models of why and how accidents occur. These can be then used to predict when accidents might occur and to direct strategies to prevent them from occurring. Interestingly, the conclusions of this study provide support for a model of accident causation developed recently by Wagenaar and colleagues[48]. Based on theoretical concepts of human error and their role in causing accidents, this model describes a general accident causation sequence as starting with management decisions that allow general failure types to occur or persist. These are factors in the situation that are incorrect or defective, may have been so for a long time, but do not become obvious until something happens to signal their existence such as an accident or 'near miss'. These then provide the setting for human actions either becoming major errors or for normally minor errors to have harmful consequences. These ideas provide converging evidence that to be most effective, accident prevention must focus on pre-existing work practices or latent failures that lie at the root of so many accidents. In practical terms this means influencing decisions at the level of the organization of the situation, for example, management for workplace accidents and road and traffic authorities for road accidents.

CONCLUSIONS

There appears to be sufficient circumstantial evidence linking rheumatic symptoms to accidents, although definitive prospective studies have not been performed that analyze how many of those persons injured in 'rheumatic sites' ultimately develop such symptoms. We believe that accident-preventive measures might also prevent the rheumatic symptoms that arise in the sites of injury. We have scrutinized the prevention of accidents in general, and more specifically, examined those areas that might lead to rheumatic disease.

Despite the definition of accidents as being 'unforeseen', they are certainly not unavoidable or unpreventable. How many fractures of the hip and associated arthritic pain could be prevented by simple strategies, for example, eliminating unnecessary steps in buildings, a trap for elderly persons wearing bifocal lenses? Although more specific preventive approaches to answering such rhetorical questions will be elaborated upon in subsequent chapters, in general terms, it is clear that strategies can be introduced in the home, in the workplace and the sports field, which can minimize accidents, their not inconsiderable co-morbidity and the health care costs that are borne by all.

ACKNOWLEDGEMENT

The authors would like to thank the management of the ACC (New Zealand) for permission to reproduce data and adapt figures for the annual reports.

REFERENCES

1. Olivieri I, Gemignani G, Christou C *et al*. Trauma and sero-negative spondyloarthropathy: report of two more cases of peripheral arthritis precipitated by physical injury. Ann Rheum Dis. 1989; 48:520–521

2. Wisniesky J. Trauma and Reiter's syndrome. Ann Rheum Dis. 1989; 43:829–32

3. Kaprio LA. Injury. In Wilson, Sir John, ed., Disability Prevention: the Global Challenge. Oxford, Oxford University Press, 1983, pp. 41–46

4. Accident Compensation Corporation. Annual Report 1989. Wellington: ACC, 1989

5. World Health Organization. Euro Reports and Studies #40: Seatbelt and Other Devices to Reduce Injuries from Traffic Accidents. Copenhagen: WHO, 1981

6. World Health Organization. Euro Reports and Studies #57: The Epidemiology of Accident Traumas and Resulting Disabilities. Copenhagen: WHO, 1982

7. Foggon G. Occupational accidents. In Wilson, Sir John, ed., Disability Prevention: the Global Challenge. Oxford, Oxford University, 1983, pp. 47–49

8. Slavin RE, Swedo J, Cartwright J Jr *et al*. Lead arthritis and lead poisoning following bullet wounds. Human Pathol. 1988; 19:223–235

9. Wilson GE, Curry A, Kennaugh JH *et al*. Severe granulomatous arthritis due to spinous injury by a 'sea mouse' annelid worm. J Clin Pathol. 1990; 43:291–294

10. Kern D, Zlatkin MB, Dalinka MH. Occupational and post-traumatic arthritis. Radiol Clin North Am. 1988; 26:1349–1356

11. Radin EL, Ehrlich MG, Chernack R. Effect of repetitive impulse loading on the knee joint of rabbits. Clin Orthop. 1978; 131:288–293

12. Felson DT. Osteoarthritis. Rheum Dis Clin North Am. 1990; 16:499–512

13. Davis MA, Ettinger WH, Niehaus JM *et al*. The association of knee injury and obesity with unilateral and bilateral osteoarthritis of the knee. Am J Epidemiol. 1989; 130:278–288

14. Klunder KB, Rud B, Hansen J. Osteoarthritis of the hip and knee joint in retired football players. Acta Orthop Scand. 1980; 51:925–927

15. Wright V. Post-traumatic osteoarthritis – A medico-legal minefield. Br J Rheumatol. 1990; 29:474–478

16. Murray-Leslie CF, Lintott DJ, Wright, V. The knees and ankles in sport and veteran military parachutists. Ann Rheum Dis. 1977; 36: 327–331

17. Mankin J. Current concepts review: the response of articular cartilage to mechanical injury. J Bone Joint Surg (Am). 1982; 64:460–466

18. Rasmussen PS. Tibial condylar fractures as a cause of degenerative arthritis. Acta Orthop Scand. 1972; 43:566–750

19. Fairbank TJ. Knee joint changes after meniscectomy. J Bone Joint Surg. 1948; 30-B:664–670

20. Tapper ER, Hoover NW. Late results after meniscectomy. J Bone Joint Surg. 1969; 51-A: 517–526

21. Johnson RJ, Kettelkamp DB, Clark W *et al.* Factors affecting late results after meniscectomy. J Bone Joint Surg. 1974; 56-A:719–729

22. Mack GR, Bosse MJ, Gilberman RH. The natural history of scaphoid non-union. J Bone Joint Surg. 1984; 66-A:504–509

23. Ruby LK, Stinson J. The natural history of scaphoid non-union. J Bone Joint Surg. 1985; 67-A: 428–432

24. Ruby LK, Leslie BM. Scaphoid Non-union. Hand Clin. 1987; 3:529–33; J Bone Joint Surg. 1984; 66-A:504–509

25. Fisk J. Osteoarthritis of the wrist. Clin Rheum Dis. 1984; 10:571–588

26. Vender MI, Watson HK, Wiener BD, Black DM. Degenerative change in symptomatic scaphoid non-union. J Hand Surg (Am). 1987; 124: 514–519

27. Burry HC. Sport, exercise and arthritis. Br J Rheumatol. 1987; 26:386–388

28. Kannus P, Jarvinen M. Osteoarthrosis of the knee due to chronic post-traumatic insufficiency of the lateral ligament compartment. Clin Rheumatol. 1988; 7:200–207

29. Funk JR. Osteoarthritis of the knee following ligamentous injury. Clin Orthop. 1983; 172: 154–157

30. Iseki F, Fujikawa K. Clinical pictures of osteoarthritis of the knee joint. J Jap Orthop Assoc. 1980; 54:563-574

31. Harrison JE, Frommer MS, Ruck EA, Blyth FM. Deaths as a result of work-related injury in Australia, 1982–1984. Med J Australia. 1989; 150:118–125

32. Heinrich HW. Industrial Accident Prevention. New York, McGraw Hill, 1959

33. Lozada-Larsen SR, Laughery KR. Do identical circumstances precede minor and major injuries? Proceedings of the Human Factors Society, 1987 pp. 200–204

34. New South Wales Road Traffic Authority, Road Safety Bureau. Seat belt and child restraint usage in NSW. October and November, 1990, Research Note RN3/91

35. Hopkins BL, Conrad RJ, Dangel RF *et al.* Behavioural technology for reducing occupational exposures to styrene. J Appl Behav Anal. 1986; 1:3–11

36. LaFlamme L. A better understanding of occupational accident genesis to improve safety in the workplace. J Occup Accid. 1990; 12:155–165

37. Haddon W. The changing approach to the epidemiology, prevention, and amelioration of trauma: the transition to approaches etiologically rather than descriptively based. Am J Public Health. 1968; 58:1431–1438

38. Tuominen R, Saari J. A model for analysis of accidents and its application. J Occup Accid. 1982; 4:263–273

39. Leplat J. Accident and incidents production: Methods of analysis. J Occup Accid. 1982; 4: 229–310

40. Johnson W. MORT Safety Assurance System. New York, Marcel Dekker, 1980

41. Corlett EN, Gilbank G. A systematic technique for accident analysis. J Occup Accid. 1978; 2:25–38

42. Hale AR, Glendon AI. Individual Behaviour in the Control of Danger. Amsterdam, Elsevier, 1987

43. Oleske DM, Brewer RD, Dan P, Hahn J. An epidemiologic evaluation of the injury experience of a cohort of automotive parts workers: a model for surveillance in small industries. J Occup Accid. 1989; 10:239–253

44. Woodcock Webb K. Ergonomics and occupational accident reporting – using accidents to obtain information about person-task-environment systems. Karwowski W, ed., Trends in Ergonomics III. Amsterdam, Elsevier, 1986

45. Kletz TA. Accident data – the need for a new look at the sort of data that are collected and analysed. J Occup Accid. 1976; 1:95–105

46. Williamson AM, Feyer A-M. Behavioural epidemiology as a tool for accident research. J Occup Accid. 1990; 12:207–222

47. Feyer A-M, Williamson AM. A classification system of the causes of occupational accidents for use in preventive strategies. Scand J Work Environ Health. 1991; 17:302–311

48. Wagenaar WA, Hudson PTW, Reason JT. Cognitive failures and accidents. Appl Cognit Psychol. 1990; 4:273–294

5. THE PRIMARY PREVENTION OF SPORT-INDUCED RHEUMATIC DISEASES

Anthony Gear

INTRODUCTION

If the elimination of injuries was our only concern, it would be proper to advise all our offspring to play snooker and croquet. Other factors dictate that everyone should be active participants in sport and exercise, which include a sense of well-being, companionship and enjoyment. The protective effects on the cardiovascular system and the skeleton, plus the secondary benefits to lifestyle, such as reduced smoking, add medical arguments to the case for physical activity. Diet and exercise are the only two physiological means that we have to control our weight. In recent years there has been a huge upsurge in sporting activity in the developed world. Jogging led the trend which has now been expanded to include cycling, aerobics, gym, canoeing and, most popular of all, walking. Unquestionably our bodies derive much benefit from this potpourri of activities, but this is countered by the numerous injuries to which our fragile frames are susceptible. There are few things so pathetic as an active sportsman rendered slothful and degenerate by injury.

In this discussion, the term 'rheumatic diseases' will be used in a broad sense to include all disorders of the musculoskeletal system resulting from sport. These include acute and overuse injuries, metabolic effects, particularly on bone, and late sequelae such as osteoarthritis. This chapter considers epidemiological and etiological factors involved in sports injuries, and discusses in general terms the measures which can be taken to prevent them. The frequency of injuries and the potential for avoiding them make sport a fertile field for preventive strategies.

Apart from the health of the individual there are important economic gains to be made from reducing exercise-related accidents. The New Zealand Accident Compensation Scheme is a comprehensive, no-fault social insurance scheme for victims of unintentional injury. In 1989, the population of about three and a half million people made 139 856 claims (at a cost of 777 million NZ dollars in pay-outs), of which 18% were for sports injuries. Of these, 7165 (28.5%) were for rugby football injuries, soccer being second highest with 1662 (66%) injuries[1].

FACTORS AFFECTING THE INCIDENCE OF SPORT INJURIES
Type of sport

Goldberg and colleagues[2] separated sport into four categories: augmented speed (e.g. skateboarding and winter-sports), collision (e.g. football and ice hockey), contact (e.g. basketball and soccer) and non-contact (e.g. tennis and golf), and suggested that at least in children there was a decreasing frequency of injuries as one moves through the categories[2,3]. Although this hypothesis seems logical, no correction was made for

Table 1 Total injury rate by sport. All figures are calculated or estimated from references 5, 6, 9, 10, 12–18 and 76

Sport	Injury rate (per 1000 hours)	% Musculoskeletal
Ice hockey		
youth	10	40
professional	140	40
Rugby		
youth matches	17.6	55
severe injuries	1.4	65
senior practices	1.3	85
senior matches	16.6	85
Soccer		
youth non-competitive	0.5/1.1 (male/female)	53
youth competitive	14/32 (male/female)	53
senior practice	7.6	76
senior matches	16.9	76
professional		64–73
Gymnastics		
club, non-competitive	0.4–0.7	
elite women	7–53	60–85
Recreational ice skating		
new rink	2.8	42
established rink	0.8	
Recreational softball	2.3	50

the number of participants and the number of player-hours. It is not surprising that in 'rugby-mad' New Zealand this sport accounts for nearly one-third of injuries requiring medical treatment[1], while in Finland winter sports are responsible for 44% of children's injuries[4]. With its huge number of players, soccer causes the most number of sports injuries throughout the world accounting for 50–60% of injuries in Europe[5].

Sex

More women are presenting with injuries as their participation in exercise increases, although males still account for about 80% of patients seen at sports medicine clinics[6]. This not only reflects the number involved, but also the higher participation by men in augmented speed and collision sports. Nevertheless, when direct comparisons are made between men and women in sports in which both take part, women may be more prone to injury. In basketball, women are more susceptible to patello-femoral problems and anterior cruciate ruptures than men[7], and female youth soccer players sustain twice as many injuries as their male counterparts[5]. Apart from patello-femoral pain syndromes and dislocations, De-Haven and Lintner found men and women to suffer similar types of injuries[6].

Age

Children generally suffer fewer mishaps than adults, but are susceptible to some specific injuries which will be considered separately. Inflammatory conditions such as tendinitis are said

44

Table 2 Involvement of joints (expressed as a percentage of the total sports injuries for that sport). All the figures are calculated or estimated from references 5, 6, 10, 11, 17–19, 20 and 76

Sport	Hand/wrist	Elbow	Shoulder	Hip	Knee	Ankle
American football	3				31	12
Rugby			7		15	14
Australian rules	24	2	10	1	6	12
Soccer	upper extremity: 8–17			3–20	12–48	8–41
Ice hockey	2–8		9–22	9–36	10–12	low
Basketball	3				55	11
Baseball	9		25		31	3
Softball	21	1	2	0	3	10
Women's gymnastics	0–7	5	1	2	14–24	27
Martial arts	upper extremity: 27			lower extremity: 47		
Tennis	7	14	9		19	5
Squash	6	7	7		24	13

to become more prevalent with advancing age[6], but this may be because mature athletes are more likely to participate in those sports associated with overuse injuries, like road running.

Weight

In team sports, such as American football and ice hockey, the injuries increase as the average weight of the players rises[7,8]. Heavier gymnasts are also more prone to injury[9].

INJURY RATES

It is difficult to present precise injury rates for different sports as the literature is inconsistent in defining injuries and in the expression of the rates. Too often rates are expressed as the number of injuries per participant without time limits; thus an incidence of 0.33 injuries per 100 gymnasts may be regarded by some as meaningless[10]. Other studies relate figures to a total population[11], which may present other difficulties in the comparison of data.

In most sports, more than half the significant injuries are to the musculoskeletal system, although there are obviously exceptions, e.g. ice hockey in which about 50% of injuries involve the head and neck region[12]. Table 1 provides a crude estimate of injury rates of some of the more popular sports, expressed as the number of injuries per 1000 player-hours. In a study of adult rugby players, Clark and colleagues found a rate of one injury every 60 hours (16.6 per 1000 hours) in matches compared with one in 780 hours (1.3 per 1000 hours) in practice; over 80% of the reported injuries were to the musculoskeletal system[13]. In his study on schoolboy rugby injuries, Davidson found an incidence of 17.6 per 1000 player-hours in matches[14], which approximates Clark's data. Ice hockey, another collision sport, also has a high injury rate, but only 20% involve the musculoskeletal system. The injury rate in young players is 10 per 1000 hours, while in professional ice hockey, this rate soars to 140 injuries per 1000 player-hours[12]. In a review of the epidemiology of the world's most popular sport, soccer, Keller and colleagues found that injuries occurred in 0.5 per 1000 hours for young non-competitive players, 14 per 1000 hours for a national youth competition and 16.9 per 1000 hours for senior competitive players[2]. In both youth studies, the injury rate for girls is about twice that for boys.

45

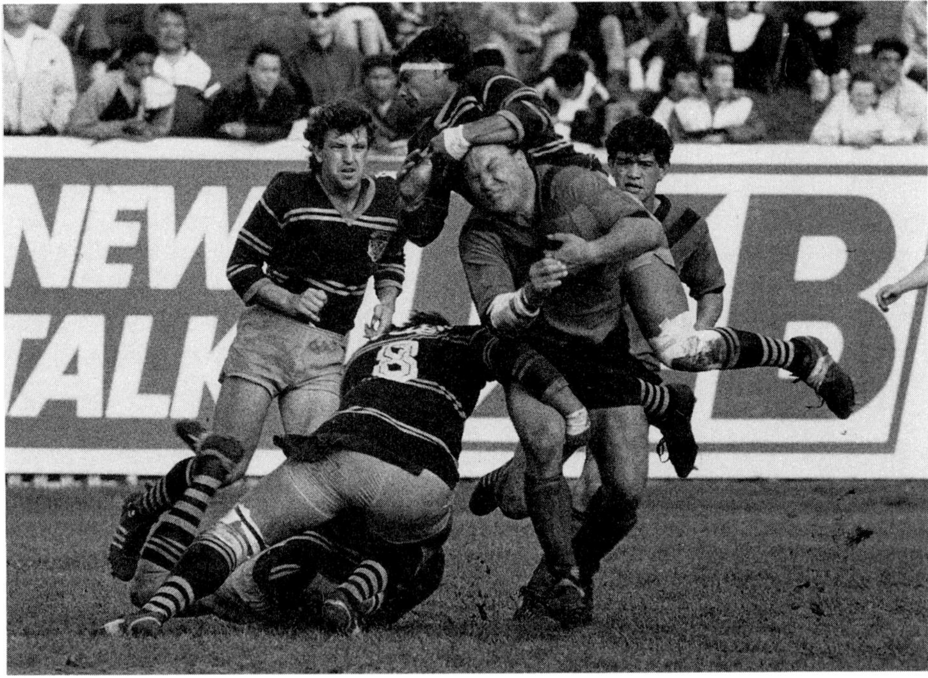

Figure 1 High tackle in rugby league. (Reproduced with kind permission from *The New Zealand Herald*)

These figures contrast sharply with non-contact sports where, for example, 2.8 injuries occurred per 1000 attendances at a newly-opened ice skating rink in Oxford, and fell to 0.8 per 1000 ten weeks after the rink opened. In this last study, upper limb fractures were the most common injury[15]. A similar (1.6 injuries per 1000) incidence was reported in an ice skating rink in Ulster[16]. Recreational softball has a comparable incidence of 2.3 injuries per 1000 players per day[17], whilst in gymnastics, the rate differs according to the sex and the level of competition, where injuries occur at a rate of 7 to 53 per 1000 hours in elite women gymnasts and 0.4 to 0.7 per 1000 hours in non-competitive club gymnasts[10].

ACUTE INJURIES

For the purposes of this discussion, acute injuries include sprains (ligaments), strains (muscles and tendons), dislocations and fractures, exclusive of the skull. Table 2 presents estimates of the proportion of various anatomical sites, expressed as a percentage of the total sports injuries, involved in a number of selected sports. In most sports, the lower limb is more prone to injury than the upper limb, even in racquet sports, e.g. tennis and squash[19]. The knee suffers the most joint injuries overall, with ankle injuries at a similar level in soccer and gymnastics. Catching sports, e.g. baseball, softball and cricket, are associated with a high proportion of hand injuries[20]. Baseball also has a high incidence of shoulder lesions. The ankle would seem to be well protected by rigid boots in winter sports. Australian rules football breaks all the rules, but then there are no games like it. Not only are ankle injuries twice as frequent as knee injuries, but the upper limb is involved more often than the lower[21]. Although many injuries are severe enough to end the sporting career of young players, it is injury to the cervical spine that has the most devastating effect. Rugby and American football put the participants at greatest risk for such an injury, but other sports in which this risk must be weighed include ice hockey, gymnastics, wrestling, diving and trampolining[22–25].

Although reports of quadriplegia appear with some regularity in the news media, in reality, such injuries are relatively uncommon. A study conducted over 18 years, which involved a total of 93 780 player games of rugby at an Australian school, revealed an incidence of 0.012 cervical spine injuries per 1000 player-hours[14]. Scher states that 'clearly these injuries, however few, are unacceptable'[26]. It is disturbing to note that the prevalence of these injuries may not be falling in rugby and may actually be rising in ice hockey. Scher reports that in the Cape Province in South Africa the incidence of injury attributed to rugby was 5 per year from 1981 to 1987 compared with 3 per year between 1964 and 1980[26]. Reports from Canada suggest that neck fractures in ice hockey are a new and disturbing problem[22,23]. On the other hand, rule changes in American football have had a very significant impact[27].

Different factors contribute to spinal cord injury in each sport. In American football, 'spearing', in which the impact in a tackle is with the top of the head, with the neck held between neutral and 30°, was the major factor[27]. In ice hockey crashing head first into the boards, often due to a push or a check from behind, is the most frequent cause of spinal cord injury[22,23]. In rugby, the two most important mechanisms are the collapsed scrum with the front row forwards being caught with their necks in flexion as a push from behind continues, and the illegal high tackle[26,28,29] (Figure 1). Sadly, in both football and ice hockey, a successful measure to prevent head injuries has contributed to more spine injuries. Improved protective gear has led to increased confidence and speed, resulting in more episodes likely to cause injuries[22].

OVERUSE INJURIES

While there is a paucity of reliable epidemiological studies on acute sports injuries, valid data are virtually non-existent for overuse injuries. The literature is replete with questionnaire-based surveys, retrospective analyses of patients attending sports medicine clinics, and reviews of injured patients without adequate control groups. Much of the current dogma is based on 'logic', guesswork and extrapolation, but little on scientific research. This section will be further influenced by the author's own prejudices.

Overuse injury can be defined as an injury to a structure or system that is due to repetitive forces beyond the capacity of that structure or system to withstand or adapt to such forces[30]. The tissues involved include muscles and related soft tissues, tendons, entheses, apophyses, ligaments, cartilage and bones. The pathology includes compartment and impingement syndromes, tendinitis, enthesitis, apophysitis and stress fractures. The development of osteoarthritis is not generally included as a sports overuse injury, although cartilage pathology in the form of chondromalacia patellae is.

Many injury studies are based on the presentation to casualty departments or acute sports medicine clinics and thus it is difficult to compare the incidence of overuse injuries and acute injuries. In collision sports, the vast majority are acute injuries13, while in road running, overuse injuries predominate31. In soccer 10–25% are overuse while in women's gymnastics approximately 40% are[10,18].

Clement has suggested five categories of aetiological factors in injury production: (a) training errors; (b) dysfunction of strength or flexibility; (c) training surfaces; (d) running shoes; and (e) biomechanical factors[7].

Because the training required for optimal performance is the same as that causing injury, namely high mileage, and hill, speed and interval training, there is a fine line between excellence and breakdown. An athlete should increase the intensity of training at a rate slow enough to allow his body to adapt[32,33]. We have to be fit before we start training. A commonly cited example of muscular dysfunction is the abnormal tracking of the patella due to a relatively weak vastus medialis, an event that would be extraordinarily difficult to prove and thus remains speculative. In other sites, 'muscle imbalance' is demonstrated only after injury and is therefore difficult to implicate as a cause.

Training on hard surfaces is no longer a problem with appropriate shoes. Indeed, it can be argued that running on surfaces that are too soft may result in increased tension on the Achilles tendon and associated muscles. Running on cambered roads may cause problems, particularly in runners who have not had time to adapt to the slope[7]. Running shoes have undergone rapid evolutionary change over the last 20 years, achieving effective shock absorption, minimizing pronation and controlling excessive foot motion[7]. 'Shin splints', most frequently caused by inflammation at the origin of tibialis posterior, are associated with increases in maximum pronation and maximum pronation velocity[33]. Others argue that prolonged pronation plays a role. Curved-last shoes may aggravate the problem. Attempts have been made to control hindfoot motion with rigid heel counters[34]. Examination of some modern running shoes suggests that manufacturers would have athletes run in blocks of concrete. Performance, which is nearly as important to many recreational runners as it is to elite athletes, is adversely affected by heavy shoes. The author believes it is more appropriate to control undesirable foot movements with wedges in lighter shoes. Another problem that can arise from anti-pronation shoes is the increased valgus stress placed on the knees which can cause an iliotibial band syndrome[34].

In addition to excessive pronation of the feet, anteversion of the hip, abnormalities of the extensor mechanism across the knee, excessive tibial varum and various foot disorders have been implicated in lower limb overuse injuries. It is beyond the scope of this chapter to discuss all of these. A group of conditions, for which there must always be a high index of suspicion, particularly in enthesitides of the hindfoot, is HLA B27-associated diseases.

The shoulder joint requires specific consideration given its unique anatomy and its susceptibility to subacromial inflammation and damage. The major pathogenic mechanism of injury seems to be an impingement, which catches the rotator cuff and other soft tissues between the humeral head and the coracoacromial arch. Impingement occurs with repetitive movements, which may be high velocity as in baseball pitching, slower as in swimming or very slow as in archery[35–37]. It has been suggested that there is a continuum which progresses from instability to subluxation to impingement to tendinitis and finally to rotator cuff tear[35]. In archery, the impingement is aggravated by small repetitive movements at the end of the draw phase. Conditioning to improve glenohumeral stability, particularly of those muscles reducing anterior subluxation, and the elimination of unnecessary movement at full abduction and extension may play a role in preventing shoulder problems in these sports.

Stress fractures are an important, albeit relatively infrequent, overuse injury in many sports. The lumbar spine may be at greatest risk in those sports that are associated with hyperextension and/or rotation. In a prospective study of young cricket fast bowlers, 11% developed lumbar stress fractures over a single season[38]! Injury was more frequent in those who bowled with a more open delivery, delivered from a greater height, and had greater upper body strength. Gymnasts are similarly at risk of lumbar stress fractures with a prevalence of pars interarticularis defects of 11% and of spondylolisthesis of 6%[39,40].

METABOLIC EFFECTS ON BONE

Generally, exercise improves bone mass. However, extreme exercise leads to amenorrhea and decreased bone density, although this is not as marked as in women with secondary amenorrhea from other causes[41,42]. The high incidence of stress fractures in these athletes confirms their reduced skeletal strength. However, many of these athletes also have a low calorie intake, and the relative role of diet in the development of decreased bone mass and stress fractures is still to be determined. Vegetarianism may aggravate the problem further. Wyshak and colleagues have indirectly assessed bone mass by retrospectively studying, by questionnaire, the prevalence of fractures in women who had been college athletes compared with non-athletes, with particular emphasis on non-alcoholic carbonated beverage consumption. First fractures after the age of 40 were more common in those with a low milk intake, non-athletes and, in athletes, those with a higher carbonated beverage consumption. They propose that the high level of phosphate in some soft drinks inhibits calcium absorption. They recognize the marked limitations of their methodology, but if this can be shown to be true, it has important epidemiological implications[43].

LATE MUSCULOSKELETAL COMPLICATIONS OF SPORT

The 'couch-potatoes' of the world have predicted that the exercise boom will spawn a generation of cripples. There are reports of sports-related activities causing osteoarthritis (OA) in virtually all joints, which are countered by articles stating such activities do not increase the incidence of OA, or that some sports may even have a protective effect, an issue recently reviewed by Panush[44]. This section briefly highlights some of the interesting points from the ongoing debate.

There is general agreement that instability and meniscectomy are factors that predispose the knee to the development of OA[44–48], although strong thigh muscles in untreated anterior cruciate ligament rupture seem to reduce the incidence of OA by increasing the knee's stability[49]. Most evidence suggests that running does not predispose to arthritis provided there are no contributory biomechanical factors[42,44,47,50–52] (some patients insist that their osteoarthritic, unstable, and painful knees are actually improved by running). While OA is not regarded as an early consequence of running, this question has been inadequately studied in former runners who are in their seventh, eighth or ninth decades, when OA most commonly becomes symptomatic.

The literature is far more contradictory regarding the development of OA in collision and contact sports, although impact alone is probably not enough to cause OA[52,53]. There are few well-controlled studies and the differing diagnostic criteria for OA add to this confusion; as an example, early studies included joints with some periarticular calcification on X-ray which do not fulfil the currently acceptable criteria for OA[44]. Although mechanical stress on normal joints is not thought to play a major role in the genesis of osteoarthritis, it should not be dismissed altogether. The Framingham OA study has shown an association between those occupations requiring frequent knee bends and OA[54]. This author believes that this should be of particular concern to cricket wicket-keepers who go through the totally unnecessary ritual of squatting and then standing before each ball is bowled (Figure 2). It is somewhat mystifying why they do not crouch slightly as the ball is bowled, which is of course what the slips do. The catchers in baseball and softball might also be wise to consider the ergonomics of their chosen position. In a controlled

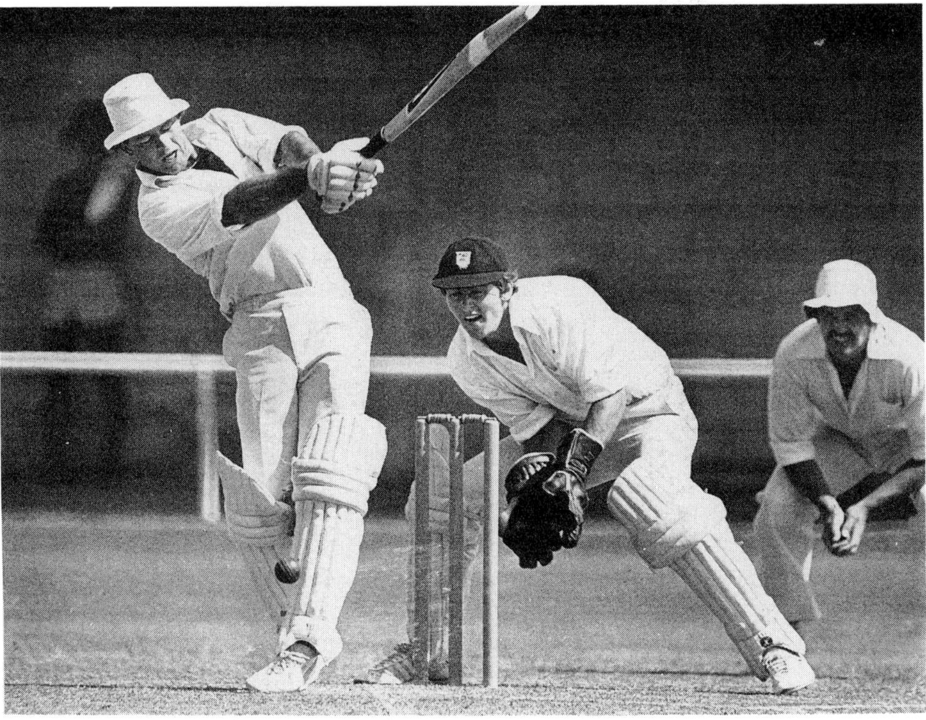

Figure 2 Wicket keeper in a crouched position having come up from a squat. (Reproduced with kind permission from *The New Zealand Herald*)

study on asymptomatic current rugby players, Scher has demonstrated a disturbing increase in degenerative disease of the cervical spine[55], which is most marked amongst the tight forwards and increases with age. Eight of the 150 players studied had radiological evidence of previous vertebral fractures! Could the common denominator to early cartilage degeneration in sport be an abnormal shearing stress while the joint is loaded?

SPORT AND THE MUSCULO-SKELETAL SYSTEM OF CHILDREN

Children and their families derive enormous enjoyment from sport and the increasing numbers participating must be lauded. Unfortunately, this growth has been accompanied by higher intensity and demands. Involvement in sport as an adult is greatly influenced by sports activities in child-

hood, and 72% of high school students' leisure time is spent on activities to which they had been introduced before the age of twelve[56]. Competition is good and provides a measure of relative skill, but there is a point where it becomes potentially harmful socially, physically and psychologically. It is discouraging to watch sane adults become maddened monsters as they roam the sidelines shouting encouragement, instructions (often contradictory) and abuse at their offspring who 'strut and fret their hour upon the stage'[57]. Most kids survive and many thrive on this primitive behavior, but it is the top few young athletes for whom we should be most concerned, as they are most at risk of becoming Maffulli's 'sacrificial lambs to a coach's or parent's ego'[58]. The controversy of children in competitive sport is widely debated and opinions, guidelines and advice abound[3,31,56,58–63]. It is some comfort to

50

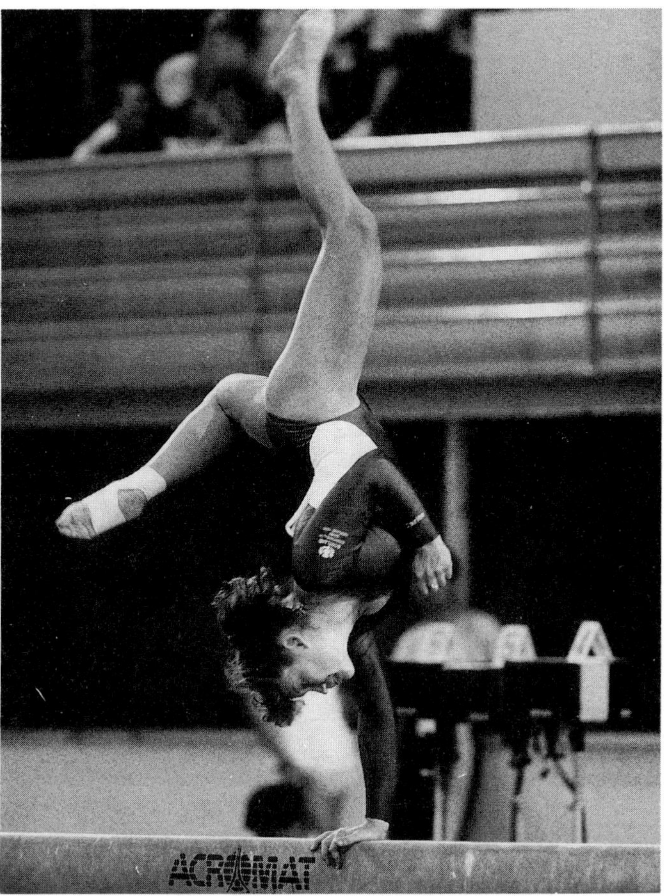

Figure 3 In gymnastics the arm becomes a weight-bearing limb. (Reproduced with kind permission from *The New Zealand Herald*)

know that the injury rate in children is proportional to age and thus lower in the younger ones[2,31].

Children's musculoskeletal systems differ from those of adults in a number of respects.

(1) They have epiphyses and epiphyseal growth plates which are susceptible to injury particularly just before they close.

(2) Their bones are relatively weaker than their tendons and ligaments, resulting in a higher proportion of fractures compared to soft tissue tears.

(3) Their weaker bones also make them more prone to overuse stress fractures.

There is concern that repetitive trauma, e.g. in road running, or pressure to the growth plate, e.g. in weight lifting, may compromise growth. In a discussion on the problem Apple quotes contradictory work[31]. It has been demonstrated experimentally that pressure applied across the growth plate in rabbits inhibits bone growth, although considerable pressure was required to stop it altogether[64]; pressure applied at right angles to growth resulted in angular deformities. This contrasts to the data presented in 1952 by Strombino and colleagues, who were unable to demonstrate an effect of pressure on epiphyseal growth[65]; nor could Peterson and Burkhart[66] find evidence in the literature or in the Mayo Clinic files that epiphyseal pressure injury causes premature or partial closure of the growth plate. Apple concludes that pressure on epiphyses due to running does not seem to induce adverse effects, although the same cannot be said for girls' gymnastics where the arm becomes a weight bearing limb (Figure 3). Albanese *et al.* present compelling evidence that premature growth plate closure occurs in the distal radius in gymnasts, resulting in a shortening of the radius vis-à-vis the ulna[67]. Roy *et al.* described stress related changes in the distal radial epiphysis, but found no premature closure[68]. With one exception these gymnasts were exercising at least two hours daily on average and in Roy's group 18 out of 21 were doing six hours five days a week or 30 hours weekly. These experiences must be rather unusual and therefore one has to wonder whether the routine in a particular gym is not to blame. Although Apple suggests that running does not produce adverse pressure effects on the growth plates themselves, he emphasizes the susceptibility of the apophyses to traction forces[31]; in his group's study on runners, apophyseal problems accounted for a mere 0.3% of adult injuries compared with 18% in children. Osgood–Schlatter's and Sever's diseases were the most common diagnoses but other apophyses were also involved. Mirbey *et al.* report on avulsion fractures of the tibial tuberosity in six adolescent athletes[69] and noted that those at greatest risk for this type of injury were adolescent boys from the age of 14, particularly if they have had Osgood–Schlatter's disease. The growth plate seems to be especially vulnerable in the preclosure period, because the stronger fibrocartilaginous elements are replaced by columnated cells. Both springing off and landing activities can cause this acute injury.

Children's bones are more susceptible to stress fractures[31]. This is particularly true for runners who suffer lower limb fractures and gymnasts who have a four-fold increase in spondylolysis[31,70,71]. Scheuerman's disease may also be due to multiple microtraumas and occurs in a number of sports including weight lifting, jumping, diving, judo and gymnastics. Sports that place stress on the spine, especially at the time of growth spurts, may also lead to other back problems[71]. Children's relatively weak bones predispose them to an increased risk of fractures relative to other injuries and this is most apparent in winter sports, particularly skiing. Sherry showed that compared with adults children have a slightly lower incidence of injuries on the ski slopes but these tend to be more serious. Children were injured more often in collisions, ski-lift accidents and failure of boot-bindings to release[72]. Dry slopes (snowless 'ski' slopes covered by a synthetic 'rug') seem to carry a similar risk of fractures to the lower limbs[73].

PREVENTION OF MUSCULO-SKELETAL SPORTS INJURIES

As with so much in sports medicine the strategies to prevent injury are based on a good deal of common sense, some good research and an element of folklore. This section considers these and examples are quoted to illustrate their application.

Research

This should be the foundation of health promotion, injury prevention and treatment. The need for good epidemiological and controlled prospective studies has been previously emphasized. One boon to the descriptive study of the mechanisms of injury has been the video camera. The study of injuries to the cervical spine has allowed steps to be taken to reduce the risks in rugby[26,28], American football[27] and gymnastics. Mechanisms of injury have now been described in ice-hockey[22,23] which should initiate the introduction of preventive measures.

Choosing appropriate sports for the individual
'His glasses are pink and white and as thick as the bottom of a Coca-cola bottle and when he puts his goggles over them they mist up'[74a]. Clearly an individual described thus should be advised by all that ski jumping is definitely not a sport that he should watch, let alone take part in. This uncomplimentary description by Chris Brasher of British ski jumper Eddie 'The Eagle' Edwards may be balanced by the view expressed by Barry Waters who commented, 'Eddie "the Eagle" has shown the world that lack of ability need be no barrier to success on the slopes'[74b]. Mr Edwards illustrates the importance of free choice in sports however inappropriate that choice may seem to others. The role of health professionals is to advise sportsmen and sportswomen and their parents about risks that may not be recognized by the participant. The post-meniscectomy middle-aged man considering road running or the young gymnast with lumbar hyperlordosis[9] are examples of relative contraindications to particular sports. Steele and White have suggested that the injury risk of an individual wishing to take up gymnastics can be predicted reasonably accurately, using a simple set of five variables. They showed positive associations between the risk of injury and lumbar hyperlordosis, weight and age; and a negative association with height and good musculature[9]; they were unable to show that hypermobility increased the chance of injury.

Environment
Many sports are dependent on good weather conditions for their safe conduct. Strong winds make hang-gliding, parachuting[75] and rock-climbing hazardous. These are also dependent on good

visibility, as are motor racing and downhill skiing. Rain adds to the risks in many sports, including cycling and equestrian sports. The topography of an area must be suitable whether it is for parachute landing or winter sports. The disappointment of cancellation puts enormous pressure on administrators to allow an event to take place despite adverse environmental conditions. Resistance to these pressures contributes to safer sport and the prevention of injury. In certain sporting events, for example motor rallies, the Trans-Alaska dog-sled race and around-the-world yacht races, extreme environmental conditions contribute to the excitement, challenge and success of the occasion.

The playing surface or area
Notice at Eton School – '*No boy may go ice-skating on any water not passed by the Headmaster*'[74c]. Surfaces that have been roughened in wet weather, and then dry out leaving holes are particulary likely to cause ankle injuries. Similarly, thick grass with a firm root system in hard ground can cause boot studs to become firmly locked, leading to knee injuries[76]. Adequate watering of dry fields will allow some give which reduces the risk of ligament or meniscus damage. Good preparation of fields is, by these two examples, tremendously important in reducing injuries[2]. Coaches and administrators must have the courage to call off games if the surface is dangerous. The provision of specific facilities contributes to safety as demonstrated by the development of skateboard parks[3].

Lighting
Common sense dictates there should be adequate lighting but this is not always possible. The athlete who likes to run to and from work, or the jogger who can only get onto the road in the early morning or late evening must train in poor light or abandon their sport, unless they have access to a treadmill or well lighted track. Running on such pedestrian and unchallenging surfaces is not es-

pecially appealing to some runners; indeed the author has known experienced club captains who derive a perverse pleasure from leading runs over the roughest terrain in the dark. Training in poor light should be done along routes well known to the runner or cyclist.

Training

It is difficult to produce convincing evidence that training reduces injuries. Nevertheless, if one were to take a group of very unfit former players and put them on a field with fit, current players, few would argue that the unfit players are more likely to suffer injury. The musculoskeletal system undergoes important adaptations with training. Muscles hypertrophy, bones, ligaments and tendons strengthen and with specific exercises, flexibility increases[77]. Training may be divided into:

(1) General conditioning. This training, undertaken by most sportspeople, is aimed at weight reduction and improving cardiovascular fitness, flexibility and muscle conditioning. A general training program is a vital component of preseason conditioning.

(2) Specific training. This is preparation for a particular sport and will be very different for a gymnast compared with a triathlete.

There should be three components to every exercise session.

(1) The warm-up. A gentle, ten minute, loosening-up jog should be followed by stretching exercises. It should be completed by gradually increasing the intensity of exercises utilizing those muscles required for the conduct of that day's activity.

(2) The day's planned training program or competition.

(3) The warm-down. Again this should be a jog followed by stretching exercises. The philosophy behind this is to allow a more controlled adaptation to the resting state. Pooling of blood is reduced with gradual redistribution to other organs preventing hypotension and allowing for more efficient removal of metabolic products. Stretching also reduces pooling and helps break any muscle spasm. The warm-down decreases muscle soreness and the injuries to which 'stiff' muscles are prone.

It is often those in most need of a warm-up who neglect it, as this author experienced when he took part in a fathers' race at a school's sports day and, although very fit for marathon running, tore his hamstring. Imagine the derision that a poor parent would receive if he or she did a proper warm-up before a parents' race. Maybe the only sensible escape in this situation is to swallow one's pride and jog the race.

Preseason preparation

The first golden rule of all training is that the build-up should be gradual. Training between seasons should continue to provide a foundation level of fitness. Some sportspeople even take the opportunity to ensure super cardiovascular fitness or to build strength. The footballer who takes up road-running and runs half-marathons or even marathons will attain a cardiovascular fitness level previously unknown to him. The concern is what adverse effect this may have on his speed.

Specific training should start weeks before a competitive season. The danger of intense late preparation is well illustrated by a 'rebel' Australian cricket team which toured South Africa. Due to the secrecy surrounding the tour, the players had no opportunity to train before their arrival. Under a very enthusiastic coach they underwent a crash fitness program and in their first match sprinting in the field and quick singles caused an epidemic of muscle strains.

Supervision

Inadequate supervision contributes to unnecessary injury. Supervisors should insist on appropriate safety equipment, and dangerous equipment not in use should be locked away. In gymnastics, most evidence indicates that injury rates are lower if a spotter is present[10], and the same person should not supervise two dangerous manoeuvres simultaneously. Informal sport also requires monitoring.

Technique

Correct technique is basic in the prevention of sports injuries. There are right ways and many wrong ways of catching and throwing, kicking a ball and tackling, dressage and show-jumping, swimming and bare-foot water skiing, parachuting and bunjee jumping, ski jumping and getting onto a ski lift. Tackling in rugby illustrates the importance of technique. The days of head down and closed-eye tackles which predispose to injury especially of the cervical spine, should be over. All players must be confident that their own coach has a full understanding of the sport, and no coach should teach manoeuvres beyond his/her level of training.

Coaching

The coach has a role, often the key role, to play in all strategies mentioned in this discussion, but possibly his or her most important influence is in forming the attitudes of players[76]. Too frequently this has been a negative attitude with platitudes like, *'rugby is not a game for nambie-pambies'*. Coaching must be directed toward making the game safe not only for their own team but for the opposition as well. The professional foul is increasingly seen on the amateur playing fields, and the coaches, along with the players, should be held accountable for unfair play causing injuries.

Rules

Most sports adapt their rules to make their sport safer. One of the more drastic measures was the removal of the trampoline from Olympic gymnastics because of the high incidence of neck injuries. Injuries to the cervical spine were markedly reduced when spear tackles (American football) and high tackles (rugby) were banned. Simply changing the rules is insufficient if they are not implemented by the referee. There must be sound rules but there must also be disciplinary action that can be taken against those who deliberately break the rules. The ubiquitous video camera has served to identify numerous incidents of foul play, and has been found useful in determining disciplinary action, while recognizing that video evidence should be viewed carefully and often needs two or more angles to give an accurate picture of the incident.

Children's sport

Although the same principles apply in the prevention of sports injury to children, there are some special considerations that warrant comment. Children are prone to injury at times of rapid growth and prior to epiphyseal closure. Unfortunately the period of most rapid growth occurs at an age when sport becomes increasingly competitive and coaches, young athletes and often their parents are pushing for more intense training[5,56]. The American Academy of Pediatrics and the Canadian Association of Sports Sciences have issued statements on the involvement of children in competitive sports[56,62,63], in which the real and potential dangers are emphasized and limitations on training are recommended.

Anthropometrically matched groups

The division into physically matched groups is particularly important in children's sport (Figure 4). In addition to chronological age, the child's height, weight, experience and skill levels should be considered[56]. Backous' group

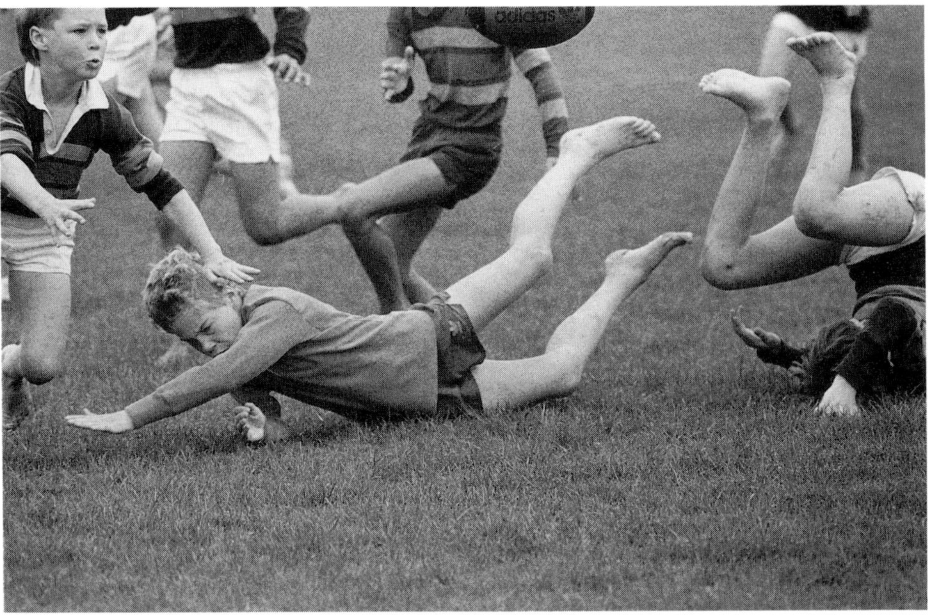

Figure 4 Physically matched groups are important in children's sport. (Reproduced with kind permission from *The New Zealand Herald*)

showed that in soccer, skeletally mature but muscularly weak boys are more susceptible to injury and suggest that hand-grip strength is a useful measure of overall strength[78]. In adult team sports, the level of competition and the different playing positions generally contribute toward a reasonable balance. For example, in rugby a 1.7 m 60 kg scrum-half can play relatively safely against a 2 m 210 kg lock-forward, provided that they have similar skill levels.

Protective gear
Simply stated, protective gear should be in good condition, the correct size, properly fitted and must always be worn.

Safe equipment
The need for adequate supervision of potentially dangerous equipment has been stressed. Footwear requires special attention; shoes must be specifically designed for each sport. A disturbing trend has been replacement of the emphasis on safety and function by fashion and marketing gimmicks. In road running and some other sports, the problem has been further exacerbated by the discontinuation of lines, forcing runners to continually experiment with new designs. Ideally, a good, light, and inexpensive running shoe which can be adapted with wedges to most individuals' needs should still be available five years after its 'launch' on the market.

Strapping and bracing
Prophylactic ankle strapping has become part of basketball and other similar sports such as netball. Strapping in other sports tends to be for secondary prevention in previously injured players. Whether prophylactic bracing of the knee reduces injuries in sports like American football, basketball and volleyball remains controversial[79].

56

Control of speed
In most motor sports, the limitations on speed are imposed mainly by restricting the engine capacity. Children have unwittingly slowed their cycling speed by buying the more fashionable, but heavier BMX bicycles which, in spite of their use for acrobatic manoeuvres, are associated with fewer serious injuries than lighter racing bikes[80,81].

Special attention to tournaments
Most teams play in competition once or twice a week. When the frequency of competition increases to once or twice each day, the players are at increased risk of injury. The warm-up before each game remains important, but the warm-down becomes imperative. Nutrition takes on a special role in optimizing glycogen stores between games. A high carbohydrate diet is essential[82,83] and some workers believe that this should be in the form of complex carbohydrates. Fluid replacement during and after games requires careful attention. In games where substitutions are allowed, a player developing cramp should be rested immediately. Cricket, with its long hours and breaks between sessions presents its own problems. Although a warm-down may not be necessary for every fielder at the end of each session, it would be beneficial to the bowlers. The warm-up before each session makes good sense but is rarely practised.

Diet
Replenishment of depleted glycogen stores while training is as important as it is during tournaments. Diet and amenorrhea appear to interact in the development of osteoporosis and stress fractures in women runners and those on vegetarian diets seem to be particularly prone to these afflictions[84,85]. *'There is no area of nutrition where faddism, misconception and ignorance are more obvious than in athletics'*[74d]. Calcium supplementation is a necessary preventive strategy for those athletes on inadequate diets.

Precautions during infections
It is a popularly held concept, to which the author adheres, that muscles and possibly tendons are more susceptible to injury at times of viral infections, especially those causing myalgia.

Ergonomics
The unnecessary crouching by wicket-keepers has already been mentioned. In striving for more power and speed, cricket fast-bowlers and tennis servers risk back injury from improper body position. Attention to posture and movement in most sports should play an increasing role in the diminution of injuries and this is a fertile field for future research.

Education
Once research has identified the causes, education becomes the key to reducing and preventing injury. The message has to be taken out with a missionary zeal and has to be directed toward the athletes, the parents, the teachers, the coaches and trainers, the administrators and perhaps even to the legislators. Fortunately most people involved with sport have seen enough accidents to make them receptive to considering and attempting to implement protective measures.

In conclusion, musculoskeletal injuries will always be a part of sport, but numerous measures are available to reduce them, even if:

No game was ever worth a rap for a rational man to play, into which no accident, no mishap, could possibly find its way

Adam L Gordon – Australian poet[74e].

REFERENCES

1. Annual report. Accident Compensation Corporation of New Zealand 1989
2. Goldberg B, Witman PA, Gleim GW *et al*. Children's sports injuries: Are they avoidable? Phys Sportsmed. 1979; 7:93–101

3. MacDonald GL. Sports injuries in children. Necessary consequence of competition? Postgrad Med. 1985; 78:279–289

4. Kvist M, Kujala UM, Heinonen OJ *et al.* Sports-related injuries in children. Int J Sports Med. 1989; 10:81–86

5. Keller CS, Noyes FR, Buncher CR. The medical aspects of soccer injury epidemiology. Am J Sports Med. 1987; 15:S105–112

6. DeHaven KE, Lintner DM. Athletic injuries: comparison by age, sport and gender. Am J Sports Med. 1986; 14:218–224

7. Taunton JE, McKenzie DC, Clement DB. The role of biomechanics in the epidemiology of injuries. Sports Med. 1988; 6:107–120

8. Gleim GW. The profiling of professional football players. Clin Sports Med. 1984; 3:185–197

9. Steele VA, White JA. Injury prediction in female gymnasts. Br J Sports Med. 1986; 20:31–33

10. McAuley E, Hudash G, Shields K *et al.* Injuries in women's gymnastics. Am J Sports Med. 1987; 15:S174–131

11. Birrer RB, Halbrook SP. Martial arts injuries. The results of a five year national survey. Am J Sports Med. 1988; 16:408–410

12. Sim FH, Simonet WT, Melton LJ, Lehn TA. Ice hockey injuries. Am J Sports Med. 1987; 15: S86–96

13. Clark DR, Roux C, Noakes TD. A prospective study of the incidence and nature of injuries to adult rugby players. S Afr Med J 1990; 77:559–62

14. Davidson RM. Schoolboy rugby injuries, 1969–1986. Med J Aust. 1987; 147:119–120

15. Williamson DM, Lowdon IMR. Ice-skating injuries. Injury. 1986; 17:205–207

16. Freeland P Implications of two newly opened ice rinks on an accident and emergency department. Br Med J. 1988; 296:96

17. Shesser R, Smith M, Ellis P et al. Recreational softball injuries. Am J Emerg Med. 1985; 3: 199–202

18. Weiker GG. Club gymnastics. Clin Sports Med. 1985; 4:39–43

19. Chard MD, Lachmann SM. Racquet sports-patterns of injury presenting to a sports injury clinic. Br J Sports Med. 1987; 21:150–153

20. Belliappa PP, Barton NJ. Hand injuries in cricketers. J Hand Surg (Br). 1991; 16B:212–214

21. Findlay D. After the final siren: Australian rules football injuries presenting to a casualty department. Aust Fam Physician. 1986; 15:267–274

22. Reid DC, Saboe L. Spine fractures in winter sports. Sports Med. 1989; 7:393–399

23. Tator CH. Neck injuries in ice hockey: a recent, unsolved problem with many contributing factors. Clin Sports Med. 1987; 6:101–114

24. Silver JR, Silver DD, Godfrey JJ. Trampolining injuries to the spine. Injury. 1986; 17:117–124

25. Silver JR, Silver DD, Godfrey JJ. Injuries of the spine sustained during gymnastic activities. Br Med J. 1986; 293:861–863

26. Scher AT. Rugby injuries of the cervical spine and spinal cord – has the situation improved? S Afr Med J. 1989; 76:46

27. Tort JS, Vegso JJ, O'Neill RJ et al. The Epidemiologic, pathologic, biomechanical and cinematographic analysis of football-induced cervical spine trauma. Am J Sports Med. 1990; 18:50–57

28. Scher AT. Rugby injuries to the cervical spinal cord sustained during rucks and mauls. S Afr Med J. 1983; 64:592–594

29. Scher AT. Rugby injuries of the upper cervical spine. S Afr Med J. 1983; 64:456–458

30. Paty JG. Diagnosis and treatment of musculo-skeletal running injuries. Semin Arthritis Rheum. 1988; 18:48–60

31. Apple DF. Adolescent runners. Clin Sports Med. 1985; 4:641–655

32. Jacobs SJ, Berson BL. Injuries to runners: a study of entrants to a 10 000 meter race. Am J Sports Med. 1986; 14:151–155

33. Messier SP, Pittala KA. Etiologic factors associated with selected running injuries. Med Sci Sports Exerc. 1988; 20:501–505

34. Sutker AN, Barber FA, Jackson DW, Pagliano JW. Iliotibial band syndrome in distance runners. Sports Med. 1985; 2:447–451

35. Jobe FW, Bradley JP. Rotator cuff injuries in baseball. Prevention and rehabilitation. Sports Med. 1988; 6:378–387

36. Richardson AB. Orthopedic aspects of competitive swimming. Clin Sports Med. 1987; 6: 639–645

37. Mann DL, Littke N. Shoulder injuries in archery. Can J Sports Sci. 1989; 14:85–92

38. Foster D, John D, Elliot B *et al.* Back injuries to fast bowlers in cricket: a prospective study. Br J Sports Med. 1989; 23:150–154

39. Ciullo JV, Jackson DW. Pars interarticularis stress reaction, spondylolysis, and spondylolisthesis in gymnasts. Clin Sports Med. 1985;4:95–110

40. Micheli LJ. Back injuries in gymnastics. Clin Sports Med. 1985; 4:85–93

41. Heath H. Athletic women, amenorrhea, and skeletal integrity. Ann Intern Med. 1985; 102:258–259

42. Lane NE, Bloch DA, Hubert HB *et al.* Running, osteoarthritis and bone density: initial 2-year longitudinal study. Am J Med. 1990; 88:452–459

43. Wyshak G, Frisch RE, Albright TE *et al.* Non-alcoholic carbonated beverage consumption and bone fractures among women former college athletes. J Orthop Res. 1989; 7:91–99

44. Panush RS. Does exercise cause arthritis? Long term consequences of exercise on the musculoskeletal system. Rheum Dis Clin North Am. 1990; 16:827–836

45. Gear MWL. The late results of menisectomy. Br J Surg. 1967; 54:270–272

46. Fairbank TJ. Knee joint changes after menisectomy. J Bone Joint Surg (Br). 1948; 30B:664–670

47. Burry HC. Sport, exercise and arthritis. Br J Rheumatol. 1987; 26:386–388

48. Allen PR, Denham RA, Swan AV. Late degenerative changes after menisectomy: factors affecting the knee after operation. J Bone Joint Surg (Br). 1984; 66:666–671

49. McDaniel WJ, Dameron TB. Untreated rupture of the anterior cruciate ligament: a follow-up study. J Bone Joint Surg (Am). 1980; 62:696–705

50. McDermott M, Freyne P. Osteoarthrosis in runners with knee pain. Br J Sports Med. 1983; 17:84–87

51. Sohn RS, Micheli LJ. The effect of running on the pathogenesis of osteoarthritis of the hips and knees. Clin Orthop. 1985; 198:106–109

52. Genti G. Occupation and osteoarthritis. Ballière's Clin Rheum. 1989; 3(1):193–204

53. Burke MJ, Fear EC, Wright V. Bone and joint changes in pneumatic drillers. Ann Rheum Dis. 1977; 36:276–279

54. Felson DT. The epidemiology of knee osteoarthritis: results from the Framingham osteoarthritis study. Semin Arthritis Rheum. 1990; 20 Suppl 1: 42–50

55. Scher AT. Premature onset of degenerative disease of the cervical spine in rugby players. S Afr Med J. 1990; 77:557–558

56. Hughson R. Children in competitive sports – a multi-disciplinary approach. Can J Appl Sport Sci. 1986; 11:162–172

57. Shakespeare W. Macbeth Act 5 Scene 5

58. Maffulli N, Helms P. Controversies about intensive training in young athletes. Arch Dis Child. 1988; 63:1405–1407

59. Rians CB, Weltman A, Cahill BR *et al.* Strength training for prepubescent males: Is it safe? Am J Sports Med. 1987; 15:483–489

60. Cowart VS. For some of the nation's young athletes, training may be too much of a good thing. JAMA. 1989; 262:735 & 739

61. Noakes TD. In Lore of Running. Oxford University Press, 1985

62. Nelson MA, Goldberg B, Harris SS *et al.* Committee on Sports Medicine. Strength training, weight and power lifting, and body building by children and adolescents. Pediatrics. 1990; 86:801–803

63. Nelson MA, Goldberg H, Harris SS et al. Committee on Sports Medicine. Risks in distance running for children. Pediatrics. 1990; 86: 799–800

64. Arkin AM, Katz JF. The effects of pressure on epiphyseal growth. J Bone Joint Surg. 1956; 38A:1056–1076

65. Strobino LJ, French GO, Colonna PC. The effect of increasing tensions on the growth of epiphyseal bone. Surg Gynecol Obstet. 1952; 95:694–700

66. Peterson HA, Burkhart SS. Compression injury of the epiphyseal growth plate. J Pediatr Orthop. 1981; 1:377–384

67. Albanese SA, Palmer AK, Kerr DR *et al.* Wrist pain and distal growth plate closure of the radius in gymnasts. J Pediatr Orthop. 1989; 9:23–28

68. Roy S, Caine D, Singer KM. Stress changes of the distal radial epiphysis in young gymnasts. Am J Sports Med. 1985; 13:301–308

69. Mirbey J, Besancenot J, Chambers RT *et al.* Avulsion fractures of the tibial tuberosity in the adolescent athlete. Am J Sports Med. 1988; 16:336–340

70. Commandre FA, Taillan B, Gagnerie F *et al.* Spondylolysis and spondylolisthesis in young athletes: 28 cases. J Sports Med Phys Fitness. 1988; 28:104–107

71. Commandre FA, Gagnerie G, Zakarian M *et al.* The child, the spine and sport. J Sports Med Phys Fitness. 1988; 28:11–19

72. Sherry E, Korbel P, Henderson A. Children's skiing injuries in Australia. Med J Austr. 1987; 146:193–195

73. Hill SA. Incidence of tibial fracture in child skiers. Br J Sports Med. 1989; 23:169–170

74. The Guinness Dictionary of Sports Quotations compiled by C Jarmao, Guinness Publishing, 1990. a. Brasher C. p. 165; b. *Ibid.* Waters B. p. 165; c. *Ibid.* anon p. 163; d. *Ibid.* Short SH, Short WR. p. 180; e. *Ibid.* Gordon AL. p. 205

75. Ellitsgaard N, Warburg F. Movements causing ankle factures in parachuting. Br J Sports Med. 1989; 23: 27–29

76. Roy SP. The nature and frequency of rugby injuries. S Afr Med J. 1974; 48:2321–2327

77. Rooks DS, Micheli LJ. Musculoskeletal assessment and training: the young athlete. Clin Sports Med. 1988; 7:641–677

78. Backous DD, Friedl KE, Smith NJ *et al.* Soccer injuries and their relation to physical maturity. Am J Dis Child. 1988; 142:839–842

79. Baker BE. Prevention of ligament injuries to the knee. Exerc Sport Sci Rev. 1990; 18:291–305

80. Worrell J. BMX bicycles: accident comparison with other models. Arch Emerg Med. 1985; 2:209–213

81. Park KGM, Dickson AP. BMX bicycle injuries in children. Injury. 1986; 17:34–36

82. Costill DL, Miller JM. Nutrition for endurance sport: carbohydrates and fluid balance. Int J Sports Med. 1980; 1:2–14

83. Costill DL, Miller JM. The role of dietary carbohydrate in muscle glycogen resynthesis after strenuous exercise. Am J Clin Nutr. 1981; 34:1831–1836

84. Van Velden DP. Stress fractures and posterior tibial syndrome in elite athletes. S Afr J Sports Med. 1987; 2:10–13 & 20

85. Marcus R, Cann C, Madvig P *et al.* Menstrual function and bone mass in elite women distance runners. Endocrine and metabolic features. Ann Intern Med. 1985; 102:158–163

6. FIBROMYALGIA

Richard Wigley

HISTORY

Fibromyalgia is a condition characterized by multiple tender points accompanied by diffuse pain that was first described by Gowers in 1904[1], and named fibrositis on the assumption that it was an inflammatory process of fibrous tissues. As this explanation was not sustained, the term 'fibromyalgia' was introduced[2], although fibrositis continues to be used in some standard textbooks[3].

Simons and Travell[4] review a large number of terms that have been used, introducing their own title, 'myofascial pain syndrome'. It appears that this term would include those cases of fibromyalgia , repetitive strain and other regional pain syndromes in which there are tender points which they call 'trigger points', which may or may not be active. Pressure on active trigger points induces persistent pain remote from the point stimulated and they describe taut muscle bands and a muscle twitch response. Wolfe and colleagues[5] comparing fibromyalgia diagnosed by rheumatologists and myofascial pain syndrome cases diagnosed by Simons, were not able to demonstrate satisfactory observer consistency in distinguishing 'tender points' from trigger points. Taut muscle bands and twitch response were found in both conditions and in controls so would be best disregarded.

Further objective research is needed to distinguish, if possible between these syndromes. The tender points of fibromyalgia were reproducibly detected.

DIAGNOSTIC CRITERIA

Yunus and co-workers[2] define fibromyalgia as having four or more tender points at characteristic (see below) musculoskeletal points, accompanied by pain. An American College of Rheumatology Committee[5], after recursive partition analysis of established clinical cases of fibromyalgia from various tertiary referral clinics, compared with routine cases attending such clinics, has recommended the following diagnostic criteria for fibromyalgia:

(1) A complaint of diffuse pain is obligatory and;

(2) Eleven or more trigger points at the following sites (Figure 1):
    (a) Occiput,
    (b) Low cervical C5 – C7,
    (c) Upper trapezius,
    (d) Supraspinatus (upper inner angle of scapula),
    (e) Second rib (above and lateral to junctions), and
    (f) Lateral epicondyle (2 cm distal),
    (g) Gluteal (upper outer quadrants),
    (h) Greater trochanters (posterior), and
    (i) Medial aspect of the knee(proximal to joint line).

These tender points *do not* include the following sites generally used by clinicians:

(a) Spine of C7 vertebra,
(b) Spines of the mid dorsal vertebrae,
(c) Sacrum,
(d) Origin of the gluteus maximus muscle, and
(e) Origin of the pectoralis minor muscle.

The last point, the origin of the pectoralis minor muscle, recently described as a 'tender point' is a site of considerable interest in routine clinical practice, as the associated anterior chest pain, if unrecognized, may lead to inappropriate hospitalization for cardiorespiratory complaints. Given this concern, the pectoralis minor 'point' may require further consideration in future definitions of fibromyalgia.

Because many features typical of fibromyalgia also occur in other rheumatic diseases such as rheumatoid arthritis, this creates problems in establishing diagnostic criteria. Although the American College of Rheumatology's diagnostic criteria[7] for fibromyalgia are valid in tertiary referral centers, and serve to distinguish fibromyalgia from other major rheumatic diseases, at the population or primary care level, diagnostic sensitivities and specificities are quite different (see below). As an example, tender points must be counted in a similar fashion for both cases and controls as the diagnoses cannot be treated as mutually exclusive. For instance, attempting to separate rheumatoid arthritis from fibromyalgia on the basis of tender point count is not appropriate as the two diagnoses should be made separately and the number of tender points counted for each should be recorded.

Yet another problem is that Simons and Travell[4] have described many more tender points using the name trigger points. Building on the work of Kellgren[8] who established the pain referral patterns of the spine and joints they have described referral patterns for most of the muscles. Simons and Travell also hold that for each of these patterns there is one or more 'trigger points'[4], which

may be latent or active. They hold that an active trigger point is a focus of hyperirritability in a muscle or its fascia which causes pain, in contrast to a latent trigger point, which is locally tender but causes pain only when palpated. These authors note that it is more difficult to induce referred pain in latent than in active trigger points, which would explain the existence of pain remote from an affected site. For instance, static contraction of the wrist extensor muscles may cause pain referred to the base of the thumb and lateral wrist. This is otherwise difficult to explain on the basis of sustained muscle contraction ischemia, as there are no muscles at that site. As already stated difficulties have been encountered in the reproducibility of the signs described by Simons and Travell[4].

The characteristic wincing and eyelid flicker on relatively light pressure at fibromyalgic tender points compared with neutral sites is easily recognized but it would be easy for an enthusiastic examiner to press a little harder or not according to his biases of the moment. The American College of Rheumatology Committee[5] endeavored to minimize this error by integrating dolorimetry into daily practice. Langley and colleagues[9] have developed a simple, accurate and low-cost dolorimeter from a plastic syringe, which could be used in the clinic and in population surveys.

EPIDEMIOLOGY

Until the criteria for diagnosing fibromyalgia are standardized, population studies will be difficult. During the course of a population survey of rheumatic disease in a village near Beijing, Wigley and co-workers[10] serially examined 141 symptomatic and 28 asymptomatic Chinese villagers for the presence of fibromyalgia and soft tissue rheumatism in order to establish a method for identifying fibromyalgia and other types of soft tissue rheumatism. In another study, Veerapen and Wigley[11] examined 312 patients with rheumatic symptoms selected from 2594 adult Malays, Chinese and

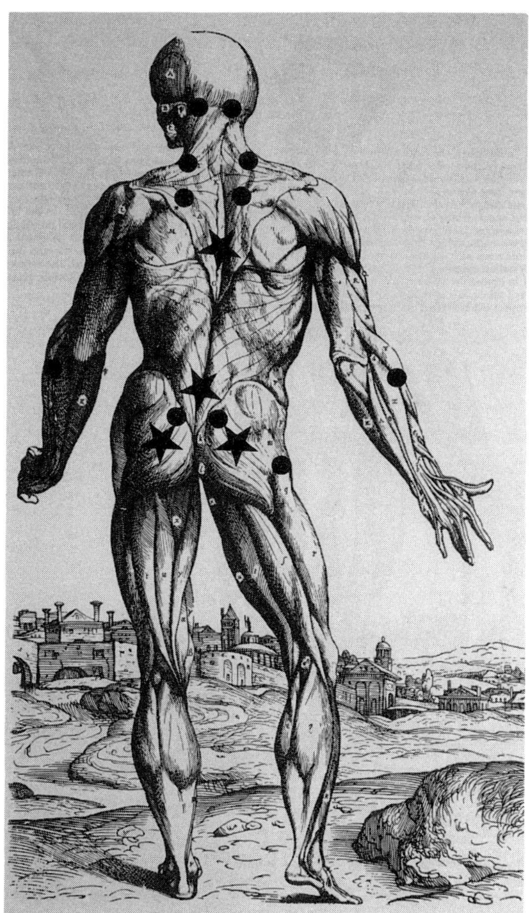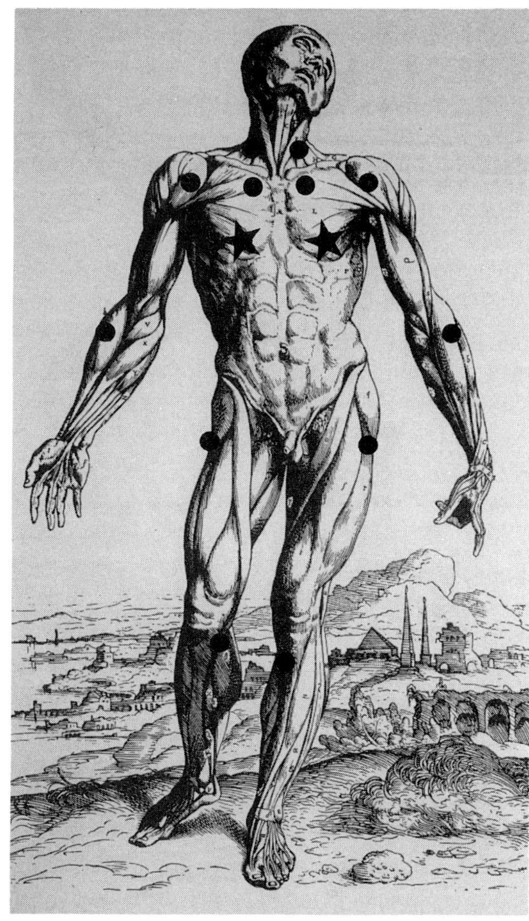

Figure 1 The tender points sites specified for the ACR definition of fibromyalgia (•) and the additional sites (★) are superimposed on the classical anatomical drawings of Versalius

Tamil Indians in rural Malaysia, counting all of the previously indicated tender points, except at the pectoralis minor origin. Fibromyalgia patients appeared to be tense, nervous, anxious, and had drawn features, which is a constellation of clinical findings that the author generally associates with fibromyalgia. Thus, recognition of fibromyalgia was not impeded by language barriers, as the major clinical features were apparent from body language. Assessment of clinical features[3] associated with fibromyalgia, e.g. irritable bowel and non-restorative sleep patterns were less easy

to determine. Of 22 patients that the author would, in routine clinical practice, have classed as having fibromyalgia, 21 had five or more tender points. In this exploratory study, fibromyalgia was diagnosed in 2.8% Indian, 1% Malay and in one in 251 Chinese women. As living conditions were similar in the three ethnic groups in this rural community, environment may be less important than genetic and cultural differences. The predominance of women was as expected from Caucasian studies. Three women and one man had definite rheumatoid arthritis.

The use of tender points as diagnostic criteria for fibromyalgia is somewhat problematic; Buskila and colleagues[12] found that 7.3% of boys and 9.4% of normal school children had more than ten tender points. If ten tender points were required for a diagnosis of fibromyalgia in the above Malaysian survey, only four women would have met the diagnostic criteria; if eight or more tender points are accepted, 11 women (two Malay) would have been diagnosed, and if five tender points were used, 21 were diagnosed. In other words the sensitivity would rise from 19% to 52% to 95% if different rheumatologists' diagnostic criteria were accepted as the gold standard. The low frequency of tender points in the other 290 in the Malaysian survey who had other rheumatic complaints may be more a reflection of a lower prevalence of inflammatory rheumatic complaints in the rest of this rural population than is seen in the clinic controls used in establishing the American College of Rheumatology criteria. Croft and co-workers[13] used dolorimetry in a general practice derived sample of 1329 adults who had reported widespread pain, and found in a subsample that the relative risk of more than ten tender points was 10.5. Clearly further studies using dolorimetry should be performed to derive suitable diagnostic criteria for population studies. This would also provide data on pain thresholds which may differ culturally, ethnically or even genetically.

In a population-based study[14] in Finland using several sets of criteria, prevalence was low at 0.75%. Associations were shown for female sex, age, low educational level, and heavier work, but not for physical or mental stress[14].

PATHOPHYSIOLOGY

Moldofsky and Scarisbrick[15] have shown that fibromyalgia patients have an abnormal non-restorative sleep pattern, and awaken feeling tired, and complaining of stiffness. Frequent waking may occur, but some patients feel that they sleep well, despite electroencephalographic abnormalities. Goldenberg and associates[16] have shown that a normal sleep pattern is restored by small doses of tricyclic sedatives and not by other sedatives. Whether this is the primary abnormality or the result of sleep disturbance is not clear. Similar symptoms were induced by sleep deprivation in volunteers[17], resolving after the volunteers had a period of undisturbed sleep. Though Clark and colleagues[18] do not support the ischemic hypothesis, Lund and co-workers[19] suggest that the pain is due to chronic muscle tension lowering tissue oxygen pressure. Most of the studies refer to active exercise when it is the effect of sustained muscle contraction that is in question. High-energy phosphates (e.g. adenosine 5'-triphosphate) are decreased in muscles affected by pain, which implies that fibromyalgic pain is indeed of muscular origin, and may be due to ischemia[20]. Although de Blecourt and colleagues[21] were unable to confirm this by *in vivo* magnetic resonance spectroscopy in the resting state, they suggest that a dynamic stress test may be needed to demonstrate changes. Simms and co-workers[22] also used magnetic resonance with leg control sites and comparable physically unfit control subjects with and without exercise, and concluded that the changes observed could be explained by deconditioning of muscle. The ischemia hypothesis is supported by Edwards and colleagues[23], who showed in healthy adults that low-load isometric contraction produces ischemia secondary to increased intramuscular pressure and subsequent impairment of blood flow.

CLINICAL

Fibromyalgia has many features in common with the repetitive strain or overuse syndrome, a clinical complex that will be discussed in Chapter 7. Indeed, Littlejohn[24] suggests that fibromyalgia and the occupational overuse syndrome are variations on the same theme, and can only be separated using arbitrary criteria. Moreover, the author has found that careful questioning may reveal that an otherwise 'typical' case of fibromyalgia may have started with asymmetrical work related pain, and that typical cases of occupational overuse syndrome may, if neglected, progress to fully symmetrical fibromyalgia. If this relation is valid, then the possibility that fibromyalgia is precipitated by occupation requires formal study. The associations with heavy physical stress, low educational level and female sex in a large Finnish population study[14] would support this contention. Despite the similarities, in fibromyalgia, the tender points are often symmetrical, while in the overuse syndromes, these points are fewer in number, often asymmetrical, and occur in an occupational setting. In both, ischemia appears to be the initiating event; in the latter, ischemic pain leads to tightening of neighbouring muscles, causing a vicious cycle of escalating pain that is described by Smythe[3] as the pain amplification syndrome. Mengshoel and colleagues[25] showed for the upper limb that both static and dynamic load endurance was lower in fibromyalgia than in healthy hospital staff controls, although aerobic capacity was normal in both groups.

The influence of internal and external stress factors needs to be further studied. Patients with fibromyalgia and the overuse syndrome may often be described as 'perfectionists'[3] (the 'type A' personality popularized in North American literature), and have a history of competitive and obsessive behavior. This feature warrants consideration as a possible diagnostic criterion for fibromyalgia or the occupational overuse syndrome, but may prove difficult to define. Formal studies of the psychological influence are needed but require the development and validation of suitable questionnaires. Despite the possible influence of a perfectionist personality, most psychological features are more credibly explained as secondary to anger, frustration and anxiety, which may exacerbate the clinical symptoms. The above-noted features are of greatest use in

distinguishing both fibromyalgia and the occupational overuse syndrome(s) from the less common cases of malingering and hysteria and the more common individuals who make the most of their symptoms for social and financial gain. Smythe notes that, in addition to an association with the irritable bowel syndrome, fibromyalgia may be accompanied by other features of hyperirritability, e.g. increased urinary frequency, noise intolerance, cold intolerance and Raynaud's phenomenon, tachycardia and hyperreflexia. These features have been cited in support of the contention that fibromyalgia is a type of psychogenic rheumatism[26], in which the pain is initially peripheral in the muscles.

PREVENTION

If as suggested above, fibromyalgia is a psychophysical (whole body) disorder that affects tense competitive perfectionist people, then it is appropriate to educate the general public in tension and anger control, concentrating especially on relaxation techniques. Haanen and co-workers[27] found hypnosis with relaxation therapy to be superior to physiotherapy in resistant cases of fibromyalgia and the author has been encouraged by relaxation therapy in management. Bolwijn and colleagues[28] were unsuccessful in treating fibromyalgia with a combination of low impact fitness training and biofeedback training. It is difficult for these subjects to learn relaxation and to practice it routinely, so that any efficacy study should include a measure of the success (or lack thereof) of the relaxation instruction. Bennett and colleagues[29] are testing the hypothesis that exercise helps in treatment. If this is true, exercise may also be of value in primary prevention. If a predisposing personality type susceptible to these conditions is identified, such an individual should be singled out for counselling. Since public education has been effective for other medical conditions, e.g. coronary artery disease, hypertension and cancer, it may be ill-advised to delay confirmation of such relations before undertaking preventive and educational activities regarding rheumatic diseases. Since prevention of fibromyalgia may involve changing certain personality traits, the challenge is not inconsiderable. Some religions such as Buddhism already practice this approach. The relaxation approach to therapy is elaborated further in the next section. If fibromyalgia is indeed a late manifestation of the occupational overuse syndrome, as contended above, then prevention of that complaint should also prevent fibromyalgia.

REFERENCES

1. Gowers WR. Lumbago: its lessons and analogues. Br Med J. 1904; 1:117–121

2. Yunus M, Masi AT, Calabro JJ, Miller KA, Feigenbaum SL. Primary fibromyalgia (fibrositis): clinical study of 50 patients with matched normal controls. Arthritis Rheum. 1981; 11:151–171

3. Smythe H. Fibrositis. In Kelley WN *et al.*, eds., Textbook of Rheumatic Diseases. Philadelphia, WB Saunders, 1985, pp. 481–489

4. Simons DG, Travell JG. Myofascial pain syndromes. In Melzack and Wall, eds., Pain. Churchill Livingstone, 1984, pp. 263–276

5. Wolfe F, Simons D, Fricton J, Bennett RM, Goldenberg DL, Gerwin RD, Hathaway D, McCain GA, Russell IJ. The fibromyalgia and myofascial pain syndromes: a study of tender points and trigger points in persons with fibromyalgia myofascial pain syndrome and no disease. Am Coll Rheum Seattle. 1990, Abstr. D22

6. Smythe H. The 'repetitive strain injury syndrome' is referred pain from the neck. J Rheumatol. 1989; 15:1604–1688

7. Wolfe F, Smythe H, Yunus MB, Bennett RM *et al.* The American College of Rheumatology 1990 criteria for the classification of fibromyalgia. Arthritis Rheum. 1990; 33:160–172

8. Kellgren JH. Deep pain sensibility. Lancet. 1949; 1:943

9. Langley GB, Fowles M, Sheppeard H, Wigley RD. A simple dolorimeter for the quantification of joint tenderness in inflammatory arthritis. Rheumatol Int. 1983; 3:109–112

10. Wigley RD, Zhang NC, Hu DW, Sheng CS. *et al.* ILAR study of rheumatic disease in China: IV: Shiao Hong Men village, Beijing. APLAR Bull. 1990; 9:72–75

11. Veerapen K, Wigley, RD. Malaysian COPCORD study. Unpublished

12. Buskila D, Press J, Gedalia A, Klein M *et al.* Assessment of nonarticular tenderness and prevalence of fibromyalgia in children. Am Coll Rheumatol Boston. 1991; Abstr. D156

13. Croft PR, Schollum J, Silman AJ. Fibromyalgia symptoms in the general population. Am Coll Rheumatol Boston, 1991; Abstr. D157

14. Mäkelä M, Heliövaara M. Prevalence of fybromyalgia in the Finnish population. Br Med J. 1991; 303:216–219

15. Muldosky H, Scarisbrick P, England R, Smythe H. Musculoskeletal symptoms and non-REM sleep disturbance in patients with 'fibrositis syndrome' and healthy subjects. Psychosomat Med. 1975; 37:341

16. Goldenberg DL, Felson DT, Dinerman H. A randomized trial of amitryptiline and naproxen in the treatment of patients with fibromyalgia. Arthritis Rheum. 1986; 59:1371–1377

17. Moldofsky H, Scarisbrick P. Induction of neurasthenic musculoskeletal pain syndrome by selective stage sleep deprivation. Psychosomat Med. 1976; 38:35

18. Clark C, Campbell SM, Forehand ME, Tindall EA, Bennett RM. Clinical characteristics of fibrositis. II. A 'blinded' controlled study using standard psychological tests. Arthritis Rheum 1985; 28:132–137

19. Lund N, Bengtsson A, Thorborg P. Muscle oxygen pressure in primary fibromyalgia. Scand J Rheumatol. 1986; 15:165–173

20. Bengston A, Henriksson KJ, Larsson J. Reduced high energy phosphate levels in the painful muscles of patients with fibromyalgia. Arthritis Rheum. 1986; 29:817–821

21. De Blecourt AC, Wolf RF, Van Rijswijk MH, Kamman RL *et al.* In vivo ^{31}P magnetic resonance spectroscopy (MRS) of tender points in patients with primary fibromyalgia syndrome. Rheumatol Int. 1991; 11:51–54

22. Simms RW, Roy S, Skrinar G, Hrovat M, *et al.* F31P-NMR spectroscopy of muscle in fibromyal-

gia syndrome patients and sedentary controls. Am Coll Rheumatol. 1991; Abstr. D155

23. Edwards RHT, Hill DK, McDonnell M. Myothermal and intramuscular pressure measurements during isometric contractions of the human quadriceps muscle. J Physiol. 1972; 224:58–59

24. Littlejohn GO. Fibrositis/fibromyalgia syndrome in the work place. Rheum Dis Clin North Am. 1989; 15:45–60

25. Mengshoel AM, Forre O, Komnaes HB. Muscle strength and aerobic capacity in primary fibromyalgia. Clin Exp Rheumatol. 1990; 8:475–479

26. Goldenberg DL. Psychiatric and psychological aspects of fibromyalgia syndrome. Rheum Dis Clin North Am. 1989; 15:105–114

27. Haanen HCM, Hoenderdos HTW, Romunde LKV, Hop WCJ, Malee C, Terwiel JP, Hekster GB. Controlled trial of hypnotherapy in refractory fibromyalgia. J Rheumatol. 1991; 18:72–75

28. Bolwijn P, Van Santen-Hoeufft M, Kleijnen J, Van der Linden SJ, Houben H, De Klerk E. Fitness training and biofeedback in fibromyalgia: a randomized controlled trial; Abstract. XII EULAR Congress, Budapest, 1991; Abstr. PD1-14. p. 265

29. Clark SR, Burckhardt CS, O'Reilly CA, Campbell SM, Bennett RM. Exercise and patient outcome in fibromyalgia. Am Coll Rheumatol. 1991; Abstr. D151

7. OVERUSE SYNDROMES (REPETITIVE STRAIN SYNDROME)

Richard Wigley

INTRODUCTION

In the seventeenth century, Ramazzini called attention to a relationship between upper arm pain, certain repetitive tasks, e.g. writing, as well as a constrained sitting position and excess mental efforts, which occurred in scribes and clerks[1]. Osler noted similar pains in telegraphers[1], and Brain[2], in describing writer's cramp, identified most of the factors now considered to be important in the repetitive strain syndrome of keyboard workers that has attracted attention in the last decade[3]. The Japanese encountered this same problem in keyboard operators during the 1950s[4], and controlled this by integrating 10-minute breaks into each working hour.

Various terms have been used for this syndrome in different countries; in the USA, the National Institute of Occupational Safety and Health (NIOSH) prefers the term 'cumulative trauma disorder' (CTD)[5]; in Australasia, 'repetitive strain injury'[6] (RSI) has been used. 'Occupational overuse syndrome'[7,8] (OOS) is favored, as repetition is thought to be a less important risk factor, and the presence of trauma and/or injury is controversial and can be misinterpreted by those with the complaint as meaning permanent injury. The disadvantage of including the adjective 'occupational' in the definition is that it ignores related problems that arise in sports and the domestic scene. Whether housewives have an occupation should not be in dispute, but as they are not paid wages, they do not have an occupa-

tion with respect to insurance legislation in many jurisdictions. Thus 'overuse syndrome' is preferable, as it would include the latter[3]. The term 'regional myofascial pain syndrome'[9] includes those overuse syndromes where trigger points are present, but excludes most of the less severe cases that lack these: this then is an unsatisfactory term, especially in prevention, where the identification of minor initial symptoms is essential. Other equivalent terms, e.g. occupational neurosis, and psychogenic rheumatism are inappropriate, as the patients may perceive that their complaints are being viewed by their physicians as nonexistent and this has a negative impact on therapy. The muscular component of this condition or 'occupational cramp'[2], is distinct from what is understood by the lay public when using the word cramp, and, as it leads to confusion in the context of the overuse syndrome, is a term that is best avoided.

Overuse syndromes have been distorted by the existence of international differences in compensation laws, and have caused confusion to the point where some appear to deny the very existence of the phenomenon despite its global distribution. The Australasian College of Physicians favors separation of the more clearly defined overuse syndromes with more objective signs, as has been done in this monograph under the heading of 'regional pain syndromes' (*see* Chapter 8). This latter group includes rotator cuff injury, tennis elbow, tenosynovitis, de Quervain's dis-

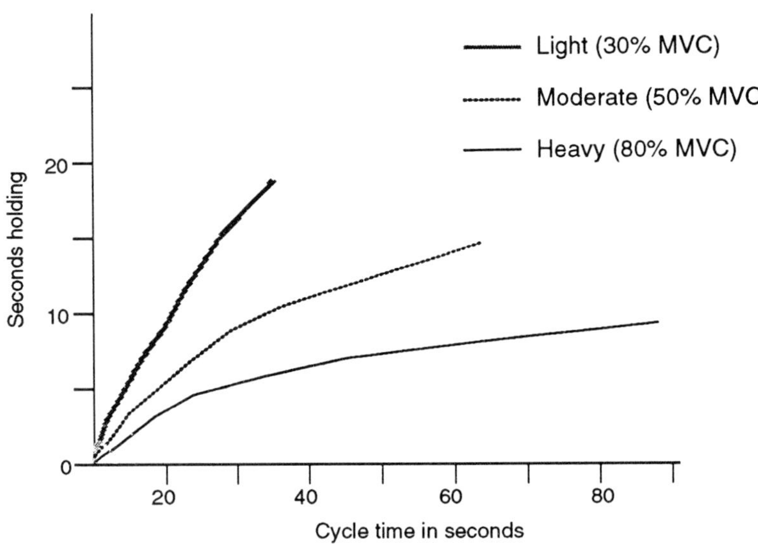

Figure 1 A diagram showing the relationship of the static holding time (vertical axis) to the cycle time to allow recovery of muscle at light, moderate and heavy percentages of maximum voluntary strength (MVC)

ease, carpal tunnel syndrome and bursitis. Although regional pain complexes may be due to overuse, they often follow single or multiple, direct or indirect injuries, often occur as isolated events, have characteristic physical signs, often respond to local therapy such as local injections and surgery, and the degree of force involved is usually greater than in the overuse syndromes described in this chapter.

Clinical features

Pain from unaccustomed loads, sustained loading, repetitive movements and poor ergonomics are so much a part of the general life experience as to be considered by some as normal. Such pain is physiological in the sense that it signals a need to rest or to change position. As this pain is compensated for without the development of 'disease', and without outside assistance, it might be called 'good' pain. When despite compensatory efforts, relief is not achieved, *disease* (or what Hadler describes as a 'dilemma' (*see* Chapter 29) develops, in which case the subject strives to continue the activity, despite the discomfort and

pain, and his state either worsens or he seeks medical advice. If he seeks medical care for what is perceived to be 'bad pain', he becomes a patient and his condition is anointed with a diagnostic label. The pain may persist after finishing the labor (Figure 1) that caused the bad pain, continue long after the initiating events have ceased, and become self-amplifying in a cycle of chronic pain which ultimately dominates the clinical picture. Many occupations give rise to similar symptoms, but the common factors are repetitive movements continued over long periods of time, with pain from sustained contraction of the supporting muscles to the part of the anatomy performing the repetitive work. Pain is at first transient, occurring only at the time of work, but later continues at rest. Well-developed cases are characterized by a burning sensation, numbness, tingling and subjective weakness. The nature of the weakness is of interest; the grip strength may initially be normal, but repeated gripping often results in a rapid fall-off in power secondary to pain. Pain often increases several minutes after testing grip strength and may persist for hours. A coarsening of fine motor skill (focal dystonia) may occur in more severe cases, but visible muscle wasting is uncommon even in over-splinted, advanced, and/or neglected cases. Also typical of advanced cases are night pain and insomnia, which escalate the self-sustaining vicious cycle of fluctuating, but increasingly intolerable pain, causing more tension, frustration and anger, leading to more fatigue and depression. Paresthesia tend to be transient and variable in the overuse syndrome, unlike those of the clearly defined entrapment syndromes referred to in Chapter 8. Some patients complain of swelling which is rarely observed by the examiner, who may then classify the condition as tenosynovitis. Skin color changes and Raynaud's phenomenon or algodystrophy[10] occur in a minority of advanced cases; these respond poorly to therapy.

Most subjects with less severe symptoms of the overuse syndrome referred to in this section respond to the improved ergonomics, modification in frequency and duration of tasks, and instruction in frequent brief muscle relaxation. With the appropriate advice, most of those suffering from overuse syndromes can be rehabilitated while continuing to work. Some will need to be placed on disability leave, and indeed most of those seen at specialist referral will already be off work, so rehabilitation efforts must be started while they are off work. Some respond negatively to conventional medication, active exercises, physiotherapy machines, non-steroidal anti-inflammatory drugs and injections, although they may report temporary improvement through the use of non-traditional modalities (massage, acupuncture and transcutaneous electrical nerve stimulation (TENS)).

Differentiating overuse from other soft tissue rheumatic syndromes is complicated by the present lack of universally accepted definitions. Fibromyalgia (Chapter 6) has much in common with overuse syndromes, but the pain in fibromyalgia is symmetrical and widespread with characteristic tender points, while these points in the overuse syndrome are usually unilateral and fewer than four in number. In the author's experience, most overuse patients have only one tender point, about 5 cm distal to the lateral epicondyle; however, severe overuse may progress to a full-blown fibromyalgia with symmetrical pain and multiple tender points. The author has also found that a detailed occupational history of patients presenting with fibromyalgia, revealed that many had had initial symptoms attributable to occupational overuse, a finding that requires confirmation by formal studies.

Some patients have tender points at the upper inner scapular angle, the occiput and/or the origin of the pectoralis minor. The myofascial pain syndrome[9] appears to include the more severe cases of overuse syndrome, although the authors do not comment on the relation of pain to occupation. Tension headaches are frequent in overuse syndrome, and like the sleep deprivation syndrome may be part of the same disease spectrum. The so-called 'thoracic outlet syndromes' may also be regarded as variants of the overuse syndrome, as sustained tension in a fixed position needed to support the shoulder girdle may adequately explain these symptoms. Quintner and Elvey[10] suggest that nerve roots may be entrapped at their exit from the cervical spine (discussed below) in overuse complexes. However, except in those rare cases where there is objective evidence of pressure on the medial cord of the brachial plexus, it is unclear whether the improvement reported following surgery in overuse is in fact the result of the associated cessation of work, rather than the surgery itself. Smythe has noted that the presence of organic disease such as rheumatoid arthritis, which may be accompanied by stiffness and the tension associated with 'guarding'-type pain, does not exclude a diagnosis of fibromyalgia[11], a point that also holds true for overuse syndrome.

The myalgic meningo-encephalitis (ME syndrome), now known as the chronic fatigue syndrome[12], may represent a variation on the same theme, regardless of whether it follows a chronic viral infection. About one-half of these subjects complain of a fibromyalgic type pain. Wood and colleagues[13] were not able to demonstrate peripheral weakness or fatiguability in this syndrome and concluded that the increased perception of effort was central. It is the author's impression that people with the chronic fatigue syndrome tend to reject a suggestion that the problem is one of overuse or inappropriate use of a normal, often supernormal, eye, mind, nerve, muscle, finger complex whereas overuse syndrome subjects usually welcome this explanation of their symptoms.

BACK AND LOWER LIMB OVERUSE

Although a similar biomechanical background[14] may underly the virtually ubiquitous problems of back, leg and foot pain in the workplace, relatively little has been published on this important subject. Fry[15] has re-discovered a description of leg overuse in women using treadle sewing machines. Marr, an occupational podiatrist, has argued that lower limb discomfort should be regarded as an overuse syndrome, presenting evidence that those with hypermobility are at greater risk[16]. As with the arm, there are both well-defined syndromes, e.g. trochanteric bursitis (which is analogous to the rotator cuff syndrome), ischial bursitis, and the tarsal tunnel syndrome[16,17] (which is analogous to the carpal tunnel syndrome), in addition to a vaguely defined group with signs of diffuse discomfort. Keyboard, checkout and factory chain workers may have similar symptoms due to unsuitable chair height, as they are forced to reach for foot pedals or to spin chairs to reduce body torsion. Carpet layers are at particular risk from repetitive work kneeling and stretching carpet with a knee kicker[18]. The author has had personal experience with long arch pain in the accelerator foot while driving long distances, which is relieved by switching on an automatic accelerator control.

Pathophysiology

The possible mechanisms by which overuse syndrome symptoms may arise are reviewed by Edwards[19]. Compression of capillaries caused by the repetitive movements leads to local ischemia, and accumulation of metabolites in the static muscle; these metabolites irritate nerve endings, and are considered to be the most likely primary source of pain[19]. Local ischemia of nerves that pass through the affected muscles may explain the frequent transient paresthesias in which there are no well-defined localizing or neurological signs. Although the ischemic hypothesis assumes biochemical rather than histological changes, there is also evidence[19,24] of minor microscopic changes that do not indicate permanent muscle damage. The weakness is often transient and although it may be ischemic in origin, it may simply represent a response to pain.

Quintner and Elvey[10], like Smythe, believe that the primary site of abnormality is at the emergence of nerve roots from the cervical spine and focus attention on the etiological role played by posture. In a critical review of this hypothesis, Wall suggests that soft tissue damage engenders hyperexcitable foci, both peripherally, and in the spinal cord, and emphasizes that all pain with overt physical causes has a mental component, and that pain without an organic basis is rare and has characteristic properties that are not seen in the repetitive strain injury (overuse) syndrome (RSI). He also deplores attempts to separate somatic from psychological factors, as they are completely interdependent '...*The subdivision of pain origin into either physical or mental is outdated and dangerous. All pains with an overt physical cause have a mental component. On the other hand, pains with no physical lesions are rare and with characteristic properties not included in RSI*'[25]. Much that has been written on the psychological aspects of this complaint has been written by those who received a highly selected subsample of referral cases with psychological features[26]. In this regard, the author of the present review considers such features to be common only in late neglected or mishandled cases, readily explained as secondary to the original symptoms. The focal dystonia hypothesis is discussed under writer's cramp.

Repetition of movement and the amount of load moved, which are significant factors in overuse in a factory setting[21], may be less important in the production of symptoms, than the sustained muscle tension typical of key board operation and certain light industries. A muscular force of 10% of maximum muscle power delays blood flow, with cessation of flow occurring at 50% power, the endurance limit being 5% in static load[14]. The recovery time to clear lactate after exertion increases with the percentage of maximum force applied[22] (Figure 1). While a 10 s contraction at 80% of maximum muscle strength requires a 70 s recovery period, as might occur in heavier production line work, minimal recovery is needed between relatively prolonged contraction periods for light, e.g. keyboard work. The working periods can be lengthened even more by frequently altering the wrist's working angle, thereby reducing the muscle strength needed and the recovery periods. It has been suggested that the rigidity of currently recommended industrial footwear, which minimizes major crush and burn injuries, may increase overuse foot pain[16], which could be reduced by redesign.

Since the above-indicated mechanisms are not mutually exclusive and probably operate in concert, prevention and management are based on controllable common themes:

(1) Pain generated by sustained bad posture, even with light loading, implying bad ergonomics;

(2) Frank overload in heavier occupations;

(3) Repetition; and

(4) Management pressure and over willing compliance.

Symptoms of overuse include paresthesias and muscle spasms arising as secondary reflexes to pain, which themselves may cause escalating pain capable of spreading to more proximal sites. Cohen and colleagues[27] suggest that the pain and dysfunction are analogous to reflex sympathetic dystrophy with hyperexcitability in the posterior horn cells of the cord to explain the prolonged pain in severe cases of this condition. Referred muscular pain may be perceived distal to the source of pain within the muscle[9]; as an example, pain perceived from the wrist tendons may in fact be referred from the forearm muscles, leading the examiner to assume that the pain is tendonous in origin. Tendinitis and tenosynovitis have been invoked as causes of the overuse syndrome[14], but convincing evidence of this mechanism seems to be confined to the obvious cases of overload in heavy work. There is some evidence that the subjective sensation of swelling, that often proves difficult to corroborate by the examiner, may not arise from often-diagnosed tenosynovitis, but may have a physiological basis arising from ischemia leading to local exudation of fluid[21].

Likewise, tender points may actually be related to diffuse muscle disease, and not indicate an optimal biopsy site. A tender point 4–6 cm distal to the external epicondyle is almost always present in the overuse syndrome of keyboard and other manual workers. Assessment without dolorimetry is hazardous since this point can be quite tender in normals. Proximal tender points may not be present in milder cases of overuse, and thus may be secondary and not primary features of this condition, arising from the neck, as suggested by Smythe[23].

All these factors suggest interrupting sustained posture when it cannot be completely avoided by frequent, brief breaks, applying anthropometrically appropriate weight handling limits and improving management procedures in addition to educating the keyboard workers. Magnetic resonance spectroscopy which is non-invasive and can be applied in actual work situations promises to elucidate the metabolic changes *in vivo*[20].

OCCUPATIONS AFFECTED
Keyboard operation
This is regarded for the present discussion as the prototypic overuse syndrome, and thus will be discussed in greatest detail, with differences between this and other forms of overuse being noted under separate categories that follow. As in fibromyalgia, many patients suffering from the overuse syndrome are regarded as highly competitive individuals with perfectionist tendencies in both work and non-work-related activities, even prior to developing overuse symptoms[3], and thus resemble other 'driven' individuals, e.g. athletes[28], 'type A' executives, and concert performers or actors, who are virtually by definition, competitive perfectionists. These characteristics may lead them to continue working, despite the pain, as they are unwilling to accept what they perceive as defeat, which is coupled to a fear of losing their job and not fulfilling their domestic and financial commitments. These people are distressed by their inability to work, and often return prematurely with recurrence of symptoms. Occupational discomfort is common, if not universal, but is normally overcome by positional readjustments and work breaks without the need for external intervention. Some seek aid for symptoms that are initially mild and recurrent, but which slowly or abruptly become acutely distressing. Exacerbation of symptoms and a call for help frequently occurs when a colleague has resigned, often with the same complaint, or when the company's management demands that a task be completed by a certain deadline, which would require working through breaks into overtime. All this may be aggravated by a heavier domestic commitment, or outside interest, e.g. competitive sport, knitting or playing a musical instrument. This may be elucidated by diligent questioning of the patient's social history. This is not a disease of the lazy.

Ergonomics
Poorly designed work stations may force a worker to sustain both an awkward posture for long periods, and to maintain sustained muscle contraction, placing pressure on blood vessels and nerves. In one office visited by the author, key punch operators had to bend their heads low to see a small vertical visual display unit (VDU) at desk height. Operators then turned to the left to read documents on a low desk; not surprisingly, pain in the back of the neck was prevalent and had not gone (as the supervisor had claimed), when roof windows were closed to eliminate draft. A simple shelf to raise the VDU was all that was needed.

Figure 2 shows a badly planned work station leading to thigh pain due to inadequate foot support and neck pain due to a small horizontal liquid crystal display (LCD) screen on the typewriter. The desk should allow the arms to be horizontal. In many cases the author has found it helpful, where there is sufficient desk space, to move the keyboard forward so that the forearms rest on the desk so that the shoulder, arm and neck muscles can relax since they are no longer required to support the hands. If the keyboard unit is not deep enough, a raised wooden board between it and the edge of the table will prevent over-extension of the wrists with dorsal wrist and forearm pain. If the keyboard is fixed close to the edge of the desk it will be cheaper to attach a 6 inch board to the front edge of the desk than to buy new equipment. Those taught to type with arms unsupported can train themselves to type with the arms supported, quite quickly regaining their original speed.

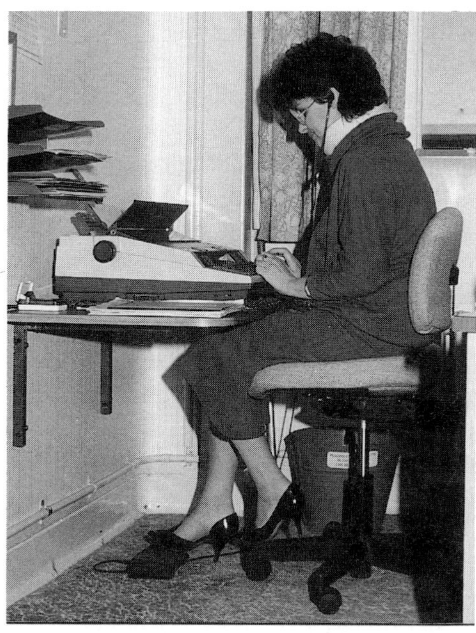

Figure 2 A poorly designed work station with excessive neck flexion to view a horizontal liquid crystal display (LCD) screen on the typewriter necessitating a neck support, excessive wrist extension and thigh pain from lack of foot support

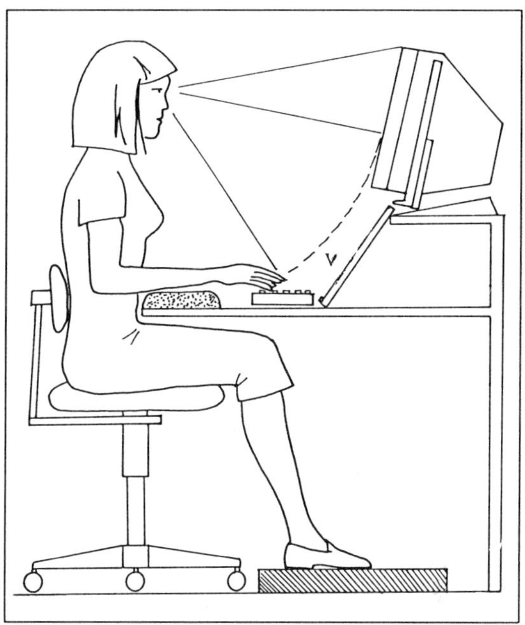

Figure 3 An idealized computer work station with arm support, to minimize wrist extension and room for a copy stand (V) between keyboard and VDU screen and a foot platform for those with short legs. (Modified with kind permission from the Pocket Ergonomist, Brown & Mitchell)

Arms supports were not shown to be helpful in one study[29] but the subjects were shown reaching a long way forward whereas a vertical position for the upper arm is usually recommended. Figure 3 shows a computer station with forearm support raised enough to allow operation of a flat keyboard without excessive wrist extension. This shows a vertical body position but many prefer to lean backward 10°. The slope for holding copying material is placed between screen and key board but some prefer to have this on either side of the screen allowing lateral rather than vertical eye movement. The latter may be more suitable for text whereas the former may be preferred for columns of figures.

Poor ergonomics alone may cause overuse syndrome but other factors described above also contribute and may cause overuse syndrome when the work station is ideal. Seating should be adjustable so that the back is supported, leaning slightly backward, the VDU directly in front of the face or 10–20° below that, at a distance appropriate for easy reading with a vertical neck posture allowing for the individual's vision and spectacles. An older person using bifocal lenses may develop neck pain from having to extend his neck to focus the VDU with the lower lens. The problem can be solved by lowering the VDU or using spectacles of appropriate focal length.

In many typing schools, the students are taught that the arms should be raised, a principle that seems to be a carry-over from the days of mechanical typewriters. There is a need to re-educate the instructors, as only light finger touch is required on electronic keyboards, and the forearms can be completely rested on the desk with complete shoulder relaxation. In this position the height of the table is less critical but adjustment of height for different operators using the same station is desirable. The use of a number pad with one hand to enter numbers from documents turned over with the other hand normally dictates working at desk level but the desk could be sloped upwards and suitable document holders on angle poise type arms are now available for this purpose. The VDU may be placed lower to minimize neck and eye movement reducing both neck and eye strain which will increase the error rate.

Placement of the writing surface is not a new problem. Five centuries ago, scribes used sloping desks to bring work closer to eye level (*see* Figure 4). The one illustrated also shows that the forearm is rested and a quite sophisticated mechanism is used to adjust the position of the writing slope. Architects still use this principle. If a telephone has to be answered intermittently, it should be placed so that reaching out and twisting to one side is not necessary. This should be done in a relaxed manner as with typing and all activity since rhythmic smooth movements minimize sustained muscular contraction.

Expensive custom-made furniture is often not ideal for a particular person and can be difficult to alter quickly if another person shares the same work station. Inexpensive modification of standard furniture can be more satisfactory as for instance shortening the legs of a wooden table or providing a foot rest for a smaller person may solve seat discomfort leading to posterior thigh discomfort and tense posture. Key boards and visual display units which can be separately moved on the desk without restriction can be better than elaborate custom built layouts which are fixed without arm support. Some manufacturers supply arm rest attachments to allow the weight of the whole arm to be carried by the

support, thus eliminating the static load from the upper-limb girdle-neck and thorax. Green and Briggs emphasize the need to ensure that operators fully understand the use of their equipment[30]. Many may be put off work when advice on rest followed by increased work load is appropriate. Typical rehabilitation for keyboard operators would include controlled work loads such as no typing or typing for 10 min/h, and gradually increasing up to a full work load. With this advice, the time off work dropped from 34% to 3.4%, and in other occupations from 91 to 31.5[31]. The overall severity of symptoms decreased, which in part may have been due to an accumulation of severe cases in the previous years. It was argued that a positive approach to prevention and rehabilitation had paid off in physiological and economic terms. One study of 1545 clerical workers at 38 work sites in Massachusetts demonstrated that VDU workers had an increased prevalence of adverse conditions pertaining to vision, musculoskeletal discomfort, and headaches. The magnitude of disabilities attributed to VDU use was directly proportional to the number of hours spent at the terminal[32], with those working 7 h or longer per day being at greatest risk.

Administrators and those dictating work who are not accustomed to keyboard work often do not appreciate the need for regular breaks to maintain sustained productivity[33] and may make staff feel guilty if they do not accept extra work. Work planning is made easier if the degree of urgency is made clear in advance on copy documents or dictation tapes since non-urgent work can be fitted in at intervals between other jobs.

Epidemiology

Lack of internationally agreed definitions is an impediment to epidemiological study of this syndrome, which has been described under different names in Japan[4], Australia[34], Britain[1], USA[35], Finland, New Zealand[3] and no doubt in other countries. Earlier literature was referred to under the term 'visual display unit' which was then considered to be the cause of the musculoskeletal as well as the eye symptoms. Reporting of the syndrome is more reflective of the availability of compensation rather than to actual occurrence of overuse syndrome(s). For example, in Great Britain compensation is only available if the diagnosis is carpal tunnel syndrome or tenosynovitis (popularly known as 'teno') providing a bias to the use of these terms. In Australia compensation depends on use of the word injury, hence the term repetitive strain injury (RSI), though demonstrable physical injury is not usually evident. These legal problems are discussed by Hadler in Chapter 29.

A total of 4891 cases of RSI were reported in Telecom Australia[36] from 1981, peaking in 1984 and remitting in 1988. Hocking was not able to explain this epidemic on workplace or legal intervention and he reports to this author that the rate is still very low in 1992.

When 10–28% of Japanese office machine operators were affected by overuse syndrome(s), legislation was introduced that limited work to 5 h/day with 10 min breaks each hour, and a limit of 40 000 keystrokes/day. These efforts, and others, e.g. job rotation in the office, was followed by a reduction of overuse symptoms[4]. The success of this Japanese 'experiment' was not appreciated in other countries, such as Australia, where the reported frequency of overuse has risen dramatically in the last decade at great cost to compensation insurance. The report of an Australian committee to investigate this epidemic[5] recommended staging of the severity of the complaint but legal inference of an inevitable progression through the stages to total permanent disablement led to criticism of staging. This has created a heated controversy which continues.

There is a clear need for definition and grading[3,5] to avoid confusion that occurs when the far more common mild cases with minimal-to-moderate disability are compared to the severe tertiary referral cases, which are a small percentage of the whole. These definitions are also necessary for epidemiological surveys and for stratifying cases in intervention trials. In view of this the following alternative is suggested:

Grade 1: Upper limb or neck discomfort of asymmetrical onset of more than 1 months' duration, increased by repetitive work, sustained or awkward posture and relieved by rest with no physical sign except tenderness;

(a) Those who do not seek medical care, and

(b) Those who seek medical care.

Grade 2: As in 1 but with pain at rest and loss of work time.

Grade 3: As in 2 but with unremitting pain and/or sleep disturbance.

This is similar to the grading system proposed for overuse syndrome of musicians by Fry[37], who includes a higher grade for the few overuse victims who are totally incapacitated.

PREVENTION OF KEYBOARD OVERUSE SYNDROME

Optimal work station design as above indicated is clearly important, and presupposes the effective collaboration of architects, engineers, ergonomists and management. Flexibility should be allowed for individual variation in height and breadth. Anthropometric tables are available for many populations but allowance should be made for ethnic differences, where for example, the shorter Asians and broader heavier Polynesians will have different requirements. Poor lighting and ventilation and other features contributing to the 'sick building syndrome'[38], will also contribute to overuse symptoms. VDU screens on older equipment are not always easily read, and environmental lighting should be such that it does not cause annoying reflection from the screen. Movable keyboards allow rapid change to suit individual work preferences; separate movable number pads are helpful for the left-handed and enable periodic change from one side to another as an alternative to breaks. If the key board is too high in relation to the forearm support it may be necessary to raise the arm support, as suggested above.

The Japanese experience[4] indicated that breaks should be taken every hour. Recent information indicates that breaks should be taken much more frequently. Even brief breaks at 40-min intervals are not effective, which would be expected based on the ischemic hypothesis, as it only takes a few minutes for ischemia to develop[14]. Work-site relaxation training using blood pressure monitoring has been used[39]. The need for short breaks (micropauses) has been demonstrated by electromyographic studies and a timing device was designed by Brown and Mitchell[40] for use in the workplace, which can be preset to signal when a break should be taken. Improvement with cognitive behavior therapy[41] including electromyography (EMG) biofeedback and relaxation was greater than with those waiting to be called for this instruction. This was more economically applied in groups than to individuals, but both were equally successful. Prescribed mid-morning, afternoon and lunch breaks must also be taken. Missing such breaks to leave early to collect the children from school is a common fault. The need for adequate sleep, is demonstrated by sleep deprivation experiments on volunteers, who eventually develop overuse type pains, and recover on restoration of a normal sleep pattern[42].

The value of frequent brief relaxation is demonstrated by athletes. One leading cricketer advocates systematic relaxation between each ball, a few seconds per minute, which enhances perfor-

mance. Such anecdotal evidence is useful in prevention, education and treatment since it implies that the goal is to achieve the best possible efficiency from the complex mind-body machine. It also shows that exercise is compatible with relaxation in alternation as in running where one set of muscles relaxes as the opposite set contracts. Evidence on the importance of the speed of repetition is conflicting. Speed may not be important if breaks are taken for positive relaxation to minimize the duration of static load. A factory study of force and frequency of loading showed significant associations of symptoms with high frequency and heavy loading, frequency being the main contributor[21] but sustained loading which is now considered the most important variable[3] was not measured in that study.

A preselection questionnaire could test the author's contention[3] that a competitive, perfectionist personality, before development of symptoms, determines which subjects are susceptible to overuse syndrome might well identify those at risk. Standard psychological questionnaires, designed to detect subnormal features, would be unsatisfactory as these people have usually been above-normal achievers before developing symptoms, and standard questionnaires such as the Minnesota Multiphasic Personality Inventory (MMPI) test would reflect present rather than premorbid states. Such individuals should not be precluded from employment but should rather be recognized as potentially becoming a company's most efficient operators, given instruction as suggested above and should work up to full speed gradually, making frequent breaks a habit. As with athletes, the workers should resume work gradually after leave of absence, as for pregnancy.

It is important to provide temporary staff to relieve those who are off work, as overuse syndrome is often precipitated by a sudden increase in work load due to the absence of a colleague, who may have left the job having similar complaints. The same instructions designed for a more relaxed rhythmic working mode with frequent breaks[43,44], should translate to daily living activities, as susceptible individuals tend to be overtense and worried while performing domestic duties, e.g. 'I can't watch television if I am not knitting'. A number of books and tapes are available on methods of relaxation but group instruction is useful in allowing discussion.

OTHER OCCUPATIONS
Writer's cramp
This complaint differs from keyboard overuse only in that the symptoms which are identical are limited to the forearm and wrist of the dominant hand. Brain's classic description of this complaint[2] needs little alteration to fit the modern scene. The tendency for the wrists or finger to spasm may be greater in this complaint than in keyboard workers, and has been called focal dystonia, which is less common in key board operators. Because Brain called writer's cramp an occupational neurosis (which at the time, implied a condition of neurological origin), the use of this term is counter productive, since 'neurosis' implies to the layman psychological inadequacy, while those with symptoms of overuse are often above average performers.

Clerks who were mostly men were commonly affected before the introduction of typewriters early this century. All documents had to be written by hand so the clerk was faced with the same problems as today's keyboard operator. To counter this, children were taught in school to write with straight relaxed fingers with the forearm well supported on a sloping desk at optimum height, the movements being made from the elbow to produce a smooth flowing script, a method that is no longer taught. Thus, one commonly sees people writing in cramped positions with the distal phalanx of the forefinger hyperextended, indicating a tight grip. Left-handed writers may hold the pen with the wrist in full flexion requiring a high static load. It is advisable that writers be retrained to write in the manner described above. For primary prevention this method should be taught in schools, and educational authorities should review current methods of teaching handwriting to school children.

Sheehy and Marsden[45] quote Poore who describes his examinations of many hundreds of patients with writer's cramp, '...the frequency of the disorder in the late Victorian era must stand as a tribute to the success of the British empire, the enormous office staff required to run it, and the difficulties of manipulating the quill pen.' These writers argue that by analogy to other dystonias attributed to hypothetical lesions in the basal ganglia that writer's cramp is a focal dystonia. Early cases do not show incoordination or involuntary muscle contractions and this hypothesis does not offer any therapeutic or preventive opportunity.

This syndrome is now more frequently encountered in those with overuse syndrome from keyboard operation who have changed to clerical work, and the symptoms occur in the dominant hand only. This problem is increased when a ball point pen must be forcefully pressed to imprint several carbon copies. Care should be taken in office design to ensure that writing is done in optimal position, as for typing. Adequate desk space should be available to ensure comfortable forearm support. Sloping desk tops, used by medieval monks (Figure 4), no doubt fitted their ergonomic requirements allowing a more upright posture. Perhaps sloping desks should be reintroduced into the modern office. These have been in constant use by architects, who use adjustable sloping desks, as catalogued by Chippendale in the eighteenth century. It would be expected that eye, neck and back strain would decline as a result.

Figure 4 An illustration from a Flemish manuscript of 1485 showing a Carmelite monk using a sloping adjustable desk, enabling him to write in an erect position with the arm resting on the slope of the desk. (Reproduced with kind permission of the British Library)

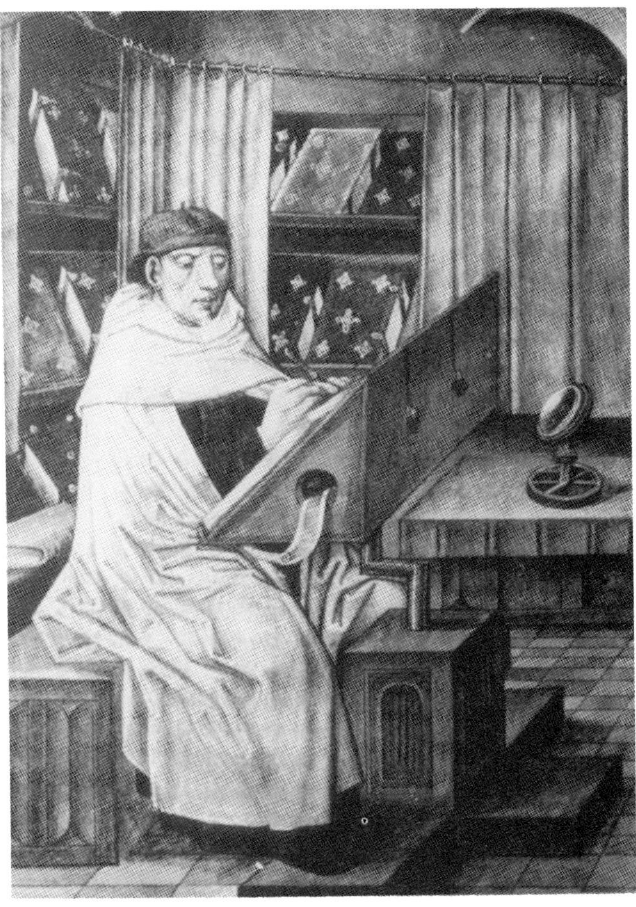

Checkout operators

Supermarkets have increased the speed of price verification and the wrapping of consumer foods by designing work stations in which groceries are passed over an electronic bar-code scanner on the left or entering prices into a cash register on the right[46]. Some workers turn even further to the left when packing the goods in bags. Those who sit, even with a suitable typist's swivel chair, repeatedly twist their neck and spine from side to side and may develop shoulder, neck and sometimes back symptoms, as well as carpal tunnel syndrome[47]. Those who stand can step around while packing groceries to avoid twisting, but may develop leg and foot fatigue symptoms. Some work stations can be arranged so that alternation of sitting and standing is possible. Rotation of tasks several times a day from checking out to wrapping, and then to stacking goods on shelves can vary the load. Stacking goods onto shelves can lead to other forms of occupational complaints, e.g. rotator cuff symptoms, especially in short people. This may be avoided by the provision of a movable double step. At peak hours in the store, a second person can do the wrapping, reducing the checkout operator's tasks. Cash register and bank teller work station adjustments to individual heights can be difficult if the station is used by more than one person.

Musicians

The overuse syndrome is common in musicians[37,48–52], and has the same symptoms as other forms of overuse. Fry[36] found 116 cases of overuse syndrome in 1249 students in seven music schools; the hand and wrist were affected in 63, the arm in 40 and the spine in 23 music students (Tables 1 and 2). Hartsell and Tata[52] reached similar conclusions in a retrospective survey in a music school in Canada. Overuse is often accompanied by cramp and loss of coordination, focal dystonia, nerve impingement, weakness and diminished precision in playing leading to depression. Lockwood[50] notes that anxiety is a major contributor to performance-related problems, and may respond to the use of β-adrenergic blocking agents. The localization of the complaint is a function of the body region required to support the instrument's static load.

The clarinet is supported with the right thumb; the muscles of the first interosseous space and radial aspect of the wrist become painful. This can be resolved by suspending the instrument from a neck strap. Orchestral violinists develop pain in the neck and left shoulder with tenderness of the rotator cuff secondary to sustained contraction supporting the instrument. Pianists tend to have hand and shoulder discomfort rather than back pain, in a fashion somewhat similar to that described in keyboard operators. Guitarists develop forearm pain and tender epicondyles which

Table 1 Frequency of overuse syndrome (OS) by instrument and sex (1249 music students)

	Female		Male		%
	n	%	n	%	with OS
Keyboard	141	4.3	268	11.2	8.8
Woodwind	98	12.2	178	13.5	13.0
Strings	167	7.8	182	8.2	8.0
Brass	104	5.8	42	7.1	6.8
Percussion	52	5.8	17	17.6	8.7

Table 2 Instruments involved in overuse syndrome

Instrument	Male	Female	Both
Keyboard	15	10	25
Woodwind	10	22	32
Strings	7	21	28
Brass	6	17	23
Percussion	2	6	8
Total	40	76	116

are often helped by moving the left arm closer to the body[48].

Prevention

Intensive practice for competitions, especially in the young should be discouraged. Well-planned practice sessions with frequent breaks and instruction in relaxation and tension reduction are recommended, in addition to attention to posture. Early reporting of symptoms is advocated, which would be facilitated by the availability of a physician interested in performance medicine. One follow-up study of occupational therapy revealed that gentle stretching exercise and warming up and cooling down routines were often helpful, although two affected individuals were definitely made worse by the exercise regimen[49]. As with other studies, the onset of symptoms usually followed a drastic increase in practice and performance time, and the authors concluded that 'Careful management of one's performance schedule may be the most effective way to manage or prevent these problems'.

Fry's recommendations for prevention are:

(1) Education,

(2) Limit practice hours per day with regular breaks,

(3) Use supports to carry the weight of wood-wind and brass instruments.

The latter is normal practice for bassoonists who support the instrument on a strap that they sit on. Although it is unlikely that an ergonomist could design an instrument that would be acceptable to players, ingenuity may succeed in developing practical support devices for violins, violas and other instruments held in awkward positions.

In addition to these measures, the author advocates teaching systematic relaxation from an early stage. Instruction of music instructors, whose conservatism may be difficult to overcome, is important, and the total number of hours per session and per day should be regulated. For most instruments, rests are written into the music itself, but violinists and pianists are often required to play for long periods without a break. Conductors should be aware that breaks for relaxation and muscle stretches during practices and rehearsals will minimize the risk of overuse syndrome. Some major orchestras maintain a consultant for this purpose.

Farming

Overuse syndromes in agriculture are largely a function of the instrument being used to perform the labor. The short handled hoe, as recorded by Van Gogh (Figure 5), has fallen into disuse in many developed nations as it causes overuse-type back pain[53]. In Indonesia this type of hoe is routinely used in cultivation of rice crops (Chapter 24), but is not associated with low back pain[55], perhaps because the laborers take frequent short breaks[56]. The carrying pole, used still in South East Asia, and in rural China, is a most efficient method of carrying weights without back flexion, twisting or shoulder strain, although some workers may develop skin thickening on the shoulders which may be painful[56]. A similar device, the European shaped yoke is no longer used. This appears to be a regrettable step backward in the

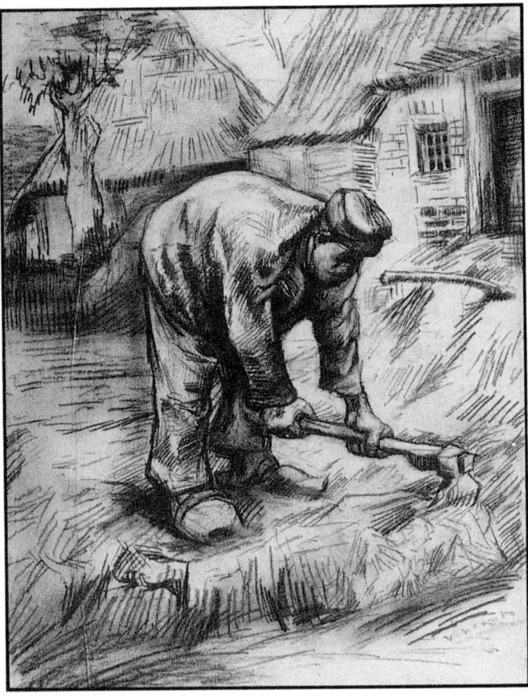

Figure 5 A Van Gogh drawing of a Dutch farmer using the short-handled hoe still used in Indonesia. (Reproduced with kind permission from Rijksmuseum, Knoller Muller, Otterloo, Holland)

modernization of the farm, as the author has seen shoulder and elbow pain in dairy farmers wives who carry milk pails. This might have been avoided by the use of such an old-fashioned tool. In Australasia where sheep shearing is a competitive occupation, indeed a competitive sport, low back pain is very common if not universal. In western farming, back pain is a major problem, contributed to by vibration in motor vehicles and tractors.

Production chain work

The rate of a conveying chain line should be controlled with regular breaks to minimize overload. As is the practice in some meat freezing works, rather than slowing the whole chain, two slaughtermen alternate for each carcass for the heavier tasks. Alternatively, heavy tasks can be

82

rotated at 15-min intervals. Stools provided to raise the level to optimum work height may need to be changed at 15-min intervals for tall and short operators to work at optimum arm height (*see also* Chapter 9).

Machinists

Women working in clothing factories are susceptible to overuse syndrome especially where bonuses are offered for increased production. Since each task takes a relatively short time a brief relaxation break can be taken between each task.

Weaving

Weavers and basket makers are susceptible to typical overuse syndrome(s). This was identified in a Philippines COPCORD study where no compensation is available. This might in other countries have been attributed to secondary gain[53].

OVERUSE COMPLEXES UNDERGOING OBSOLESCENCE

Telegraphists cramp

This is analogous to writer's cramp, and thus need not be detailed further. As electronic keyboards replace Morse code, the problems will now be those of all keyboard operators. One study of rate of keying-in telegraphists[57] failed to show an association with rate and symptoms though the comparability of groups was in question especially since the severely affected would have resigned leaving only a survivor population.

Telephone exchange operation

Old manual exchanges caused problems as long reaches were needed, longer for left handers. These have been supplanted by electronic keyboards in developed countries so operators are now exposed to the same risks as other keyboard operators[36].

Other occupations

These are too numerous to detail, as any repetitive sustained activity can produce the symptoms. The reader is referred to texts on occupational disease for detail[1]. Bakers filling pastries, carpenters, builders, panel beaters, electricians, television repairmen and innumerable others may develop overuse syndrome(s). Observation of the workplace often aids in determining suitable preventive measures, for example those experiencing difficulties with screw drivers may be able to use an electric tool. In a large white ware factory, engineers designed a clip to replace screws so eliminating a major cause of pain, disability, inefficiency and loss of work. Builders who have difficulty in hammering large nails may be able to use a mechanical hammer. Visual artists are susceptible to back, neck and shoulder complaints[58].

There has been remarkably little basic work on the epidemiology of occupational overuse syndromes. Thompson, Bacon and Harrington have examined people in 18 workplaces in Birmingham, England[59]. In some workplaces, symptoms were so common that insufficient controls were available for a planned case–control study. Thoracic/neck joint dysfunction was noted in nearly half the subjects despite the fact that most of the jobs involved repetitive movement of the upper limb beyond the elbow. Clearly postural factors as well as movement factors were involved in the resulting syndrome. As stated by Thompson, Bacon and Harrington:

The point we wish to make is that a careful and thorough review of workplace activities will often provide a logical explanation for the resulting clinical features, and in addition paves the way for preventive action by modification of the workplaces.

MEASURES FOR MINIMIZING OVERUSE SYNDROMES

Educational materials to be targeted to the interested medical, managerial and governing bodies are discussed in Chapter 31. The New Zealand Occupational Health and Safety section of the Government Department of Labour have prepared general guidelines and a series of booklets and leaflets for the prevention and control of overuse syndrome[8] and its management[60], which are to be distributed to the schools and polytechnical colleges, to managers, supervisors, workers and unions, as well as to general medical practitioners, therapists and the appropriate specialists.

The author has found that it takes considerable time to explain all the details in the consultation situation, and has prepared an audiotape (now also available in print[61]) that discusses general relaxation techniques, and recommends three second break periods following three minute work periods. General advice is also offered on rationalization of work patterns at home and at work and on coping with social problems. These have been found to be helpful in otherwise resistant cases and though not formally evaluated may have preventive value if made available to work groups at risk such as factory staffs and typing pools. Queries about this are discussed at two further visits and the subject is encouraged to lend the tape to colleagues, management and spouses. Visits to the workplace by the medical adviser, although desirable, are often impractical, in which case the relevant occupational health specialist, factory doctor or occupational safety and health (OSH) officers may be requested to visit. The victims of overuse would then be advised on appropriate ergonomics and job planning to prevent the development of symptoms in remaining staff.

The need to take a detailed occupational history cannot be overemphasized. Too often this has not been done by specialists who have neither taken an adequate history nor visited the workplace but do not hesitate to give far-reaching opinions for medico-legal purposes.

FUTURE DIRECTIONS

There is a clear need for good quality epidemiological studies with high response rates and case control studies to define risk factors. Controlled intervention studies are needed, for instance, the computer programs, e.g. WordPerfect or Lotus 1,2,3, that the keyboard operators work with, could be programed to set breaks of differing length and frequency. Questionnaires to assess symptoms could also be included in the software and sequentially analyzed. The operators, being keyboard trained, should have no difficulty with this. Worry that management would respond unfavorably to some answers could be eliminated by confidential questionnaires. Little has been written on overuse syndrome type problems with the low back and overuse syndromes affecting the feet but this should be a fruitful field for future research.

GENERAL PREVENTION

The following general suggestions are made for the prevention of overuse syndrome:

Education

(1) General public education to increase awareness of the problem and the risks of overload;

(2) Education for schools, teachers, employers, unions;

(3) Pre-employment education in work methods to all staff;

(4) Additional instruction to identified susceptibles, and those with previous overuse syndrome;

(5) Teach how to live and work in relaxed optimum posture;

(6) Increase activity gradually for new personnel or those returning from leave, i.e. maternity leave;

(7) Employ temporary replacements for those off work to prevent overuse symptoms in remaining staff; and

(8) Use EMG feedback, videotapes and audiotapes on the work site to teach relaxation to groups and individuals.

Work station planning

(1) Improve the ergonomic design of work stations by consultation with ergonomists, architects, engineers, management, user and labor organizations;

(2) Improve the ergonomics of work practices where feasible; and

(3) Continually communicate with equipment acquisition staff.

Task design and work organization

(1) Match physical and psychological factors to the job;

(2) Avoid bonuses for extra production;

(3) Adjust work rates and frequency and duration of breaks to the optimum for production chain work; and

(4) Rotate duties where possible to minimize duration of sustained activity and boredom.

Social factors

(1) Promote self-coping methods;

(2) Avoid negative influences such as iatrogenic factors, overdependency on treatment providers and the martyr role;

(3) Foster employer/staff/union rapport; and

(4) Reduce monotony by varying tasks.

CONCLUSION

The overuse syndrome is a common disorder causing much distress and inefficiency in the workplace with considerable scope for prevention. Many of the conclusions reached above are based on clinical observations. There is clearly a need for further work on the definition of syndromes and for controlled trials of various measures aimed to prevent and improve the control of overuse syndrome. We could also profitably relearn some of the lessons learned by trial and error in the past.

REFERENCES

1. Dalton S, Hazelman B. In Raffle Lee, McCallum, Murray, eds., Hunter's Diseases of Occupations. London, Hodder and Stroughton, 1987, pp. 620–633
2. Brain WR. Diseases of the Nervous System. London, Oxford University Press, 6th edn, 1962, pp. 853–854
3. Wigley RD. Repetitive strain syndrome. Fact not fiction. NZ Med J. 1990; 103:75–76
4. Ohara H, Nagagiri S, Itani T et al. Occupational health hazards resulting from elevated work rate situations. J Human Ergon. 1976; 5:173–182
5. Silverstein B. Hand-wrist disorders among investment casting plant workers. J Hand Surg. 1987; 12A:838–844
6. Browne CD, Nolan BM, Faithful DK. Occupational repetition strain injuries. Med J Aust. 1984; 1:329–332
7. Brooks P. Regional pain syndrome: the importance of nomenclature. Br J Rheumatol. 1989; 28:180–182
8. Guidelines for the Prevention and Management of Occupational Overuse Syndrome. New Zealand Dept of Labour, Wellington, 1991
9. Simons DG, Travell JG. Myofascial pain syndromes. In Wall R, Melzack G., eds., Pain. Churchill Livingtone, 1984, pp. 263–276
10. Quintner JL, Elvey RL, Thomas AN. Regional pain syndrome. Med J Aust. 1987; 146:230–231
11. Smythe HA. Fibrositis. In Kelley et al., eds., Textbook of Rheumatic Disease. 1985, pp. 481–489

12. Stokes MJ, Cooper RG, Edwards RHT. Normal muscle strength and fatiguability in patients with effort syndrome. Br Med J. 1988; 297:1014–1017

13. Wood GC, Bentall RP, Gopfert MA, Edwards RHT. comparative psychiatric assessment of patients with chronic fatigue syndrome and muscle disease. In press, 1991

14. Chaffin DB, Andersson G. Occupational biomechanics. New York, John Wiley, 1984

15. Fry HJH. Overuse syndrome in musicians: 100 years ago. An historical review. Med J Aust. 1986; 145:620–625

16. Marr SJ. Overuse syndrome of the lower limbs. J Occup Health Safety ANZ. 1985; 1:130–134

17. Forst L, Hryhorczuk D. Occupational tarsal tunnel syndrome. Br J Indust Med. 1988; 45:277–278

18. Thun M, Tanaka S, Smith AB, Halperin WE, Lee ST, Luggen ME. Morbidity from repetitive knee trauma in carpet floor layers. Br J Indust Med. 1987; 44:611–620

19. Edwards RH. Hypotheses of peripheral and central mechanisms underlying occupational muscle pain and injury. Eur J Physiol. 1988; 57: 275–281

20. Griffiths RD, Edwards RH. Magnetic resonance spectroscopy in the recognition of metabolic disease. J Inherit Metab Dis. 1987; 10 Suppl. 147–158

21. Armstrong TJ, Fine LJ, Goldstein SA, Lifshitz YR, Silverstein BA. Ergonomics considerations in hand and wrist tendinitis. J Hand Surg. 1987; 12A:830–837

22. Rodgers SH. Recovery time needs for repetitive work. Semin Occup Med. 87; 2:19–24

23. Smythe H. 'Repetitive strain injury syndrome' is referred pain from the neck. J Rheumatol. 1988; 15:1604–1606

24. Fry HJH. Regional pain syndrome. Br Med J. 1989; 28:452

25. Wall PD. Neurogenic hypothesis of RSI. Bammer G, ed. Australian National University, Canberra, 1991, p. 50

26. Lucire. Neurosis in the work place. Med J Aust. 1986; 145:877–881

27. Cohen ML, Arroyo JF, Champion GD, Browne GD. Evidence for neuropathic mechanisms in diffuse upper limb (occupational cervicobrachial disorder) and diffuse musculoskeletal (fibromyalgia) pain syndromes. Pain. 1990; 32:89–94

28. Hartley LH. In Sports Medicine. WB Saunders, 1984, pp. 42–53

29. Bendix T, Jessen F. Wrist support during typing – a controlled, electromyographic study. Appl Ergon. 1986; 17.3:162–168

30. Green RA, Briggs CA. Effect of overuse injury and the importance of training on the use of adjustable work stations by keyboard operators. J Occup Med. 1989; 31:557–562

31. Oxenburgh MS, Rowe SA, Douglas DB. Repetitive strain injury in keyboard operators. Successful management over a two year period. J Occup Health Safety ANZ. 1985; 1:106–112

32. Rossignol AM, Morse EP, Summers VM. Video display terminal use and reported health symptoms among Massachusetts clerical workers. J Occup Med. 1987; 29:112–118

33. Baidya KN, Stevenson MG. Local muscle fatigue in repetitive work. Ergonomics. 1988; 31: 227–239

34. McDermott FT. Repetition strain injury: a review of current understanding. Med J Aust. 1986; 144:196–200

35. Parniapour M, Nordin M, Skovron ML, Frankel VH. Environmentally-induced disorders of the musculoskeletal system. Med Clin North Am. 1990; 74:347–349

36. Hocking B. 'Repetition strain injury' in Telecom Australia. Med J Aust. 1989; 154:724

37. Fry HJH. Prevalence of overuse (injury) syndrome in Australian music schools. Br J Indust Med. 1987; 44:35–40

38. Letz GA. Sick building syndrome: acute illness among office workers-the role of building ventilation, airborne contaminants and work stress. Allergy Proc. 1990; 11:109–116

39. Fiedler N, Vivona-Vaughan E, Gochfield M. Evaluation of a work site relaxation training program using ambulatory blood pressure monitoring. J Occup Med. 1989; 31:595–627

40. Brown DA, Mitchell R. How to use the fresh muscles trainer. A simple tool for learning to relax at home and at work. Group Occupational Health Centre. Sydney, 1986

41. Spence SH. Cognitive-behavior therapy in the management of chronic occupational pain of the upper limbs. Behav Res Ther. 1989; 27:435–436

42. Moldofsky P, Scarisbrick P, England BA, Smythe H. Musculoskeletal symptoms and non-REM

sleep disturbance in patients with 'fibrositis syndrome' and healthy patients. Psychosomat Med. 1975; 37:341–351

43. Sundelin G, Hagberg M. The effects of different pause types on neck and shoulder EMG activity during VDU work. Ergonomics. 1989; 32: 527–537

44. Henning RA, Sauter S, Salvendy G, Krieg EF. Microbreak length and performance in data entry task. Ergonomics. 1989; 32:855–864

45. Sheehy MP, Marsden CD. Writer's cramp – a focal dystonia. Brain. 1982; 105:461–480

46. Slappendill C. Study of check out operators. Report to ACC and Clerical Worker's Union. Massey University Palmerston North, New Zealand

47. Barnhart S, Rosenstock L. Carpal tunnel syndrome in grocery checkers. Western J Med. 147: 37–40

48. Owen E. Instrumental musicians and repetition strain injury. J Occup Health Safety ANZ. 1985; 12:135–139

49. Goodman G, Staz S. Occupational therapy for musicians with upper extremity overuse syndrome; patient perceptions regarding effectiveness of treatment. Med Probl Perform Arts. 1989; 9:14

50. Lockwood AH. Medical problems of musicians. N Engl J Med. 1989; 230:221–225

51. Middlestadt SE, Fishbein M. Health and occupational correlates of perceived occupational stress in symphony orchestra musicians. J Occup Med. 1988; 30:687–692

52. Hartsell HD, Tata GE. A retrospective survey of music-related musculo-skeletal problems occurring in undergraduate music students. Physiother Can. 1991; 43:13–18

53. Wigley RD, Manahan L, Caragay R, Muirden KD, Valkenburg The Philippine COPCORD Study Phase 2&3. Rheumatol. Internat., 1991; 11: 157–61

54. Zenz C. Developments in Occupational Medicine. Year Book Publishers, Chicago, 1980, pp. 159–168

55. Darmawan J. Indonesian COPCORD. Doctoral thesis, Erasmus University, Rotterdam, 1987

56. Suzuki S. Conjunctivitis due to cultivation work observed among Indonesian peasants. Proc 10th Asian Conference on Occupational Health. Singapore 1982. pp. 187–189

57. Ferguson D. An Australian study of telegrapher's cramp. Br J Indust Med. 1971; 28:280–285

58. Chang WS, Bejjani FJ, Hyan D, Bellgarde M. Occupational musculoskeletal disorders of visual artists: A questionnaire and video analysis. Ergonomics. 1987; 30:33–46

59. Thompson D, Bacon PA, Harrington JM, Nayak USL. Occurrence and mechanism of occupational repetition strain injuries. University of Birmingham, 1990. p. 188

60. Guidelines for Occupational Overuse Syndrome. OSH, Dept of Labour, New Zealand Government Printer. Wellington, 1991

61. Wigley RD, Turner WED, Blake BL, Darby FW, McInnes R, Harding P. Occupational overuse syndrome. Treatment and rehabilitation: a practitioner's guide. OSH, Department of Labour, Wellington, 1992

8. REGIONAL PAIN SYNDROMES

Anders Bjelle and Richard Wigley

INTRODUCTION

This section includes the more clearly defined and localized overuse and/or occupational or sports-induced pain syndromes which were not discussed in the chapter on overuse syndromes (Chapter 7), although most cases are induced by occupational overuse. In the most common of these conditions, the pain arises from the shoulder, causing the so-called 'rotator cuff syndrome', which is followed in frequency by epicondylitis (tennis and golfer's elbow), carpal tunnel syndrome and trochanteric bursitis. Less common is the tarsal tunnel syndrome, and a long list of complaints, including occupational bursitis, entrapment neuropathies, tendinitis, tenosynovitis, and stenosing tenovaginitides such as de Quervain's disease. These syndromes may also be due to single injuries, and if related to other diseases such as arthritis, they are classified accordingly. Back pain is dealt with separately in Chapter 9.

Regional pain syndromes include a wide variety of conditions and diseases, which are difficult to classify given the lack of generally accepted criteria for establishing their diagnoses. Epidemiological studies of these syndromes will thus have inherent differences, which impede comparison of data. Regional pain may be caused by inflammatory conditions, as well as non-inflammatory soft tissue rheumatic conditions. Since soft tissues play an important role in the stability and function of the large joints, it is important to consider the multifactorial nature of regional complaints with an interplay between diseases, predisposition and mechanical factors.

Regional pain in the general population has been inadequately studied from an epidemiological standpoint, and most surveys are largely confined to manual workers, since these problems are a major health hazard in industry and the workplace. Data from developing countries have slowly emerged, indicating a high prevalence of regional soft tissue complaints largely related to poor ergonomics in the workplace (Chapter 3). Regional pain may originate from a variety of anatomical sites. Figure 1 is a flow diagram showing the likely sequence of events leading to overuse syndromes[1], and Figure 2 indicates the overlap of risk factors, predisposing factors and the disease state itself.

This chapter reviews available data on regional pain syndromes in the general population, in some patient groups and in populations of workers, with an emphasis on primary prevention.

EPIDEMIOLOGY

In the absence of internationally accepted classifications, some authors have introduced their own *ad hoc* definitions for these complaints, which makes the comparison of different studies a precarious exercise (Table 1). A number of methodologic difficulties are involved in studies of regional pain syndromes. As yet, there is no

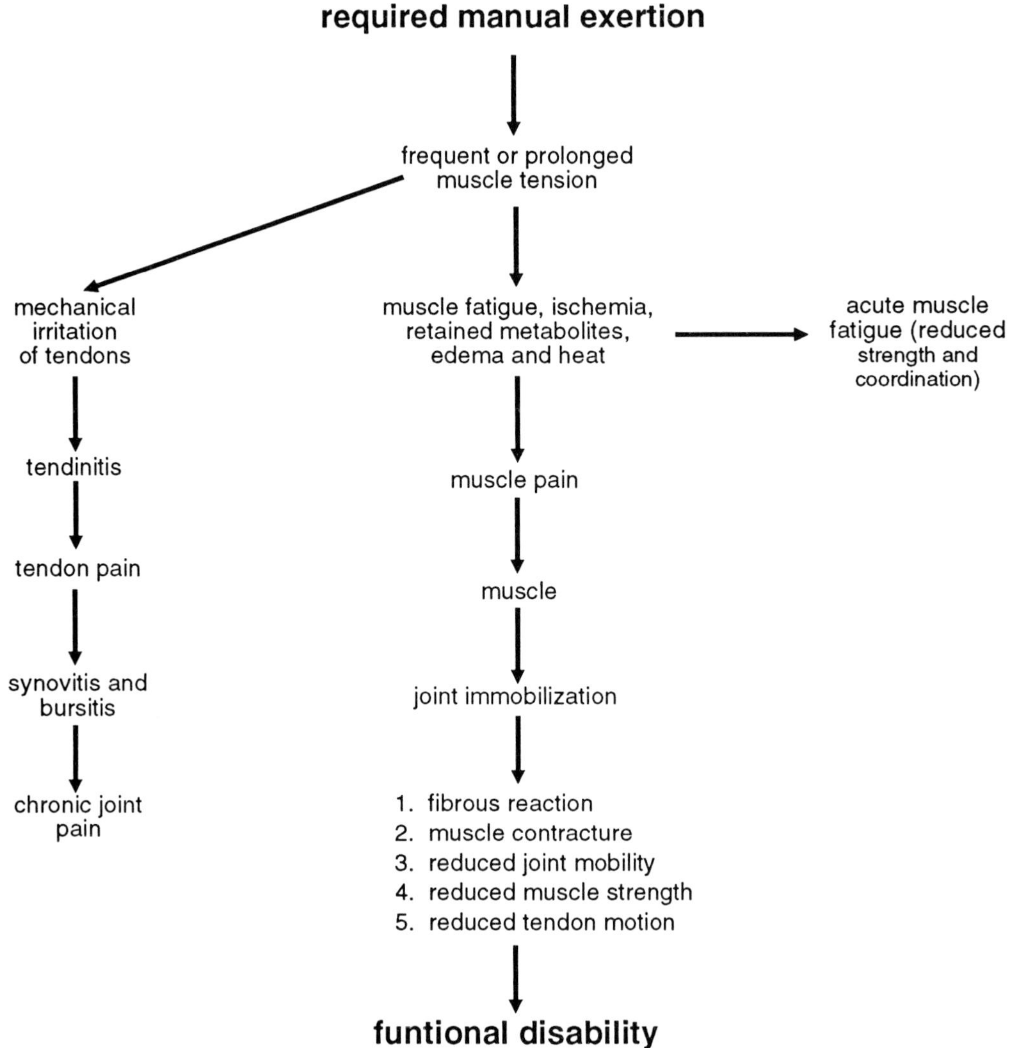

Figure 1 The sequence of events producing musculoskeletal pain and functional disability because of frequent or prolonged muscle tension. (Reproduced with kind permision from reference 1)

generally accepted method for examining the shoulder[2] or hip regions. The diagnostic terminology is heterogeneous and classification and epidemiological criteria are not established. The complex interaction between the large joints and adjacent areas, as well as the frequent occurrence of referred pain, further complicates epidemiological surveys.

Presently available laboratory tests and radiographic examinations have been disappointing regarding the understanding of disease processes in regional pain[3]. New methods for examining regional structures and their function(s) are desperately needed. More systematic evaluation of available methodology and concepts for diagnosis and classification are also necessary.

Epidemiological data can be gathered in many ways (Table 2). The classical cross-sectional epidemiological studies of musculoskeletal disorders have been mainly concerned with arthritis and not soft tissue regional pain complaints. Knowledge of the prevalence and incidence in well-defined populations is of great interest, although the information gained from cross-sectional studies is limited regarding the understanding of risk factors. Unfortunately the considerable costs involved often prevent cross-sectional surveys from being performed. Longitudinal studies of cohorts overcome some of the drawbacks of cross-sectional studies when one is, for example, studying possible risk factors. Although the attrition rate of participants in longitudinal studies may be an obstacle, especially in industries where there is a high rate of worker turnover and although the expense, efforts and time involved in such studies are not inconsequential, they do provide valuable data and must be encouraged.

Table 1 Areas of difficulty in studying the epidemiology of shoulder complaints

Criteria and classification

Diagnostic procedures

Study design

Methods of measuring risk factors

Table 2 Epidemiological information on shoulder complaints

Cross-sectional surveys

Longitudinal cohort studies

Case–control studies

Interventive studies

Health care registers

Insurance and other registers

Common knowledge

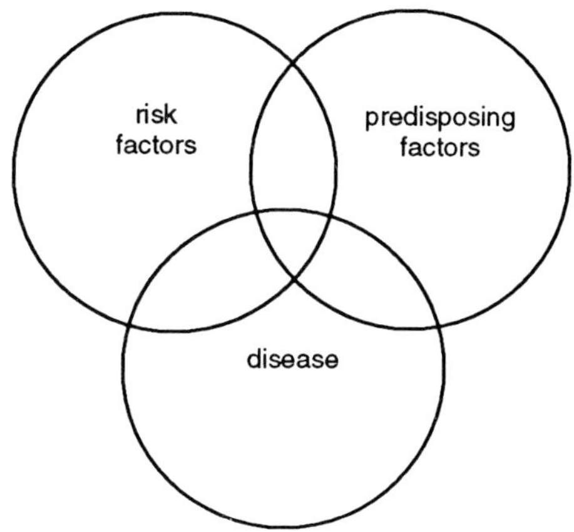

Figure 2 Venn diagramm showing the multifactorial nature of work-related musculoskeletal complaints in industrial workers. The stress from work may not ony be physical. Diseases affecting the musculoskeletal system are many-fold, and predisposing factors, like age and anthropometric factors rendering the individual unsuitable for the task, must be considered

The case–control design is a less expensive and less time consuming way to study risk factors. The selection and definition of cases and controls is crucial, but case–control data allow relatively efficient detection of possible risk factors. These can also serve as pilot studies before starting more extensive surveys. Understanding the effects of preventive intervention or treatment requires data generated by both case–control and longitudinal studies. The results from intervention studies on shoulder complaints in industrial and other workers are now gradually appearing. Occasionally, such studies focus on overly simplistic questions, e.g. the issue of load only, and do not consider other environmental or individual factors. Despite the ready availability of health care or insurance data, they are often of limited usefulness in studying disorders in the locomotor system. The information gained from such studies could be an important start before expanding into more expensive and extensive surveys. Often risk factors may be 'common knowledge' or 'anecdotal', in sportsmen and in industrial workers, but such sources of information are often not used for taking preventive measures. Finally, the notes of a person's occupational history in routine medical practice is usually inadequate since it is time consuming for the doctor.

SHOULDER PROBLEMS
General population
In a Swedish population survey conducted during the 1960s, painful shoulder was defined as 'a clinically confirmed restricted movement, manifested as insufficient passive abduction and inward rotation with concomitant pain'[4]. A higher prevalence of painful shoulder was found in males than in females in age groups 56–60 years (27 and 20%, respectively) and 70–74 years (21 and 16%, respectively). The prevalence of painful shoulder was similar in males and females between ages 31–35 (7–8%) and 42–46 (15%), and lower than in age groups 56–60 and 70–74 years. The annual incidence peaked significantly in the age group 42–46 years (2.5% and 2.2% in males and females, respectively), compared to around 1% in both sexes in both age groups 31–35 and 56–60 years, and 0.9 (females) and 1.6 (males) in the oldest age group of 70–74 years.

In the United States, the Health and Nutrition Examination Survey (HANES) between 1971 and 1975[5], studied the adult population ages 25–74 years[6], and found that 6.7% had suffered from shoulder complaints of more than 1 month's duration, and almost 40% had associated neck complaints. In over 80%, the complaints had occurred during the year before the survey, although only a few of the over 6000 persons studied reported that their shoulder complaints had caused absence from work. Physician-observed abnormalities in the shoulder were found in 3.0%.

In an interview survey from Finland performed in 1973–1974[7], shoulder pain was either common or occurred continuously during the year preceding the interview. In women, right-sided shoulder and upper arm region pain was present in 11% of those under the age of 50 and in 25% of those over the age of 50 years; left-sided pain was less common at 9% and 20%, respectively. In men, the prevalence was 11% under 50 and 22% over 50 years of age, the left and right side being similar. A threefold increase of shoulder symptoms was found in probands reporting 'psychiatric symptoms' compared with those not reporting such symptoms by a psychiatric screening tool.

A similar survey in a Philippine village[8] revealed that 1.7% in men and 2.8% of women over age 15 had shoulder pain; the pain was located in the trapezius area in 7.7 and 5.6% in males and females, respectively, and in the neck in 7.5 and 6.2%, both being regions that are more affected in farmers than in non-farmers, suggesting an association between working conditions and pain in the neck/trapezius area. A survey of the inhabitants in an Indonesian village showed that 10.7% of the population over 15 years of age had past complaints in the shoulder[9] (see Chapter 3).

Elderly populations
In a study of the elderly in Sweden[10], shoulder complaints of both sides were reported by 16% of female and 15% of male 79-year-olds; rotator cuff tenderness on palpation was noted in the dorsal aspect in 6% of females (0% of males), in the anterior aspect in 10% of females (0% of males), and in the upper part of the right shoulder in 12% of females (8% of males). The range of motion was normal in 61%. Active internal rotation was decreased in one third of the individuals, passive internal rotation was decreased in only 16%. The frequency of restricted range of motion in individuals reporting shoulder complaints was 50%[11]. There was no difference regarding complaints in individuals with either active or passive restricted range of motion regarding the frequency of complaints, although both forms of

restricted movement were significantly associated with difficulty in entering public transport, positive 'ear-lobe' test, 'hands above head' test and 'difficulty with clothes' test. A study from England[12] of 100 geriatric in-patients revealed various shoulder complaints in 21 patients, only three had sought medical attention for their complaints. This calls for more attention to shoulder complaints in elderly hospitalized individuals since it may be of importance for their general rehabilitation potential.

Working populations

Technical developments have created many new work situations during recent years for both blue and white collar workers. There is often a prolonged learning curve required to understand and adapt technical and organizational innovations to the capacity of the human body and mind. Shoulder pain is not a single entity but rather a symptom caused by a constellation of etiologies; despite the multifactorial nature of shoulder disorders, only one factor is frequently considered in the clinical situation. Geographical variations of the magnitude of the problem related to insurance policies may be encountered[13–15]. Economic and other interests from the employees or their counterparts sometimes interfere with a scientific approach[16]. An important reminder of a World Health Organization (WHO) committee[17] is that physical work usually has a positive effect on the individual and may be associated with an improvement in physical capacity. Furthermore, goal achievement and self-fulfilment in one's work are sources of satisfaction and enhanced self-esteem.

Terminology

A WHO expert committee recommends the term 'occupational disease' when there is a direct cause-and-effect relationship between work-related activities and rheumatic complaints[17]. Work-related diseases are conditions in which the working environment and the performance of work both contribute significantly to a multifactorial disease (Figure 1).

TECHNIQUES FOR MEASURING ENVIRONMENTAL FACTORS

Interview and questionnaire

A major problem is the lack of relevant parameters for quantitating risk factors (Table 3). Our studies[18,19] have illustrated information obtained by interviews or questionnaires. In workers with chronic shoulder complaints[17], the ergonomic evaluation was based on three factors:

(1) The workers' opinion of whether their present work load was heavy;
(2) The worker's opinion about the work load in their previous jobs; and
(3) Their present work situation regarding work with their hands at or above shoulder level.

Workers with chronic shoulder and neck complaints reported significantly more work with their hands at or above shoulder level than control workers (Table 4). Previous heavy work was not more common among cases than among controls.

Film recordings

These provide more objective estimates of work load, as films are recorded under actual working conditions. Ergonomic factors in acute cases[19] were studied by a technician, who then filmed the

Table 3 Ergonomic methods of measuring the load on the musculoskeletal system

Subjective estimates, e.g. scales or other gradings
Filming or other objective registrations
Biomechanical calculations
Electromyography
Biochemical tests, e.g. serum creatinine phosphokinase
Invasive methods, e.g. biopsy or measurement of oxygen tension

Table 4 Ergonomic factors in chronic shoulder complaints (in percent of affirmative answers to a questionnaire). NS, non-significant

Workers' reports of heavy load in	Patients	Controls	Significance of difference
Present job	76%	70%	NS
Previous job	41%	32%	NS
Work with hands at or above shoulder level	65%	15%	$p < 0.05$

patients and control subjects during several work cycles, which allowed quantification of the number of times and the length of time during the day that the workers lifted their hands to or above shoulder level. The results showed that the duration of forward flexion or abduction of both arms was significantly longer, and the number of times significantly higher, compared to the controls (Table 5).

Electromyography (EMG)

EMG signs of shoulder muscle fatigue develop rapidly in elevated arm positions[3,20]. The shoulder load in workers with acute shoulder pain was investigated by EMG recordings using surface electrodes on shoulder muscles during sev-

Table 5 Ergonomic factors in acute shoulder complaints

	Patients ($n = 13$)	Controls ($n = 26$)	Significance of difference
Duration of abduction and forward flexion (hours/day)			
right side	1.03	0.52	$p < 0.01$
left side	1.22	0.51	$p < 0.05$
Frequency of abduction and forward flexion			
right side	1258	639	$p < 0.00$
left side	1096	498	$p < 0.01$

eral work cycles[19]. The results suggested that, in workers with acute shoulder complaints, the median load on the descending part of the trapezius muscle exceeded the normal threshold values.

Other tests

The load on muscles or joints can also be calculated biomechanically (Figure 3), and is reflected by biochemical tests, e.g. serum creatinine kinase levels[21]. Invasive methods like measuring oxygen tension could also be used. There is, however, a great need for improved techniques. The application of test methods appropriate to the workplace necessitates close contact with the individual worker and management at the workshop level. The need for collaboration with trade unions and employers must also be recognized fully.

Cross-sectional studies of work-related diseases

These studies are often invalidated by the selection process by the individual researcher, which targets only certain types of jobs for study. Although less demanding tasks, which are often used for comparison, do not create selective influence, they may be of great value for quantifying a problem and promoting further studies[22]. In a questionnaire study of assembly-line workers who had not attended the health care center for shoulder complaints, over a third reported having suffered from such complaints during the previous year[23,24]. In another production industry, the prevalence of shoulder complaints in all employees was 20% in females and 12% in males[25]. A higher female/male ratio of workers, higher age, heavier work load, shorter body height and more work with vibrating hand-tools were important differences between workers with and those without shoulder complaints.

Longitudinal studies of cohorts

As above noted, these studies are time-consuming, expensive and often invalidated by high at-

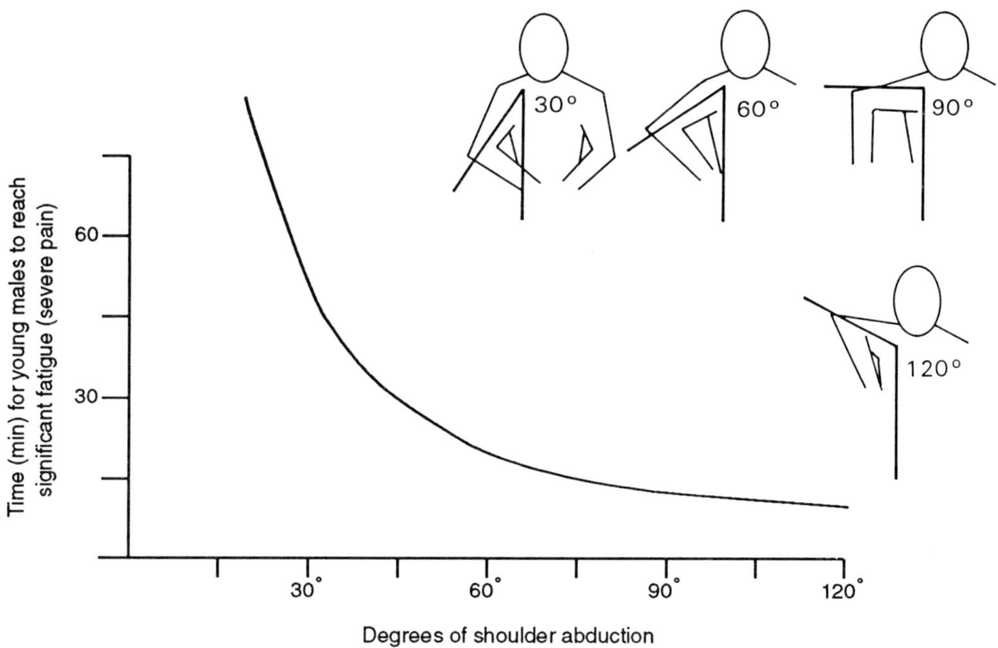

Figure 3 The time for developing significant shoulder muscle fatigue at varied arm abduction angles. (Modified with kind permission from reference 1)

trition rates, and, while they promise to yield much information in the future, to date they have not fulfilled their claimed potential.

Case–control studies

This design has many advantages in the present stage of development, and given its relatively low cost, it is unfortunate that more data from completed studies are not available. The complexity of shoulder complaints requires careful consideration of confounding factors in the study of work conditions, therefore the selection of cases and controls is crucial. In one study[18], 20 consecutive workers with complaints for more than 3 months were examined. Another 20 consecutive workers attending the industrial health care center for the first time because of non-traumatic shoulder–neck pain were selected for a study of acute complaints[19]. Rheumatological and radiographic examinations and extensive laboratory tests were performed to exclude other diseases, which were found in three and seven of the samples, respectively; two controls were selected for each of the workers, and matched for age, sex and workplace. Anthropometric variables did not differ between cases and controls, nor when compared to the means for Swedish industrial workers. Ergonomic evaluation showed that the shoulder load was significantly higher in workers with acute and chronic shoulder complaints than in their controls.

Interventive studies

Both case–control and longitudinal interventive studies of work-related shoulder pain are few but important. One study of Finnish assembly line workers showed that the introduction of 'micro-pauses' resulted in fewer complaints of muscle

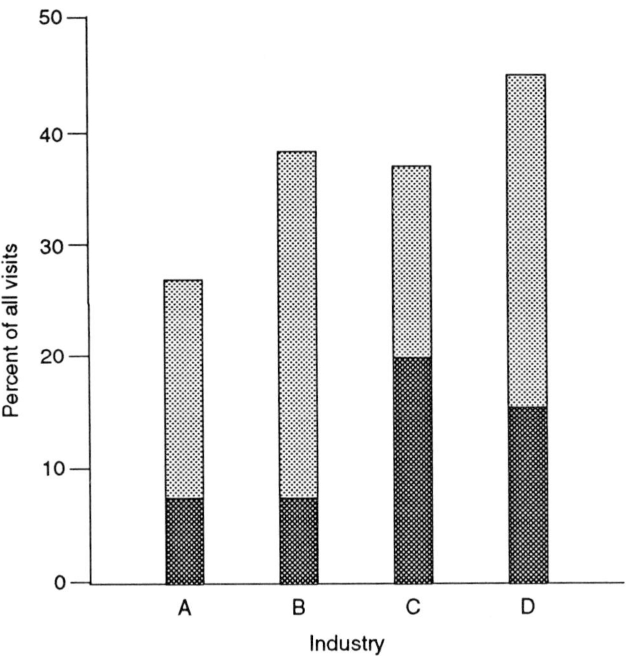

Figure 4 The frequency of shoulder complaints and other musculoskeletal complaints in four different production industries (dark tint, shoulder; light tint, other)

fatigue at the end of the work day[26]. In a Norwegian study, redesign of the production line resulted in a lower load on workers' shoulders as measured by EMG[27], and a reduced rate of sick-leave among the workers.

Occupational health care registers

These data sets may reveal differences in the patterns of locomotor complaints between industries. Such data must be interpreted with care[28], but may, as a minimum, heighten the awareness of actual or potential ergonomic problems[23,24] specific to an industry or to a specific workplace (Figure 4). In one Swedish manufacturing industry, 19% of cases of prolonged (greater than 4 weeks) sick leave among blue collar workers were attributed to shoulder–neck disorders[29], which ranged between 10 and 23% in heavy manufacturing and 12–27% in light assembly. Prolonged sick leave due to shoulder–neck com-

plaints was unusual among salaried staff but 10 times more frequent in female than in male (hourly) wage-earners. Prolonged sick leave was most frequent in die-casters with a heavy load on their shoulders during a limited period of time and in spray-painters and assembly line operators with a moderate to low load on the shoulders during a prolonged period of time. Assemblers had less prolonged sick leave due to shoulder–neck complaints than workers on the assembly line, possibly because of shorter work cycles.

Insurance register data

While such data are readily available, they must also be interpreted with some caution, given certain biases or the lack of certain types of information[30]. Despite these caveats, such data may not only indicate problem areas[31], but also emphasize the economic consequences[10,32]. In a Finnish study of reports on occupational disorders in

96

which repetitive tasks were mentioned as an associated factor, periarthritis of the shoulder accounted for 9% of all cases[33]. It was more frequent in females than in males and correlated to age. Butchers and workers in the food-processing industry had the highest risk of developing painful shoulders.

Common knowledge

This can be illustrated by anecdotal terms like 'chauffeur's shoulder'[34]. It is regrettable that little respect may be paid at the workplace to the workers' and foremen's own knowledge of an increased risk of shoulder pain after specific working operations. Surprisingly, conservatism in attitudes to work situations among both employers and employees frequently prevents a change of obviously unsuitable working positions, even though they are well recognized by either or both parties. Lessons could be learned from sports medicine and music performers where preventive measures for known risks of developing overuse syndromes are implemented.

INDIVIDUAL RISK FACTORS

Age was significantly higher (mean, 53 years) in production workers with chronic shoulder pain, than the mean age of 38 years in all workers in the factory studied (and in industrial workers in Sweden in general)[18]. Health care[25,29] and insurance data[33] corroborate the role played by age in the development of shoulder complaints by production workers. The influence of age may partly be due to the frequency of degenerative changes of the rotator cuff[35], which is a tissue highly vulnerable to trauma after the age of 40 years.

Sex Regardless of the study design, most evidence suggests that females run a higher risk than males of developing shoulder complaints when working in production industries, a suggestion that is supported by health care data[29], insurance registers[33] and cross-sectional studies[25].

Anthropometric variables are obviously important, as was found in cross-sectional analysis[25]. The fact that this was not observed in case–control studies[18,19] may be due to job selection, the relatively small numbers of cases included in such studies, the availability of the option for adjusting the working height for the tall and short workers in these industries and other variables.

Muscle strength was lower in shoulder muscles of workers with shoulder complaints than in their matched controls[18,19, 23,33]. Whether this is a cause or an effect can only be determined through longitudinal studies, although the fact that muscles other than the shoulder muscles are not weaker[18,19,23] favors the theory of an effect rather than a cause. Here too, job task selection is probably important.

Psychological factors were not regarded as having a major impact on the pathogenesis of periarthritis in the workers studied by Wright and Hag[36]. Undeniably, workers with chronic shoulder complaints suffer socially when they are absent from work for prolonged periods[18], but the effect would be difficult to measure objectively. The finding that immigrants are at a greater risk of developing shoulder complaints than Swedish citizens[25,33] may be related to psychosocial factors, although this remains unproven. The influence of stress on the load on the shoulder muscles demonstrated by EMG is an important observation[37] that should be accorded more attention in future studies among production industry workers. Another factor rarely considered is the distribution of periods of work and rest during the working day[38] (Figure 5), which could be addressed through collaboration by the workers and their trade unions, foremen, and employers, and with the advice from ergonomists and health care centers.

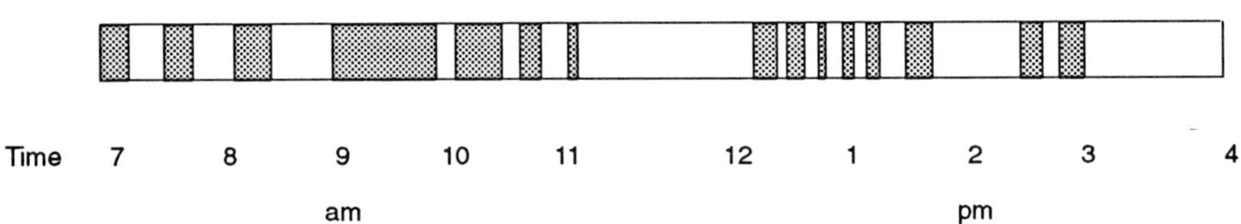

Figure 5 Work (hatched) and rest (white) periods during full working day in production industry worker with shoulder complaints, as recored by filming

CHRONIC SHOULDER DISEASES

In one study of chronic shoulder complaints, previously undetected inflammatory rheumatic diseases were diagnosed in three workers out of 20[18], two of whom suffered from Reiter's syndrome, while the third had atypical rheumatoid arthritis that presented with muscular involvement before the joints were affected. In seven workers among 20 with acute shoulder complaints[19], various signs of other rheumatic complaints were identified, but the diagnoses were far less clinically distinct than in the group of workers with chronic shoulder complaints. Two patients had myopathies, four had reactive tenosynovitis, and in the seventh worker signs of a systemic rheumatic disease with a positive rheumatoid factor test were found. The main conclusion drawn from such studies is that disorders of the shoulder or neck in industrial workers are multifactorial, and that rheumatic complaints are among the causative factors, while this association is less common in health care center data or in cross-sectional studies[25,30]. The higher prevalence in the case–control studies may stem from the different examination settings, the type of workers in the former studies[18,19] being brought to a university department of rheumatology, with its special interest and experience in diagnosing systemic rheumatic diseases and other diseases that impact on the musculoskeletal system. Nevertheless, the finding of reactive arthritis in two out of 20 workers with chronic shoulder complaints[18] and the observation of lower resistance to shoulder load in patients with

inactive forms of ankylosing spondylitis[37] underscore the importance of subclinical rheumatic diseases in shoulder pain.

ENTHESITIS (ENTHESOPATHY)

Enthesitis may affect the origins or insertions of any muscle into bone, and cause local tenderness that must be differentiated from the tender points of fibromyalgia. These points coincide at the upper inner angle of the scapula, the insertion of the neck muscles into the occiput, the origin of the gluteus maximus and its insertion into the greater trochanter. Strain of the insertion of the rotator cuff into the humeral tuberosity can also be classed as an enthesitis but is considered separately in this chapter. Epicondylitis and rotator cuff strains are common in all communities[39–41]; the former frequently arises out of hobby activity such as gardening and sport, while the latter is more commonly occupational or accidental in nature. Enthesitis is also a feature of the spondylarthropathies (Chapter 19).

Lateral epicondylitis

Lateral epicondylitis (tennis elbow) can be viewed as a prototype for problems arising from strain of muscles at their origins from or insertion into bones, which are usually the weakest point of the muscles most likely to be strained when biomechanically stressed. Medial epicondylitis (golfer's elbow) is pathogenically similar, but affects the flexor muscle origin from the medial epicondyle. Such lesions may arise at almost any

98

site. Only the common syndromes will be detailed.

Sport-induced epicondylitis[42] is discussed in further detail in Chapter 5, and may result from single or multiple direct or indirect injuries and from sustained overload. In the typical case, pain on the lateral epicondyle arises during overuse and extends towards the wrist. Acute tenderness is present over the origin of the wrist and finger extensors, and pain can be reproduced by loading the muscles concerned. Forced extension of the wrist, then the fingers separately and then supination will reproduce the pain. In some cases only part of the muscle is affected so that only wrist extension or extension of only one finger will produce pain, indicating the relevant part of the muscle that is affected. This complaint may be difficult to separate from the diffuse overuse syndrome (Chapter 7), where tenderness is more distal, over the neck of the radius and beyond. The pain occurs after a fall, direct injury or sustained overuse and is aggravated by any task involving the movements listed above. Weakness from pain may lead to light loads being unexpectedly dropped, as for example the dropping of a hot pot. Precise movements required in sport and industry may not be possible, and pain may persist indefinitely if the affected muscle continues to be loaded.

Pathology
Small tears in muscle have been demonstrated in cases severe enough to come to surgery and thermography shows increased heat at the site of tenderness[42].

Prevention
Primary prevention of the complaint and secondary prevention of recurrence of symptoms are achieved by avoiding overload of the affected muscle. Weights should be lifted with the wrists in supination to deliver the weight to the wrist flexors which arise from the medial condyle. If the complaint has been induced by repeated supination, as in using a hand screwdriver in the manufacture of electronics, its replacement by an electric screwdriver may be effective. Electric screw drivers in heavier industry may create new problems, as sustained pressure must be retained till the correct torque is reached, or alternatively, if the screw driver suddenly stops at the end of its travel, the wrist and forearm may be suddenly wrenched. This problem occurs on a much larger scale with motorized post hole diggers. If these suddenly lock, the considerable torsion force is suddenly transferred to the operators arms. There are many variations on this theme, so that in each occupational situation, the work pattern must be studied to see if finger and wrist extension and supination can be reduced. If one elbow is affected, care must be taken not to overload the other elbow, thereby inducing bilateral epicondylitis. Transferring the load onto the forearm flexors, and lifting with the hand in supination reduces the extensor load, but may give rise to medial epicondylitis. In one washing machine factory, replacing screws with clips eliminated this problem (Griffiths, personal communication). Vibration control is also desirable, and is discussed in Chapter 22. For a detailed analysis of biomechanical problems in the workplace, the reader is referred to the monograph by Chaffin and Andersson[1].

Medial epicondylitis (Golfer's elbow)
This condition is analogous to tennis elbow, albeit less common, and affects the finger and wrist flexors and the pronators. Loading the affected muscles is the cause of the problem, and can be used in a diagnostic setting to identify the site of damage. The same considerations are applicable to the lateral form and hold for the prevention of medial epicondylitis.

Other sites of enthesitis
The gluteus maximus may be affected at the origin from the sacrum or iliac crest and the insertion into

the greater trochanter. This pain not infrequently follows acute strain and overuse, and although it is often interpreted as pain of spinal origin, as there is usually pain on stooping, the localization of tenderness, the lack of restriction of back movement and a negative straight leg raise test suggest a local disorder. Trochanteric pain is common in women engaged in heavy work such as cleaning, house work and gardening which require frequent stooping. Pain at the gluteal insertion into the trochanter can be difficult to differentiate from trochanteric bursitis, in which the tenderness is distal to the top of the trochanter. Inflammation of the two bursae between the three gluteal muscles above their insertion into the trochanter may not be distinguishable from enthesitis. Such nuances are in fact academic, as each of these regional complaints arise from overuse and resolve with appropriate rest. Steroid injection relieves up to 90% of cases of trochanteric bursitis[43], but in the author's experience, the bursitis usually recurs unless the activity pattern can be modified. Adductor magnus origin pain and local tenderness where this muscle is attached to the pubis and ischio-pubic ramus can be distressing, causing pain on abduction of the thigh and in females, dyspareunia.

Plantar fasciitis with local tenderness at the origin of the plantar fascia from the os calcis has long been associated with prolonged walking and standing, and has been dignified as 'policeman's heel', a condition that is prevented by adding sponge rubber cushioning to the shoe and/or use of shoes patterned after athletic footwear. Levator scapulae insertion pain and tenderness can be due to enthesitis at this site, and is often accompanied by a history of shoulder overload[1], the mechanism of which is evident in Figure 6. With lateral downward rotation of the scapula (curved arrows), the superior medial angle of the scapula moves the insertion of the levator scapulae muscle (V-S1 to V-S2). The muscle under the traction becomes ischemic, inflamed, and thus

tender and painful at the tender point[42]. This can be difficult to distinguish from the trigger spot tenderness of fibromyalgia but in that condition tender points are multiple (Chapter 6).

Prevention of enthesitis requires control of the working, domestic and sporting conditions, so that muscles and tendons are not overloaded in an abrupt or single strain, through direct injury or by repetitive situations[42]. Dimberg and colleagues[39,40] studied of 2814 workers in a Swedish automobile factory. Symptoms from the neck and arms were strongly correlated with physical stress, and those who used vibrating hand tools had a twofold increase in risk. Mental stress at the onset of symptoms has been associated with an increased incidence of trapezius myalgia, lateral epicondylitis and carpal tunnel syndrome in the dominant limb; women had double the baseline rate and short stature and overweight increased the rate. Playing racquet sports decreased the prevalence, and possibly the risk, of neck and arm symptoms. This may be related to muscle strength and endurance.

TENOSYNOVITIS AND TENDINITIS

Tenosynovitis and tendinitis are discussed by Rowe[44]. Tenosynovitis may be part of an overuse syndrome, or may be secondary to a number of other conditions such as rheumatoid arthritis and tuberculosis, in which swelling is usually palpable. Achilles tendinitis and peritendinitis, and patella tendinitis are most commonly associated with sports and are discussed in Chapter 5, but may also be occupational. Tenosynovitis of the wrist flexor tendon sheaths may present as pain on wrist flexion, but more often with median nerve pressure in the carpal tunnel and therefore is discussed below under the carpal tunnel syndrome. Palpable swelling moving proximally with finger flexion is more likely to be due to an underlying disease, such as rheumatoid arthritis, than to overuse. Tenosynovitis of the wrist extensor tendons is usually due to rheumatoid arthritis,

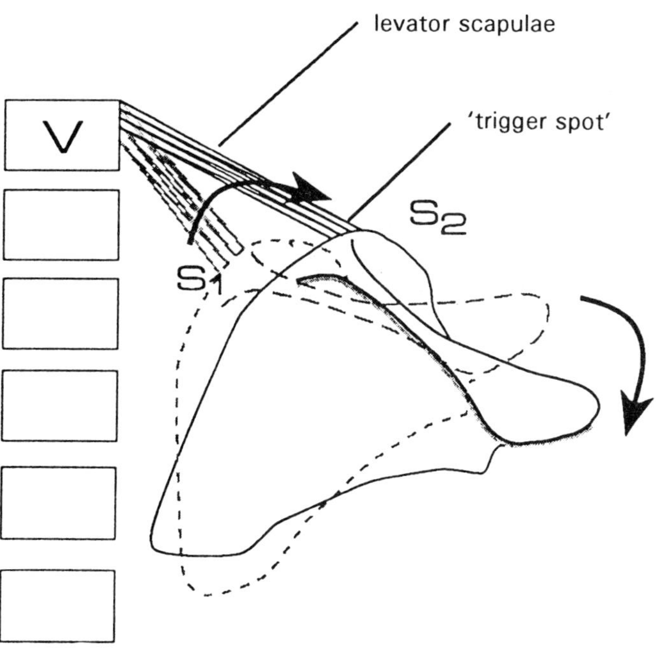

Figure 6 Levator scapulae 'trigger' zone in the postural fatigue syndrome. With lateral downward rotation of the scapular (curved arrows), the superior medial angle of the scapula moves the insertion of the levator scapulae muscle (V-S1 to V-S2). The muscle under traction becomes ischemic, inflamed, and therefore tender and painful at the 'trigger' site. (Modified with kind permission from Cailliet, R. *Shoulder Pain* (2nd edn.). Philadelphia, FA Davis Co., 1981)

but may result from inappropriate use, e.g. hammering at awkward angles[45]. Swelling pain and crepitus around the tendons proximal to the sheaths is due to overuse and is more correctly called peritendinitis crepitans[46]. Thumb abductor tenosynovitis (de Quervain's disease) causes pain along the medial aspect of the lower radius which is aggravated by thumb abduction, and most frequently follows repetitive thumb abduction, as in using pruning shears in fruit growing or scissors in cutting material for clothing. This may be prevented by using spring-loaded scissors and shears. Similar syndromes may arise in any of the other tendon sheaths, i.e. the finger flexor, posterior tibial, peroneal, and ankle extensor sheaths.

Prevention hinges on minimizing the effects of causative factors, i.e. allowing micropauses in manufacturing cycles, improving the design of tools such as slaughtermen's knives[1], which have three blades designed to reduce the wrist deviation and the knife's tendency to fall out of the hand while the worker is de-boning turkey carcasses, or introducing alternative methods (i.e. using clips instead of screws or automation or the use of machines such as hydraulic lifts or forklifts for bales of hay and for building materials. Tenosynovitis of the long head of the biceps is usually associated with the rotator cuff syndrome.

Tendinitis

Numerous studies during the last 100 years show that tendinitis is a major cause of occupational disability and workman's compensation in intensive hand work[47]. Highly repetitive and forceful jobs carry a 29-fold greater risk than low force low repetition jobs, which may be explained by viscous deformation of tendons and adjacent tissue[47].

Stenosing tenovaginitis

Narrowing of tendon sheaths is often associated with nodular swelling of tendons, which results in 'triggering', and most commonly occurs in the fingers. Stenosing tenosynovitis typically occurs in those with rheumatoid arthritis or overuse and may, for example, affect the thumb abductor subjected to heavy loads, such as demanded by pruning shears and large scissors, as well as the thumb flexor, finger flexor, posterior tibial and peroneal tendons . This syndrome may in fact be a tendinitis[47], in which the tendon structure is distorted, which may be likened to a partially untwisted rope with a localized expansion. Finkelstein's test is positive, i.e. pain is induced by holding the thumb under the fingers and then flexing the wrist to the ulna side if the thumb abductor tendon is affected.

Prevention

As with tenosynovitis, prevention is effected by controlling any underlying disease, most commonly overuse syndrome, or other conditions, such as tuberculosis. Work situations should be studied and abnormal postures eliminated when possible. Excess wrist extension and/or lateral flexion may be corrected by changing the design of the tool used[1,45].

Bursitis commonly arises from repeated minor or fewer major injuries but may be part of any other disease causing synovitis such as rheumatoid arthritis, gout or tuberculosis. Subdeltoid bursitis frequently complicates rotator cuff injuries.

Trochanteric bursitis is common, and is analogous to subdeltoid bursitis at the shoulder, and can prove difficult to distinguish from enthesitis. There are two bursae on the lateral aspect of the trochanter where the fascia lata rides over the bone and inserts into the superior tibio–fibula joint region. Pain occurs on stooping or rising from a chair, and on resting the weight on the affected side at night. The pain is often referred along the course of the tendon and may simulate sciatica[48], as may subgluteal bursitis[49]. In the elderly, this condition is often associated with spine, hip or knee degenerative conditions which may alter the load on the bursa.

As was previously advised in Chapter 7 on minimizing overuse syndrome, prevention of inflammation of the bursa hinges on correcting posture, avoiding stooping in gardening and other activities, and the use of such expediencies as heel lifts, higher chairs, and more frequent work breaks.

Olecranon bursitis follows local pressure, often related to occupation and is prevented by wearing pads on the elbows and or covering working surfaces with sponge rubber. Ischial bursitis (weavers' bottom) is controlled by suitably padded seats. Prepatella bursitis is a risk for all who kneel or squat frequently in their occupation, e.g. house maids (and housewives), miners, and carpet layers, or as in South East Asians, as part of their life-style. Infrapatella bursitis is said to be a risk for parsons who kneel with the knee flexed at a right angle, which places more weight on the bursae in relation to the patella ligament. Anserine bursitis causing pain and swelling over the upper tibia medially is more likely to occur in overweight women with genu valgum, and is often precipitated by unaccustomed exercise such as jogging. Achilles bursitis also results from unaccustomed exercise, often when the region is confined by new, too tight shoes. Bunions over the first metatarso-phalangeal joint in hallux valgus result from pressure from narrow shoes and are prevented by wearing shoes that are roomy enough to accommodate the wide forefoot of metatarsus primus varus which predisposes to hallux valgus. Prevention of bursitis requires avoidance of overuse injuries, or pressure causing the inflammation in the bursa, and if not possible, the use of protective padding, such as commonly used by carpet layers.

ENTRAPMENT NEUROPATHIES
Carpal tunnel syndrome

Pressure on the median nerve as it passes through the carpal tunnel with ten flexor tendons is the most common entrapment syndrome. In the prototypic entrapment, there is pain along the course of the flexor aspect of the forearm and wrist with variable paresthesiae ('pins and needles') over the palm and undersurface of the thumb to the fourth fingers, which is characteristically most intense at night, causing its victim to awaken, and shake his arms or hang them over the side of the bed for relief. In late neglected cases, there is numbness and diminished pinprick sensation over the thumb to third fingers and wasting of the thenar eminence. When the diagnosis of carpal tunnel is in doubt, nerve conduction studies may be performed. Most patients have a history of overuse, and those with definite signs are discussed below. The more common subjective, often variable and diffuse symptoms from overuse with paresthesiae of the fourth and fifth fingers are discussed in Chapter 7. Some have nerve pressure secondary to another disease such as rheumatoid tenosynovitis or arthritis of the radio-carpal joint. In some cases, the underlying disorder may in fact be an overuse tenosynovitis leading to swelling sufficient to cause nerve pressure without being visible or palpable.

Prevention

The prevention of overuse in general is detailed in Chapter 7. For the rest, prevention demands treatment of the underlying diseases which range from tuberculosis to myxedema. Repetitive wrist flexion and extension, strong gripping with external rotation, impact forces on the palm and vibratory forces were found to predispose to carpal tunnel syndrome[50]. A case study[51] showed that both hand-held vibrating tools and repetitive work were common etiological factors. In the electronics industry[52], the permanent employment of ergonomists is urged for prevention. Grocery checkout operators[53,54] and garment machinists[55], and many other workers, are susceptible to occupational overuse and the carpal tunnel syndromes, both of which are related to repetitive movement, for which improved ergonomics plays a critical role in prevention. Chiang and co-workers[56] found both repetitive work and exposure to cold to be risk factors in carpal tunnel syndrome in frozen food factory employees so that cold exposure should be controlled also. Prevention of this syndrome requires control of any underlying disease(s), overuse, vibration, cold exposure and improving work ergonomics and tool design, where feasible. In secondary prevention, it is important to minimize these risk factors in treated patients returning to work or in whom relapse is probable[57].

Other entrapment syndromes

For a detailed description of these much less common complaints the reader is referred to Nakano[58] and Mandel[59]. Involvement of the cervical nerve roots is discussed in Chapter 7, as some workers offer this as an explanation for the arm and neck symptoms in the repetitive strain syndrome.

Ulnar nerve

Entrapment of the ulnar nerve in Guyon's tunnel at the wrist affects sensation only on the palmar surface of the fourth and fifth fingers, without affecting the flexor carpi ulnaris and flexor digiti pollicis to these fingers. This has been attributed to occupation[60], and has been reported in motorcycle and bicycle riders[61]. When entrapment occurs at the elbow in the cubital tunnel, the fourth and fifth fingers are weakened.

Anterior interosseus nerve entrapment may cause weakness in flexion of the thumb and fingers, which is accompanied by pain at the elbow, without corresponding sensory symptoms. Compression of the posterior interosseus branch of the radial nerve as it enters the supinator muscle impedes finger extension, and causes extensor carpi ulnaris weakness with radial deviation on extension.

This may be caused by trauma or synovitis around the elbow including rheumatoid arthritis. Suprascapular nerve neuropathy may result from the use of crutches[62].

Lower limb
In the lower limb the sciatic nerve may become entrapped as it passes the piriformis muscle or becomes compressed by habitual squatting, as is common practice in India[63], and other parts of South East Asia. The sciatic, peroneal or tibial nerves may be entrapped by a Baker's cyst at the knee[64]. The peroneal nerve is vulnerable as it rounds the fibula neck. Compression results in foot drop and sensory reduction.

The tarsal tunnel syndrome (posterior tibial nerve entrapment) which causes burning feet especially at night, may be secondary to synovitis or ganglion, both of which may be due to overuse[59]. Femoral nerve entrapment is rare but the lateral femoral cutaneous nerve is affected more often (meralgia paresthetica) with sensory alteration on the lateral aspect of the thigh attributed to obesity, and thus requires weight loss.

SUMMARY
Regional pain syndromes are common in populations, but the functional consequences to its victims have been accorded lower priorities than other complaints. Methodological difficulties contribute to the absence of widely accepted classifications and criteria, which in turn hinders comparisons of prevalence among various groups across geographical lines and in different occupational, domestic and sports scenes. Regional pain and dysfunction are often an accompanying feature of common rheumatic disorders, as well as non-rheumatic disorders such as diabetes and are common among elderly hospitalized patients. Under-reporting of regional pain

may be a hindrance for the general prevention and rehabilitation of many patients. The relationship of work to regional pain syndromes has attracted much attention in recent years. Due to the important economic, social, legal and insurance interests involved, the problem has often been oversimplified, the multifactorial origins of regional pain syndrome(s) in workers has been overlooked, thereby losing the opportunity for prevention. Many of these syndromes result from occupational or sports-related abuse, the primary prevention of which is delineated in Chapters 5 and 7.

REFERENCES
Shoulder
1. Chaffin DB, Andersson G. Occupational biomechanics. New York, John Wiley, 1984
2. Bjelle A, Jensen EM. Guidelines for the diagnosis and therapy of shoulder pains. Läkartidningen. 1983; 80:2984–2988
3. Hagberg M . Shoulder pain – pathogenesis. In Hadler NM (ed.). Clinical Concepts in Regional Musculoskeletal Disease. Orlando, Grune and Stratton, 1987, pp. 191–200
4. Allander E. Prevalence, incidence and remission rates of some common rheumatic diseases or syndromes. Scand J Rheumatol. 1974; 3:145–153
5. Miller HW. Plan and operation of the health and nutrition examination survey; United States 1971–1973. Vital and Health Statistics Series 1, No. 10. Washington: Public Health Service, US Department of Health Service, 1973
6. Cunningham LS, Kelsey JL. Epidemiology of musculoskeletal impairments and associated disability. Am J Public Health. 1984; 74:574–579
7. Takala J, Sievers K, Klaukka T. Rheumatic symptoms in the middle-aged population in southwestern Finland. Scand J Rheumatol. 1982; Suppl. 47:15–29
8. Manahan L, Caragay R, Muirden KD, Allander E, Valkenburg HA, Wigley RD. Rheumatic pain in a Philippine village. A WHO-ILAR COPCORD study. Rheumatol Int. 1985; 5:149–53

9. Darmawan J. Rheumatic conditions in the northern part of central Java. An epidemiological survey. Thesis. Rotterdam: Erasmus University, 1985

10. Bergström G, Bjelle A, Sorensen LB, Sundh V, Svanborg A. Prevalence of symptoms and signs of joint impairment at age 79. Scand J Rehabil Med. 1985; 17:173–182

11. Bergström G, Aniansson A, Bjelle A *et al.* Functional consequences of joint impairment at age 79. Scand J Rehabil Med. 1985; 17:183–190

12. Chard MD, Hazleman BL. Shoulder disorders in the elderly (a hospital study). Ann Rheum Dis. 1987; 46:684–687

13. Brown CD, Nolan BM, Faithful DK. Occupational repetition strain injuries. Guidelines for diagnosis and management. Med J Aust. 1984; 40:329–332

14. Ellard J. Compensation neurosis. Leading article. Med J Aust. 1985; 142:535

15. Hadler NM. Industrial rheumatology. The Australian and New Zealand experiences with arm pain and backache in the workplace. Med J Aust. 1986; 144:191–195

16. Hadler NM. The roles of work and of working in disorders of the upper extremity. Baillière's Clin Rheumatol. 1989; 3:121–141

17. WHO. Identification and control of work-related diseases. Report of a WHO expert committee. World Health Organization Technical Report Series No. 714. Geneva: World Health Organization, 1985

18. Bjelle A, Hagberg M, Michaelsson G. Clinical and ergonomic factors in prolonged shoulder pain among industrial workers. Scand J Work Environ Health. 1979; 38: 205–210

19. Bjelle A, Hagberg M, Michaelsson G. Occupational and individual factors in acute shoulder–neck disorders among industrial workers. Br J Indust Med. 1981; 38:356–363

20. Herberts P, Kadefors R. A study of painful shoulder in welders. Acta Orthop Scand. 1976; 47:381–387

21. Hedberg GE. Physical strain in Swedish lorry drivers engaged in the distribution of goods. J Human Ergol. 1985; 14:33–40

22. Hagberg M, Wegman DH. Prevalence rates and odd ratios of shoulder–neck diseases in different occupational groups. Br J Indust Med. 1987; 44:602–610

23. Bjelle A, Hagberg M, Michaelsson G. Sjukdom, Hålder och belastning på muskulaturen orsaken till skulder–nackbesvär hos industriarbetare. (Distinct connection between the load on the muscles and shoulder–neck symptoms in industrial workers). Läkartidningen. 1984; 81:1419–1422

24. Bjelle A, Hagberg M, Michaelsson G. Work related shoulder–neck complaints in industry. A pilot study. Br J Rheumatol. 1987; 26:365–369

25. Dimberg L (ed). Symptoms from the neck and upper extremities – an epidemiological, clinical and ergonomic study. Gothenburg, Volvo, 1985

26. Loupajärvi T, Kourinka I, Kukkonen R. The effects of ergonomic measures on the health of the neck and the upper extremities of assembly-line packers – a four year follow-up study. In Proceedings of the 8th Congress of the International Ergonomics Association, Tokyo, 1982, pp. 515–516

27. Westgaard RH, Aarås A. The effect of improved workplace design on the development of work-related musculoskeletal illness. Appl Ergon. 1985; 16:91–97

28. Harrington JM. Epidemiologic study of work-related diseases. Scand J Work Environ Health. 1984; 10:353–359

28. Kvarnström S. Occurrence of musculoskeletal disorders in a manufacturing industry with special attention to occupational shoulder disorders. Scand J Rehabil Med. 1983; 8 (Suppl 8):1–114

30. Hadler NM. The recognition of the illness of work incapacity: An exercise in diagnosis or adjudication? In Hadler NM, Gillings DB (eds.), Arthritis and Society. The Impact of Musculoskeletal Diseases. London, Butterworths 1985, pp. 75–88

31. Westgaard RH, Aarås A. Postural muscle strain as a causal factor in the development of musculoskeletal illnesses. Appl Ergon. 1984; 15:162–174

32. Anderson JAD. Shoulder pain and tension neck and their relation to work. Scand J Work Environ Health. 1984; 10: 435–442

33. Kivi P. Rheumatic disorders of upper limbs associated with repetitive occupational tasks in Finland 1975–1979. Scand J Rheumatol. 1984; 13:101–107

34. Huskisson EC, Dudley Hart F. Joint Disease: All the Arthropathies. 3rd edn, Bristol, John Wright, 1978, pp. 85–86

35. Post M. The Shoulder. Surgical and Non-surgical Management. Philadelphia, Lea, Febiger, 1978, pp. 306–310

36. Wright V, Hag AM. Periarthritis of the shoulder. I. Aetiological considerations with particular reference to personality factors. Ann Rheum Dis. 1976; 35:213–219

37. Weber A, Fassler C, O'Hanlon JF, Gierer R, Grandjean E. Psychophysiological effects of repetitive tasks. Ergonomics. 1980; 23:1033–1046

38. Hagberg M, Hagner I-M, Bjelle A. Shoulder muscle strength, endurance and electromyographic fatigue in ankylosing spondylitis. Scand J Rheumatol. 1987; 16:161–165

Enthesitis

39. Chard MD, Hazelman BL. Tennis elbow; a re-appraisal. Br J Rheumatol. 1989; 28:186–109

40. Dimberg L, Olafson A, Stephansson E, Aagaard H, Oden A, Andersson GB. The correlation between work environment and the occurrence of cervico-brachial symptoms. J Occup Med. 1989; 31:447–453

41. Dimberg L. The prevalence and causation of tennis elbow lateral humeral epicondylitis in a population of workers in an engineering industry. Ergonomics. 1987; 30: 573–579

42. Chard MD, Lachman SM. Racquet sports – patterns of injury presenting to sports injury clinic. Br J Sports Med. 1987; 21:21: 150–153

Tenosynovitis

43. Schapira D, Menachem N, Scharf Y. Trochanteric bursitis: A common clinical problem. Arch Phys Med Rehabil. 1986; 67:815–817

44. Rowe ML. The diagnosis of tendon and tendon sheath injuries. Semin Occup Disorders. 1987; 2:1–6

45. Schoenmarklin RW, Marras WS. Effects of hand angle and work orientation on hammering. Hum Factors. 1989; 31: 397–411

46. Barton N. Repetitive strain disorder: Often misdiagnosed and often not work related. Editorial. Br Med J. 1989; 299:405–406

47. Armstrong TA, Fine LJ, Goldstein SA, Lifshitz YR, Silverstein BA. Ergonomics considerations in hand and wrist tendinitis. J Hand Surg. 1987; 12:830–837

Bursitis

48. Doherty M. Common regional pain syndromes. Practitioner. 1989; 233:1467

49. Swezey RL. Pseudo-radiculopathy in subacute trochanteric bursitis of the sub-gluteus maximus bursa. Arch Phys Med Rehabil. 1976; 57:387–390

Entrapment

50. Schenck RR. Carpal tunnel syndrome the new industrial epidemic. AAOHN J. 1989; 37: 226–231

51. Wieslander G, Norbäck D, Gothe C-J, Juhlin H. Carpal tunnel syndrome (CTS) and exposure to vibration. repetitive wrist movements, and heavy manual work: a case referent study. Br J Indust Med. 1989; 46:43–47

52. Morse LH. Repetitive motion musculo-skeletal problems in the microelectronics industry. State Art Rev Occup Med. 1986; 1:167–174

53. Barnhart S, Rosenstock L. Carpal tunnel syndrome in grocery checkers. Western J Med. 1987; 147:27–40

54. Margolis W, Kraus JF. The prevalence of carpal tunnel symptoms in female supermarket checkers. J Occup Med. 1987; 29:953–956

55. Sokas RK, Spiegelman D, Wegman DH. Self reported musculoskeletal complaints among garment workers. Am J Indust Med. 1989; 15: 197–206.

56. Chiang HC, Chen SS, Yu HS, Ko YC. The occurrence of carpal tunnel syndrome in frozen food factory employees. Kao Hsiung I Hsueh Ko Hsueh Tsa Chih. 1990; 6:73–80

57. Hagberg M, Nystrom A, Zetterlund B. Recovery from carpal tunnel syndrome hand surgery in

males in relation to vibration exposure. J Hand Surg (Am). 1991; 16:66–71

58. Nakano KK. Entrapment neuropathies. In Kelley *et al.*, eds., Textbook of Rheumatology. Philadelphia, WB Saunders, 1989, pp. 1844–1859

59. Mandel S. Neurologic syndromes from repetitive trauma at work. Postgrad Med. 1987; 82:87–92

60. Hunt JR. Occupational neuritis of the deep branch of the ulnar nerve. J Nerv Ment Dis. 1958; 35:676

61. Eckman PB, Perlstein G, Altrocci PH. Ulnar neuropathy in bicycle riders. Arch Neurol. 1975; 32:130–131

62. Shabas D, Scheiber M. Suprascapular neuropathy related to the use of crutches. Am J Phys Med. 1986; 65:298–300

63. Ansari AH. Osteoarthritis of knee joint amongst squatters. 6th SEAPAL Congress Rheumatol, Tokyo, 1988; Abstr. F11 5:p 210

64. Wigley RD, Paterson DE. Calf haematoma following anticoagulants in synovial rupture. NZ Med J. 1982; 95:630–632

9.   BACK PAIN

John A.D. Anderson

INTRODUCTION

The 'back' extends from the skull to the coccyx and comprises the spinal column, scapulae, posterior aspects of the rib cage and the nerves, muscles, ligaments and tendons associated with these structures. The back's contribution to the agony of the human condition is extensive, especially if one considers that many painful complexes arise from spinal lesions and present with symptoms predominantly, or even exclusively, in the upper or lower limbs. While many painful backs result from lesions of the cervical or lumbar intervertebral discs, others have no demonstrable pathology, even though the precipitating event in such cases is indistinguishable from those that trigger disc lesions[1]. A widely accepted and unifying theme is that most episodes of back pain, whether acute or chronic, can be linked to physical stress either during work, recreational activities or household chores (including 'do-it-yourself' activities and gardening). And yet, 'back pain' is a symptom, not a diagnosis.

Prevention of any disease hinges on both reducing environmental risks and improving personal resistance. Advice on preventing back pain would thus be aimed, on the one hand at modifying hazards in the occupational, recreational or domestic environment, and on the other by inducing individuals to reduce their personal risk by appropriate evasive action. A third measure, based on the principle of secondary prevention, is to identify any person who might have a special risk factor, e.g. by screening methods, and then persuading him to avoid environmental situations which, though not particularly hazardous to normal individuals, might constitute a danger (in terms of the onset of back pain) to those with an impairment. In this chapter, these three approaches will be considered in relation to lumbosacral (lower back) pain and cervicoscapular (upper back) pain.

LUMBOSACRAL PAIN

The lower back may be simplistically defined as the area between the lower edge of the rib-cage and the gluteal folds. Painful conditions may arise directly from the lower back or, as in sciatica and cruralgia, which are intimately linked to this region, originate in lesions of the nerve roots.

Environmental factors

Most epidemiological evidence has linked lumbosacral pain to the lifting of heavy or poorly positioned loads, an association that has been largely confirmed by well-designed biomechanical studies. The acceptance of such compelling evidence by responsible legislative bodies may provide one avenue of prevention. It is thus disappointing that the recommendations of the International Labour Organization in the 1960s[2] suggesting maxima of 25 kg (compact load) for youths and 58 kg overall have not been adopted as statutory requirements in the countries represented at that conference.

An approach to this issue exists in some countries that introduced legislation couched in vague general terms, e.g. the Health and Safety at Work Act of the UK[3], in which allowable weight maxima in the working environment are not specifically addressed. Under the terms of this Act, employers have a duty to provide and maintain a system of work that is safe and without risk to the health of their employees, so far as is *practicable* in reasonable terms. These requirements, of course, cover manual lifting and handling and the Act requires that employers provide information, instruction, training and supervision to ensure the health and safety of the employees, again 'so far as is reasonably practicable'. It is claimed (with some justification) that such generalizations are preferable to arbitrarily defining weight maxima, since a weight that might be hazardous to an otherwise normal worker with poor physique, presents no such hazard to a more muscular individual who indulges in weight lifting as a form of recreation.

There are other considerations: if the weight has to be lifted beyond chest height, or at a distance from the vertical axis of the trunk, then smaller

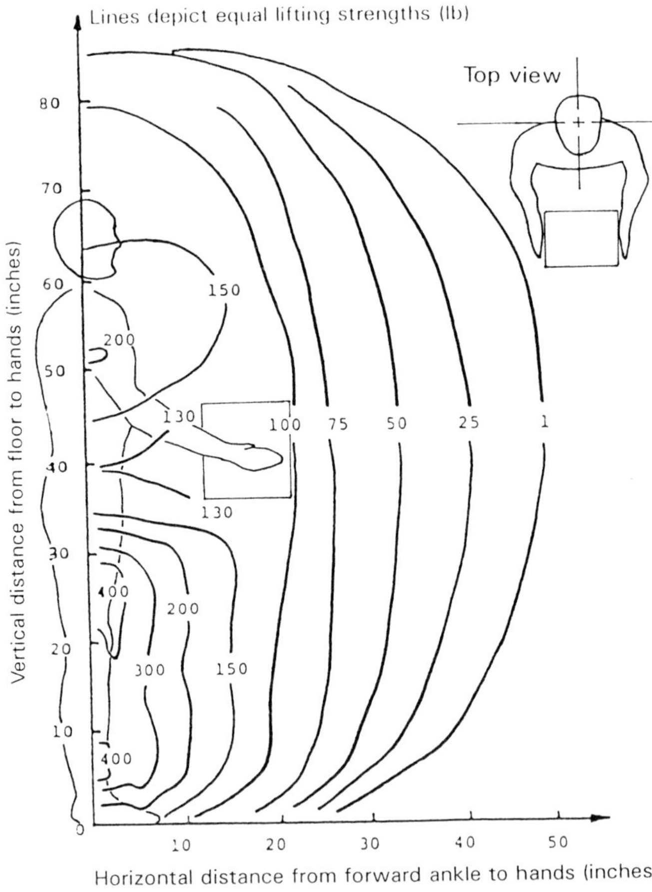

Figure 1 Equal strength requirements for lifting weights (in pounds). (Reproduced with kind permission from Chaffin DB. J Environ Pathol Toxicol. 1979; 2: 31–66)

110

maximum loads should apply; in the case of shared weight lifting, if one of the partners is poorly trained and lets his side of the load slip, then the other will have an unexpected excessive weight to control. It would seem reasonable, therefore, that responsible employers should ensure that the design of the workplace and the tasks involved in any job should not only limit the absolute weight but the position of that weight relative to the worker's body in accordance with the principles outlined by Chaffin[4] for what was described as the lift-strength ratio (LSR), i.e. the maximum load required to be lifted, divided by the predicted strength of a large, strong male in the same position (Figure 1). The author points out that the graph used in this evaluation assumes slow, well-controlled handling of large loads (i.e. tote boxes) with both hands nearly symmetric in front of the body. Thus it applies to only perhaps 50–70% of materials-handling activities in industry. Complementary to this definition, Chaffin has produced schematic lines similar to contours, which depict equal lifting strengths at various heights above ground level and at various distances in front of the body. The precise figures may be open to debate but the principle is generally accepted by most workers concerned with preventing back strain from lifting excessive weights.

Against this background, environmental prevention may be achieved, either by reducing the size and weight of the load itself or, if this is not practicable, by requiring two-man lifts, or the use of mechanical aids, e.g. straps or handles. In addition, attention should be paid to other aspects of the working environment, e.g.:

(1) Storage of items at a convenient height;

(2) Designing the work area to ensure that there is enough space to enable the operator to approach easily, move into a position of maximum comfort and safety for the lifting process and face directly the object to be lifted rather than working at an angle;

(3) There should also be enough environmental light to enable hazards associated with the lift to be assessed easily; and

(4) No roadway between the point of origin and the destination should be obstructed in any way; steps on the route should be replaced by ramps whenever possible.

Preventive measures of this nature are obviously easier to achieve in large factories, particularly if trade unions or other workers' representatives have a powerful voice and their views are respected. Unfortunately, hazardous situations may often prevail in places of work where few people are employed, the space is restricted, and the union voice may be minimal or completely absent. Although factories employing ten or fewer workers comprise less than 10% of the total work force in the United Kingdom, the sheer number of such workplaces overwhelms the bodies responsible for the health and safety of workers, e.g. the Health and Safety Executive, making it impossible to check on such places of work with any frequency. Court actions may be lengthy, indecisive and tend to be of greater benefit to the legal profession than the work force.

Two other environmental factors in relation to workplace merit consideration. The first is the posture which the worker must adopt while performing various tasks associated with his job. Reference has already been made to lifting and posture and the fact that where heavy weights are involved posture may be critical. However, even without unduly heavy weights Andersson, Nachemson and their co-workers[5,6] have assessed the effects on intradiscal pressure of lifting associated with asymmetrical movement and also the relationship between intradiscal pressure and intra-abdominal pressure measured

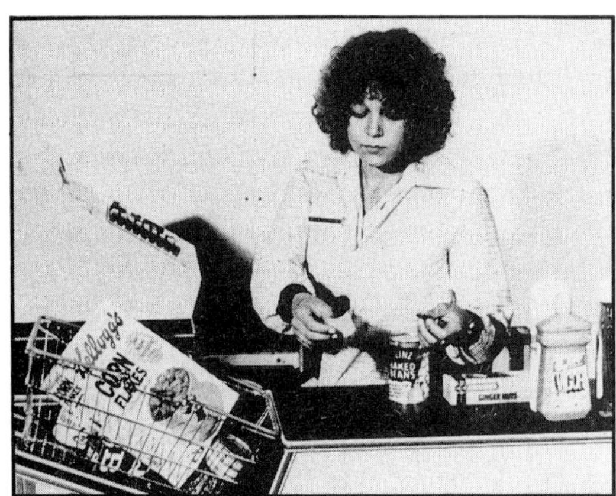

Figure 2 A check-out cashier in a confined space having to rotate to her right repeatedly to operate the cash register

by the radio pill developed by Davis[7]. Subsequently, Sweetman and colleagues[8] and Otun and co-workers[9] have combined the intra-abdominal pill with electromyographic measurement of the lumbar muscle masses and vertebral posture in the antero–posterior and lateral axes, for continuous monitoring at the place of work. These and other studies have indicated that posture at work is a contributory factor to back pain. Indeed, even when minimal weights are involved, posture may be a factor as in, for example, the positions adopted by check-out cashiers in supermarkets[10] (Figure 2). Here, it is desirable to keep the cash drawer as far away as possible from the conveyor belt, in order to avoid snatch thefts, which causes the cashier, sitting in a confined space, to adopt an awkward, semi-rotated posture.

Such observations have implications in machine design in factories, chair design in offices and in the design of workspaces. Redesigning equipment may be expensive, and employers are often reluctant to undertake these measures for what may appear, at first sight, to be trivial complaints. Furthermore, competition among related industries often militates against optimal design. Rivalling commercial concerns related, for example, to car seating, make cooperation across company lines uncommon; manufacturers rarely admit that their seats contribute to back pain, and yet each wants to develop the optimum seat for a particular vehicle. Such myopic thinking contrasts sharply with the overwhelming cooperation that is achieved during times of war, where issues such as optimal seating design for pilots and other service personnel are a national priority Thus, a peacetime 'dividend' is the existence of back pain clinics, often populated by patients who drive for long distances, who are well-aware that the seating arrangement in a particular vehicle may be better for their backs than another. What appears to be important is the maximum flexibility in seating position to suit the needs of the driver on a daily basis, with or without the use of special back supports for car seats available on the market.

Another environmental factor, also related to seating, is that of vibration. The jarring effect of substandard suspension may well be relevant in those occupations which require a higher than average exposure to this hazard. Vibration has been studied in general terms by Griffin and colleagues[11], and may be a relevant factor in the back pain of tractor drivers[12–14], a concept supported by Stayner and co-workers[15], who used vibration simulation studies to aid in tractor design. Confounding variables affecting tractor drivers include secondary movements carried out while ploughing, where the driver may sit with a rotated spine, spending much of his time looking backwards to check furrow alignments. Also, the nature of the work implies a variable exposure to cold and damp environmental conditions. Thus, climate, posture and vibration operate simultaneously, although attention to the latter two factors provides strategies for preventive intervention in some cases of lumbosacral pain.

In domestic working environments, similar hazards are found, but there are no unions or inspecting bodies to monitor potential hazards. The virtual standardization of the heights of various kitchen and laundry appliances, and the counter-sinking of wash-tubs below a standard worktop height has forced housewives, ranging in height from the smallest to the tallest, to adapt themselves to the same working level, whilst storage cabinets and shelves are seldom designed at heights or with spacious approaches which have now become a requirement of the factory scene. The same principles of ergonomic design apply in both the domestic and occupational workplace. Regrettably, the major health priorities, e.g. smoking-related diseases, alcohol, acquired immune deficiency syndrome and cancer, have minimized the resources left for such bodies as the Health Education Authority to devote to the problem of lumbosacral pain, even though the illness and misery caused thereby would justify greater attention to this aspect of domiciliary advice. For these and other reasons, consumer-oriented bodies such as the Back Pain Association in Britain have been established and they have helped to focus attention on these and related problems.

Lastly, on the sports field and particularly in relation to contact sports, the laws of the different games and their enforcement are supposed to be one way of reducing environmental hazards. Unfortunately, due to the competitive nature of some sports, e.g. weight-lifting, there are no maxima which might serve to protect the backs of competitors.

Personal factors in preventing lumbosacral pain

Even if ideal circumstances could adequately control all environmental hazards, it would still be necessary to train individuals in the best use of their bodies in order to avoid lumbosacral pain. It is axiomatic that good general health and exercise of both the lumbar and abdominal muscles, which provide support for the lumbosacral region, will afford some protection against the in-

juries of daily life. 'Back Schools' concentrate on these aspects for both the fit and those who have already developed problems, and some claims for successful prevention of lower back pain have been made[16]. What is, more doubtful is whether or not the adoption of erect posture at all times, or the avoidance of the slouched position when sitting, are as beneficial as some enthusiasts maintain. There is moreover, some evidence that hypermobility of the lumbar spine itself may be a risk factor in back pain[17], and over-indulgence in exercises designed to increase mobility may be less protective than is sometimes believed.

Training in lifting techniques is a complementary measure to the environmental approaches at the workplace and elsewhere, which have been mentioned above. It is clearly impracticable for every member of the work force to receive personal instruction from a fully trained ergonomist. However, the importance of the issue has led to the development of a simple course for instructors, who are themselves members of the work force in different organizations. In an outline plan for one such training scheme Bickley[18] has suggested three rules for lifting (the so-called 'GRASP' approach). This is based on Getting Ready (mentally), Assessing the Situation (in terms of the weight, size and position of the object to be lifted as well as any obvious hazards in the path to be traversed during the lifting process) and the Positioning of the body (so that wherever possible the thigh muscles are used in the lifting process rather than the back muscles, as in bending the knees rather than bending the back). The idea is that those who have attended a training course will receive a diploma which conforms to the standards laid down by the Royal Institute of Public Health and Hygiene. They then return to their places of work to instruct others and to spot hazards. An important part of the short course deals with the law and the responsibilities of both employers and employees. Although, at first sight, a training program for what appears to be the simple act of lifting might be regarded as over elaborate, an important part of the training is to influence the attitude of individuals with regard to the lifting process so that, hopefully, the stages in the GRASP process become second nature. Arguably, by the time the person has entered the work force it may be too late to teach a person how to lift heavy objects, and therefore approaches to lifting should be taught to school children in order to achieve a habit reaction in the same way as instruction on crossing roads or hand-washing after going to the toilet. Such instruction at school could also mean that housewives, whose 'workplace' is the home, would receive the same personal preventive instruction as their working husbands. Notably, lift-training lays great emphasis on *avoiding* unilateral or rotational lifts, but not on coping with one-sided loads. Such instruction does not help the executive with an overloaded briefcase or the housewife with a heavily laden shopping basket, each of whom carry their burdens unilaterally, often on the side of the dominant hand. While the use of a rucksack or similar carrying device may be less attractive aesthetically, it might go some way towards preventing low back problems in these two groups.

Identification of those at special risk

It has been suggested that an underlying lumbar spine abnormality predisposes one to episodic back pain more readily than those without such impairments. Indeed there is general agreement that many cases of low back pain are associated with spondylolisthesis[19], and that those involved in heavy manual work are at greater risk from such impairments than those engaged in lighter activities. This seemingly logical conclusion suffers from the paucity of reliable clinical signs indicating the presence of such defects. Furthermore, the routine use of X-rays as part of a pre-employment examination schedule, particularly with the oblique views needed to detect such conditions as spondylolysis, appears to be unjus-

tified at the present time[20]. There is an added complication in the United States, where employers can be held responsible for allowing those with known defects to undertake potentially hazardous activities, as employees with such impairments would qualify for higher compensations from their employers in the event of an injury. Knowledge about the spine's status would either cause an employer to reject more potential employees than might be necessary, or, were the employer to accept an employee with possible defects, might result in increased liability. The same interpretation might apply in the UK in relation to the Health and Safety at Work Act.

There is, in addition, a lack of specificity of X-ray examinations which applies equally to both ultrasonic examinations and to magnetic resonance imaging. An example of lack of specificity in this respect was demonstrated by one attempt to reduce litigiously-associated spinal impairments where 1181 of a total of 4103 potential employees were rejected for production work following routine X-rays[21]. Although this reduced the number of successful claims[22], it resulted in an unacceptably high proportion of the work force being branded with the stigma of being potential 'back' cases, thus being rejected for many types of employment thereafter. This lack of specificity in relation to X-rays of the lumbar spine is further exemplified by the fact that almost all clinicians whose interests require them to study radiographs of the trunk have come across unexpected spinal defects in the plates of patients who are completely free from lumbosacral pain.

Claims have also been made that those with a narrowing of the lateral aspects of the spinal canal's lumen (trefoil outline) are more likely to suffer from back pain than those with wider canals[23]. It has been argued that this particular defect allows minimal additional intrusion, e.g. by a disc prolapse, prior to nerve root compress-

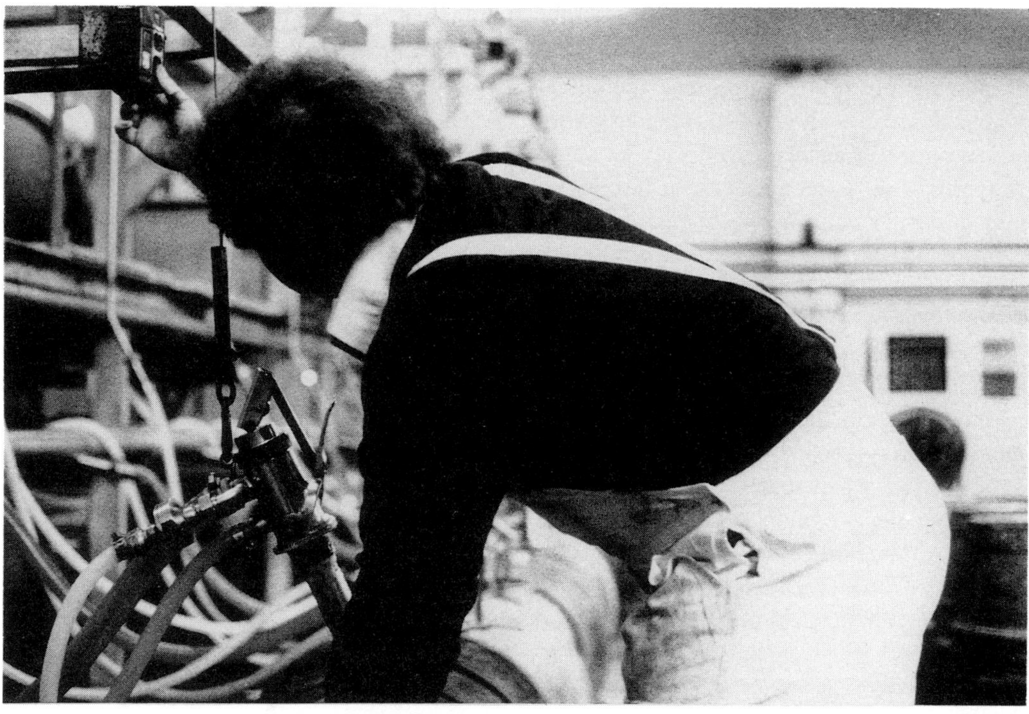

Figure 3 A man having to operate a machine with a flexed lumbar spine and extended neck to maintain eye contact with the part of the machine worked on

ion. Despite these uncertainties and the lack of specificity, the general consensus among occupational physicians is that it is advisable to warn those with repeated history of short episodes of back pain (regardless of X-ray or other investigative findings), to avoid seeking employment at the heavier end of the work spectrum. Furthermore, it is usually possible to obtain this sort of information from a self-completed questionnaire administered to potential employees.

CERVICOSCAPULAR PAIN
Environmental factors
Studies of West Indian women who carry weights on their heads suggest that they are at greater risk of suffering spondylosis of the cervical spine than those who do not[24], although the development of cervicoscapular pain appears to be less dependent on the absolute weight borne, than the head's

position itself. Working for prolonged periods with the arms raised to or above shoulder level was shown in the electronics industry to be associated with a higher than average sick leave for cervicoscapular pain[25], which was reduced by changing the arm position, or providing for rest periods when positional changes were not possible. Cervical pain is also associated with shorthand typing, an activity in which a notebook placed on the desk at the side of the typewriter requires the typist to hold the neck in a position of semi-flexion and lateral rotation for long periods. The use of a notebook holder, mounted at eye level above the typewriter, allows the typist to adopt a more natural sitting posture. A similar principle applies to music stands for members of orchestras; in general these are adjustable to the height of maximum comfort for the performer. There is less flexibility for pianists, and for organists, who have the added difficulty of reaching for stops, which increases the awkwardness of their playing positions. Since redesigning an organ panel is likely to be as costly as redesigning complex industrial machinery, it may be some time, (perhaps only after a test case in the courts), before designers may be persuaded to adopt preventive measures for what is a minority group.

Because lower back pain is more common than upper back pain, it often receives more attention in formal studies of occupational posture. Figure 3 shows a workman operating a machine that requires both forward flexion of the lumbar spine and compensatory hyperextension of the cervical spine to retain eye-level visual contact with the machine. Although this employee's main complaint was of cervicoscapular pain rather than lumbosacral pain, the neck and upper back complaint was resolved by redesigning the work station so as to reduce the flexion required of the lumbar spine.

Another example of controlling back pain by modifying the work, is exemplified by a worker in a slaughter house, who removed sheep skins by pulling backwards and using a closed fist to separate the pelt (Figure 4), a task that carried a high risk of back pain and painful 'pelter's knuckles'. Both of these were eliminated by suspending the carcass from all four legs so that the operator could use his body weight to separate the pelt (Figure 5). Another important preventive means for reducing cervicoscapular pain is the use of head rests in cars, which can reduce the incidence of whiplash injury on rear impact, and also (particularly to passengers) provide head support during long journeys.

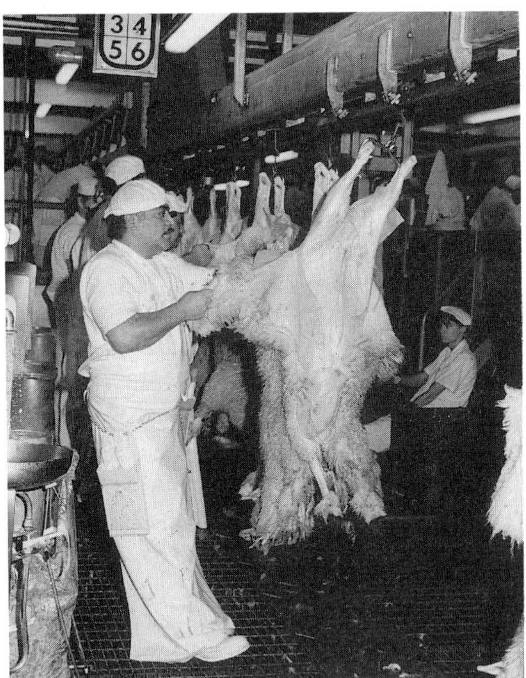

Figure 4 A slaughter house worker using back extension and a fist to separate sheep pelts with a high rate of back pain and 'pelter's knuckles'

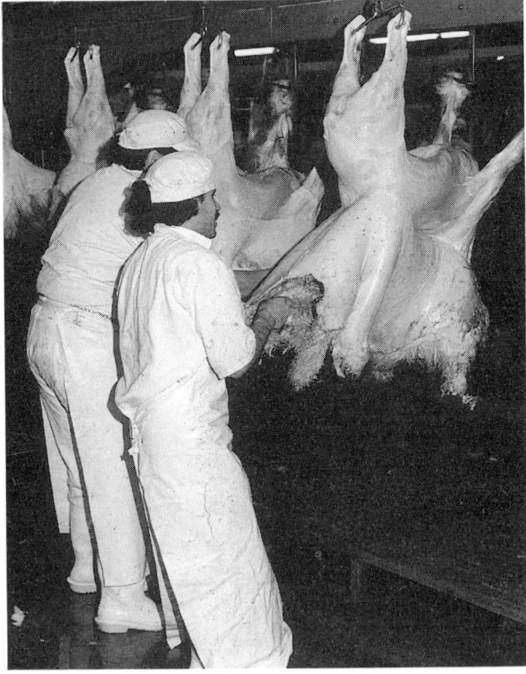

Figure 5 A successful modification to the task by suspending the carcass by both hind and forelimbs

PERSONAL PREVENTIVE MEASURES

Public education, identification of hazards to the cervical spine, and the use of preventive devices in the environment are equally applicable to those already discussed in relation to problems of the lumbar spine. Because complaints of cervicoscapular pain are less common, there are correspondingly fewer formal preventive measures. One simple measure for cervicoscapular pain is to ensure that the pillow height in bed is not excessive. Ideally, a single firm pillow is best to ensure the maintenance of the occipito-cervical contour. Regrettably as people get older, the need for a higher pillow for cardiovascular reasons may present difficulties to an age group most susceptible to the effects of cervical spondylosis and a compromise may be necessary, such as raising the head of the bed by 4–6 inches. Other devices for those with cervicoscapular pain include special mirrors in motor vehicles, which assist driving in reverse, as the full rotation of the neck required for this process may aggravate symptoms considerably.

Identification of those at special risk

Routine examinations, patient screening and examination of the neck specifically for the presence of asymptomatic cervical spondylosis or cervical ribs usually bear little fruit, given the non-specificity of the symptoms. Nevertheless, certain factors place a person at increased risk of suffering upper back and neck pain. Such factors include obesity and the habit of holding the neck forward from its axis and semi-flexed, particularly in the working situation where resting becomes difficult. Those undertaking jobs that require certain types of repetitive and/or 'unnatural' movements, should weigh their ongoing risk of frank lumbosacral pain, cervicoscapular pain as well as the carpal tunnel syndrome, which is discussed elsewhere.

SUMMARY AND CONCLUSIONS

(1) The back extends from the occiput to coccyx and the common sites for the symptom complex of back pain are the lumbosacral and cervicoscapular regions. Preventive measures in each site require different strategies.

(2) Environmental risk factors for lumbosacral pain (often including sciatica and cruralgia) are the weights to be handled and the workspace design that may force the adoption of awkward posture. The distance of the load from the body axis and the contribution of other 'exogenous' factors, e.g. vibration, particularly found in tractor seats with sagging springs, may also constitute risk factors.

(3) Absolute weight is a less important risk factor for cervicoscapular pain than posture, especially in tasks that require anterior and lateral flexion of the cervical spine for long periods, or those associated with hyperextension of the neck. Another important risk factor is working for prolonged periods with the arms above shoulder level.

(4) Legislation and complementary inspection to enforce weight limits, hazardous posture and seat design are important preventive measures in the working environment. When tasks cannot be altered to allow the arms to be below shoulder height, then the provision of arm rests (adjustable for height) may be helpful.

(5) Personal preventive measures include health education on handling and posture as well as encouragement to improve general fitness through exercises and attendance at back schools.

(6) In general, pre-employment screening by a physical examination, X-rays or ultrasound etc. for spinal defects is unproductive. However, a self-completed questionnaire designed to explore any history of repeated spells of lumbosacral pain or cervicoscapular pain may alert employers and the physicians

advising them against taking such individuals on to the payroll for heavy work – particularly if awkward posture is also involved.

(7) Evaluation of anatomical structure and functional capacity in relation to the back are equally unlikely to be helpful to employees, although those who complain of back pain should be examined for evidence of degenerative changes and, if found, should be offered the possibility of a change in their working routine or alternatively, the environment in which the job is performed, in order to prevent further deterioration.

REFERENCES

1. Anderson JAD. Epidemiological aspects of back pain. J Soc Occup Med. 1986; 36:90–94
2. International Labour Organization. Maximum Weight Recommendation (128). Geneva: ILO.1976
3. Great Britain. Health and Safety at Work Act. London, HMSO, 1974
4. Chaffin DB. Human strength capability and low back pain. J Occup Med. 1974; 16:248–254
5. Andersson GBJ, Ortengren R, Nachemson A. Intradiscal pressure, intraabdominal pressure and myoelectric back muscle activity related to posture and loading. Clin Orthop Rel Res. 1977; 129:156–164
6. Nachemson A. Lumbar intradiscal pressure. In Jayson MIV, ed., The Lumbar Spine and Back Pain. 2nd edn, Tunbridge Wells, Pitman Medical, 1980, pp. 341–358
7. Davis PR. The use of intra-abdominal pressure in evaluating stresses on the lumbar spine. Spine, 1980; 6:90–93
8. Sweetman BJ, Moore CS, Jayasinghe WJ, Anderson JAD. Monitoring work factors relating to back pain. Postgrad Med J. 1976; 52 (Suppl. 7): 151–155
9. Otun EO, Heinrich I, Anderson JAD, Crooks J. 'PADAS' an ambulatory electronic system to monitor and evaluate factors relating to back pain at work. Ergonomics. 1984; 27: (Suppl. 10): 268–271
10. Kiernan PJ, Anderson JAD. Monitoring spinal movement relating to back pain: observations on check-out operatives. Report to Guy's Hospital (unpublished): London Guy's Hospital. 1980
11. Griffin MJ, Witham EM, Parsons KC. Vibration and comfort I. Transitional seat vibration. Ergonomics. 1982; 25:142–162
12. Matthews J. Ride comfort for tractor operators. I. Review of existing information. J Argric Engin Res. 1964; 9:3–31
13. Matthews J. Ride comfort for tractor operators II. Analysis of ride vibrations of pneumatic tyred tractors. J Agric Engin Res. 1964; 9:147–158
14. Sjoflot L. The tractor as a place of work. Ergonomics. 1982; 25:11–18
15. Stayner R, Collins TS, Lines JA. Tractor ride vibration simulation as an aid to design. J Agric Engin Res. 1984; 29:345–355
16. Hall H, Iceton JA. Back school. Clin Orthop. 1983; 179:10–17
17. Grahame R, Jenkins JM. Joint hypermobility, asset or liability. Ann Rheum Dis. 1972; 31: 109–113
18. Bickley P. Training for hospital personnel to prevent back strain. Memorandum to Royal Institute of Public Health and Hygiene (Unpublished) London
19. Wiltse JJ. Surgery for intervertebral disk disease of the lumbar spine. Clin Orthop. 1977; 129: 22–24
20. Epstein BS, Epstein JA, Jones MD. Degenerative spondylolisthesis with an intact neural arc. Radiol Clin North Am. 1977; 15:275–287
21. Kosiak M, Aurelius JR, Hartfiel WF. Backache in industry. J Occup Med. 1966; 8:51–58
22. Kosiak M, Aurelius JR, Hartfiel WF. Backache in industry. J Occup Med. 1968; 10: 588–593
23. Porter R, Wicks M, Ottewell D. Measurement of the spinal canal by diagnostic ultrasound. J Bone Joint Surg. 1978; 60(B):481–484
24. Lawrence JS. Rheumatism in Populations. London, Heinemann, 1978
25. Westgaard RH, Aaras A. The effects of improved work place design on the development of musculoskeletal illnesses. Appl Ergon. 1985;16: 91–97

10. OSTEOARTHRITIS – PATHOGENESIS, ETIOLOGY AND PREVENTION

W. Watson Buchanan and Peter Lee

INTRODUCTION

Osteoarthritis, also known as osteoarthrosis or degenerative joint disease, is the oldest disease known to have affected humans. It is, moreover, one of the most widespread diseases of the animal kingdom and has been identified in birds, mammals and even in dinosaurs. Osteoarthritis (OA) occurring without apparent cause is referred to as 'primary' OA, and when it follows an injury or congenital or pathological condition, such as fractures, hip dysplasia, leg length discrepancy, Paget's disease and joint infection or inflammation, it is called 'secondary' OA. Subsets of OA have been described, including generalized OA[1] and erosive OA[2–7] but the validity of these entities have yet to be established. Monarticular involvement is exceptional; most patients having several joints involved and a bilateral and symmetrical distribution is not uncommon[8].

PATHOGENESIS

Osteoarthritis can be regarded as a 'failure' of the tissues comprising a joint[9,10], and is a combination of two processes: cartilaginous attrition and the formation of osteophytes[11]. The earliest changes consist of flaking and pitting of the surface of articular cartilage, which is followed by the development of deep fissures and clumps of chondrocytes. These chondrocytes have been shown to be metabolically active with an increased uptake of ^{35}S isotope[12], which reflects an increased synthesis of proteoglycans and collagen in an attempt to repair cartilage damage. Nevertheless, the half-life of newly formed proteoglycans in osteoarthritis has been shown to be reduced[13] and there is an overall reduction in the concentration of matrix components. Intrinsic enzymes, e.g. acid phosphatase, neutral protease, cathepsin D and collagenase, produced by chondrocytes, participate in the normal turnover of articular cartilage by a continuous process of breakdown and regeneration. However, when these enzymes are produced in excess, a net loss of cartilage occurs resulting in progressive destruction of the joint[14–20]. This process may be triggered or accelerated by the presence of synovium derived interleukin-1 (IL-1) or a cytokine similar to IL-1, which is capable of stimulating enzyme production by chondrocytes[21–24]. Contrary to the previously held belief that the synovium was a relatively inert tissue, the synovium may actually play an important role in the pathogenesis of osteoarthritis.

As the cartilage progressively undergoes attrition, changes begin to occur in the underlying bone. The normally smooth surface is replaced with rough and shaggy rugosities, known as fibrillation. Erosion of the cartilage then ensues until, in severe cases, the underlying subchondral bone is denuded. New bone formation occurs so that the subchondral tissues become sclerosed or eburnated. Ultimately, as cartilage breakdown continues, chondrocyte necrosis ensues, leaving only ghost outlines of the cells. Subchondral cysts (géodes) develop when the articular cartilage degenerates and synovial fluid is forced through defects in the articular cortex into the subchondral bone marrow. These lesions may in some instances regress and eventually disappear[25]. There is an alteration in appearance of the bone end through remodeling, collapse of the joint surface and the development of marginal osteophytes by endochondral ossification.

While the cartilage and bone bear the brunt of the damage in osteoarthritis, abnormalities often occur in soft tissues, and consist of fibrosis and thickening of the capsule, atrophy of adjacent muscles, entrapment of debris in the synovium and a mild to moderate synovitis with infiltration by lymphocytes and plasma cells. The latter is seen in up to 20% of surgically resected osteoarthritic specimens[26]. The changes may resemble those in rheumatoid arthritis but a severe inflammatory cell infiltrate and pannus formation are not usually seen[8,26,27]. The synovial fluid in osteoarthritis may show the presence of mild inflammatory changes but the total white cell count is rarely greater than 2×10^9/l (2000/mm^3).

ETIOLOGICAL FACTORS

While the histological and biochemical changes occurring in OA are well documented, the precise causative factors that initiate the events leading to cartilage degeneration are not as yet well defined. It is likely that both the primary and secondary forms of OA are multifactorial in origin and result from the interaction of several etiological or risk factors.

Crystal deposition

The synovitis typical of osteoarthritis has been attributed to an immunologic reaction to debris, such as from cartilage and bone degradation, or to hydroxyapatite or calcium pyrophosphate dihydrate crystals released into the joint. Fifty percent of osteoarthritic synovial fluids have been shown by electron microscopy to contain hydroxyapatite crystals[28,29]. Chondrocalcinosis often co-exists with osteoarthritis, but whether crystal deposition leads to premature cartilage degeneration or their presence is secondary to cartilage damage has not been established[30,31].

Immunological factors

Immunoglobulins and complement component C3 have been demonstrated in osteoarthritic cartilage[32] and anticollagen antibodies have been found in patients with OA[33,34]. The significance of these immunological factors in the pathogenesis of osteoarthritis is uncertain[35] but they are believed to play a minor role in OA, if at all. However, once cartilage damage has occurred, a secondary immune process may contribute to or enhance further destruction[36].

Ligamentous laxity and bone density

Although most research has concentrated on the molecular structure and functional relationships of articular cartilage in the pathogenesis of osteoarthritis[37,38], there is increasing evidence that the quality of joint ligaments and juxta-articular bone may also be important. Indeed a higher prevalence of osteoarthritis has been observed in patients with joint laxity[39,40], the most common example of which is recurrent dislocation of the patella[41]. Increased bone density has been shown to be associated with a greater frequency of osteoarthritis of the hip[42–44]. Radin and colleagues[45,46] demonstrated that repeated impact loading of a joint resulted in microfractures of the subchondral bone which heal by microcallus formation. This results in a loss of bone resilience and ability to absorb forces transmitted across the joint, thereby predisposing the overlying articular cartilage to degeneration.

Climate

Climactic factors have not been shown to have any influence whatsoever on the prevalence of osteoarthritis[47–49], but involvement of the interphalangeal joints of the hands may follow frostbite[50].

Sex and hormones

Middle aged and elderly females have not only more severe, but also more widespread osteoarthritis than males of the same age group[51,52]. Erosive inflammatory osteoarthritis tends to involve the interphalangeal joints of women soon after the menopause, which begs the possibility that estrogens may have a protective effect during a woman's youth[6]. Nonetheless, in postmenopausal females with OA, the levels of urinary gonadotrophins were not different from those in subjects without the disease[53]. Subsequent laboratory studies indicated that estrogens have an adverse effect on the metabolic functions of chondrocytes, depressing proteoglycan synthesis while increasing quantities of proteoglycanase[54–56]. Estradiol treatment has been associated with more severe articular cartilage damage[57]; the amelioration of experimental OA in rabbits with tamoxifen, an estrogen antagonist, raises the possibility that this disease may be modified effectively through hormonal manipulation[57,58].

Genetic factors

Heredity clearly plays a role in the pathogenesis of OA in such conditions as ochronosis, Ehlers–Danlos syndrome, congenital dislocation of the hip, Legg–Perthes' disease and in epiphyseal dysplasias. In some of these entities, the disease results from a biochemical alteration, for example ochronosis (alkaptonuria), where a deficiency of homogentisic acid oxidase results in the deposition of homogentisic acid in cartilage and subsequent chondrocyte toxicity. In others, such as the Ehlers–Danlos syndrome, OA is attributed to mechanical factors. However, in most genetic disorders that predispose to the development of

OA, the underlying mechanism remains uncertain[59].

The role of genetic factors in the etiology of primary OA is far less clear. Stecher[60] first suggested that Heberden's nodes, which are threefold more common in the sisters of affected patients, are inherited as an autosomal dominant trait in women, but recessive in men, a view accepted by McKusick[61]. Lawrence[62] found a concordance of osteoarthritis in 60% of monozygotic compared to 39% of dizygotic twins, which supports a genetic role, albeit not particularly strongly. The recent developments in this field have been recently reviewed by Jiminez[63]. No correlation has been found with either blood groups or tissue types[64], but Heberden's nodes and osteoarthritis of the hip and first metatarsophalangeal joints appear to be rare in African–Americans, and in Native Americans[47,60,64]. Recently, Knowlton and colleagues[65] demonstrated a genetic linkage between polymorphism in the type II procollagen gene and primary generalized osteoarthritis, with mild chondroplasia, in a large family.

Aging

The prevalence of OA increases with age and virtually the entire population will develop it, provided that they live long enough. This disease not only has a major socioeconomic impact in persons still at work, but is the commonest cause of functional impairment in those of retirement age[66]. It is now evident that age related changes in joints can begin even in the second decade of life, and by age 40 years, all people will have developed such abnormalities[67]. But the question remains: what is the nature of the relationship between aging and osteoarthritis? Does biochemical aging of cartilage occur, predisposing to surface failure with 'normal' use, or are single or multiple injuries, sustained overuse or misuse, abnormal loading or other factors also required? Despite the damning evidence suggesting that age is a risk factor for OA, specific changes occur in cartilage with aging that differ substantially from those of osteoarthritis[68]. The density of chondrocytes decreases with age and may be responsible for the altered biochemical composition of the matrix in articular cartilage[69]. Chondroitin-4-sulfate and keratan sulfate are both increased with age, while there is a reduction in chondroitin-6-sulfate, and in the length of the glycosaminoglycan chains[70,71]. The result is that aging cartilage binds less water, is less resilient and has less tensile strength[72]. Mechanical factors may then lead to fatigue fractures of the collagen network, weakened by changes in the supporting matrix[73–74]. Evidence that cartilage becomes more susceptible to mechanical breakdown with age requires confirmation, and available data are insufficient to conclude that OA is due to biological aging of articular cartilage, although age related changes resulting in altered joint mechanics may be of import in the pathogenesis of osteoarthritis.

Mechanical stress

There is substantial evidence that OA is more common in those joints subjected to the greatest physical stress[77], and conversely, OA rarely develops in paralysed limbs[78,79]. Obesity might be expected to predispose to OA in weight-bearing joints, a theory that appears to be supported by data from the obese female knee[80], although this is less true in the hip[81] if, indeed, at all[82]. Patients with morbid obesity, however, do not appear to be at an increased risk of osteoarthritis in the lower limb joints[83]. A confounding factor is that while Heberden's nodes occur with increased frequency in obese females, it is difficult to explain why some weight-bearing joints, such as the ankle, are spared. Smythe has observed that thickening of the insertion of the extensor tendon precedes the development of both Heberden's and Bouchard's nodes[84,85], and suggests that the tendon is also shortened, thereby restricting flexion. Contraction of the powerful flexor muscles, acting against this resistance produces compressive forces across the joint which results in 'crush' fractures of the subchondral bone. Subsequently, there is healing of the bone with stiffening and degeneration of the overlying articular cartilage.

Occupation

There is overwhelming evidence that the mechanical stresses associated with certain occupations and sporting activities are linked with a higher incidence of OA. Those who are engaged in mining[86,88], use of pneumatic drills[45,89], heavy industry[88,90–3] and agricultural manual labor[48,92,94] are at an increased risk for OA in those joints that are repeatedly stressed or traumatized. Lawrence[95] found distal interphalangeal joint OA to be more common in cotton pickers, which is, moreover, related to handedness[96,97]. However, not all studies have shown an increased prevalence of osteoarthritis in these occupational groups. Burke and colleagues[89] found no increase in OA of the elbow in pneumatic drill operators, and a similar lack of increased risk was observed in other joints of workers involved in heavy manual labor[98–100]. Despite the widely held opinion that sportsmen, especially those in contact sports such as football and wrestling[101–109] (but not running[110–114]) are at an increased risk for suffering OA, contrasting studies have reached the opposite conclusion that there is no increased incidence of OA in athletes, including gymnasts[115], football players[116,117], and parachutists[105]. The discrepancies reported by different workers in the development of OA in certain occupations and sporting activities have been well reviewed by Genti[118], who noted that the results of many of these studies rested solely on the presence of osteophytes. In addition, those subjects who had previously suffered trauma, for example meniscal damage, were not excluded[119]. Injuries to menisci and other soft tissue injuries can ultimately lead to cartilaginous degeneration[120,121].

Mechanical stress alone does not appear to cause OA, whether chronic as in running or in high-impact activities such as parachute jumping, while joints that are repeatedly subjected to abnormal stresses, as in cotton sorters, may suffer OA. Nevertheless, the question remains: why is the ankle joint spared from osteoarthritis even when it is unduly stressed[122]? The recent finding of Felson and co-workers[123] in the Framingham study strongly supports the contention that occupational 'wear and tear' is a major factor in the development of OA. These authors found that members of the cohort who were employed in occupations which were demanding, both in physical work and knee bending, were more likely to develop osteoarthritis of the knee joint. This raises the possibility that job modification might prevent such disease. It has been suggested (Chapter 3) that OA of the knee, especially of the medial compartment, is more common in eastern cultures where squatting is a necessary part of daily living activity. While acute injuries to joints should receive prompt and proper attention, prevention of osteoarthritis in the workplace or in the sports arena may prove impossible until more information is available[112].

Diet

There is no evidence that any particular diet can prevent osteoarthritis[124], with the possible exception of Kashin–Beck disease[125] which is endemic in Manchuria, North Korea and other parts of North East Asia, and which has been variously related to the ingestion of grain infected with the fungus *Fusaria sporotrichiella* or to a selenium deficiency[126]. Obesity is best avoided for various reasons, although there is no proof that this will lessen the likelihood of developing OA.

Smoking

Felson and colleagues recently reported the results of an American Health and Nutritional Examination Survey, showing that cigarette smokers had *less* osteoarthritis than non-smokers[127].

Those who were heavy smokers (more than 40 cigarettes per day) were almost five times less likely to have osteoarthritis. The reduced risk remained after adjustment for age, sex and body weight. However, a recent British study failed to find any association between smoking and a reduced incidence of osteoarthritis[128].

PREVENTION

Preventive measures have not played an important role in the routine management of osteoarthritis. The main reason is that the disease, at least the primary form, was considered to be a simple degenerative process. There was little understanding of the underlying factors and mechanism involved. The recent advances in knowledge with regard to the pathogenesis of osteoarthritis provide some hope that new therapeutic approaches may prevent or at least retard the progressive cartilage attrition occurring in this disease.

In many forms of secondary OA, progressive cartilage breakdown and eventual development of the full-blown disease may be prevented or slowed down through the early recognition and treatment of any potentially causative underlying abnormalities. Thus, inflammatory arthropathies such as rheumatoid arthritis require effective suppression of the synovitis with anti-inflammatory and other drugs; septic arthritis requires early diagnosis and treatment with the appropriate antibiotics; fractures of the long bones should be properly reduced with correct alignment; excess joint laxity with recurrent subluxation requires surgical stabilization, and leg length discrepancy may benefit from correction with orthotics. Nonetheless, certain anatomic or metabolic abnormalities such as congenital hip dysplasia and ochronosis, which may lead to secondary osteoarthritis, have not proven amenable to successful surgical correction or medical treatment.

Table 1 Risk factors for osteoarthritis. (Reproduced with kind permission from reference 139)

Age
Gender
Mechanical stress
Repetitive joint (mis)usage
Joint trauma
Obesity
Congenital /developmental bone and joint disorders
Prior inflammatory joint disease

The major problem with disease prevention in primary osteoarthritis is that the initiating cause or causes are not clearly defined. Recent studies indicate, however, that certain therapeutic approaches show some potential in slowing down if not preventing the progressive articular cartilage degeneration. This could theoretically be achieved either through the inhibition of the enzymes responsible for cartilage breakdown or stimulation of chondrocytes to increase the rate of proteoglycan production. In several animal models, treatment with low dose corticosteroids significantly reduces the incidence and severity of cartilage lesions and osteophytes[129–132]. These results may have been achieved through the inhibition of metalloprotease synthesis by both chondrocytes and synovial cells. In addition, the synthesis of possible activators of metalloprotease such as plasminogen activators[133] and cytokines (for example IL-1) which may stimulate enzyme production by chondrocytes[134], are both depressed. It may be possible to prevent the development of OA through hormonal manipulation, given the apparent amelioration of experimental osteoarthritis in rabbits by use of the estrogen antagonist, tamoxifen[57,58].

Recent studies indicate that certain non-steroidal anti-inflammatory drugs (NSAIDs) including tiaprofenic acid, diclofenac sodium and piroxicam, may also have a chondroprotective effect by inhibition of metalloprotease production[135,136].

Sodium salicylate in therapeutic concentrations was found to suppress proteoglycan synthesis[137], which begs the question of whether salicylates should be avoided in treating OA. On the other hand, benoxaprofen and sulindac may increase the rate of proteoglycan synthesis by chondrocytes[138]. Current evidence has been found from *in vitro* experiments or animal models only, and the relevance of these observations to the treatment of osteoarthritis in humans is uncertain. Whether NSAIDs have the ability to influence significantly the course of this disorder in the long term needs to be determined by controlled studies.

PRIMARY PREVENTION

Hochberg[139] reviewed the epidemiology of osteoarthritis, and listed the established risk factors that are amenable to intervention (Table 1). Although aging is inevitable, certain hereditary conditions may ultimately be diagnosed or even manipulated through gene engineering. Hereditary gout responds to drug therapy, thus removing one cause of osteoarthritis. Mechanical stress, injury and vibration, as well as repetitive joint abuse are all factors amenable to modification of work stations, equipment and work practices, on the roads and sports fields, as elaborated in Chapters 4, 5, 9, 22 and 28. Obesity control (Chapter 25) although difficult, and not definitively proven to reduce the incidence of osteoarthritis or its severity is indicated for many other reasons, so should be generally recommended. The early control of predisposing conditions of congenital origin, due to bone disease or inflammatory arthritis merges with secondary prevention discussed above.

REFERENCES

1. Kellgren JH, Moore R. Generalised osteoarthritis and Heberden's nodes. Br Med J. 1952; 1: 181–187
2. Crain DC. Interphalangeal osteoarthritis. JAMA. 1961; 175:1049–1053

3. Peter JB, Pearson CM, Marmor L. Erosive osteoarthritis of the hands. Arthritis Rheum. 1966; 9:365–388

4. McEwen C. Osteoarthritis of the fingers with ankylosis. Arthritis Rheum. 1968; 11:734–744

5. Marmor L, Peter JB. Osteoarthritis of the hand. Clin Orthop. 1969; 64:164–174

6. Ehrlich GE. Osteoarthritis beginning with inflammation: definition and correlations. JAMA. 1975; 232:157–159

7. Utsinger PD, Resnick D, Shapiro RF, Wiesner KB. Roentgenologic, immunologic and therapeutic study of erosive (inflammatory) osteoarthritis. Arch Intern Med. 1978; 138:693–697

8. Huskisson EC, Dieppe PA, Tucker AK, Cannell LB. Another look at osteoarthritis. Ann Rheum Dis. 1979; 38:423–428

9. Sokoloff L. The Biology of Degenerative Joint Disease. Chicago: University of Chicago Press,. 1969

10. Christensen SB. Osteoarthrosis; changes in bone, cartilage and synovial membrane in relationship to bone scintigraphy. Acta Orthop Scand. 1985; 56 (Suppl. 214):1–43

11. Hernborg J, Nilsson BE. The relationship between osteophytes in the knee joint, osteoarthritis and aging. Acta Orthop Scand. 1973; 44:69–74

12. Collins DH, McElligott TF. Sulphate (35S04) uptake by chondrocytes in relation to histological changes in osteoarthritic human articular cartilage. Ann Rheum Dis. 1960:. 19:318–330

13. Teshima R, Treadwell BV, Tranan CA, Mankin HJ. Comparative rates of proteoglycan synthesis and size of proteoglycans in normal and osteoarthritic chondrocytes. Arthritis Rheum. 1983; 26:1225–1230

14. Ehrlich MG, Mankin HJ, Treadwell BV. Acid hydrolase activity in osteoarthritic and normal human cartilage. J Bone Joint Surg. 1973; 55A:1068–1076

15. Sapolsky AI, Howell DS, Woessner JF Jr. Neutral proteases and cathepsin D in human articular cartilage. J Clin Invest. 1974

16. Sapolsky AI, Matsuta K, Woessner JF Jr, Howell DS. Metal-dependent neutral proteoglycanase from normal and ulcerated human articular cartilage. Trans Orthop Res Soc. 1978; 3:71

17. Lahey PJ, Ehrlich MJ, Mankin HJ. Neutral protease activity vs. severity of osteoarthritis. Trans Orthop Res Soc. 1979;4:46

18. Fessel JM, Chrisman OD. Enzymatic degradation of chondromacroprotein by free-cell extracts of human cartilage. Arthritis Rheum. 1964; 7:398–405

19. Ali SY. The degradation of cartilage matrix by an intracellular protease. Biochem J. 1964; 93: 611–618

20. Sandy JD, Brown HL, Lowther DA. Degradation of proteoglycan in articular cartilage. Biochem Biophys Acta. 1978; 543:536–544

21. Deshmukh-Phadke K, Nanda S, Lee K. Macrophage factor that induces neutral protease secretion by normal rabbit chondrocytes. Eur J Biochem. 1980; 104:175–180

22. Gowen M. Wood DP, Ihrie EJ *et al.* Stimulation by human interleukin-1 of cartilage breakdown and production of collagenase and proteoglycanase by human chondrocytes but not by human osteoblasts in vitro. Biochem Biophys Acta. 1984; 799:186–193

23. Ridge SC, Oronsky AL, Kerwer SS. Induction of the synthesis of latent collagenase and latent neutral protease in chondrocytes by a factor synthesised by activated macrophages. Arthritis Rheum. 1980; 23:448–454

24. Ehrlich MG, Armstrong AL, Treadwell BV, Mankin HJ. Degradative enzyme systems in cartilage. Clin Orthop Rel Res. 1986; 213:62–68

25. Macys JR, Bullough PG, Wilson Jr PD. Coxarthrosis: a study of the natural history based on a correlation of clinical, radiographic and pathologic findings. Semin Arthritis Rheum. 1980; 10:66–80

26. Meachim G, Whitehouse GH, Pedley RB, Nichol FE, Owen R. An investigation of radiological, clinical and pathological correlations in osteoarthrosis of the hip. Clin Radiol. 1980; 31:565–574

27. Salvati EA, Granda JL, Mirra J, Wilson PD. Clinical, enzymatic and histological study of synovium in coxarthrosis. Int Orthop. 1977; 1:39–42

28. Schumacher HR. Arthritis associated with apatite crystals. Ann Intern Med. 1977; 81–411

29. Malemud CJ, Moskowitz RW. Physiology of articular cartilage. Clin Rheum Dis. 1981; 7:29–55

30. McCarty DJ. Pyrophosphate dihydrate crystal deposition disease (pseudogout syndrome). Clinical aspects. Clin Rheum Dis. 1977; 3:61–69

31. Dieppe P. Calcium phosphate crystal deposition and clinical subsets of osteoarthritis. In Peyron

JG, ed., Epidemiology of Osteoarthritis. Paris, Geigy, 1981, pp. 71–80

32. Cooke TD, Bennet EL, Ohno O. Identification of immunoglobulins and complement components in articular collagenous tissues of patients with idiopathic osteoarthritis. In Nuki G, ed., Aetiopathogenesis of Osteoarthritis. Tunbridge Wells, Pitman Medical, 1980, pp. 144–155

33. Golds EE, Cooke TDV, Poole AR. Immune regulation of collagenase secretion in rheumatoid and osteoarthritic cell cultures. Coll Relat Res. 1983; 3:125–140

34. Jason HE. Autoantibody specificities of immune complexes sequestered in articular cartilage of patients with rheumatoid arthritis and osteoarthritis. Arthritis Rheum. 1985; 28:241–248

35. Cooke TDV, Scudamore RA. Immunological aspects of osteoarthritis. EULAR Bull. 1988; 17:17–18

36. Cooke TDV. Significance of immune complex deposits in osteoarthritic cartilage. J. Rheumatol. 1987; 14 (Suppl.): 77–79

37. Mow van C. Molecular structure and function relationships for articular cartilage. EULAR Bull. 1988; 17:9–13

38. Muir H. Osteoarthritis; biochemical aspects. EULAR Bull. 1988; 17:14–16

39. Kirk JA, Ansell BM, Bywaters EGL. The hypermobility syndrome. Ann Rheum Dis. 1967; 28:419–425

40. Bird HA, Tribe CR, Bacon PA. Joint hypermobility leading to osteoarthritis and chondrocalcinosis. Ann Rheum Dis. 1978; 37:203–211

41. Sutro CJ. Hypermobility of knees due to overlength capsular and ligamentous tissues. Surgery. 1947; 21:67–78

42. Foss MLV, Byers PD. Bone density, osteoarthrosis of the hip and fracture of the upper end of the femur. Ann Rheum Dis. 1972; 31:259–264

43. Roh YS, Dequeker J, Mulier JC. Bone mass in osteoarthrosis, measured by in vivo photon absorption. J Bone Joint Surg. 1974; 56:587–591

44. Solomon L. Osteoarthritis of the hip and femoral neck fracture. In Studies in Joint Diseases. London, Arthritis and Rheumatism Council. 1978

45. Radin EL, Aul IL, Rose RM. Role of mechanical factors in the pathogenesis of primary osteoarthritis. Lancet. 1972; 1:519–522

46. Townsend PR, Rose RM, Radin EL, Raux P. The biomechanics of the human patella and its implications for chondromalacia. J Biomech. 1977; 10:403–407

47. Bennett PH, Burch TA. Osteoarthrosis in the Blackfeet and Pima Indians. In Bennett PH, Wood PHM, eds., Population Studies in the Rheumatic Diseases. Amsterdam. Excerpta Medica, 1968, pp. 407–412

48. Bjelle A. Osteoarthrosis and back disorders in Sweden. In Peyron JG, ed., Epidemiology of Osteoarthritis. Paris, Geigy, 1981, pp. 17–29

49. Lawrence JS, Sebo M. The geography of osteoarthritis. In Nuki G, ed., The Aetiopathogenesis of Osteoarthrosis. Tunbridge Wells: Pitman Medical, 1981, pp. 155–183

50. Tishler JM. The soft tissue and bone changes in frost bite injuries. Radiology. 1972; 102:511–513

51. Mikkelsen WN, Duff IF, Dodge HJ. Age and sex specific prevalence of radiographic abnormalities of the joints of the hands, wrists and cervical spine of adult residents of the Tecumseh, Michigan, community health study area. 1962–1965. J Chronic Dis. 1970; 23:151–159

52. Acheson RM, Collart AB. New Haven survey of joint diseases XVII. Relationship between some systemic characteristics and osteoarthrosis in a general population. Ann Rheum Dis. 1975; 34:379–487

53. Rogers FB, Lansbury J. Urinary gonadotrophin excretion in osteoarthritis. Am J Med Sci. 1956; 232:419–420

54. Rosner IA, Goldberg VM, Getzy L, Moskowitz RW. Effects of estrogen on cartilage and experimentally induced osteoarthritis. Arthritis Rheum. 1979; 22:52–58

55. Rosner IA, Manni A, Malemud CJ, Boja BA, Moskowitz RW. Estradiol receptors in articular chondrocytes. Biochem Biophys Res Commun. 1982; 106–1379

56. Kent L, Malemud C, Moskowitz BW. Differential response of articular chondrocyte populations to thromboxane B2 and analogs of prostaglandin cyclic endoperoxides. Prostaglandins. 1980; 19: 391–406

57. Rosner IA, Malemud CJ, Goldberg VM, Papay RS, Getzy L. Moskowitz RW. Pathologic and metabolic responses of experimental osteoarth-

126

ritis to estradiol and an estradiol antagonist. Clin Orthop. 1982; 171:286–290

58. Colombo C, Butler N, Hickman L, Selwyn W, Chart J, Steinetz B. A new model of osteoarthritis in rabbits. Evaluation of anti-osteoarthrosic effects of selected anti-rheumatic drugs administered systemically. Arthritis Rheum. 1983; 26:1132–1139

59. Stanescu R, Stanescu V, Maroteaux P. Peyron JG. Constitutional articular cartilage dysplasia with accumulation of complex lipids in chondrocytes and precocious arthrosis. Arthritis Rheum. 1981; 24:965–968

60. Stecher RM. Heberden's nodes. A clinical description of osteoarthritis of the finger joints. Ann Rheum Dis. 1955; 14:1–10

61. McKusick V. Genetic factors in disease of connective tissue: a survey of the present state of knowledge. Am J Med. 1959; 2:283–302

62. Lawrence JS. Rheumatism in Populations. London, William Heinemann Medical, 1977

63 Jiminez SA. Molecular biological approaches to the study of heritable osteoarthritis. J Rheumatol. 1991;18 (Suppl.) 27:7–9

64. Kellgren JH, Lawrence JS, Bier F. Genetic factors in generalised osteoarthritis. Ann Rheum Dis. 1963; 22:237–255

65. Knowlton RG, Katzenstein PL, Moskowitz RW, Weaver EJ, *et al.* Genetic linkage of a polymorphism in the type II procollagen gene (COL2A1) to primary osteoarthritis associated with mild chondroplasia. N Engl J Med. 1990; 322:526–530

66. Wood PHN. Rheumatic complaints. Br Med J. 1971; 27:82–88

67. Lowman EW. Osteoarthritis. JAMA. 1955; 157:487–488

68. Brandt KD, Fife RS. Aging in relationship to the pathogenesis of osteoarthritis. Clin Rheum Dis. 1986; 12:117–130

69. Vignon E, Arlot M, Patricot LM, Vignon G. The cell density of human femoral head cartilage. Clin Orthop. 1976; 121:303–308

70. Buckwalter JA, Kuettner KE, Thonar EJ-M. Age related changes in articular cartilage proteoglycans: electronmicroscopic studies. J Orthop Res. 1985; 3:251–257

71. Roughley PJ, White RJ. Age-related changes in the structure of the proteoglycan subunits from human articular cartilage. J Biol Chem. 1980; 255:217–224

72. Weightman B. In vitro fatigue testing of articular cartilage. Ann Rheum Dis. 1975; 34 (Suppl.): 108–110

73. Weightman BO, Freeman MAR, Swanson SAV. Fatigue of articular cartilage. Nature. 1973; 244:303–304

74. Freeman MAR. The fatigue of cartilage in the pathogenesis of osteoarthrosis. Acta Orthop Scand. 1975; 47:323-328

75. Gardner DL, Elliott RJ, Armstrong CG, Longmore RB. The relationship between age, thickness, surface structure, copliance and composition of human femoral head articular cartilage. In Nuki G ed., The Aetiopathogenesis of Osteoarthrosis. Tunbridge Wells, Pitman Medical, 1980, pp. 65–83

76. Kempson GE. The mechanical properties of articular cartilage. In Sokoloff L, ed., The Joints and Synovial Fluid. New York, Academic Press, 1980, pp. 177–238

77. Jermain RD. Stress and the etiology of osteoarthritis. Am J Phys Anthropol. 1977; 46:353–366

78. Glynn JH, Sutherland I, Walker JF, Young AC. Low incidence of osteoarthritis of hip and knee after anterior poliomyelitis: a late show. Br Med J. 1966; 2:739–742

79. Burke MJ, Roman V, Wright V. Bone and joint changes in lower limb amputees. Ann Rheum Dis. 1978; 37:252–254

80. Hartz AJ, Fischer ME, Bril G *et al.* The association of obesity with joint pain and osteoarthritis in the Hanes data. J Chronic Dis. 1986; 39:311–319

81. Solomon L, Schnitzler C, Browett J. Osteoarthritis of the hip. The patient behind the disease. In Peyron JG, ed., Epidemiology of Osteoarthritis. Paris, Geigy, 1981, pp. 40–52

82. Saville PD, Dickson J, Age and weight in osteoarthritis of the hip. Arthritis Rheum. 1968; 11:635–644

83. Goldin RH, McAdam L. Louie JS *et al.* Clinical and radiological survey of the incidence of osteoarthritis among obese patients. Ann Rheum Dis. 1976; 35:349–353

84. Smythe HA. Digital extensor thickening - the primary lesion of Heberden's and Bouchard's nodes. Arthritis Rheum. 1980; 23:749

85. Smythe HA. The mechanical pathogenesis of generalised osteoarthritis. In Peyron JG, ed., Osteoarthritis: Current Clinical and Fundamental Problems. Paris, Ciba-Geigy, 1985, pp. 66–70

86. Lawrence JS. Rheumatism in coal miners III. Occupational factor. Br Med J. 1955; 12:249–251

87. Kellgren JH, Lawrence JS. Osteoarthrosis and disc degeneration in an urban population. Ann Rheum Dis. 1958: 17:388–397

88. Lindberg H. Montgomery F. Heavy labour and the occurrence of gonarthrosis. Clin Orthop Rel Res. 1987; 214:235–236

89. Burke MJ, Fear EC, Wright V, Bone and joint changes in pneumatic drillers. Ann Rheum Dis. 1977; 36:276–279

90. Partridge REH, Duthie JJR. Rheumatism in dockers and civil servants: a comparison of heavy manual and sedentary workers. Ann Rheum Dis. 1968; 27:559–568

91. Maulwald G. Kniegelenksveranderungen bei Schweissen im Schiffbau Beitrage. Orthop Traumatol. 1981; 27:181–185

92. Frank O. Klemmayer K. Die Coxarthrose bei der landbevolkerung. Z Rheumatol. 1968; 27:317–319

93. Mintz G. Saga A. Severe osteoarthritis of the elbow in foundry workers. Arch Environ Health. 1973; 27:78–80

94. Louyot P, Savin P. Le coxarthrose chez l'argiculteur. Rev Rheum Malad Osteo-articulaires. 1966; 33:625–632

95. Lawrence JS. Rheumatism in cotton operatives. Br Med J. 1961; 18:270–276

96. Acheson RM, Chan YK, Clemett AR. New Haven survey of joint diseases. XII. Distribution and symptoms of osteoarthrosis in the hands with reference to handedness. Ann Rheum Dis. 1970; 275–286

97. Hadler NM, Gillings DB, Imbus HR et al. Hand structure and function in an industry setting. Influence of three patterns of stereotypes repetitive usage. Arthritis Rheum. 1978: 21:210–220

98. Lawrence JS, Brenner JM, Bier F. Osteoarthritis: prevalence in the population and relationship between symptoms and X-ray changes. Ann Rheum Dis. 1966; 25:1–24

99. Sairanen E, Brushhaber L, Kaskinen M. Felling work, low back pain and osteoarthritis. Scand J Work Environ Health. 1981; 7:18–30

100. Lindberg H. Danielsson LG. The relation between labor and coxarthrosis. Clin Orthop Rel Res. 1984; . 191:159–161

101. Brodelius A. Osteoarthrosis of the talar joints in footballers and ballet dancers. Acta Orthop Scand. 1961; 30:309–314

102. Ambre T, Nilsson BE. Degenerative changes in the first metatarsophalangeal joints of ballet dancers. Acta Orthop Scand. 1978; 49:317–319

103. Solonen KA. The joints of the lower extremity of football players. Ann Cher Gyn Fenn. 1966; 55:176–180

104. Oderkekerhen JC, Chantraine A, Bernard A. Arthrosis and axis deviation of the knee joint in old soccer players. J Belge Rheum Med Phys. 1973; 2:874

105. Murray-Leslie CK, Lintott DJ, Wright V. The knees and ankles in sport and veteran military parachutists. Ann Rheum Dis. 1977; 36:327–331

106. Klunder KD, Rud B, Hansen J. Osteoarthritis of the hip and knee joint in retired football players. Acta Orthop Scand. 1980; 51:925–927

107. Boyer T, Delaire M, Beranck L et al. Un antécédent de practique sportive est-il plus fréquent chez les subjets attends d'arthrose? Une étude controlée. In Peyron JG, ed., Epidemiology of Osteoarthritis. Paris, Geigy, 1981, pp. 156–3

108. Frey A, Muller W. Heberden-Arthrosen bei Judo-Sportlern. Schweiz Med Wochenschr. 1984; 114:40–47

109. Moran JM, Hemman JH, Grenwald AS. Finger joint contact areas and pressures. J Orthop Res. 1985; 3:49–55

110. Puranen J, Ala-Ketala L, Peltokallio P et al. Running and primary osteoarthritis of the hip. Br Med J. 1975; 1:424–425

111. Kraus JF, D'Ambrosie RD, Smith EG et al. Epidemiological study of severe osteoarthritis. Orthopedics. 1978; 1:37–42

112. Shon RS, Micheli LJ. The effects of running on the hip and knees. Clin Orthop Rel Res. 1985; 198:106–109

113. Lane NE, Bloch DA, Jones HH et al. Long-distance running, bone density and osteoarthritis. JAMA. 1986; 255:1147–1151

114. Panush RS, Schmidt C, Caldwell JR, Is running associated with degenerative joint disease? JAMA. 1986; 255:1152-1154

115. Estmond CJ, Hudson A, Wright V. A Radiological survey of the hips and knees in female specialist teachers of physical education. Scand J Rheumatol. 1979; 8:264–268

116. Roas A. Degenerative phenomena in the joints of football players. Geneeskunde Sport. 1975; 8: 32–34

117. Wright V. Biomechanical factors in the development of osteoarthrosis; epidemiological studies. In Peyron JG, ed., Epidemiology of Osteoarthritis. Paris, Geigy, 1981, pp. 140–146

118. Genti G. Occupation and osteoarthritis. Baillières Clin Rheumatol. 1989; 3:193–204

119. Altman RD. Hochberg MC. Degenerative joint disease. Clin Rheum Dis. 1983; 9:681–693

120. McDermott M. Freyne P. Osteoarthrosis in runners with knee pain. Br J Sports Med. 1983; 17:84–87

121. Moretz JA, Harlan SD, Goodrich J et al. Long-term follow-up of knee injuries in high school football players. Am J Sports Med. 1984; 12: 298–300

122. Funk FJ Jr. Osteoarthritis of the foot and ankle. In Symposium on Osteoarthritis. American Academy of Orthopic Surgeons, eds., St. Louis, CV Mosby, 1976, pp. 287–301

123. Felson DT, Hannan MT, Anderson JJ, Naimark A. Occupational physical demands (PHYS), knee bending (BEND) and X-ray knee osteoarthritis (OA): the Framingham Study (Abstract). 1990; 33 (Suppl.), 10

124. Kirwan JR, Silman AJ. Epidemiological, sociological and environmental aspects of rheumatoid arthritis and osteoarthritis. Baillières Clin Rheumatol. 1987; 1:467–489

125. Nesterov AI. Clinical course of Kashin-Beck disease. Arthritis Rheum. 1964; 7:29–40

126. Sokoloff L. Endemic forms of osteoarthritis. Clin Rheum Dis. 1985; 11:187–202

127. Felson DT, Anderson JJ, Naimark A, Hannan MT, Kannel WB, Meenan RF. Does smoking protect against osteoarthritis? Arthritis Rheum. 1989; 32:166–172

128. Spector TD, Hart DJ, Doyle DV. Are cigarette smoking and HRT protective for osteoarthritis? Br J Rheumatol. 1989; 28(Suppl):11

129. Moskowitz RW, Goldberg VM, Schwab W, Berman L. Effects of intraarticular corticosteroids and exercise in experimental models of inflammatory and degenerative arthritis. Arthritis Rheum. 1975; 18:417

130. Butler M, Colombo C, Hickman L et al. A new model of osteoarthritis in rabbits: III. Evaluation of anti-osteoarthritic effects of selected drugs administered intraarticularly. Arthritis Rheum. 1983; 26:1380–1386

131. Williams JM, Brandt KD. Triamcinolone hexacetonide protects against fibrillation and osteophyte formation following chemically induced cartilage damage. Arthritis Rheum. 1985; 28:1267–1274

132. Pelletier J-P, Martel-Pelletier J. Protective effects of corticosteroids on cartilage lesions and osteophyte formation in the Pond-Nuki dog model of osteoarthritis. Arthritis Rheum. 1989; 32:181–193

133. Hamilton JA, Bootes A. Phillips PE, Slywka J. Human synovial fibroblast plasminogen activator: modulation of enzyme activity by antiinflammatory steroids. Arthritis Rheum. 1981; 24:1296–1303

134. Larrick JW, Kunkel SL. The role of tumor necrosis factor and Interleukin-1 in the immunoinflammatory response. Pharmaceut Res. 1988; 5: 129–139

135. Verbruggen G, Veys, EM, Schatteman L et al. Proteoglycan metabolism in tissue-cultured human articular cartilage: influence of piroxicam. J Rheumol. 1989; 16:355–362

136. Pelletier J-P, Martel-Pelletier J. The therapeutic effects of NSAID and corticosteroids on OA: to be or not to be. J Rheumatol. 1989; 16:266–269

137. Brandt KD. Effects of nonsteroidal anti-inflammatory drugs on chondrocyte metabolism in vitro and in vivo. Am J Med. 1987; 83 (Suppl.), 29–34

138. Hess EV, Herman JH. Cartilage metabolism and antiinflammatory drugs in osteoarthritis. Am J Med. 1986; 81 (Suppl. 5B):36–43

139. Hochberg HC. Epidemiology of arthritis; current concepts and new insights. J Rheumatol. 1991; 18 (Suppl.) 27:4–6

Readers interested in further reading are encouraged to read the recent publication of Moskowitz RW, Howell DS, Goldberg VM, Mankin HJ. Osteoarthritis Diagnosis and Medical/Surgical Management, 2nd edn, Philadelphia, WB Saunders, 1992

11. PRIMARY PREVENTION OF RHEUMATIC FEVER AND RHEUMATIC HEART DISEASE

Richard Talbot

INTRODUCTION

It has been observed that the importance of this disease is out of proportion to its incidence for three reasons; first, in many cases it is completely preventable; second, it is largely a disease of children; and third, many cases have cardiac damage, producing years of compromised cardiac function.

Epidemiology

In developing countries, rheumatic fever and rheumatic heart disease continue to be major problems. Available information suggests incidence rates for rheumatic fever of about 100/100000 in younger age groups[1]. It has been observed that these figures are often an underestimation as less severe cases frequently go unreported. The mean prevalence for rheumatic heart disease in school children appears to be about 10/1000 [1].

In the developed world, incidence rates slowly declined between 1900 and 1940. This is thought to be due to improved standards of living with smaller families, better housing, and therefore less crowding. With the advent of antibiotics in the 1940s, the decline in incidence accelerated. It has been suggested that secondary prevention, to prevent recurrences, played a major role in this decline initially, while effective primary prevention projects took a further decade or so to be developed. In many countries, incidence rates are now well below 1/100000 [2]. This subject is excellently reviewed by Markowitz and Kaplan[3].

Between these two extremes, pockets of higher incidence of rheumatic fever are seen in the developed world[4]. These largely consist of ethnic minority groups – Australian Aborigines[5], New Zealand Maoris[6], Navajo Indians[7] etc. (Table 1). However, between 1984 and 1988, focal areas of resurgence were seen in civilian populations in the United States[8–24] – the largest being in the Intermountain area, where an eightfold increase was observed during an 18-month period[8]. There has been reasonable support for the observation that the majority of cases in these recent outbreaks came from white, middle class, rural or urban communities where crowding did not ap-

Table 1 Diagnoses recorded at monthly cardiac clinics (1973–1981) held in the Indian Health Service Hospital, Sells, Arizona. (Reproduced with kind permission from reference 7)

Total visits	962
Rheumatic fever and rheumatic heart disease	794*
Cardiomyopathy, toxic and idiopathic	92
Hypertensive heart disease	32
Congenital heart disease	30
Coronary heart disease	12

*Includes periodic examination of patients following documented rheumatic fever

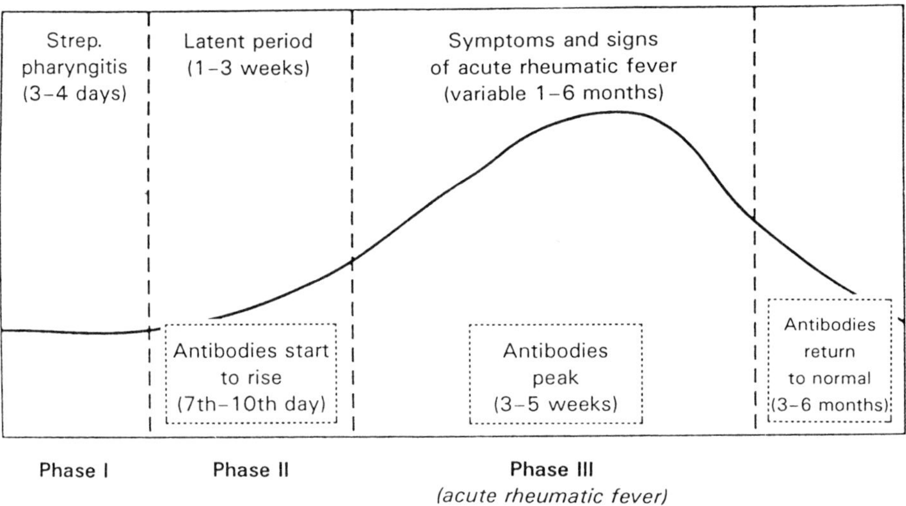

Figure 1 The course of acute rheumatic fever. Latent periods of over 35 days have been reported but these may be possibly due to reinfection

pear to be a major factor, and where preceding epidemics of streptococcal infections were not seen[4]. The explanation for these is not entirely clear although probably multifactorial, including an increase in streptococcal virulence[25–27] and a relaxation of the medical communities approach to diagnosis and treatment[4]. It has been suggested by Karey and Kaplan[20] that these may have been part of a more general increase in incidence rates in the United States. In addition to these civilian outbreaks, there were also at least two episodes in military establishments[28–32] – the first for many years – involving preceding epidemics of streptococcal pharyngitis in crowded conditions.

Etiology

Rheumatic fever is initiated by a Group A β-hemolytic streptococcal infection of the upper respiratory tract – usually pharyngitis. This typically lasts 3–4 days[34], although symptoms are recalled by only 35–50% of patients[34]. This is followed by a variable 'latent period' (1–3 weeks in the majority)[34] before the picture of rheumatic fever is seen in a relatively small proportion –

estimated at 3–30/1000 cases (endemic and epidemic situations, respectively) (Figure 1).

Rheumatic fever results from a dynamic interaction between the Group A β-hemolytic streptococcus, the host, and the environment[33] (Figure 2). There is strong support for the hypothesis that only some streptococci are 'rheumatogenic' and that this depends on the antigenic propensity of the M protein in their cell wall[35–39]. Only some M types, sharing a specific epitope with components of cardiac and joint tissue, appear to evoke the formation of cross-reacting antibodies[40–43]. Although this is the favored autoimmune mechanism, several cross reacting systems have been described, including a cross reaction between Group A streptococcal polysaccharide and glycoproteins from heart valves[44].

Rheumatogenicity may not be based entirely on autoimmunity[3,45,48]. It has been observed that rheumatogenic streptococci tend to be more virulent (with a greater capacity to invade the host), frequently with a mucoid growth form produced by large hyaluronic capsules, while they tend to

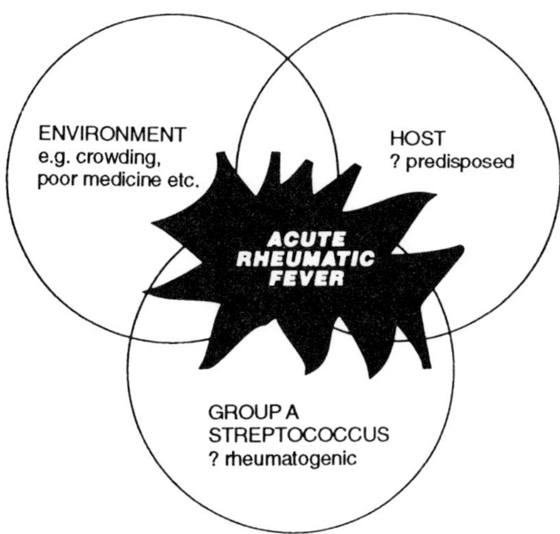

Figure 2 Dynamic interaction between Group A streptococcus, the host and the environment to produce acute rheumatic fever

be resistant to phagocytosis (a property largely conferred by M protein which masks complement receptors on the streptococcal cell surface, inhibiting opsonization and phagacytosis)[46,49]. This promotes longer convalescent carriage which is necessary to stimulate the immune reaction[48,50]. The streptococcus may also become more virulent with rapid passage from host to host[51].

Considering the host, rheumatic fever typically occurs between the ages of 6 and 15 years with a peak at about 8 years[33]. Although the disease incidence decreases after this period, this is thought to be at least partly due to the decreased exposure to streptococcal infection. Certainly, in conditions of crowding such as military camps, the incidence remains high until at least 22 years of age[52,53].

First, there appears to be a familial susceptibility to the acquisition of Group A streptococcal infections[51,58]. In an excellent study of 15 apparently susceptible and 15 non-susceptible families, conducted by Zimmerman and Wilson[51] it was shown that once a strain was introduced into susceptible families, it tended to 'ping pong' among family members, while in non-susceptible families, the infection tended to be self-limiting (Table 2). Cultures of all family members showed striking differences. Group A β-hemolytic streptococci were seen in almost all members of susceptible families but only 50% of non-susceptible families, while a significantly higher proportion of the susceptible group were M typable. Second, a familial tendency has been observed[54–57]. Surfaces of the peripheral blood non-T cells from individuals with a history of rheumatic fever have been demonstrated by the use of monoclonal antibodies to be antigenically distinct from the majority of the population[59,60]. This characteristic has also been shown to be present in a significantly higher proportion of relatives of rheumatic fever patients[61,62].

The lower incidence of rheumatic fever in adults is likely to be explained largely by the presence of antibodies to M proteins. Secretory IgA and IgG in saliva directed against streptococcal strep

Table 2 Results of throat cultures in 'susceptible' and 'non-susceptible' patients, showing higher proportion of Group A β-hemolytic streptococci in 'susceptible' families and higher proportion that were M typable. (From Zimmerman and Wilson[51] with permission)

Category of family	Total cultures	β-Hemolytic (%)	β-Hemolytic Group A (%)	Group A (%)	Typability (%) M Type	T Type
Carrier	722	45.7	92.7	42.4	57.8	94.1
Non-carrier	578	5.5	50.0	2.8	31.0	87.5

133

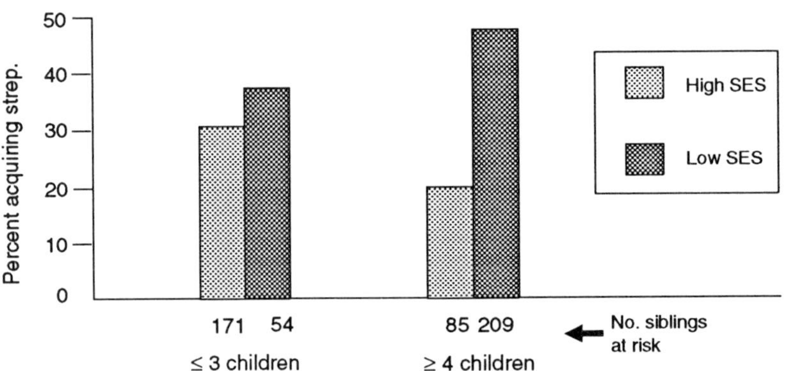

Figure 3 Risk of sibling streptococcal acquisition by socioeconomic status (SES) and size of family. (Reproduced with kind permission from reference 33)

C5a peptidase has recently been described and may also contribute[64].

Considering the environment, there is no doubt that rheumatic fever is a disease of poorer socio-economic groups. Urbanization and crowding are likely to be very important factors explaining both the epidemics during the industrial revolution in the West, and contributing to the apparent increase now seen in the underdeveloped world[63,143] (Figure 3). Lack of medical services in these situations is undoubtedly also important.

A seasonal variation in the prevalence of streptococcal pharyngitis is also frequently seen, e.g. an increase in the Fall in North America – probably due to poorer ventilation and greater crowding with the cooler weather, and the start of a new school year[33].

DIAGNOSIS AND TREATMENT OF STREPTOCOCCAL PHARYNGITIS
Diagnosis
A red throat is non-specific and the majority of cases of pharyngitis are non-streptococcal. Group A streptococci are found in about 35% of cases of pharyngitis in children. Only about half this group is accompanied by the antibody rise which signifies the tendency to develop suppur-

ative complications and the risk of rheumatic fever (the other half being carriers with little or no risk of spreading the disease and with symptoms for some other reason)[46,65–68](Figure 4).

An experienced physician makes a correct diagnosis of streptococcal pharyngitis on clinical grounds in about 50% of cases (75% if culture results are available from other patients)[67].

The predictive value of individual clinical manifestations is disappointing. Pharyngeal exudate is frequently seen in viral infections (Table 3), especially in infants and younger children. Anterior cervical adenitis is the best sign available, although only 30% of children in Wannamaker's study[66] with cervical adenitis had the combination of a positive culture and antibody response. From this study, its positive predictive value was 61%.

The keystone of diagnosis is the throat culture. This has to be carefully performed by an experienced operator. The technique is important. With the use of a tongue depressor and good lighting, a cotton or Dacron swab is vigorously rubbed over each tonsillar area without touching the tongue or lips[69–71]. Despite the desire of parents to be involved, in a series of 98 paired throat

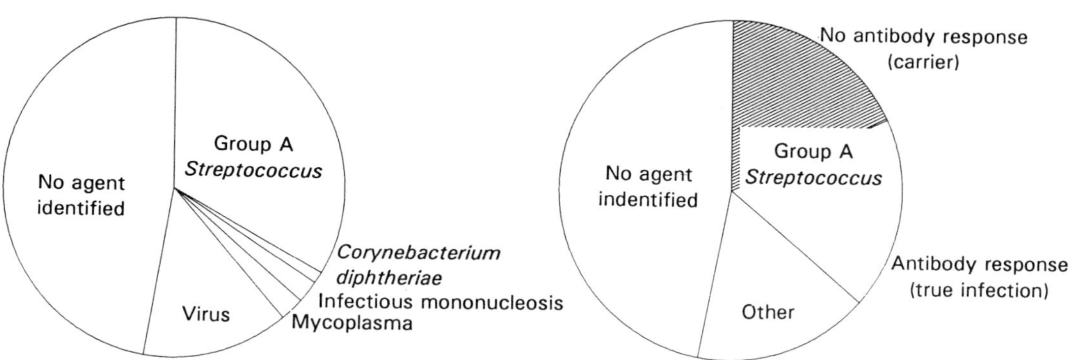

Figure 4 At left, estimated proportion of acute pharyngitis associated with various microbial agents. At right, proportion of children with clinical pharyngitis who develop a streptococcal antibody response. (Modified with kind permission from reference 66)

swabs, taken by doctors and parents, a 32% incidence of false negatives was shown with parents' throat swabs. This is clearly unreliable[72]. The solution in some situations may be to use skilled paramedical staff rather than abandon this idea completely.

With regard to the culture, a dry swab with silica gel can be used for postage. Streptococci may be kept for several days by this technique, indeed Taplin and Landsell isolated streptococci up to 1 month after sampling[21]. The swab is then inoculated onto a blood agar plate, streaked with a wire loop, and incubated at 37 °C for 24 h. β-Hemolytic streptococci are recognized by an area of clear hemolysis. Confirmation (in particular, differentiation from hemolytic staphylococci and gram-negative cocci) may need to be made by a gram stain. Group A streptococci are usually identified by their bacitracin sensitivity, employing a bacitracin disc on the culture plate[33].

A recent discussion of culture methods[34] suggests that an increase in yield of positive cultures may be obtained by the use of selective blood agar plates containing sulfamethoxazole trimethoprim inoculated anaerobically for 24 h and aerobically in the presence of 10% CO_2 for the second 24 h. In this study, 27% of their positive cultures were detected after 40 or more hours of

Table 3 Common features of streptococcal and viral pharyngitis. (Reproduced with kind permission from Dodu and Böthig[1])

	Streptococcal	*Viral*
Season	cool, rainy months	varies
Age	5–15 years	all ages
Onset	often abrupt	more gradual
Initial symptoms	painful to swallow	mild sore throat
Other symptoms	tender, cervical lymph nodes	runny nose hoarseness, cough
Pharyngeal appearance	redness, edema, exudate	redness, ulcers, vescicles

incubation. Obviously this adds considerably to the expense. Usually the only important organisms to identify are Group A β-hemolytic streptococci which so far are all sensitive to penicillin. If cost is a limiting factor in the performance of throat cultures, one may consider requesting the laboratory to perform a less expensive service by omitting identification of all bacterial species and sensitivity testing[73]. If there is no access to laboratory facilities, it is quite practicable for doctors to perform their own cultures with a small incubator, provided culture medium can be obtained[7,33].

Is one throat culture sufficient? Kaplan and colleagues studied paired cultures and showed that if only one culture had been obtained, 10% of patients with a positive culture would have been missed. The great majority of these exhibited only a light growth of streptococci on their second culture[65]. It could not be shown that this subgroup consisted mostly of carriers – one-third developed a significant serological response.

A 'bona fide infection' can be distinguished from a carrier only by the presence of Group A streptococcal antibodies[68]. The ASO titer is the most useful, being readily available and performed by most laboratories with reliable results. The normal value varies with age, geographical area etc.[74]. However, in the 6–14 year age group, a titer of 333 is considered borderline, while 500 indicates a recent streptococcal infection. Seventy-five to eighty percent of patients with an untreated streptococcal infection will show a rise in this titer, while increased accuracy may be obtained by the addition of antihyaluronidase and antistreptokinase titers, increasing the accuracy to 90% and 95% respectively[33]. Anti-DNAse B is also widely used – possibly its main advantage being that it is elevated longer than other streptococcal antibodies. It is of particular use in chorea for this reason[75]. The 'streptozyme' test, combin-

ing five antibodies in a single test is less accurate and is not recommended[76].

Because of the importance of starting treatment promptly, the decision is made on the basis of the clinical picture and the throat culture, accepting the fact that roughly half the cases treated are 'bona fide infections'[68], while the other half are carriers.

Reculturing following a course of treatment is not usually performed unless special circumstances exist, e.g. during an outbreak of acute rheumatic fever or acute nephritis in the community, following close contact with a known rheumatic fever case (on the assumption one is dealing with a 'rheumatogenic' strain), when the patient remains ill with signs and symptoms suggesting streptococcal pharyngitis[68], in known cases with rheumatic heart disease or a past history of rheumatic fever, or when there is *any* doubt about compliance with a full course of oral therapy.

Rapid streptococcal detection kits have been available for more than a decade. The technique depends on extraction of Group A carbohydrate from the cell wall and identification by one of a number of specific reactions. There are several good reviews[77,78].

Proponents argue that throat swabs processed by conventional means in the USA have little impact on patient management[77,79–81]. In a survey of Rhode Island physicians, Holmberg and Faich[79] pointed out that 87% of physicians prescribed antibiotics before the result of throat cultures were known, while 40% continued antibiotics for 10 days regardless of throat culture results. In another study[80], a negative culture caused 58% of physicians to discontinue antibiotics while 42% continued treatment. The major reason throat swabs were not used more effectively seemed to be the delay in obtaining the result.

136

The major argument against rapid detection kits is their lack of sensitivity. Although a specificity rate in the 'high nineties' is generally reported, there is a large problem with false negatives – the sensitivity varying from over 90% with 4+ cultures taken by conventional means to less than 50% with 1+ cultures[82]. A positive result from a rapid detection kit may be regarded as a reliable indication to start antibiotics, but a negative result *must* be confirmed by a conventional culture. From the point of view of epidemiological studies, this lack of sensitivity makes the rapid detection systems unacceptable while lack of isolation of the streptococcus prevents subsequent M typing[78].

M typing is not employed in the routine diagnosis of streptococcal pharyngitis, but becomes important in the epidemic situation and the development of a vaccine.

TREATMENT OF STREPTOCOCCAL PHARYNGITIS FOR PRIMARY PROPHYLAXIS OF RHEUMATIC FEVER

Recommended management of the individual

Having made a clinical diagnosis of streptococcal pharyngitis, one really has three choices[66]:

(1) Administer intramuscular benzathine penicillin immediately. This is the treatment of choice in a febrile, toxic patient with severe pharyngitis, in 'emergency room practices' or where there is any doubt whether the patient will be seen again for follow-up and in the patient with a past history of rheumatic fever or known rheumatic heart disease.

(2) Defer administration of penicillin until the results of the throat culture are known, and then give benzathine penicillin or a 10-day course of oral penicillin, depending on the reliability of the patient.

(3) Begin treatment with oral penicillin immediately. If the culture confirms a streptococcal infection, the time course of treatment may be abbreviated by giving benzathine penicillin. Oral penicillin could be discontinued in those with a negative culture.

For the recommended dose regimens, see Table 4[83].

Penicillin is the drug of choice. A single injection of benzathine penicillin (1.2 million units in adolescents and adults and 600 000–900 000 units in children) provides effective eradication of the streptococcus in the majority of cases. It has the advantage of prolonged action, preventing re-infection for several weeks[84]. Although the early studies of Chamovitz and co-workers[85] claimed a 99% success rate as determined by throat cultures at 21 days, this would seem over optimistic today. Several later series demonstrated a failure to eradicate the streptococcus from up to 18% of cases on repeat culture[86,87], while Kaplan[88] reported a failure rate of 25–30% recently. It is unclear how much of this problem is due to poor compliance, re-exposure to homologous streptococci in the household etc., and how much is due to penicillin tolerance, with failure of the antibiotic to eradicate the organism[86,87,89]. It is also unclear what proportion of these cases where failure to eradicate the organism has been demonstrated are, in fact, carriers, and therefore of little consequence.

The main disadvantage of benzathine penicillin is the local discomfort at the injection site. In one large series, three-quarters of the patients complained of discomfort, lasting 24–48 h[85]. Pain at the time of injection can be reduced by drawing up 1–2 ml of 1% lignocaine following the penicillin and then injecting the former slowly, first. A small amount of procaine penicillin mixed with the benzathine penicillin will also help. Care

Table 4 Recommended treatment for streptococccal pharyngitis (WHO Technical Report Series[83])

Antibiotic	Delivery route	Dose
Benzathine benzylpenicillin	intramuscular	1 200 000 units for adults & children weighing > 30 kg; 600 000–900 000 units for children weighing < 30 kg (given as a single injection)
Phenoxymethylpenicillin[a, b]	oral	250 mg , q.i.d. for 10 days; children weighing < 20 kg, 125 mg q.i.d.

The following drugs are effective, but usually not recommended: amoxycillin, ampicillin, cephalosporins, clindamycin, dicloxacillin; the following are not effective or are contraindicated: chloramphenicol, sulfonamides, tetracyclines, trimethoprim. (a) Phenoxymethylpenicillin is the preferred oral formulation because of its more reliable absorption; if it is not available, benzylpenicillin may be used. (b) For patients allergic to penicillin, oral erythromycin is an accepted alternative; the recommended dose is 250 mg, 4 times daily. For children weighing less than 25 kg, 40 mg kg^{-1} day^{-1}, not to exceed 1 g, divided into two to four doses. In regions with erythromycin resistance, cephalosporins are acceptable, bearing in mind that patients sensitive to penicillins may also be allergic to cephalosporins

must be taken that the full dose of benzathine penicillin is, however, given.

A 10-day course of oral penicillin is a reasonable alternative *provided* it is taken reliably. The problem of non-compliance of patients on oral therapy is *very* large and is a powerful argument against this form of treatment unless the physician is extremely confident of the reliability of the patient and/or family. Many reviews of this subject report disappointing results. Bergman and Werner[90] reported 56% of their patients had discontinued penicillin by the 3rd day and 82% by the 9th day. Leistyna and Macaulay[91], in a series from private practice, reported that 89% of 162 children completed the course. For this reason it is recommended that a follow-up visit and repeat throat culture is performed in all patients who have been prescribed oral therapy.

Allergic reactions to penicillin have been reported in between 0.7% and 8% of treatment courses. The main danger is immediate hypersensitivity (type I) reactions. Anaphylactic reactions occur in 0.015% to 0.004% penicillin treatment courses[92]. The incidence of fatality from a single course of penicillin lies between 0.0015% and 0.002% – roughly one death per 50 000–100 000 treatment courses[92]. Youth and middle-aged adults are reported to have the greatest risk for an acute allergic reaction, which is rather less frequent in children[92,93]. Orally administered penicillin produces fewer allergic reactions than parenteral penicillin[94]. Sullivan and colleagues[94] in a search of the literature, discovered only nine anaphylactic deaths after oral penicillin – a comparatively minute number compared with those reported after parenteral administration[50]. Although reactions of any kind to benzathine penicillin are reported to be more common (2.24% injections given)[95], serious allergic reactions or death are extremely uncommon, and this risk is justified by the long-term advantages of prophylaxis.

In patients allergic to penicillin, erythromycin 125–250 mg four times daily for 10 days is the drug of choice. However, resistant streptococcal strains have been reported[96]. Tetracycline, given in a similar dose, is very much a third choice as an increasing number of resistant Group A streptococci have been encountered – exceeding 40% in some series[97].

Table 5 Recurrent cases of rheumatic fever with same M-type on throat culture (signifying failure to eradicate infection). (Reproduced with kind permission from reference 98)

	Total	Same M-type	Different M-type	No growth
Recurrences rheumatic fever	76	46 (61%)	16 (21%)	14 (18%)
Treated (recurrences and non-recurrences)	5 198	1 040 (20%)	520 (10%)	3 638 (70%)

As discussed previously, even with good management, treatment failures do occur[98]. Catanzaro and co-workers[98], reviewing 5198 cases of Group A streptococcal pharyngitis treated in a military establishment, showed that rheumatic fever subsequently developed in 76 (1.46%). Most of these were felt to be explained by the failure to eliminate the infecting streptococcus. Despite apparently adequate therapy 61% of cases continued to harbor the original infecting organism (Table 5).

Although, in the epidemic situation, such as that described by Catanzaro and colleagues, a further course of antibiotic treatment was definitely indicated, a positive result on reculturing presents a far lower danger in the endemic situation. As shown by Kaplan and co-workers[65], these children are likely to be 'carriers' who infrequently spread the organism to other individuals. Typically, they have non-typable organisms with absence of the typical antibody response. It has been suggested that this carrier state may be important in the development of type-specific antibodies and should not be interfered with by repeat courses of antibiotics. Although theoretically attractive, this has not been demonstrated to be a problem in long-term primary prevention projects.

An important contribution to the subject of carriers versus 'bona fide infections' has recently been published by Gray and associates[99] and commented on by Denny[100]. In a 12-week study of 736 US Marine Corps recruits, hyperendemic streptococcal infection is reported despite treatment of 93% with benzathine penicillin at 30–39-day intervals. A total of 42% of treated cases were demonstrated by a rise in antibodies to have a streptococcal infection and could not be regarded as simply carriers. To prevent this, it was concluded that an appropriate antibiotic such as erythromycin had to be administered to recruits with penicillin allergy, to prevent a 'bacterial reservoir' within the population.

Amoxycillin with clavulanate (Augmentin®) can also be used. Boschi and co-workers[103], in an uncontrolled trial of amoxycillin with clavulanate as initial therapy in 162 children with streptococcal pharyngitis, showed it to be 'efficacious and well-tolerated'. A total of 77.6% remained bacteriologically cured 26 days after the course of therapy. Side-effects severe enough to necessitate discontinuation of therapy were seen in three (diarrhea, rash, edema). In those patients with streptococcal pharyngitis who failed penicillin therapy[101] or with recurrent acute streptococcal pharyngitis[102,103], amoxycillin–clavulanate therapy appears to be substantially superior to penicillin although it should be noted a similar course costs about twice as much as oral penicillin. Kaplan and Johnson[101] reported a series of 131 patients with Group A streptococcal throat

Table 6 A comparison of retreatment of upper respiratory tract persistence of Group A streptococci after oral penicillin V with a second course of oral penicillin V and with amoxycillin plus clavulanate potassium (Augmentin). (Reproduced with kind permission from reference 101)

Treatment	Total no. treated	No. treated with antibiotic	Treatment failures	
			No.	%
Initial treatment	131	oral penicillin V	50	38
First treatment*	45	oral penicillin V (24)	17	71
retreatment		Augmentin (21)	2	9
Second treatment	19	Augmentin (17)	3	18
retreatment		oral penicillin V (2)	1	50

* Total course of retreatment: Augmentin 38, with five (13%) treatment failures; oral penicillin V 26, with 18 (69%) treatment failures ($p < 0.01$)

infections, of whom 45 continued to harbor Group A streptococci after an initial 10-day course of penicillin. Significantly more successful eradication was achieved with a course of Augmentin than a further course of penicillin (Table 6).

In Brook's relatively small series of 37 patients, the infecting organism was eradicated by penicillin in 70% of patients and by amoxycillin-clavulanate potassium in 100% of patients[102]. At 1-year follow-up, 11 of the 19 penicillin-treated patients and two of the 18 amoxycillin–clavulanate-treated patients had suffered recurrent streptococcal tonsillitis[104]. However, in another small series reported by Tanz and colleagues[104] β-lactamase production was seen in only a quarter of treatment failures, suggesting that amoxycillin–clavulanate is likely to have a relatively small advantage over penicillin. Other suggested reasons for penicillin failure in this series were; poor compliance, inadvertent inclusion of chronic carriers, and re-infection with a new T type. Further work is needed here, incorporating streptococcal antibodies to assess the role of streptococcal carriers in this group of apparent treatment failures on penicillin therapy.

Another argument against prompt initiation of penicillin therapy is that it has no influence on the symptomatic course of the acute pharyngitis[66]. In fact, two carefully conducted, placebo-controlled, randomized, double-blind trials show otherwise[105,106]. In the study of Krober and colleagues[106] (Figure 5), it was observed that the penicillin-treated patients were all afebrile within 24 h. Most displayed significantly symptomatic improvement and as their throat cultures were negative, they were presumably no longer contagious and could return to school. This was in contrast to the control group where symptoms, fever and positive throat cultures persisted for 48 h – a small difference but worth considering.

Crowe and co-workers[107] performed *in vivo* studies, observing the inhibitory action of normal throat flora for Group A streptococci, suggesting this as a mechanism for the apparent resistance to infection in adults and some children. More recently[108,109] the practical application of this has been demonstrated in patients with recurrent streptococcal pharyngitis. Grahne and colleagues[108] showed a significantly lower incidence of relapse or new infection in patients treated with antibiotic and α-streptococcal

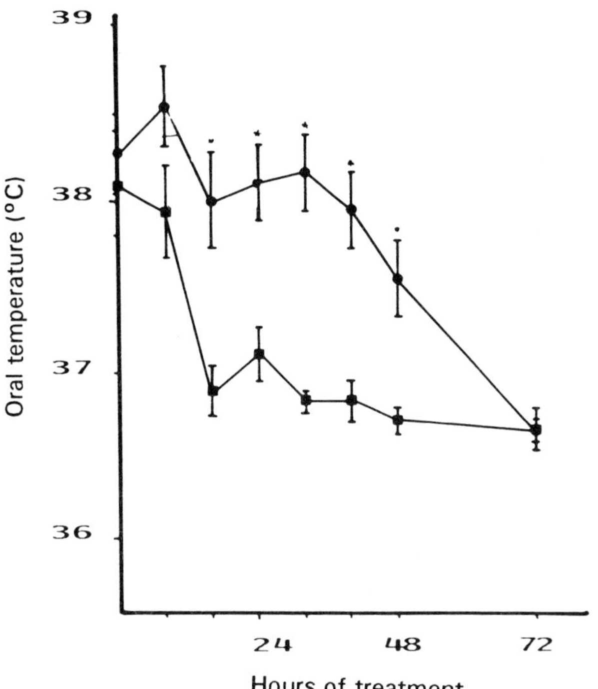

Figure 5 Comparison of persistence of fever (mean temperature of each group) in penicillin- (squares) and placebo-treated (circles) culture-positive patients during initial 72-h period of observation. Significance (asterisks), determined by Student's *t*-test ($p < 0.01$). (Reproduced with kind permission from reference 106)

strains sprayed in their mouth, compared with those treated with antibiotic alone.

Before invading the pharyngeal tissue, streptococci bind to fibronectin on epithelial cells via surface lipotheicoic acid with local cytotoxicity produced by streptolysin. This initial adhesion and cytotoxicity has been shown to be markedly reduced by pretreatment with lipotheicoic acid[110]. β-Lactamase production by upper respiratory tract flora may prevent penicillin from being effective[102]. As discussed above, amoxycillin-clavulanate may inhibit this action.

It has also been suggested that penicillinase-producing staphylococci may interfere with penicillin treatment of streptococci. Quie and associates[111] were unable to demonstrate that this was particularly important.

Antistreptococcal vaccine remains a hope for the future. Although work proceeds on this, as observed by Markowitz and Kaplan[3], it has not been high on the research agendas of developed countries due to the disappearance of rheumatic fever. The recent resurgence in the United States may give further encouragement to work in this area[39]. Major obstacles to the development of a vaccine have been the many serological types and the risk of allergic reactions[35,36]. The problem is that streptococcal M-protein is the antigen that is necessary to evoke the production of type-specific antibodies but this also evokes cross-reacting antibodies damaging cardiac tissue. Work proceeds on the identification and purification of an M-protein epitope that is able to evoke type specific antibodies without producing cross-reactive antibodies[40]. It has recently been observed that Group A streptococci can be divided into two major classes, depending on the presence or absence of antigenic epitopes within the 'C repeat' region of the M-protein, and that the vast majority of 'rheumatogenic' serotypes appear to fall into Class I[42,43].

COMMUNITY STUDIES
Historical basis and early work, including military studies

Sulfonamides were shown to be effective in preventing streptococcal infections in rheumatic subjects during the 1940s[112]. However, they were not effective in the treatment of established streptococcal pharyngitis[113]. Goerner, Massell, and Jones[114] were the first to demonstrate the effectiveness of a 10-day course of oral penicillin in reducing the incidence of recurrences in a group of rheumatic subjects.

Subsequently, Denny and colleagues[115] in the classic study at Warren Airforce Base, demonstrated that a depot preparation of procaine penicillin G in oil with 2% aluminum monostearate given to patients with streptococcal pharyngitis, would almost completely prevent the subsequent attack of rheumatic fever. Only two cases of definite rheumatic fever were seen in 798 treated streptococcal infections in contrast to 17 cases in 804 controls. These results were confirmed in subsequent studies and the dosage regimen refined by Wannamaker and associates[116]. Dibenzylethylenediamine (DBED) penicillin G ('benzathine') was introduced soon afterwards. The first reports of its use in treatment of streptococcal pharyngitis were from Stollerman and Rusoff[117] and Chamovitz and co-workers[85]. Compared with procaine penicillin it had the advantage of needing only a single injection and was at least as effective.

It has been demonstrated that streptococci must be eradicated from the pharynx for rheumatic fever to be prevented[98] and that penicillin administered as late as 9 days after the onset of streptococcal pharyngitis will be successful[118]. Another successful, early, large scale military program was reported much later[84]. Here, either mass prophylaxis (to stop epidemics) or treatment of new recruits only (to prevent epidemics) was used. By giving the latter in the 2nd week of a 9-week course, only two episodes of rheumatic fever among 58 000 recruits were seen over a 1-year period. It was observed that if the training period was greater than 9 weeks, probably more than one injection of benzathine penicillin was needed. However, the situation is unlikely to be as straightforward as this, considering the recent

study of Gray and colleagues[99]. (*See* comments in 'Treatment' section.)

Applicability of military approach to civilian populations

Following the success of the military studies, applicability of the same strategies to civilian populations was investigated. It was obvious one was dealing with a very different situation. Although the military situation had the advantage of excellent organization for case finding and efficient treatment, allowing very accurate epidemiological reporting, the age and sex distribution of the population was very limited, the period of observation relatively short, and living conditions regimented and unnaturally crowded. Furthermore, the military studies dealt with epidemics of streptococcal pharyngitis or scarlet fever with a high rheumatic fever attack rate of about 3%. Could one apply similar control strategies to school children? Early studies showed that in the endemic situation, streptococcal pharyngitis tended to be milder with a low incidence of rheumatic fever[119–121]. The only controlled study of streptococcal pharyngitis in a pediatric population was conducted by Siegel and colleagues[49]. Here, no cases of rheumatic fever were seen in 605 treated children, while two cases of rheumatic fever and one case of glomerulonephritis was seen in 608 controls – an insignificant difference. Comparisons between episodes of streptococcal pharyngitis seen in this study and at Fort Warren Airforce Base are interesting (Table 7). In general, civilian episodes were much milder with shorter convalescent carriage, while the multiplicity of M types differed from the few seen during a military epidemic. It was concluded that 'all streptococcal disease cannot be equated with the risk of rheumatic fever and acute glomerulonephritis but must be defined in terms of the virulence and epidemicity of the infecting strains.' To have any impact on the civilian population, it was concluded that much larger numbers would need to be screened and

Table 7 Comparison of streptococcal pharyngitis at the Children's Memorial Hospital (CMH) and the Warren Airforce Base (WAFB). (Reproduced with kind permission from reference 49)

	CMH	WAFB
Pharyngeal exudate (%)	40	100
Temperature >101°F (%)	30	80
White cell count >12 000 (%)	21	75
Group A streptococci (%)	86	80
Typable Group A streptococci (%)	52	92
Convalescent carrier state for 21 days (%)	29	80
Initial antistreptolysin O titer (U/ml)	285	126
Magnitude of rise (U/ml)	165	248
Patients with significant rise (%)	45	85

treated, leading to an expansion of civilian programs to relatively large population groups with screening and treating of large numbers of children via the classroom[122–128]. Taken to the extreme, programs were very demanding. As noted by Cornfeld and associates[125], to be effective in the endemic situation, over half the children in the school and many family contacts had to be treated each year with penicillin while, if children were excluded from school until cultures were negative, this might involve 50% or more of the school population at some time during the year. A more realistic approach, perhaps, is reported by Jackson and colleagues[128] – an enthusiastic program based on a private general practice in a rural area of high endemicity concentrating on efficient culturing and treatment, with reculturing of patients and also treatment of household contacts. Cooperation was excellent.

At least six successful, sustained programs, targeting school children in areas of high endemicity and using mass culturing techniques, have been reported. These have been successful in impressively reducing the prevalence of streptococcal pharyngitis. Their impact on the incidence of rheumatic fever is more difficult to assess, espe-

cially superimposed on the national decline, although several programs have suggested that this was also achieved. The first of these was established in 1954 in Casper, Wyoming by Phibbs and colleagues[129,130]. This was a legally enforced mass culture program. Symptomatic children were located daily in the schoolroom by questioning. These children and one row of asymptomatic children were sent daily to a central nursing station where their throats were examined and a culture taken of all cases with a red throat, exudate, adenopathy or fever. Children with a positive culture were sent home and were not permitted back until they had a physician's letter saying that adequate treatment had been started. If repeat throat swabs were positive or siblings had positive cultures, the family was also encouraged to have cultures. Benzathine penicillin was encouraged as the treatment of choice. With this very enthusiastic program, a marked fall in the prevalence of Group A streptococcal pharyngitis was seen, compared with neighboring communities (Figure 6). In an impressive follow up of the 10-year period 1973–1982[130] an average of 1.7 cases of rheumatic fever per 100 000 population was seen annually in the treatment area compared with 6.4/100 000 in the rest of Wyoming. Two similar programs were reported in Colorado. Zimmerman and co-workers[131] were able to show a significant reduction in streptococcal prevalence despite a simpler design, concentrating on parent education, procurement of throat swabs, even if no obvious pharyngitis, voluntary (rather than enforced) treatment, and the employment of volunteers to keep expenses down (Figure 7).

Jackson and colleagues[128] and Jackson[132], also in Colorado, experimented with various strategies and found a less vigorous program with monthly throat cultures of all pupils, using volunteers (and exclusion of children with positive cultures from school) also gave satisfactory results with regard to the streptococcal population. Successful programs involving Alaskan na-

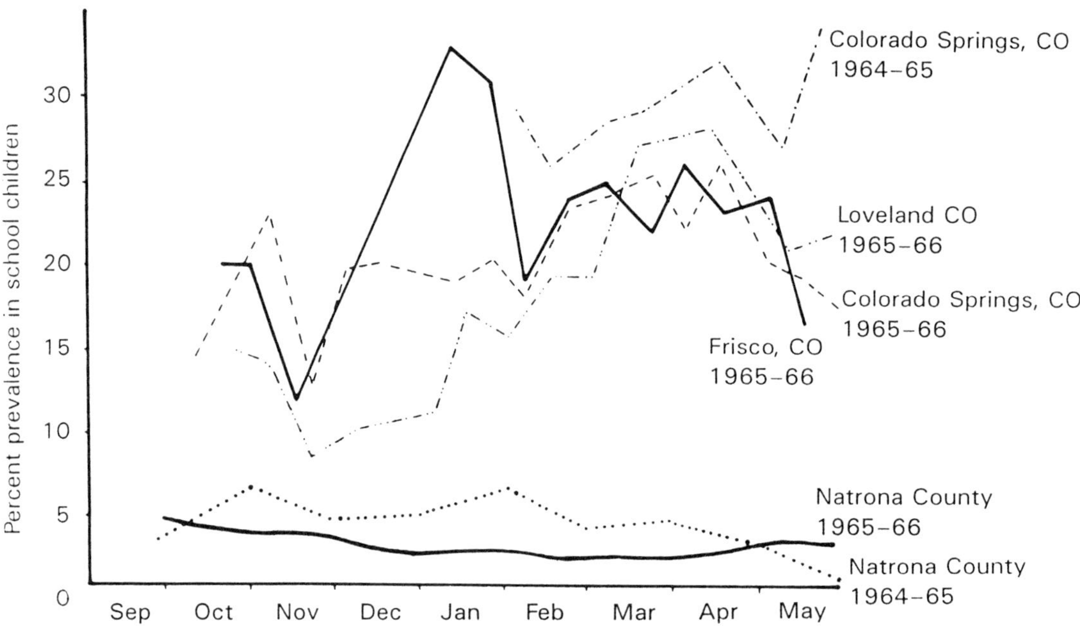

Figure 6 Streptococcal isolation rates in school children, Casper, Natrona County, Wyoming, during school years 1964–65 and 1965–66, compared with rates in children in three Colorado communities. (Adapted with kind permission from reference 129)

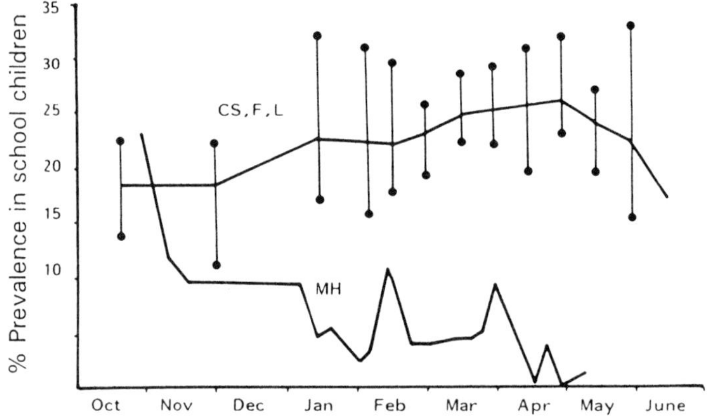

Figure 7 Comparison of prevalence of Group A streptococcus in Mosca-Hooper (M-H), 1969–70, with rates in Colorado Springs, Frisco and Loveland (CS,F,L). The vertical lines represent minimum and maximum prevalence rates observed. (Reproduced with kind permission from reference 131)

tives[133,134] and native Indians of Arizona[7] have also been reported. This last program is particularly noteworthy for the practical contribution of tribal members including running their own bacteriology laboratory. The claim was made that 'streptococcal detection and treatment are simple and inexpensive and could be implemented on a large scale in any country in the world.'[7].

144

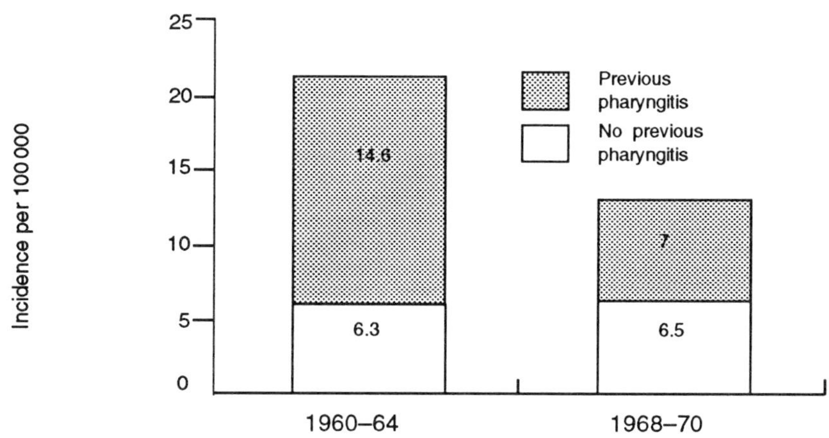

Figure 8 Change in the annual incidence of first attacks of rheumatic fever in relation to preceding clinical respiratory infection. (Reproduced with kind permission from reference 135)

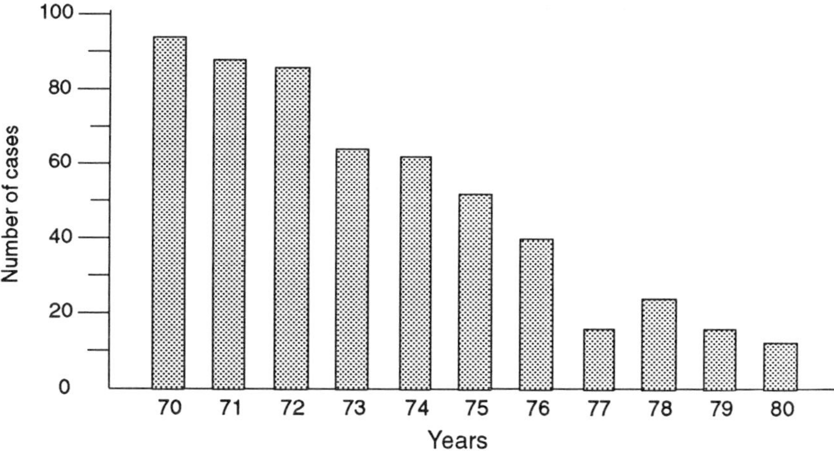

Figure 9 Decline in new cases of rheumatic fever admitted to the Children's Hospital, Costa Rica. (Reproduced with kind permission from reference 137)

The most compelling argument for targeted primary prevention of rheumatic fever is the study of Gordis[135]. Here, Blacks in poor census tract areas of inner city Baltimore, eligible or ineligible for comprehensive care programs, were compared. The incidence of first attacks of rheumatic fever in the comprehensive care tracts decreased by 60% between the two study periods but remained unchanged in the rest of Baltimore (Table 8). The decline was limited to those who gave a retrospective history of a respiratory infection and was unchanged in other cases, suggesting the critical factor was medical care rather than other factors such as improved housing (Figure 8).

Targeting of programs on high-incidence groups is important. Chun and co-workers[136] reported a

Table 8 Change in incidence of rheumatic fever in the study population eligible for comprehensive care programs as compared with non-eligible predominantly Black tracts and all of Baltimore. (Reproduced with kind permission from reference 135)

| | 1960–64 | | | 1968–70 | | | |
| | No. of cases | 1960 population | Annual incidence/ 100 000 | No. of cases | 1970 population | Annual incidence/ 100 000 | Net change (%) |
Tract							
Eligible	51	38 022	26.8	11	34 609	10.6	− 60.4
Non-eligible: >90% Black	15	21 466	14.0	20	37 433	17.8	+ 27.0
All tracts	77	73 518	20.9	42	104 086	13.5	− 35.4

primary streptococcal control program in Hawaiian schools over a 4-year period. Methods were very similar to those of Phibbs and colleagues[129]. Children were excluded from school until they had been treated. Despite this, rheumatic fever occurred with equal frequency in participating and non-participating schools. It was observed that rheumatic fever was very much more frequent in Samoan children and it was suggested that 'further school-based primary prevention efforts . . . should be intensive in nature and targeted on high risk populations'.

Where there is a very high overall incidence, one obviously has no need to target certain groups. With the extension of ambitious primary care programs, Costa Rica claims an enormous fall in the incidence of rheumatic fever over the decade 1970–1980, attributed to the 'increased general use of benzathine penicillin throughout the country for streptococcal infection.' An 87% reduction in new cases of rheumatic fever was noted during this period[137] (Figure 9).

OBSTACLES TO SUCCESSFUL PRIMARY PREVENTION

This subject is conveniently approached by considering the figure from Gordis and colleagues[138] (Figure 10). About two-thirds of all cases of

rheumatic fever are theoretically preventable by attention firstly to public education and medical facilities, and secondly by appropriate investigation and management by the doctor.

Markowitz[63] lists five main obstacles to the prevention of first attacks:

(1) The size of the population at risk;

(2) The lack of public awareness that sore throats may lead to heart disease;

(3) Inaccessibility of adequate primary care facilities for the groups that need it most;

(4) Imperfect methods for diagnosing streptococcal pharyngitis; and

(5) Ignorance on the part of many physicians that prompt treatment of a 'strep throat' can prevent rheumatic fever.

The problem is eloquently summarized by Phibbs and co-workers[129]; 'Children with streptococcal pharyngitis usually do not receive adequate diagnosis or treatment for the following reasons:

(1) Antigenically significant streptococcal phar-

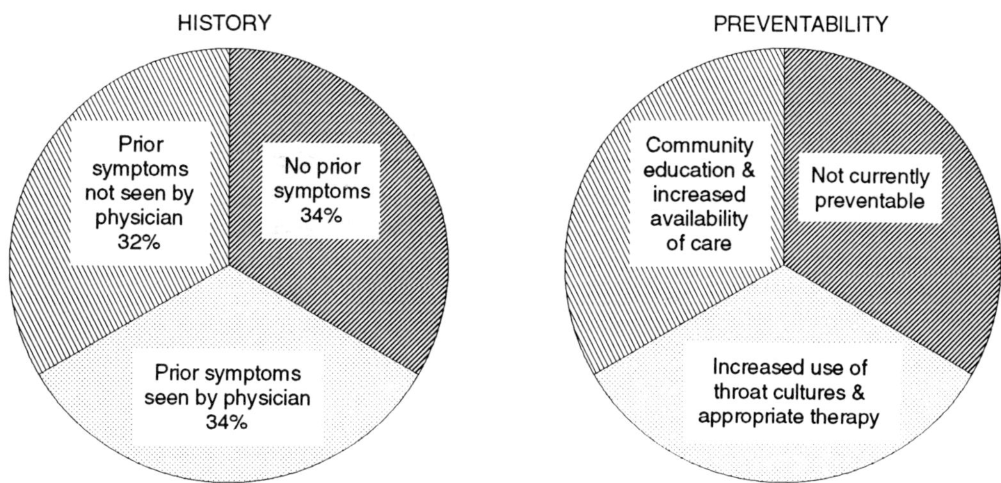

Figure 10 History (percentages) of preceding respiratory infection in 261 patients with first attacks of rheumatic fever in Baltimore (1960–64). (Reproduced with kind permission from reference 138)

yngitis is often so mild that the victim never brings it to anyone's attention;

(2) Most parents, when informed of symptoms of pharyngitis, do not call a physician but rely on throat lozenges, gargles and aspirin for any of the milder forms of the disease;

(3) Most physicians do not take throat cultures routinely on all cases of pharyngitis, and a great many do not treat streptococcal pharyngitis adequately even after it has been diagnosed; and

(4) Conventionally, therefore, the only victims of streptococcal pharyngitis who will receive adequate diagnosis and treatment will be children with severe symptoms who describe these symptoms to unusually well educated, medically orientated parents, who in turn call an exceptionally alert physician.'

Attention to these obstacles necessitates a three-pronged approach:

(1) Efficient and knowledgeable medical and paramedical staff able to diagnose and treat streptococcal pharyngitis.

In the western world, the main problem is often 'bridging the gap' between what we know (or should know) and what we actually practice. Three early studies from the USA[139–141] emphasized this – in the majority of cases with acute rheumatic fever who had visited a doctor previously with upper respiratory infections, only a small number were treated appropriately. Perhaps surprisingly, an analysis of cases from four recent outbreaks in the USA show very similar figures[3] (Table 9).

In the underdeveloped world, the main problem is insufficient trained doctors and medical facilities. Success relies therefore on a large network of nurses, paramedics, teachers and lay health workers – focusing efforts on areas of high incidence, especially via schools.

(2) Health education leading to appropriate behavior by parents and children when a sore

Table 9 Failure to prevent acute rheumatic fever. A comparison of observations from early studies with the recent resurgence in the United States. (Reproduced with kind permission from references 3, 140, 141)

	Czoniczer 1961	Grossmen, Stamler 1963	Salt Lake City 1985–86	Columbus 1984–86	NE Ohio 1986	Pittsburgh 1985–86
Number or rheumatic fever patients for whom some data available	105	110	50	40	23	17
History of sore throat respiratory illness	89 (84.8%)	94 (85.5%)	NA* (33%)	27 (67%)	18 (78%)	6 (35%)
Seen by doctor	36	62	11	6	11	4
Culture taken	—	17	11	6	NA*	2
Treated appropriately	0	10	8	6	11	2

*NA = not available

throat occurs. This is an essential part of any project. In the western world, it tends to be forgotten – an inappropriately large proportion of the health budget going to hospitals and 'high technology.' Parents and teachers must be involved. Children can transmit information to parents[142]. Television should be used more. Even the illiterate in an underdeveloped country can often be reached by this means.

(3) Policy change and support from health authorities at local and central government level. In the western world, the recent resurgence in the USA reminds us that this is not a problem that can be disregarded. Continued financial support is necessary to maintain an efficient primary prevention policy and, hopefully, for the eventual development of the vaccine. 'Pockets' of high incidence must also be targeted with appropriate use of health facilities.

In developing countries, governments often need to give higher priority to primary prevention, linking this with education and appropriate health care facilities. Massive social and financial obstacles have to be overcome with programs combining courage, originality and compromise[7,19,142].

REFERENCES

1. Dodu SR, Böthig S. Rheumatic fever and rheumatic heart disease in developing countries. World Health Forum. 1989; 10:203–212
2. Hoffman S, Henrichsen J, Schmidt K. Incidence and diagnosis of acute rheumatic fever in Denmark, 1980 and 1983. A retrospective analysis of the fulfillment of the Jones criteria in hospitalized patients. Acta Med Scand. 1988; 224:587–594
3. Markowitz M, Kaplan EL. Re-appearance of rheumatic fever. Adv Pediatr. 1989; 36:39–65
4. Talbot RG. Pockets of rheumatic fever in the developed world. XI World Congress of Cardiology. Plenary session I. Rheumatic Fever. Manila, Phillipines, February. 1990
5. Brennan RE, Patel MS. Acute rheumatic fever and rheumatic heart disease in a central Australian aboriginal community. Med J Aust. 1990; 153:335–337
6. Talbot RG. Rheumatic fever in the Hamilton health district: a nine year prospective study. NZ Med J. 1988; 101:406–408
7. Atha M, Enos E, Frank C et al. How an American

148

Indian tribe controlled the streptococcus. World Health Forum. 1982, 3:423–428

8. Veasey LG, Wiedmeier SE, Orsmond GS *et al.* Resurgence of acute rheumatic fever in the intermountain area of the United States. N Engl J Med. 1987; 316:421–427

9. Centers for Disease Control. Acute rheumatic fever – Utah. MMWR. 1987; 36:108–115

10. Odio A. Resurgence of acute rheumatic fever (letter). N Engl J Med. 1987; 317:507

11. Hosier DM, Craenen JM, Teske DW, Wheller JJ. Resurgence of acute rheumatic fever. AJDC. 1987; 141:730–733

12. Marcon MJ, Hribar MM, Hosier DM, Powell DA, Brady MT, Hamoudi AC, Kaplan EL. Occurrence of mucoid M18 *Streptococcus pyogenes* in a central Ohio pediatric population. J Clin Microbiol. 1988; 26:1539–1542

13. Congeni B, Rizzo C, Congeni J, Sreenevasan VV. Outbreak of acute rheumatic fever in northeast Ohio. J Pediatr. 1987; 111:176–179

14. Wald ER, Dashefsky B, Feidt C, Chiponis D, Byers C. Acute rheumatic fever in western Pennsylvania and the Tristate area. Pediatrics. 1987; 80:371–374

15. Burns DL, Ginsburg CM. Recrudescence of acute rheumatic fever in Dallas, Texas (abstract). Pediatric Res. 1987; 496:256

16. Giardina AC. Resurgence of acute rheumatic fever (letter). N Engl J Med. 1987; 317:507–508

17. Giardina AC, Heaton S. Acute rheumatic fever in New York city. N Engl J Med. 1988; 88:385–386

18. Hosier DM. Resurgence of acute rheumatic fever. NY State J Med. 1988; 88:352–353

19. Quinn RW. Comprehensive review of morbidity–mortality trends for rheumatic fever, streptococcal disease and scarlet fever: the decline of rheumatic fever. Rev Infect Dis. 1989; 6:928–953

20. Karey REW, Kaplan EL. Resurgence of acute rheumatic fever. Results of a survey of pediatric cardiologists. Pediatr Res. 1989; 25: 101A

21. Taplin D, Landsell L. Value of dessicated swabs for streptococcal epidemiology in the field. Appl Microbiol. 1973; 25:135

22. Leggiadro RJ, Birnbaum SE, Chase NA, Myers LK. A resurgence of acute rheumatic fever in a mid-south children's hospital. South Med J 1990; 83:1418–1420

23. Mason T, Fisher M, Kujala G. Acute rheumatic fever in West Virginia – not just a disease of children. Arch Intern Med. 1991; 151:133–136

24. Westlake RM, Graham TP, Edwards KM. An outbreak of rheumatic fever in Tennessee. Pediatr Infec Dis J. 1990; 9:97–100

25. Bartter T, Dascal A, Carroll K, Curley FJ. 'Toxic strep syndrome' A manifestation of Group A streptococcal infection. Arch Intern Med. 1988; 148:1421–1424

26. Cone LA, Woodard DR, Schlievert PM, Tomory GS. Clinical and bacteriological observations of a toxic shock-like syndrome due to *Streptococcus pyogenes*. N Engl J Med. 1987; 317:146–149

27. Stevens DL, Tanner MH, Winship J, Swarts R *et al.* Severe Group A streptococcal infections associated with a toxic shock-like syndrome and scarlet fever toxin A. N Engl J Med. 1989; 321:1–7

28. Centers for Disease Control. Acute rheumatic fever at a naval training centre – San Diego, California. JAMA. 1988; 259:1786–1787

29. Wallace MR, Garst PD, Papadimos TJ, Oldfield EC. The return of rheumatic fever in young adults. JAMA. 1989; 262: 2557–2561

30. Papadimos T, Escamilla J, Garst P, Oldfield E *et al.* Acute rheumatic fever at a navy training center. MMWR 1988; 37

31. Centers for Disease Control. Acute rheumatic fever among army trainees – Fort Leonard Wood, Missouri, 1987–1988. MMWR 1988; 37: 519–522

32. Sampson GL, Williams RG, House MD, Wetzel NE. Acute rheumatic fever among army trainees – Fort Leonard Wood, Missouri. JAMA. 1988; 260:2185–2188

33. Markowitz M, Gordis L. Rheumatic Fever. 2nd edn, Philadelphia: WB Saunders, 1972

34. Rammelkamp CH Jr, Stolzer BL. The latent period before the onset of rheumatic fever. Yale J Biol Med. 1961; 34:386

35. Stollerman GH. Nephritogenic and rheumatogenic streptococci. J Infect Dis. 1969; 120:258–263

36. Stollerman GH. The relative rheumatogenicity of strains of Group A streptococci. Mod Concepts Cardiovasc Dis. 1975; 44:35–40

37. Johnson DR, Kaplan EL. Type specific bactericidal antibody prevalence supports hypothesis that multiple serotypes are associated with US rheumatic fever resurgence. XI Lancefield In-

ternational Symposium on Streptococci and Streptococcal Diseases 1990. Siena, Italy

38. Johnson DW, Wlazlo A, Kaplan EL. Group A streptococci isolated from uncomplicated pharyngitis during a resurgence of suppurative sequelae in the United States: comparison with serotypes associated with sepsis. XI Lancefield International Symposium on Streptococci and Streptococcal Diseases. 1990. Siena, Italy

39. Stollerman GH. Rheumatogenic strains of group A streptococci (*S. pyogenes*). XI Lancefield International Symposium on Streptococci and Streptococcal Diseases. 1990. Siena, Italy

40. Dale J, Beachey E. Multiple heart cross-reactive epitopes of streptococcal M proteins. J Exp Med. 1985; 161:113–122

41. Dale JB, Baird RW, Bronze MS, Beachey EH. Tissue cross-reactive epitopes of streptococcal M-proteins. XI Lancefield International Symposium on Streptococci and Streptococcal Diseases. 1990. Siena, Italy

42. Bessen DE, Fischetti VA. Molecular characterization of two evolutionarily divergent classes of Group A streptococci and their relationship to pathogenicity: M protein structure and IgG-Fc and IgA-Fc receptors. XI Lancefield International Symposium on Streptococci and Streptococcal Diseases. 1990. Siena, Italy

43. Sriprakash KS, Relf W. A Polymerase chain reaction based classification suggests that there are two main classes of M proteins. XI Lancefield International Symposium on Streptococci and Streptococcal Diseases. 1990. Siena, Italy

44. Goldstein I, Halpern B, Robert L. Immunologic relationship between streptococcus A polysaccharide and the structural glycoproteins of heart valve. Nature. 1967; 213:44

45. Stollerman GH, Pearce IA. The changing epidemiology of rheumatic fever and acute glomerulonephritis. Adv Intern Med 1968; 14:201–239

46. Wannamaker LW. Virulence factors in streptococci. Scand J Infect Dis [Suppl.] 1982; 14(3): 22–27

47. Markowitz M. The decline of rheumatic fever: role of medical intervention. J Pediatr. 1985; 106:545–550

48. Stollerman GH. Changing Group A streptococci: The reappearance of streptococcal 'toxic shock'. Arch Intern Med. 1988; 148: 1268–1270

49. Siegel AC, Johnson EE, Stollerman GH. Controlled studies of streptococcal pharyngitis in a pediatric population. I. Factors related to the attack rate of rheumatic fever. N Engl J Med. 1961; 265: 559–566

50. Weiss ME, Adkinson NF. Immediate hypersensitivity reactions to penicillin and related antibiotics. Clin Allergy 1988; 18:515–540

51. Zimmerman RA, Wilson E. familial susceptibility to acquisition of group A β-hemolytic streptococci. Am J Dis Child. 1968; 116:292–300

52. Coburn AF, Young DC. The epidemiology of hemolytic streptococcus during World War II in the United States Navy. Baltimore, Williams and Wilkins, 1949

53. Johnson EE, Stollerman GH, Grossman BJ. Rheumatic recurrences in patients not receiving continuous prophylaxis. JAMA. 1964; 190: 407

54. Cheadle WB. The various manifestations of the rheumatic state as exemplified in childhood and early life. Lancet. 1889; 1:821, 921

55. Wilson MG, Schweitzer M. Pattern of hereditary susceptibility in rheumatic fever. Circulation. 1954; 10:699–704

56. Wilson MG, Schweitzer M, Lubsche R. The familial epidemiology of rheumatic fever: genetic and epidemiologic studies. J Pediatr. 1943; 22: 468–492, 581–611

57. Taranta A, Torosdag S, Metrakos JD, Jegier W, Uchida I. Rheumatic fever in monozygotic and dizygotic twins (Abstract). Circulation. 1959; 20:778

58. Johnson S, Streamer CW, Williams PM. An evaluation of a streptococcal control program. Am J Public Health. 1964; 54:487–500

59. Patarroyo ME, Winchester RJ, Vejerano A *et al*. Association of a B cell allo-antigen with susceptibility to rheumatic fever. Nature. 1979; 278:173–174

60. Zabriskie JB, Lavenchy D, Williams RC Jr, Fu SM, Yeadon CA, Fotino M, Braun DG. Rheumatic fever – associated B-cell alloantigens as identified by monoclonal antibodies. Arthritis Rheum. 1985; 28:1047–51

61. Regelmann WE, Talbot R, Cairns L, Martin D *et al*. Distribution of cells bearing 'rheumatic' antigens in peripheral blood of patients with rheumatic fever/rheumatic heart disease. J Rheumatol. 1989; 16:931–5

62. Rich SS, Grey ED, Talbot R, Martin D, Cairns L *et al.* Cell surface markers and cellular immune response associated with rheumatic heart disease: complex segregation analysis. Genet Epidemiol. 1988; 5:463–470

63. Markowitz M. Prevention of acute rheumatic fever and rheumatic heart disease. In Julian DF, Humphries J, eds., Preventive Cardiology. International Medical Reviews, Cardiology 2. London, Butterworths, 1983

64. Cleary P, Kaplan E, Darip M. Secretory IgA antibody directed against the Group A streptococcal C5a peptidase. XI Lancefield International Symposium on Streptococci and Streptococcal Diseases. 1990. Siena, Italy

65. Kaplan EL, Top FH, Dudding BA, Wannamaker LW. Diagnosis of streptococcal pharyngitis: differentiation of active infection from the carrier state in the symptomatic child. J Infect Dis. 1971; 123:490–501

66. Wannamaker LW. Perplexity and precision in the diagnosis of streptococcal pharyngitis. Am J Dis Child. 1972; 124:352–358

67. Wannamaker LW. A penicillin shot without culturing the child's throat. JAMA. 1976; 235: 913–914

68. Kaplan EL. The Group A streptococcal upper respiratory tract carrier state: an enigma. J Pediatr. 1980; 97:337–345

69. Taranta A, Moody M. Diagnosis of streptococcal pharyngitis and rheumatic fever. Symposium on laboratory diagnosis. Pediatr Clin North Am. 1971; 18:125

70. Di Sciasio G, Taranta A. Rheumatic fever in children. Am Heart J. 1980; 99:635–658

71. Ross PW. Swabbing technique and the isolation of beta-hemolytic streptococci from the throat. XI Lancefield International Symposium on Streptococci and Streptococcal Disease 1990. Siena, Italy

72. Fragoso MA, Manning L, Frenkel LD. Can parents do a throat culture? Pediatr Infect Dis. 1989; 8:845–847

73. Catanzaro FJ, Rammelkamp CH JR, Chamovitz R. Prevention of rheumatic fever and rheumatic heart disease. Circulation. 1970; 41: A-I

74. Rantz LA, Randall E, Rantz HH. Antistreptolysin 'O': a study of this antibody in health and disease and the hemolytic streptococcus respiratory disease in man. Am J Med. 1948; 5:3

75. Ayoub EM, Wannamaker LW. Streptococcal antibody titers in Sydenham's chorea. Pediatrics. 1966; 38:946

76. Evaluation of the streptozyme test for streptococcal antibodies. Bull WHO. 1986; 64:504

77. Facklam RR. Specificity study of kits for detection of Group A streptococci directly from throat swabs. J Clin Microbiol. 1987; 25:504–508

78. Kaplan EL. The rapid identification of Group A beta-hemolytic streptococci in the upper respiratory tract: current status. Pediatr Clin North Am. 1988; 35 535–542

79. Holmberg SD, Faich GA. Streptococcal pharyngitis and acute rheumatic fever in Rhode Island. JAMA. 1983; 250:2307–2312

80. Cochi SL, Fraser DW, Hightower AW, Facklam RR, Broome CV. Diagnosis and treatment of streptococcal pharyngitis: survey of US medical practitioners. 'Management of Pharyngitis in an Era of Declining Rheumatic Fever.' Report of the 6th Ross Conference on Pediatric Research. 1984. Ross Laboratories, Columbus, Ohio

81. Fischer PM. Rapid testing for streptococcal pharyngitis. Primary Care. 1986; 13:657–665

82. Gerber MA, Randolph MA, Chanatry J *et al.* Antigen detection test for streptococcal pharyngitis: evaluation of sensitivity with respect to true infections. J Pediatr. 1986; 108:654–658

83. WHO Technical Report Series, No. 764, 1988 Rheumatic Fever and Rheumatic Heart Disease: Report of a WHO Study Group

84. Frank PF, Stollerman GH, Miller LF. Protection of a military population from rheumatic fever. JAMA. 1965; 193:119–127

85. Chamovitz R, Catanzaro FJ, Stetson CA, Rammelkamp CH Jr. Prevention of rheumatic fever by treatment of previous streptococcal infections: I. Evaluation of benzathine penicillin G. N Engl J Med. 1954; 251:466–471

86. Stillerman M, Bernstein SH. Streptococcal pharyngitis therapy. Am J Dis Child. 1964; 107:35–46

87. Green JL, Ray SP, Charney E. Recurrence rate of streptococcal pharyngitis related to oral penicillin. J Pediatr. 1969; 75:292

88. Kaplan EL. Benzathine penicillin for treatment of Group A streptococcal pharyngitis: a re-appraisal in 1985. Pediatr Infect Dis. 1985; 4:592–596

89. Kim KS, Kaplan EL. Association of penicillin tolerance with failure to eradicate Group A strep-

tococci from patients with pharyngitis. J Pediatr. 1985; 107:681–684

90. Bergman AB, Werner RJ. Failure of children to receive penicillin by mouth. New Engl J Med. 1963; 268:1334

91. Leistyna JA, Macaulay JC. Therapy of streptococcal infections. Am J Dis Child. 1966; 111:22

92. Idsoe O, Guthe T, Willcox RR, De Weck AL. Nature and extent of penicillin side-reactions with particular reference to fatalities from anaphylactic shock. Bull WHO. 1968; 38:159–188

93. Sogn DD. Prevention of allergic reactions to penicillin. J Allergy Clin Immunol. 1987; 78: 1051–1052

94. Sullivan TJ, Yecies LD, Shatz GS, Parker CW, Wedner HJ. Desensitization of patients allergic to penicillin using orally administered b-lactam antibiotics. J Allergy Clin Immunol 1982; 69: 275–282

95. Adkinson NF Jr, Wheeler B. Risk factors for IgE-dependent reactions to penicillin. In Kerr JW, Ganderton MA eds., XI International Congress of Allergology and Clinical Immunology. London: MacMillan, 1983 pp. 55–59

96. Sanders E, Foster MT, Scott D. Occurrence of infections due to Group A β-hemolytic streptococci resistant to erythromycin and lincomycin. N Engl J Med. 1968; 278:538–540

97. Bergner-Rabinowitz S, Davies AM. Sensitivity of *Streptococcus pyogenes* types to tetracycline and other antibodies. Israel J Med Sci. 1970; 6:393

98. Catanzaro FJ, Rammelkamp CH, Chamovitz R. Prevention of rheumatic fever by treatment of streptococcal infections II. Factors responsible for failures. N Engl J Med. 1958; 259:51–57

99. Gray GC, Escamilla J, Hyams KC, Struewing JP *et al*. Hyperendemic *Streptococcus pyogenes* infection despite prophylaxis with penicillin G benzathine. N Engl J Med. 1991; 325:92–97

100. Denny FW. The streptococcus saga continues. N Engl J Med. 1991; 325:127–128

101. Kaplan EL, Johnson DR. Eradication of Group A streptococci from the upper respiratory tract by amoxycillin with clavulanate after oral penicillin V treatment failure. J Pediatr. 1988; 113:400–403

102. Brook I. Treatment of patients with acute recurrent tonsillitis due to Group A beta-hemolytic streptococci: a prospective randomized study comparing penicillin and amoxycillin/clavulanate

potassium. J Antimicrob Chemother. 1989; 24:227–233

103. Boschi G, Zanacca C, Carmeli G, Capatti C *et al*. Streptococcal pharyngitis treated by amoxycillin with clavulanate. XI Lancefield International Symposium on Streptococci and Streptococcal Diseases. 1990. Siena, Italy

104. Tanz R, Yogev R, Chadwick EG, Shulman ST. What accounts for apparent failure of penicillin in acute Group A streptococcal pharyngitis? XI Lancefield International Symposium on Streptococci and Streptococcal Diseases. 1990. Siena, Italy

105. De Meyere M, Blondeel L, Verschraegen G, Mervielde I. Streptococcal pharyngitis. Randomized, double-blind and placebo controlled evaluation of the clinical response to penicillin in general practice. XI Lancefield International Symposium on Streptococci and Streptococcal Diseases. 1990. Siena, Italy

106. Krober MS, Bass JW, Michels GN. Streptococcal pharyngitis. I. Placebo controlled double-blind evaluation of clinical response to penicillin therapy. JAMA. 1985; 253:1271–1274

107. Crowe CC, Sanders WE Jr, Longley S. Bacterial interference. II. Role of the normal throat flora in prevention of colonization by Group A streptococcus. J Infect Dis. 1973; 128:527–532

108. Grahne E, Holm SE, Roos K. An alternative treatment of recurrent streptococcal tonsillitis. XI Lancefield International Symposium on Streptococci and Streptococcal Diseases. 1990. Siena, Italy

109. Yamada T, Rouf MA, Shitara M *et al*. Specific growth inhibitory activity of an isolate of oral streptococcus for beta-hemolytic Group A streptococci. XI Lancefield International Symposium on Streptococci and Streptococcal Diseases. 1990. Siena, Italy

110. Ofek I, Zafriri D, Baird RW, Dale JB. Consequences of streptococcal adhesion to tissues: colonization and cytotoxicity. XI Lancefield International Symposium on Streptococci and Streptococcal Diseases. 1990. Siena, Italy

111. Quie PG, Pierce HC, Wannamaker LW. Influence of penicillinase-producing staphylococci on the penicillin treatment of Group A streptococci. Pediatrics. 1966; 37:467–476

152

112. Coburn AF. Prevention of respiratory tract bacterial infections by sulphadiazide prophylaxis in United States Navy. JAMA. 1944; 126:88–92

113. Morris A, Chamovitz R, Catanzaro FJ, Rammelkamp CH Jr. Prevention of rheumatic fever by treatment of previous streptococcic infections. Effect of sulphadiazine. JAMA 1956; 160:114

114. Goerner JR, Massell BF, Jones TD. Use of penicillin in treatment of carriers of beta-hemolytic streptococci among patients with rheumatic fever. N Engl J Med. 1947; 237:576–580

115. Denny FW, Wannamaker LW, Brink WR, Rammelkamp CH, Custer EA. Prevention of rheumatic fever. Treatment of the preceding streptococcal infection. JAMA. 1950; 143: 151–153

116. Wannamaker LW, Rammelkamp CH Jr, Denny FW *et al.*. Prophylaxis of acute rheumatic fever by treatment of the preceding streptococcal infection with various amounts of depot penicillin. Am J Med. 1951; 10:673–695

117. Stollerman GH, Rusoff JH. Prophylaxis against Group A streptococcal infections in rheumatic fever patients; use of new repository penicillin preparation. JAMA. 1952; 150:1571–1575

118. Catanzaro FJ, Stetson CA, Morris AJ, Chamovitz R, Rammelkamp CH Jr, Stolzer BL, Perry WD. The role of the streptococcus in the pathogenesis of rheumatic fever. Am J Med. 1954; 17:749

119. Dingle JH, Badger GF, Feller AE, Hodges RG, Jordan WS, Rammelkamp CH Jr. A study of illness in a group of Cleveland families. Am J Hygiene. 1953; 58:16–40

120. Breese BB, Disney FA. Accuracy of diagnosis of beta-hemolytic streptococcal infection on clinical grounds. J Pediatr. 1954; 44:670–673

121. Miller JM, Stancer SL, Massell BF. Controlled study of beta-hemolytic streptococcal infection in rheumatic families. I. Streptococcal disease among healthy siblings. Am J Med. 1958; 25:825–844

122. Bunn WH, Bennett HM. Community control of rheumatic fever. JAMA. 1955; 157:986–989

123. Hubbard JP. Prevention of first attack of rheumatic fever. Ann Intern Med. 1955; 43:504–510

124. Poskanzer DC, Feldman HA, Beadenkopf WG, Kuroda K *et al*. Epidemiology of civilian streptococcal outbreaks before and after penicillin. Am J Public Health. 1956; 46:1513–1524

125. Cornfeld D, Werner G, Weaver R, Bellows MT, Hubbard JP. Streptococcal infection in a school population: preliminary report. Ann Intern Med. 1958; 49:1305–1319

126. Cornfeld D, Hubbard JP, Harris TN, Weaver R. Epidemiologic studies of streptococcal infection in school children. Am J Public Health. 1961; 51:242–249

127. Cornfeld D, Hubbard JP. A four year study of the occurrence of beta-hemolytic streptococci in 64 school children. N Engl J Med. 1961; 264: 211–215

128. Jackson H, Cooper J, Mellinger WJ, Olsen AR. Streptococcal pharyngitis in rural practice. Rational medical management. JAMA. 1966; 197: 385–388

129. Phibbs B, Taylor J, Zimmerman RA. A community-wide streptococcal control project. JAMA. 1970; 214:2018–2024

130. Phibbs B, Lundin SR, Watson WB, Corbett JJ. Experience of a Wyoming county streptococcal control project. West J Med. 1988; 148:546–550

131. Zimmerman RA, Biggs BA, Bolin RA, Wilson E *et al*. An effective program for reducing Group A streptococcal prevalence. Pediatrics. 1971; 48:566–572

132. Jackson H. Streptococcal control in grade schools. Am J Dis Child. 1976; 130:273–279

133. Zimmerman R.I. Streptococcal surveillance and control in Alaskan natives. International Congress Series No 317. Amsterdam, Excerpta-Medica, 1974

134. Brant LJ, Bender TR, Bross DS. Evaluation of an Alaskan streptococcal control program. Importance of the program's intensity and duration. Prevent Med. 1986; 15:632–642

135. Gordis L. Effectiveness of comprehensive-care programs in preventing rheumatic fever. N Engl J Med. 1973; 289:331–335

136. Chun LT, Reddy V, Rhoads GG. Occurrence and prevention of rheumatic fever among ethnic groups of Hawaii. Am J Dis Child. 1984; 138:476–478

137. Mohs E. Infectious diseases and health in Costa Rica. The development of a new paradigm. Pediatr Infect Dis. 1982; 1:212–216

138. Gordis L, Lilienfeld A, Rodriguez R. An evaluation of the Maryland rheumatic fever register. Public Health Reports 1969; 84:333–339

139. Zagala JG, Feinstein AR. The preceding illness of acute rheumatic fever. JAMA. 1962; 179: 863–866

140. Grossman BJ, Stamler J. Preventability in first attacks of acute rheumatic fever in children. JAMA. 1963; 183: 985–988.

141. Czoniczer G, Lees M, Massell BF. Streptococcal infection. The need for improved recognition and treatment for the prevention of rheumatic fever. N Engl J Med. 1961; 265:951–952

142. Rhode JE, Sadjimin T. Elementary school pupils as health educators: role of school health programmes in primary health-care. Lancet. 1980; 1:1350–1352

143. Gordis L, Lilienfeld A, Rodriguez R. Studies in the epidemiology and preventability of rheumatic fever – II. Socio-economic factors and the incidence of acute attacks. J Chron Dis. 1969; 21: 655–666

12.   BACTERIAL CAUSES OF RHEUMATIC DISEASE

David Barraclough and Richard Wigley

INTRODUCTION

This chapter deals with non-sexually transmitted bacterial infections that are capable of causing arthritis and/or musculoskeletal symptoms. Subsequent chapters deal with viral, rickettsial, tropical, and sexually transmitted causes of rheumatic disease.

The clinical picture of bacterial arthritis is variable[1]. In an infant, the infected joint is irritable and accompanied by fever, while in older children and adults, articular pain and stiffness are present, and are associated with local signs of inflammation and joint effusion. In most patients there are also general signs of infection, including fever, rigors, and leukocytosis. The systemic response and local inflammatory response may be markedly attenuated in immunocompromised hosts, those with an underlying connective tissue disease, or those being treated with anti-inflammatory drugs or systemic steroids. Previous antibiotic therapy may also modify the systemic response and the local signs of infection. A clinical suspicion of a bacterial arthritis should trigger aggressive investigation, with aspiration of joint fluid for cell count, microscopy and culture, as well as blood cultures to rule out the possibility of septicemia and acute bacterial endocarditis.

PREDISPOSING FACTORS AND ASSOCIATED CONDITIONS

Compromised host defenses and previous joint damage predispose to bacterial arthritis. In rheumatoid arthritis, both of these factors are present, and may be enhanced by the use of corticosteroids, although septic arthritis may occur in the absence of corticosteroid therapy[2]. Entry of organisms into a joint may be by direct inoculation during surgery, secondary to penetrating trauma, or rarely as a complication of intra-articular injection. More commonly, however, the organisms reach the joint by hematogenous spread. Occasionally, blood spread may be from a focus such as a boil on the skin or by local invasion from osteomyelitis of a neighboring bone. However, often there is no evident preceding lesion. Other conditions that may predispose to bacterial arthritis are intravenous drug abuse with recurrent bacteremia, severe osteoarthritis, tropical pyomyositis[3] and other chronic diseases in which there is impaired resistance to infection because of phagocytic deficiencies or immunosuppressive medication[1]. Crystal arthritis and septic arthritis may co-exist[4,5].It appears that the bacterial infection develops first and that the crystal arthritis is a secondary phenomenon.

Gram-positive bacterial arthritis

Staphylococcus aureus accounts for the majority of cases of bacterial arthritis. Although still uncommon in infections acquired outside hospitals, methicillin-resistant staphylococci are sometimes present. The normally saprophytic *Staphylococcus epidermidis* may infect prosthetic joints and may cause septic arthritis in immunocompromised hosts[2]. Streptococcal arthritis may occur. Group B and group G streptococcal bacteremias[6–9] are more common in immunocompromised hosts. Pneumococcal arthritis is relatively uncommon, but may also occur in immunocompromised hosts and in alcoholics[2]. The onset of gram-positive coccal arthritides is usually acute. The diagnosis is confirmed by finding cloudy yellow joint fluid and recovering the causal organism from joint fluid or blood cultures. Meningococcal infection is discussed below and gonococcal infection in Chapter 18.

Gram-negative bacterial arthritis

These infections mainly occur in neonates, the elderly, intravenous drug users and in immunocompromised hosts. In neonates, umbilical vein catheters and femoral venipunctures may predispose to gram-negative infections[10]. The organisms include *Pseudomonas aeruginosa*, *Escherichia coli*, *Enterobacter* species, *Haemophilus influenzae* and *Klebsiella pneumoniae*. In elderly patients, *E. coli* is the most common gram-negative organism, but others may occur.

In the elderly, gram-negative organisms isolated from joint infections are shown in Table 1[11]. In immunocompromised hosts, *E. coli* has been the most common cause but *Serratia marcescens*, Enterobacter and *P. aeruginosa* have been common in heroin users in the USA[12]. Staphylococci were the cause in 37 heroin users in Spain[13].

Anaerobic bacterial arthritis

Cultures for anaerobes may be negative unless appropriate isolation techniques are used for anaerobic, as well as mycoplasma species, both of which may cause pyogenic arthritis. These organisms have increased as causes of septic arthritis in recent years as postoperative infections, or in immunocompromised hosts, and include *Bacteroides fragilis* and *Corynebacterium* species[14]. Clostridial infection may occur from direct trauma to a joint. Occasionally infections may be due to more than one organism[15].

Treatment

Initial treatment is with parenteral antibiotics. The antibiotics used, the dose, and the duration of parenteral treatment will depend on the organism involved. If bacterial arthritis is suspected, treatment should commence as soon as cultures have been taken; prompt treatment is critical, given the rapid development of joint damage in untreated or inadequately treated patients. Prolonged parenteral antibiotics are needed with most organisms or if there is associated septicemia, and must be accompanied by adequate drainage[16]. This may sometimes be performed by repeated needle aspiration, but often via arthroscopy or open surgical drainage.

Pyogenic infections of rheumatoid joints

The clinical signs of sepsis may be less pronounced than expected in rheumatoid arthritis, perhaps because of non-steroidal anti-inflammatory drugs or steroid treatment and also because of impaired host responses and previous damage to joints. Kraft and colleagues[17] have reviewed the problem of unrecognized staphylococcal infection in rheumatoid joints. One author (RDW) has seen four similar cases, in which injection into the joint was a possible cause in one and contrast injection into the knee for arthrography

Table 1 Organisms causing gram-negative bacillary septic arthritis. (Reproduced with kind permission from reference 11)

Organism	Patients (%)
Escherichia coli	7 (32)
Pseudomonas aeruginosa	4 (18)
Polymicrobial	4 (18)
Serratia marscesans	2 (9)
Enterobacter species	2 (9)
Proteus mirabilis	2 (9)
Citrobacter diversus	1 (5)

in another; each required prolonged high-dose antibiotic therapy. Such cases may be complicated by bacterial endocarditis[18].

Children

In children, *Staphylococci, Haemophilus influenzae* and gram-negative organisms predominate. Welkon and co-authors[19] review 95 cases of pyogenic arthritis in children, most of whom were under 6 years of age. The causative organism was not identified in one-third of the cases. Sacroiliac joint pyogenic arthritis may occur in infants[20]. Arthritis often complicates osteomyelitis. Infantile infectious sacroiliitis, childhood discitis, endocarditis and osteomyelitis due to *Kingella kingae* have been reported but are rare[21].

Prevention

The skin is normally inhabited by staphylococci and other organisms. It must be sterilized with antiseptic preparations containing alcohol, iodine and/or detergents before joint aspiration or any surgical procedure. If possible, these procedures should not be carried out if there is any infection such as a furuncle present. The use of factory sterilized material with a 'no touch' technique has minimized the risk of bacterial infections. In uncontrolled settings, e.g. drug abusers sharing needles, infective arthritis is a more common event. In many countries, exchange programs have been implemented, in which clean needles are made available to these individuals to minimize the introduction of pyogenic organisms as well as the transmission of hepatitis and human immunodeficiency virus (Chapter 18).

Control and prompt treatment of skin infections and improved general hygiene will lessen the risk of infection. Particular care should be taken with invasive procedures when the immune system is previously compromised by human immunodeficiency virus (HIV) infection, immunosuppressive therapy, radiotherapy and chemotherapy.

Control of methicillin-resistant staphylococci in hospitals is a difficult problem[22]. Routine nasal and other swabs to identify carriers, careful hand washing by staff, and appropriate barrier nursing, help to prevent the spread of this organism.

GRAM-NEGATIVE COCCI
Gonococcal arthritis

This is the most common form of septic arthritis seen in some centers[23], and is covered in detail in Chapter 18. Gonococcal arthritides may be due to direct bacterial infection of the joints, but often the joint is sterile on culture and the arthritis may be due to immune complex formation.

Meningococcal arthritis

Meningococccal infection is clinically similar to disseminated gonococcal infection[24–26]. Organisms may be identified by blood or joint cultures. However, joints are commonly sterile, and the arthritis attributed to immune complex deposition. One or a number of joints may be affected, but sometimes there is only a transient arthralgia. A second cause of joint sterility is the use of antibiotics prior to hospital admission[27]. There are often associated skin lesions: only 25% of patients have meningitis at the time of diagnosis of meningococcal arthritis. Meningococci reside in the throat and are transmitted by contact and droplets. Local epidemics occur in 10–15-year cycles, and are caused by one of five strains of meningococci. There is a high infection rate in contacts of carriers, and young children are most susceptible, as are those of lower socioeconomic strata. For example, meningococcal arthritis is endemic in the western Cape provinces of South Africa[28]. Culture-positive septic arthritis was seen early in the disease; sterile allergic arthritis was seen later. Primary isolated infection of a joint was seen and also arthritis in the course of chronic meningococcemia. Meningococcal urethritis and endometritis can occur simulating gonococcal infection[29].

Prevention

Prophylactic treatment of close family members and other contacts of patients with meningococcal infection with penicillin is essential; or if there is allergy to this antibiotic, sulfonamides or rifampicin should be used to prevent spread of the disease by contacts or carriers or for prophylaxis for those entering an epidemic area. Prevention with vaccines is feasible for types A, C, Y, and W but not yet for type B[22]. Treatment is usually with a high-dose parenteral penicillin.

Brucella arthritis

This form of arthritis is rare in temperate climates. Transmission of *Brucella abortus* is via unpasteurized milk, cheese or infected meat, although veterinary surgeons, farmers and meat handlers may be directly infected. Single joint infection or an asymmetrical peripheral oligo-arthritis[30] or sacroiliitis may occur. Arthritis is more common in chronic brucellosis. Bursitis, tenosynovitis, and a rheumatoid-like arthritis, as well as pseudopodagra, have been reported[1] as has osteomyelitis of the spine. Treatment is usually with tetracycline with additional streptomycin if the patient is seriously ill. Goat brucellosis (*Brucella melitensis*), which causes Malta fever, is endemic in the Middle East, and commonly involves the joints[31]. Brucellosis is prevented by pasteurizing milk and destroying animals (cattle, goats, sheep and swine) that test positive for *Brucella* species. Wild animal reservoirs continue to frustrate preventive efforts in some countries.

Mycoplasma arthritis

Mycoplasma pneumoniae is spread by droplet from throat infection and close contact. Monarticular arthritis is a rare complication. Davis and colleagues[32] reported isolating *M. pneumoniae* from synovial fluid in a patient with pneumonia and polyarthritis. The organism does not grow in conventional media and so must be sought where initial cultures are negative in septic arthritis.

Evidence of *M. arthritidis*, *M. fermentans* and *Ureoplasma* infection in adult and juvenile rheumatoid patients suggest to some workers a possible causative role[33] although previous reports have been difficult to interpret because of the possibility of accidental contamination of cultures by *Mycoplasma* organisms. Erythromycin and tetracycline are effective therapeutic agents. The only preventive measure available is by routine care to avoid droplet spread from patients with known mycoplasmal infection.

Tuberculous arthritis and osteomyelitis

Arthritis caused by *Mycobacterium tuberculosis* is now rare in countries where this organism is controlled but is still a common problem in developing countries. Approximately 5% of mycobacterial infections occur in bones or joints[34]. Malignant disease, immunosuppressive therapy and other illness in which immunosuppression occurs, such as HIV infection, predispose to mycobacterial infection. Large joints are usually affected and the vertebrae are susceptible to bone infection, which when advanced results in Pott's disease[35,36]. The diagnosis is suspected from the chronic course, a history of contact, tuberculin testing, radiology, culture and histology. Erythema nodosum, as with other infections, may herald primary tuberculous infection. The nodular eruption over joints may simulate arthritis. Poncet's disease is a rare sterile polyarthritis complicating tuberculosis[37].

Atypical mycobacterial infections may occur in joints. *Mycobacterium marinum* can be an occupational hazard for fish workers and has been reported to cause a nodular lesion on the wrist[38].

Prevention

Prevention of tuberculosis relies on such measures as the pasteurization of milk and milk products such as cheese and yoghurt. Tuberculin testing of cattle with the slaughtering of positive reactors has been an expensive but effective

158

Table 2 Fungi causing infections of bones and joints. (Reproduced with kind permission from reference 42)

Fungus	Mode of infection	Geographical distribution	Frequency of septic joint involvement
Superficial			
'maduromycoses'	fungus enters via local injury to uncovered foot	worldwide, especially in tropical climates where inhabitants do not wear shoes; rare in US	usual; soft tissue infection leading to osteomyelitis
Sporothrix schenckii	fungus enters via local injury to skin – direct implantation of plant material carrying fungus; alcoholism and myeloproliferative diseases are predisposing factors	worldwide, especially areas of high humidity; South Africa France, and Mexico are most common areas	80% of cases of systemic sporotrichosis
Candida albicans and rarely *C. stellatoidea* *C. tropicalis* *C. guilliermondi* *C. parapsilosis*	endogenous: in premature infants and other compromised hosts having *malignancies, indwelling* catheters, hyperalimentation, immunosuppressive therapies, multiple antibiotics; drug addicts (especially heroin)	worldwide	rare
Actinomyces israelii (anaerobic bacterium)	endogenous – host may or may not be compromised; focal cervicofacial disease or disseminated bacteremia; may follow oral trauma such as tooth extractions	worldwide	common in facial bones
Deep			
Aspergillus fumigatus	inhalation or endogenous infection in a compromised host; dissemination via respiratory tree and blood; rarely via gastrointestinal tract	worldwide	rare
Histoplasma capsulatum	inhalation; aerosol from soil rich in bird droppings (especially chickens, starlings) and bat feces	worldwide; in USA most concentrated in the Mid-West, Ohio and Mississipi River valleys	rare
H. duboisii	uncertain	Africa	about 66% with disseminated disease
Cryptococcus neoformans	inhalation, often compromised host as well as normal persons	worldwide; no regional concentration in US	5–10%
Coccidioides immitis	inhalation, especially during dry, dusty months	southwestern US, Central and South America especially arid dusty regions	10–20% cases with disseminated disease
Blastomyces dermatitidis	usually inhalation; very rarely inoculation into traumatized skin; most common among persons repeatedly exposed to soil. 9 males : 1 female	USA: Mississipi and River Ohio basins, middle Atlantic states, Canada, Africa, Europe, northern South America	25–50% disseminated blastomycoses cases

means of eliminating the organism. Spread of the organism to other species may constitute a major risk to cattle and humans as in New Zealand, where a large population of opossums is infected[39], and in Britain where badgers are infected by *M. bovis*[40]. This constitutes a hazard not only to those involved in controlling these animals but also of a risk of reintroduction of this organism to cattle. Control of human infection has been by close follow-up and treatment of cases and contacts. A large study has shown that isoniazid treatment for one year (considered safe in those under 35 years) of tuberculin-positive susceptible populations controls the disease. Isoniazid may also be used prophylactically in immunocompromised patients. The value of BCG vaccination is controversial but may reduce the incidence of fatal generalized infections[41].

Fungal infections (see Table 2)

The most common form of musculoskeletal involvement with fungal organisms is osteomyelitis. Occasionally there may be direct, or less often, hematogenous spread to joints. *Candida* species, *Coccidioides*, cryptococci, maduramycosis, *Sporothrix* and blastomycotic infections may cause arthritis secondary to skin infection[42]. The course of fungal infections is usually indolent and may be misdiagnosed as non-specific synovitis. Immunocompromised hosts, diabetics, intravenous drug users, those treated with multiple antibiotics or on prolonged parenteral nutrition are at special risk. Avoidance of exposure is usually not practicable as fungi are ubiquitous. Bird, especially pigeon, droppings should be avoided. Resiting of intravenous cannulas at regular intervals may help reduce the risk in hospital patients.

CONCLUSIONS

The risk of acquiring bacterial arthritis can be lessened in some situations. Particular care should be taken where host resistance is impaired, with joint injections or following joint surgery; in patients on immunosuppressive treatment for malignant and autoimmune disease and in those with HIV.

REFERENCES

1. Goldenberg DL. Bacterial arthritis. In Kelley *et al.*, eds., Textbook of Rheumatology, WB Saunders, 1989, 3rd edn., pp. 1567–1585
2. Goldenberg DL, Reid J. Bacterial arthritis. N Engl J Med 1985; 312:764–761
3. Andrew JG, Gzyz WM. Pyomyositis presenting as septic arthritis. a report of 2 cases. Acta Orthop Scand. 1988; 59:587-588
4. Heinicke M, Gomez-Reino JJ, Gorevic PD. Crystal arthritis as a complication of septic arthritis. J Rheumatol. 1981; 8:529–523
5. Gordon TP, Reid C, Rozenbilds MA, Ahern M. Crystal shedding in septic arthritis: case reports and in vivo evidence in an animal model. Aust NZ Med J. 1986; 16:336–340
6. Pischel KD, Weisman MH, Cone RO. Unique features of group B streptococcal arthritis in adults. Arch Intern Med. 1985; 145:97–102
7. Marsh L, Needs CJ, Webb J. Streptococcus group G septic polyarthritis. Aust NZ Med J. 1985; 15:647–649
8. Bramadathan KN, Koshi G. Importance of group G streptococci in human pyogenic infections. J Trop Med Hygiene. 1989; 92:35–38
9. Pittard WB, Thullen JD, Fanaroff AA. Neonatal septic arthritis. J Pediatr. 1976; 88:621
10. Bayer AS, Chow AW, Louie JS *et al.* Gram negative bacillary septic arthritis. Semin Rheumatol. 1977; 7:123–132
11. Newman ED, Davis DE, Harrington TM. Septic arthritis due to gram negative bacilli: older patients with good outcome. J Rheumatol. 1988; 15:659–662
12. Goldenberg DL. Bacterial arthritis. In Kelley *et al.*, eds. Textbook of Rheumatology. WB Saunders, 1989, p. 1573
13. Lopez-Longo FJ, Ménard HH, Carreño L, Cosin J, Ballesteros R, Monteagudo I. Primary septic arthritis in heroin users: early diagnosis by radioisotopic imaging and geographic variations in the causative agents. J Rheumatol. 1987; 14:991–994

14. Nakata M, Lewis RP. Anaerobic bacteria in bone and joint infections. Rev Infect Dis. 1984; 6S: 165–170

15. Petty BG, Sowa DT, Charache P. Polymicrobial, polyarticular septic arthritis. JAMA. 1983; 249:2069–2072

16. Broy SB, Schmid FR. A comparison of medical drainage (needle aspiration) and surgical drainage (arthrotomy or arthroscopy) in the initial treatment of infected joints. Clin Rheum Dis. 1986; 2:501–522

17. Kraft SM, Panush RS, Longley S. Unrecognised staphylococcal pyarthrosis in rheumatoid arthritis. Semin Rheumatol. 1985; 14:196–201

18. Rowe IF, Deans AC, Keat AC. Pyogenic infection and rheumatoid arthritis. Postgrad Med J. 1987; 63:19–22

19. Welkon CJ, Long SS, Fisher MC, Alburger PD. Pyogenic arthritis in infants and children; a review of 95 cases. Pediatr Infect Dis. 1986; 5:669–676

20. Sueoka BL, Johnson JF, Enzenauer N, Kolina JS. Infantile infectious arthritis. Pediatr Radiol. 1985; 15:403–405

21. Woolfery BF, Lally RT, Faville RJ. Intervertebral diskitis caused by *Kingella kingae*. Am J Clin Pathol. 1986; 85: 745–749

22. Gardiner P, Klimek JJ. Hospital acquired infections. In Wilson *et al.*, eds., Harrison's Principles of Internal Medicine. New York, McGraw-Hill, 12th edn, 1989; pp. 468–472

23. O'Brien JP, Goldenberg DL, Rice PA. Disseminated gonococcal infection; a prospective analysis of 49 patients and a review of pathophysiology and immune mechanisms. Medicine. 1983; 62:395–406

24. Schaad UB. Arthritis in disease due to *Neisseria meningitidis*. Rev Infect Dis. 1980; 2:880–888

25. Kidd BL, Hart HH, Grigor RR. Clinical features of meningococcal arthritis: A report of four cases. Ann Rheum Dis. 1985; 44:790–792

26. Flaegstaed T, Johnsen K, Avidsten D, Kristiansen BE. Benign meningococcemia with IgG and IgM anti-meningococcal antibodies measured by ELISA. Scand J Infect Dis. 1987; 19:629–633

27. Voss L, Lennon D, Sinclair J. The clinical features of paediatric meningococcal disease in Auckland. NZ Med J. 1989; 102:243–245

28. Christensen C. Meningokoksygdom og arthritis. Vgeskr Laeger. 1990; 152:1357–1359

29. Salmeron C, Marty M, Richet H, Escabde MC, Besancon F, Lagrange HP. Primary meningococcal arthritis. J Infect Dis. 1986; 13:281–283

30. Hall WH, Khan MY. Brucellosis. In Hoeprich PD *et al.*, eds., Infectious Disease. Philadelphia, JB Lippincott, 4th edn, 1989, pp. 1282–1288

31. Khateeb MA, Araj GF, Majeed SA, Lulu AR. Brucella arthritis: a study of 96 cases in Kuwait. Ann Rheum Dis. 1990; 49:994–998

32. Davis CP, Cochran S, Lisse S, Buck G, Di Nuzzo AR, Weber T, Reinarz JA. Isolation of *Mycoplasma pneumoniae* from synovial fluid in a patient with pneumonia and polyarthritis. Arch Intern Med. 1988; 148: 969–970

33. Gorina LG, Vulfovich IV, Zilfian AV, Rakovskaia IV, Pronin AV, Hooper J. Mycoplasma arthritis in man and mechanisms of its pathogenesis. Vestn Akad Med Nauk. SSR. 1989; 13:84–87

34. Butorac R, Littlejohn GO, Hooper J. Mycobacterial disease in the musculoskeletal system. Med J Aust. 1987; 147:388–391

35. Garrido G, Gomez-Reino JJ, Fernandez-Dapica P *et al.* A reveiw of peripheral tuberculosis. Semin Rheumatol. 1988; 18:142–149

36. Martini M, Adjrad A, Boiudjemaa A. Tuberculous osteomyelitis. A review of 125 cases. Int Orthop. 1986; 10:201–207

37. Dall LL, Ong L, Stanford J. Poncet's disease is a rare sterile polyarthritis complicating tuberculosis. Rev Infect Dis. 1989; 11:105–107

38. McLain EH. Case study: Mariner's TB. AAOHN J. 1989; 37:329–332

39. Collins DM, De Lisle GW, Gabric DM. Geographic distribution of restriction types of *Mycobacterium bovis* isolates from brush-tailed possums (*Trichosuris vulpecula*) in New Zealand. J Hyg (London). 1986; 96:431–438

40. Cheeseman CL, Wilesmith JW, Stuart FA. Tuberculosis; the disease and its epidemiology in the badger, a review. Epidemiol-Infect. 1989; 103:113–125

41. Harris HW. In Hoeprich *et al.*, eds., Infectious Diseases. Philadelphia, JB Lippincott, 4th edn, 1989; pp. 430–432

42. Hoffman GS, Sentochnik DE. Mycobacterial and fungal infections. In Kelley *et al.*, eds., Textbook of Rheumatology. WB Saunders, 3rd. edn, 1989, pp. 1586–1601

13. LYME DISEASE

Angelina Blaauw and Sjef van der Linden

INTRODUCTION

Lyme borreliosis, which is caused by the tick-borne spirochete *Borrelia burgdorferi*, often begins with a characteristic skin rash, erythema migrans, and may be followed by neurological, cardiac, or joint abnormalities of variable duration[1]. Erythema migrans is reported in 50–60% of patients. In 15–20% of patients in the United States, this is followed within several weeks to months by frank neurological involvement, which may be accompanied by radicular pain, pleocytosis in the cerebrospinal fluid and meningitis with superimposed cranial nerve involvement or peripheral neuropathy[2]. Cardiac involvement occurs in up to 8% of patients, most commonly in the form of fluctuating atrioventricular block. From 2 weeks to 2 years (usually 6 months) after the onset of the disease, often after intermittent episodes of arthralgia or migratory musculoskeletal pain, nearly 80% of patients begin to have brief attacks of asymmetric, oligoarticular arthritis, primarily in the large joints, especially of the knee[3]. Chronic arthritis, defined as a year or more of continual joint inflammation, begins during the 2nd or 3rd year after the onset of the disease. In severe cases, chronic Lyme arthritis may lead to the erosion of cartilage and bone and, sometimes, though rarely, to permanent joint disability[3]. The pattern of joint involvement is similar in the United States and Europe, but has been described less commonly in the European literature, possibly due to a lack of awareness[4,5]. Acrodermatitis chronica atrophicans is a late skin disorder of the disease which has been described primarily in Europe[6].

PATHOGENESIS

The Lyme disease spirochete is transmitted by Ixodes ticks that are part of the *Ixodes ricinus* complex. They include *I. dammini* in the northeastern and midwestern United States, *I. pacificus* in the western United States, *I. ricinus* in Europe and *I. persulcatus* in Asia. Ixodid ticks are also indigenous to Africa and South America, but it is not clear whether Lyme borreliosis occurs on those continents.

Carrier rates in the ticks may vary. For *I. dammini* ticks in the United States infection rates vary from 10 to 35% and even to 50% on Shelter Island, New York[7]. Only 1–3% of *I. pacificus* ticks are infected[8]. The range of infection rates of *I. ricinus* in Europe varies from 2.2 to 40%[9,10]. The infection rate of adult ticks exceeds that of nymphal and larval ticks. Infection rates of *I. persulcatus* are not exactly known, but *Borrelia burgdorferi* has been isolated from these ticks in China and Russia[11,12]. Larvae and nymphs of *I. dammini* feed on at least 31 different species of mammals and 49 species of birds[13]. White-footed mice, *Peromyscus leucopus*, are a particularly important host, but other animals such as the short-tailed shrews (*Blarina brevicauda*), raccoons (*Procyon lotor*), gray squirrels (*Sciurus carolinensis*), and white-tailed deer (*Odocoileus virginianus*) may also be parasitized by many juvenile ticks. Birds are a natural vehicle for dispersing ticks into new areas[14]. Adult ticks are more restricted, and are known to feed on 13 species of mammals; they do not feed on mice or birds. Deer are essential for the maintenance of dense tick populations. All postembryonic stages also feed on humans.

The infection is usually acquired when nymphal ticks feed between May and July, but only a minority of the patients remember the bite, probably because of the small size of the ticks. Adult ticks transmit the disease when they feed in the autumn. The disease affects people of all ages and both sexes.

In 1982, Burgdorfer and Barbour and co-workers isolated a previously unrecognized spirochete, now called *Borrelia burgdorferi*, from *I. dammini* ticks[15]. The spirochete was subsequently recovered from patients with Lyme borreliosis[6,7,16,17]. The *Borrelia* species are fastidious, microaerophilic bacteria that grow best at 33 °C in a complex, liquid medium called Barbour–Stoenner–Kelly medium[18]. *B. burgdorferi* has a length of 20–30 µm and a width of 0.2–0.3 µm, and it has 7–11 flagella. *B. burgdorferi* contains at least 30 different proteins, but the functions of only a few of them are currently known. These include the two major outer surface proteins called outer surface protein A (30–32 kDa) and outer-surface protein B (34–36 kDa)[19,20]. The 41-kDa antigen is located on the flagellum[21]. The 58- or 60-kDa antigen appears to be a heat-shock protein that is cross-reactive with an equivalent antigen in a wide range of bacteria[22]. Certain differences in morphology, outer surface proteins, plasmid and DNA 'homology' have been noted between American and European isolates of *B. burgdorferi*[23].

CLINICAL EVOLUTION OF LYME ARTHRITIS

To determine the clinical evolution of Lyme arthritis, Steere and colleagues conducted a longitudinal study of 55 patients who had not received antibiotic therapy for erythema chronicum migrans, and followed them for a mean duration of 6 years[3]. Of the 55 patients, 11 (20%) had no subsequent manifestations of Lyme borreliosis. From 1 day to 8 weeks after disease onset, 10 of the patients (18%) began to have brief episodes of joint, periarticular, or musculoskeletal pain lasting as long as 6 years, but none developed objective joint abnormalities. From 4 days to 2 years after disease onset, 28 (51%) had one episode or began to have intermittent attacks of arthritis, primarily in large joints. The duration of these episodes ranged from 3 days to 11.5 months, with a mean of 3 months. Episodes of arthritis were often separated by months or even years of complete remission. The total number of these patients who continued to have recurrences decreased by 10–20% each year. Six patients (11%) developed chronic synovitis.

PREVENTION

Humans encounter ticks in forests, transitional vegetative zones, pastures, parks, lawns surrounding homes, brushwood and woodland areas bordering lawns, and even in houses after domestic animals have carried ticks inside. Reducing the incidence of tick bites is one of the first goals to attempt in preventing Lyme arthritis. Control methods can be divided into four categories:

(1) Personal protection,

(2) Biological control,

(3) Environmental modification and physical control, and

(4) Chemical control[24].

Personal protection

Efforts made by the individual to prevent tick bites and to locate and promptly remove attached ticks may be the most effective measures that can

164

be taken to reduce the risk of contracting Lyme disease.

Repellents Repellents applied to outer clothing, including the insides of pant cuffs and socks, prevent tick bites. The acaricide permethin kills ticks[25]. Standard repellents that do not kill but repel ticks when impregnated into clothing include deet, Indalone, dimethylcarbate, benzylbenzoate and M-1960. Treated clothing may be protected for several weeks and after several washings. Other personal measures to prevent tick bites are: taping the trouser cuffs, tucking the trousers into footwear, wearing one-piece zippered suits, wearing light colored clothing which makes it easier to observe ticks and wearing clothes made of a smooth weave rather than clothes of a coarse fabric.

Tick removal Ticks attach to their hosts by cutting the skin with a pair of chelicerae and inserting the toothed hypostome. Ticks may be removed by grasping the tick as close to the skin as possible with a pair of forceps or tweezers. An antiseptic should be applied to the skin where the tick was attached. Humans should inspect their bodies after they have visited tick-infested areas and promptly remove ticks.

Avoidance of tick-infested areas Avoiding visits to known tick-infested areas during the seasonal peak feeding of nymphs from May to mid-July can reduce the risk of acquiring Lyme borreliosis.

Biological control

Efforts should be made to introduce and to establish natural enemies of ticks. Until now, none of the known microbial pathogens and invertebrate or vertebrate predators have been used successfully to control ticks[24].

Environmental modification and physical control

Altering vegetation Controlled burning of vegetation may be useful by destroying the ticks active at the time of burning, reducing the abundance of suitable animals, and making the habitat inhospitable for ticks[26]. Removal of trash piles and removal of bird feeders may help to reduce the number of ticks in the immediate vicinity of the home.

Denying ticks access to host animals Reduction in tick numbers may be achieved by eliminating the number of infected animals such as deer, but the killing of these animals will probably not be widely accepted by the public[27].

Chemical modification

Acaricides are used for treating tick-infested animals. Domestic animals may be dipped or fitted with a collar impregnated with acaricide. Nesting material treated with an acaricide has been used.

Residual sprays Residual application of acaricides for control of ticks may be effective and practical when applied to relatively small areas frequented by humans, but will be too costly when applied to larger areas.

Treatment of white footed mouse burrows

Control of subadult *Ixodes dammini* has been reported by the placement of the acaricide permethin directly on and in the burrows of white-footed mice. Studies have reported a marked reduction in numbers of larvae feeding on mice in treated versus untreated areas [28].

PREVENTION OF LYME ARTHRITIS

There are no data to support the common practice of treatment of tick bites with antibiotics, even in areas known to be endemic for Lyme borreliosis[29,30]. In a study comparing penicillin V and placebo, the risk of acquiring Lyme borreliosis was found to be lower than one would expect, given the infection rate in ticks, and it was similar to the risk of an adverse reaction to penicillin[30]. Patients should be counselled about the early symptoms of Lyme borreliosis[29].

Recognition and adequate antibiotic treatment of the early stages of Lyme borreliosis is of paramount importance in preventing Lyme arthritis[29]. Approximately 50% of the patients have the erythema migrans which is a characteristic of Lyme borreliosis. Individuals and doctors should be well aware of this skin lesion. Prompt antibiotic treatment should be started to prevent the later complications of this disease[31]. The optimal dose and duration of antibiotic treatment have not been established for any antibiotic agent[29]. Despite adequate antibiotic treatment, chronic signs and symptoms of Lyme borreliosis may occur[3]. Even in untreated patients, erythema migrans lesions fade within 3 to 4 weeks and other manifestations of the disease may occur only months later. A relationship with subsequent signs and symptoms may pass unnoticed. Adequate history taking and showing pictures of erythema migrans can be helpful in establishing the diagnosis[32]. Since only 50% of the patients with Lyme borreliosis have erythema migrans preceding other signs and symptoms, a diagnosis of Lyme borreliosis can be difficult to make. Because the culture or direct visualization of *B. burgdorferi* from patient specimens is difficult, serology is currently the only practical laboratory aid for diagnosis. Antibody titers to *B. burgdorferi* are present after 4–6 weeks in almost all patients with Lyme borreliosis. Serological results, however, should be interpreted with caution. False-positive results and inter- and intralaboratory variation have been reported[33–35]. In addition to this problem, there are a large number of patients who have asymptomatic *B. burgdorferi* infections[36]. At present, it is impossible to differentiate between asymptomatic infections and false-positive serology. The discriminative value of reporting tick bites as part of the clinical history is low[32,36]. Even the presence of antibodies to *B. burgdorferi* in the absence of typical features of Lyme borreliosis such as erythema migrans has a very low impact on a definite diagnosis of Lyme borreliosis in the normal population[32].

Lyme arthritis has been treated successfully with both oral and parenteral antibiotics[37,38]. The optimal therapy remains to be established. The response rate to oral doxycycline has been reported to be 72%[38]. In cases of persisting Lyme arthritis other factors such as immunogenetic factors and autoimmunity may play a role[39,40]. The response to antibiotics may occur 3 months or longer after completion of the therapy. In all cases of arthritis of unknown origin the diagnosis of Lyme borreliosis should be considered[41]. Progression of joint damage or other manifestations which occur in the later stages of the disease may be prevented if appropriate treatment is provided immediately after the diagnosis of Lyme borreliosis has been established.

SUMMARY

Lyme arthritis may be avoided by preventing tick bites, by recognizing the early signs and symptoms of Lyme borreliosis, such as erythema migrans and by timely antibiotic therapy. Antibiotic treatment of Lyme arthritis may prevent chronic arthritis.

REFERENCES

1. Steere AC. Lyme disease. N Engl J Med. 1989; 321:586–595
2. Logigian EL, Kaplan RF, Steere AC. Chronic neurologic manifestations of Lyme disease. N Engl J Med. 1990; 323:1438–1444
3. Steere AC, Schoen RT, Taylor E. The clinical evolution of Lyme arthritis. Ann Intern Med. 1987; 107:725–731
4. Blaauw AAM, Nohlmans MKE, van den Berg-Loonen E *et al.* Lyme arthritis in the Netherlands: a nationwide survey among rheumatologists. J Rheumatol. 1991; 18:1819–1822
5. Herzer P. Lyme arthritis in Europe: comparisons with reports from North America. Ann Rheum Dis. 1988; 47:789–791
6. Asbrink E, Hovmark A, Hederstedt B. The spirochetal etiology of acrodermatitis atrophicans Herxheimer. Acta Derm Venereol. 1984; 64: 506–512

166

7. Steere AC, Grodzicki RL, Kornblatt AN *et al*. The spirochetal etiology of Lyme disease. N Engl J Med. 1983; 308:733–739

8. Lane RS, Lavoie PE. Lyme borreliosis in California. Ann NY Acad Sci. 1988; 539:192

9. Nohlmans MKE, de Boer R, van den Bogaard AEJM *et al*. Voorkomen van Ixodes ricinus in Nederland. Ned Tÿdschr Geneeskd. 1990; 134:1300–1303

10. Aeschlimann A, Chamot E, Gigon H, Jeanneret JP, Kesseler D, Walther C. *Borrelia burgdorferi* in Switzerland. Zentralbl Mikrobiol Hyg (A). 1987; 263:450–458

11. Kriuchechnikov VN, Korenberg EI, Shcherbakov SV, Kovalevski IV, Levin ML. (Identification of *Borrelia* isolated in the USSR from *Ixodes persulcatus* ticks). Zh Mikrobiol Epidemiol Immunobiol. 1988; 12:41–44

12. Ai CX, Wen YX, Zhang YG *et al*. Clinical manifestations and epidemiological characteristics of Lyme disease in Hailin county. Ann NY Acad Sci. 1988; 539:302–313

13. Anderson JF. Mammalian and avian reservoirs for *Borrelia burgdorferi*. Ann NY Acad Sci. 1988; 539:180–191

14. Anderson JF, Magnarelli LA. Avian and mammalian hosts for spirochete-infected ticks and insects in a Lyme disease focus in Connecticut. Yale J Biol Med. 1984; 57:617

15. Burgdorfer W, Barbour AG, Hayes SF, Benach JL *et al*. Lyme disease – a tick borne spirochetosis? Science. 1982; 216:1317–1319

16. Snydman DR, Schenkein DP, Berardi VP et al. *Borrelia burgdorferi* in joint fluid in chronic Lyme arthritis. Ann Intern Med. 1986; 104: 798–800

17. Benach JL, Bosler EM, Hanrahan JP *et al*. Spirochetes isolated from the blood of two patients with Lyme disease. N Engl J Med. 1983; 308:740–742

18. Barbour AG. Isolation and cultivation of Lyme disease spirochetes. Yale J Biol Med. 1984; 57:521–525

19. Barbour AG, Tessier SL, Todd WJ. Lyme disease spirochetes and ixodid tick spirochetes share a common surface antigenic determinant defined by a monoclonal antibody. Infect Immun. 1983; 41:795–804

20. Benach JL, Coleman JL, Golightly MG. A murine Ig monoclonal antibody binds an antigenic determinant in outer surface protein A, an immunodominant basic protein of the Lyme disease spirochete. J Immunol. 1988; 140:265–272

21. Barbour AG, Hayes SF, Heiland RA et al. A Borrelia specific monoclonal antibody binds to a flagellar epitope. Infect Immun. 1986; 52: 549–554

22. Hansen K, Bangsborg JM, Fjordvang H, Pedersen, NS, Hindersson P. Immunochemical characterization of and isolation of the gene for a *Borrelia burgdorferi* immunodominant 60-kilodalton antigen common to a wide range of bacteria. Infect Immunun. 1988; 56:2047–2053

23. Barbour AG, Heiland RA, Howe TR. Heterogeneity of major proteins in Lyme disease borreliae: a molecular analysis of North American and European isolates. J Infect Dis. 1985; 152: 478–484

24. Anderson JF. Preventing Lyme disease. Rheum Dis Clin 1989; 15:757–766

25. Schreck CE, Snoddy EL, Spielman A. Pressurized sprays of permethrin or Deet on military clothing for personal protection against *Ixodes dammini*. J Med Entomol. 1986; 23:396

26. Wilson ML. Reduced abundance of adult *Ixodes dammini* following destruction of vegetation. J Econ Entomol. 1986;79:693

27. Wilson ML, Telford SR III, Piesman J *et al*. Reduced abundance of immature *Ixodes dammini* following elimination of deer. J Med Entomol. 1988; 25:224

28. Mather TN, Ribeiro JMC, Moore S. Reducing transmissions of Lyme disease spirochetes in a suburban setting. Ann NY Acad Sci. 1988; 539:402

29. Rahn DW, Malawista SE. Lyme disease: recommendations for diagnosis and treatment. Ann Intern Med. 1991; 114:472–481

30. Costello CM, Steere AC, Pinkerton RE, Feder HM. A prospective study of tick bites in an endemic area for Lyme disease. J Infect Dis. 1989; 25:136–139

31. Steere AC, Bartenhagen NH, Craft JE *et al*. The early clinical manifestations of Lyme disease. Ann Intern Med. 1987; 197:725–731

32. Blaauw AAM, Nohlmans MKE, van den Bogaard A, van der Linden Sj. Diagnostic Tools in Lyme borreliosis: the clinical history compared with serology. J Clin Epidemiol. 1992; 11:1229–1236

33. Hedberg CW, Osterholm MT. Serologic tests for antibody to *Borrelia burgdorferi*. Another Pandora's box for medicine? Arch Intern Med. 1990; 150:732–733. Editorial

34. Luger SW, Krauss E. Serologic tests for Lyme disease. Interlaboratory variability. Arch Intern Med. 1990; 150:761–763

35. Schwartz BS, Goldstein MD, Ribeiro JM, Schulze TL, Shaheid SI. Antibody testing in Lyme disease. A comparison of results in four laboratories. JAMA. 1989; 262:3431–3434

36. Fahrer H, van der Linden SjM, Sauvain MJ, Gern L, Zhioua E, Aeschlimann A. The prevalence and incidence of clinical and asymptomatic Lyme borreliosis in a population at risk. J Infect Dis. 1991; 163:305–310

37. Steere AC, Green J, Schoen RT *et al*. Successful parenteral penicillin therapy of established Lyme arthritis. N Engl J Med. 1985; 312:869–874

38. Liu NY, Dinerman H, Levin *et al*. Randomized trial of doxycycline versus amoxicillin/probenecid for the treatment of Lyme arthritis: treatment of the non-responders with I/V penicillin or ceftriaxone. Arthritis Rheum. 1989; 32:S32

39. Sigal LH. Lyme disease, 1988: Immunologic manifestations and possible immunopathogenetic mechanisms. Semin Arthritis Rheum. 1989; 18:151–167

40. Steere AC, Dwyer E, Wichester R. Association of chronic Lyme arthritis with HLA-DR4 and HLA-DR2 alleles. N Engl J Med. 1990; 323:219–223

41. Kryger P, Hansen K, Vinterberg H, Pedersen FK. Lyme borreliosis among Danish patients with arthritis. Scand J Rheumatol. 1990; 19:77–81

14. VIRUSES AND RICKETTSIAE IN RHEUMATIC DISEASES OF TEMPERATE CLIMATES

Robert Fraser and James Gear

INTRODUCTION

In this chapter, viral and rickettsial infections more commonly seen in temperate climates will be discussed. Those mainly affecting tropical populations are described in the Chapter 15.

Diffuse pain in the limbs is an accompaniment of many febrile illnesses, although it is more common and more intense in viral than in bacterial infections. This pain may be specifically localized by the patient to muscles, as in coxsackievirus infections, equally to joints and muscles as in influenza, or to neither in dengue fever (*see* Chapter 15). In general, the genesis of this pain is obscure, and as the pain simply accompanies the fever, preventive and therapeutic measures must address the viral infection itself, rarely warranting consideration as a distinct rheumatic condition. Nonetheless, viral infections may present as an acute or less commonly as a chronic rheumatic syndrome. In some infections, e.g. herpes simplex, rheumatic pain is rare; in others, e.g. coxsackie viruses, it is so common that this pain has diagnostic value. In still others, rheumatic pain may be more common than presently appreciated, but its true incidence is obscured by the subjective nature of a discomfort misinterpreted by the patient or examiner as being that of arthralgia.

The term 'arthralgia' (joint pain) suffers from linguistic laxity of usage. Arthralgia can be caused by arthritis that is manifest as increased pain on movement and synovial tenderness which is often localized[1], but without synovial swelling, effusion, overlying heat or redness. It can also arise from involvement of surrounding tendons, ligaments and their attachments. This can easily be overlooked if, as is commonly the case, there is no swelling or other sign of inflammation. Pain in a single joint can be referred from a more proximal lesion, for example, from bone. Finally, arthralgia is often used in a literal but restricted sense, to describe pain in a joint without objective evidence of inflammation. Involvement of a single joint or disproportionately severe signs in one joint raise the possibility of secondary bacterial infection, which must be recognized and treated aggressively to prevent or minimize permanent damage (Chapter 12).

Diagnostic perspectives

Population surveys have shown that ill defined and relatively mild forms of polyarthritis are common in temperate climates, and that many of those affected do not seek medical attention. In case-recognition studies, where other causes have been excluded, those who consult physicians may present with an acute disease that is indistinguishable from a proven viral infection. Some viral infections almost invariably present specific features that simplify diagnosis. The appearance of arthritis before other characteristic signs is a problem in epidemics, as the recognition of an outbreak and the measures needed to

Table 1 Viruses that can cause arthritis. (Modified with kind permission from reference 2)

	Pattern of arthritis	*Comment*
Herpesviruses		
Epstein–Barr virus	usually one or a few	usually brief arthritis,
Cytomegalovirus	large joints	minor feature of illness.
Varicella, Zoster		*See* text for exceptions
Herpes simplex[31,32]		
Hepadenavirus		
Hepatitis B[8–10]	usually polyarticular	highly variable with severe
		systemic disease
Adenoviruses		
Adenovirus type 7[37]	polyarticular	associated with erosive disease
Adenovirus type 1[33]		and 'acquired' immunodeficiency
Paramyxovirus		
Mumps[23]		
Parvovirus [25]	polyarticular	erythema infectiosum, rash often
		absent in adults
Picornaviruses		
Echovirus[44]	polyarticular or a	
Coxsackie B[45]	few large joints	
Togaviruses		
Rubivirus	polyarticular or a	arthritis most common in
Rubella	few large joints	young adult women
Alphaviruses		
Chikungunya	all broadly similar	Africa, Asia
O'nyong-nyong		Africa
Mayaro		South America
Ockelbo, Pogosta		Sweden, Finland (Sindbis-related)
Ross River virus		Australia, South Pacific
Sindbis virus		Africa, Asia, Australia
		(very low morbidity rate)
Barmah Forest virus		Australia

contain it may be delayed. Such a delay also frustrates attempts to avoid its spread to high-risk patients, e.g. immunocompromised patients with varicella, pregnant women at risk from rubella, or erythema infectiosum (parvovirus B19), or health-care workers in contact with hepatitis B. Preventive measures might therefore be appropriate in suspected cases of virus arthritis before a definitive diagnosis can be made.

VIRUSES INCRIMINATED IN RHEUMATIC DISEASE

The pathogenic role played by many viruses is uncertain in specific rheumatic conditions, e.g.

rheumatoid arthritis and lupus erythematosus, although Epstein–Barr virus has been variously considered to have a primary or secondary role. Virus infections for which there is persuasive or definite evidence of arthritogenic potential are listed in Table 1[2]; the most conspicuously arthritogenic viruses are parvovirus, hepatitis B, and certain togaviruses. Others are rarely associated with arthritis and provide few opportunities for prevention. Variola and vaccinia[3] are largely of historical interest. Nevertheless, even rare infections require early recognition, in order to institute public health control measures.

The case for primary prevention

With the exception of variola and vaccinia arthritis, and possibly, chikungunya[4,5], even the most persistent cases of viral arthritis rarely cause permanent joint dysfunction unless it is through secondary contracture from unwarranted immobilization, or the result of a secondary bacterial infection. In addition to personal distress, however, and the risk of serious non-rheumatic effects in the patient or contacts, the epidemic forms of virus arthritis can cause extensive disruption of community life, and economic loss. In some instances, effective primary prevention is already available; in others, prevention consists of public health measures to interrupt infective cycles including vectors, though these are often of limited or unproven efficacy.

Specific attributes of viral diseases

A striking feature of viral infections is the enormous variation of rheumatic complaints caused by any one virus. Although some of the rarer forms of viral arthritis were first described as being typically pauciarticular or polyarticular, increased experience has proven these diagnostic distinctions to be of limited value. In general, a purely monoarticular arthritis requires that a bacterial infection or other cause be considered. Recognizing the viral origin of acute polyarthritis is also hampered by variability in the other diagnostic signs of viral infection, such as lymphadenopathy, pyrexia and rash, and in their temporal relationship to the onset of arthritis, which is best exemplified by togaviruses and hepatitis B. The cytology of synovial effusions is of considerable help, as a synovial fluid virtually devoid of neutrophils is rarely seen in other conditions[6]. Unfortunately several viruses cause effusions, with and without neutrophils[7], although the total white cell count is often lower than in bacterial arthritis. It is of interest that rheumatoid factor(s) may be elevated in certain viral infections including rubella, parvovirus and Ross River virus, but the peripheral white cell count may show no changes, or any of those generally found in virus disease. Prominent mononuclear cells and reactive ('atypical') lymphocytes are common in Epstein–Barr virus and cytomegalovirus infections, although the latter cell type is well described in other infections. Lymphogranuloma venereum and human immunodeficiency virus (HIV) infection are discussed under sexually transmitted diseases (Chapter 18), Epstein–Barr virus under rheumatoid arthritis (Chapter 20) and chikungunya and o'nyong-nyong fevers in Chapter 15.

COMMON VIRAL CAUSES OF ARTHRITIC COMPLAINTS
Hepatitis B

The usually self-limited arthritis of hepatitis B infection is similar to that of serum sickness and may be induced by circulating immune complexes to the virus[1]. The arthritis is often accompanied by polyarthritis, morning stiffness, urticarial, erythematous, maculopapular or petechial rash, and fever in less than half the cases. Arthritis precedes jaundice, the appearance of which signals hepatitis B in about two-thirds of cases, at which time the arthritis begins to improve[8]. In non-icteric cases, deranged laboratory measures of disturbed liver function tests suggest the diagnosis of hepatitis, which must be confirmed by serology. Exposure to potential sources of infection should be critically reviewed in the interim. An association with polyarteritis nodosa has been described[9,10] (*see* Chapter 21). Since in a prospective study of 1400 hepatitis surface antigen (HB$_s$Ag)-positive natives of Alaska, no polyarteritis was found[11], it has been suggested that polyarteritis nodosa only occurs in those who develop hepatitis and not in carriers[12].

Prevention

Hepatitis B infection is transferred in a similar manner to HIV infection so that the same control measures are needed. These measures include prevention of needle stick injuries, hygiene in direct contact with patients and drug addicts, protection in sexual contact ('safe sex') and eliminating HB$_s$Ag-positive subjects from the pool of blood and blood product donors by checking all transfusion materials prepared from human blood for antigen. For those at occupational risk, effective vaccines are in widespread use in developed countries.

Parvovirus virus

First isolated in 1975, the B19 parvovirus is a single-stranded DNA virus that in 1981 was etiologically linked to the so-called 'fifth disease' (erythema infectiosum), which may also cause hemolytic and aplastic crises[13]. B19 has been reported in Britain, the USA and Germany[14]; Reid and colleagues[15] reported an outbreak of B19 erythema infectiosum in 1985 in which 42 patients had joint pains and 30 were studied in detail. All three children in the study, but only 13 of 27 adults had a rash. The arthritis affected the small joints of the hands, wrists and knees in a symmetrical fashion, and resolved in a month in all but one child, in whom the arthritis lasted for seven months. White and co-workers[16] found that 19 of 153 patients attending an early synovitis clinic had evidence of recent parvovirus infection, with peripheral joint arthropathy of sudden onset and moderate severity. In 17 patients, the symptoms persisted more than 2 months and in three, for more than 4 years. Cohen

and associates[17] found serological evidence of parvovirus infection in two mild cases of rheumatoid arthritis and four cases that had been classified as inflammatory arthritis. Shirley and colleagues[18] studied 627 cases with rubelliform rash and joint symptoms, and found evidence of rubella infection in 229, measles in seven, and parvovirus infection in 43. In nine adult cases reported in midwestern USA[19], most were rheumatoid factor-negative and none had articular erosions though many met the American Rheumatism Association criteria for rheumatoid arthritis. The mode of transmission of parvovirus infection is unknown; volunteers have been successfully infected nasally[20], and symptoms developed after an incubation period of 13–18 days; there is also evidence of intrauterine infection[21], but these data merely suggest possible control measures aimed at halting the transmission of parvovirus.

Rubella

Osler's description of rubella arthritis was so prosaic as to imply that it was a well-recognized clinical phenomenon at the time he wrote about it in 1902. The by-now respectable body of literature on both natural and vaccine-induced rubella arthritis will be briefly reviewed. Natural rubella arthritis is more severe in adults and, before vaccination, was much more common in women, affecting up to 89% of those exposed[22]. Where vaccination programs have been directed to women, the incidence is now lower and thus it is relatively more common in men, in older patients of both sexes, and may occur as late as the 6th decade, typically consisting of symmetrical polyarthritis of peripheral rather than central joints. Many mild cases do not reach medical attention, but some may be severe enough to immobilize the patient for a week or more, requiring intense analgesics. After the arthritis peaks, persistent or recurrent joint pain, tenderness and stiffness may last for a year or longer. In general, arthritis occurs before the rash but may appear as

172

late as 6 days after. It must be emphasized that mild, atypical and subclinical rubella infections occur and the rash may be slight or absent. Post-auricular and suboccipital lymphadenopathy are diagnostically more reliable signs[23,24], but are not always present with arthritis. Some cases may be associated with the carpal tunnel syndrome, and a few patients may be disabled to the point of calling rheumatoid arthritis in question[25]; all recover completely over time. The possibility that rubella may initiate rheumatoid arthritis is discussed by Phillips[26].

Immunization for rubella is motivated by the teratogenic effect of the virus on the fetus, and is recommended for prepubertal girls who are less susceptible to the joint symptoms. A total of 5–10% of those receiving the live attenuated rubella vaccine develop a mild arthritis that appears 2–4 weeks after vaccination, evoking effusions, affecting only one or two large joints merely with tenderness and painful restriction of movement. Such symptoms can however last for years so the relationship might be forgotten or be unrecognized. Adult women are more frequently and more severely affected[27]. Certain early vaccine strains that were found to provoke a distinctly higher incidence of rheumatic complications than others were abandoned and currently approved vaccines now have an acceptably low incidence[28] of arthritis. Tingle and colleagues[29] were unable to correlate antibody levels to arthritis in vaccinated cases. In a cooperative program to examine all cases of acute polyarthritis in an area subject to Ross River virus infection, only cases of natural rubella arthritis were found. The currently used rubella vaccine has greatly reduced the incidence of rubella arthritis.

LESS COMMON VIRAL CAUSES OF ARTHRITIC COMPLAINTS

This group includes arthritis associated with pox viruses, varicella herpes zoster complex, herpes simplex, cytomegalovirus, Epstein–Barr virus, adenovirus, hepatitis A and non-A, non-B hepatitis, mumps, alphaviruses in temperate climates, the Sindbis virus, Ross River viruses, coxsackie and echoviruses, which are briefly discussed below.

Pox viruses

The last case of smallpox (variola) was reported in Somalia in 1977, the battle against this great scourge of humanity was declared as won by United Nations Resolution 33.3 in 1980; joint involvement was rare and followed a viral osteomyelitis; septic arthritis was also described. The vaccinia virus itself has been reported to cause arthritis but this has only been well documented in one case[1,3].

Varicella and herpes zoster

The varicella zoster virus is a rare cause of aseptic or, less commonly, septic arthritis that most commonly appears (up to 5 days) after the rash, but may precede it. Fierman[30] reviewed the 20 reported cases of arthritis, which inluded three with bacterial arthritis, and most often affected the knee. Two further cases were reported in herpes zoster[31,32]. The possibility that live vaccine may lead to herpes zoster later in life has discouraged the use of an attenuated varicella vaccine, so that varicella control hinges on minimizing direct contact between varicella or zoster cases and susceptibles.

Herpes simplex

The few reported cases of rheumatic complaints related to these viruses have been of brief monoarticular arthritis[33,34]. Herpes simplex (HS) type 1 is usually an oral infection and HS-2 is predominantly a genital infection, and both are very rare causes of arthritis, with two cases being attributed to HS-1[33]. Most of reports of an association between these viruses and arthritis are related to secondary infection of immunosuppressed patients receiving cytotoxic therapy[35].

173

Cytomegalovirus

This virus most often affects immunosuppressed hosts, and only rarely causes rheumatic symptoms.

Epstein–Barr virus (infectious mononucleosis)

Although brief episodes of severe pain, tenderness and restricted movement of one, two, or more joints is relatively frequent, the incidence of overt arthritis is distinctly uncommon in this complaint[36].

Adenoviruses

Arthritis of limited duration has been reported with adenovirus type 7[37]; this same serotype was also isolated in a patient at the onset of juvenile rheumatoid arthritis. Serotype 1 was isolated repeatedly from the joint of a patient with immunodeficiency and chronic erosive polyarthritis[38]. The incidence of arthritis in adenovirus infection appears to be low, but confirmation of the infection in practice outside hospitals is not commonly undertaken.

Hepatitis A

Arthralgia occurs in 10–14% of hepatitis A infections, which are not generally accompanied by frank articular inflammation[1]. This disease is best controlled by general hygiene as for other diseases transmitted by fecal contamination of food and water supplies. Non-A, non-B hepatitis does not appear to cause arthritis.

Mumps virus

Mumps is a paramyxovirus, transmitted by saliva and possibly urine, which is endemic worldwide, has an incubation period of 16–18 days, and is asymptomatic in 20–40% of cases. Arthritis is uncommon (Maisondieu[39] reported arthritis in six of 1334 cases of mumps), may be accompanied by tenosynovitis, and result from a direct infection of the synovium[1], most often affecting males in the 3rd decade[40]; myalgia is much more common. Direct transfer in crowded communities is difficult to control by isolation. A live attenuated vaccine providing 70–95% protection can be used after 1 year of age. This may be accompanied by parotitis.

Alphaviruses in temperate regions

Five of these single-stranded RNA mosquito-borne viruses may cause a fever with rash and arthritis. Chikungunya and o'nyong-nyong mosquito-borne viruses causing arthritis in tropical countries are discussed in greater detail in Chapter 15. Mayaro virus causes a similar disease in the north of South America.

It must be emphasized that in some regions these diseases can no longer be considered uncommon. In temperate regions of Australia, for example, wider recognition of the clinical syndrome combined with improved methods for serological diagnosis, together with the reduced incidence of rubella following vaccination programs, has shown Ross River virus disease to be a far more common cause of clinically significant polyarthritis than rubella. Similar patterns may well unfold in other regions.

Sindbis virus

This virus, which normally affects animals, may also cause arthritis in humans, and is a very common infection in certain parts of southeast Australia, yet disease attributable to it has been very difficult to find. In South Africa, Sindbis virus (Chapter 15) is an important cause of arthritis which, in some cases may persist for several weeks to months with swelling of the joints and painful movement, a clinical picture very similar to that of Ross River virus, to which the Sindbis virus is closely related serologically. This regional comparison strongly suggests that genetic variation in the strain of virus can play a large role in determining pathogenicity for humans. Of the viruses listed in Table 1, Ockelbo/Pogosta[41] disease is restricted to Scandinavia and the Karelian peninsula, although it is related to the Sindbis and west Nile viruses. Sindbis, Barmah Forest and Ross River viruses are endemic in both tropical and temperate zones; Sindbis is endemic in several continents and the latter two to the Oceanic region.

Ross River virus

Epidemic polyarthritis was the first alphavirus disease to be described, and was subsequently shown to be caused by the Ross River virus. This well-studied condition resembles the other alphavirus arthritides, although it is rarely as severe as chikungunya (Chapter 15). Its varied geographical distribution illustrates the range of problems presented in control.

The history of epidemic polyarthritis underscores the difficulty in identifying a 'new' disease as a major public health problem. Although it was first clearly recognized as an unusual epidemic infection, it was seemingly forgotten for another 15 years, despite its distinct clinical presentation. It was later proven to be caused by an alphavirus by cross-reactivity with other alphaviruses, and by isolation from patients and mosquitoes. The pattern is now complete with the finding that a similar clinical syndrome is associated with Barmah Forest virus, which shares the same habitats[42]. The triad of constitutional effects, rash and rheumatic symptoms, in varied combinations, is shared with similar infections on other continents and rubella, with which it may be virtually identical[43]. A primarily maculopapular, vesicular and/or purpuric rash is present in about 60% of cases, which tends to spare the face. The rash may precede or follow the rheumatic and constitu-

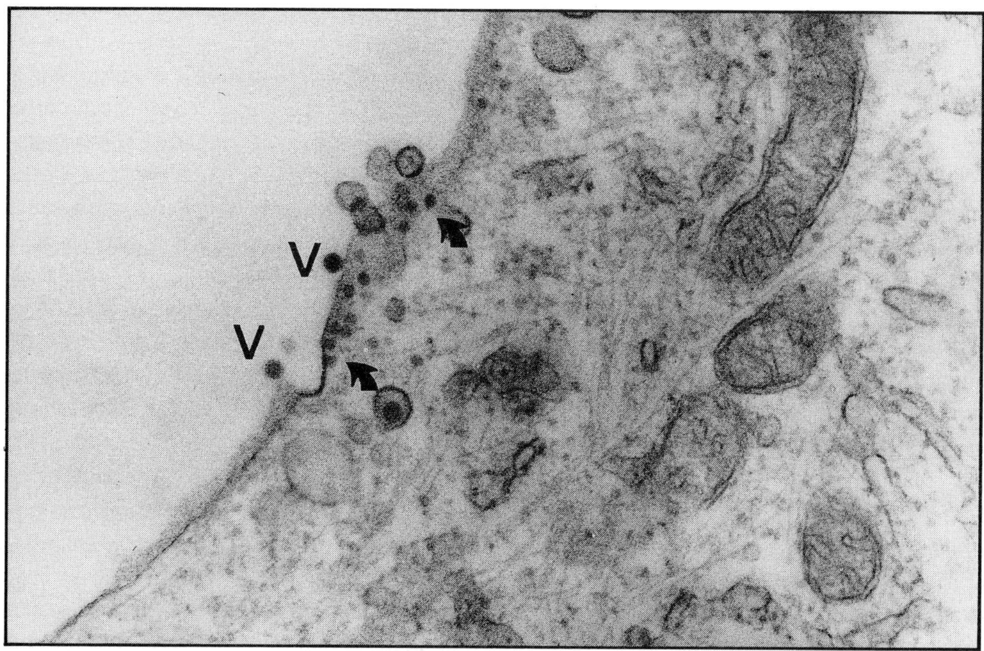

Figure 1 Ross River virus infection of human synovial cells. Virions (V), diameter 50–60 nm, are enveloped when nucleocapsids (arrows) bud through vesicular or cytoplasmic membranes. Direct virus infection of synovial tissues is often difficult to demonstrate, and not the only mechanism responsible for arthritis. (Reproduced with kind permission from Dr Daine Alcorn and Mrs Rosemary Van Driel, Dept. of Anatomy, University of Melbourne)

tional symptoms by 2 weeks and last for weeks or rarely, months, and may be the only manifestation. These features facilitate the differential diagnosis from rubella and other exanthems. Pyrexia and other symptoms are often absent or slight, but can be severe. Epidemic polyarthritis is typically peripheral and polyarticular. Affected proximal or centraxial joints recover more quickly. The full range from arthralgia to arthritis can be expressed, reaching a gout-like intensity in some cases. Synovial effusions are common, with cytology similar to that of rubella. Tendons and ligamentous structures, for instance the Achilles tendons and plantar fascia are often affected, and may be the site of present or relapsing symptoms. For further details, the reader is referred to Fraser[2], and Fraser and Marshall[44].

This condition does not permanently damage joints or tendons, but may cause complete incapacity for 1–8 weeks and lesser degrees of restriction for a year or more, even though most of those affected can resume all but the most strenuous activity after 3 months. Nonetheless, the economic burden of the acute phase alone justifies vigorous efforts at primary prevention. Although the development of a vaccine is feasible, the epidemiological patterns make field testing of such a vaccine a formidable task. Present measures are therefore directed at interrupting the infective cycle. For various reasons animal reservoirs of virus cannot be eliminated and attention is directed toward the mosquito vector, the species of which differ according to the geographic region, and determine the type of personal protection and mosquito control. For example, in Australia the main vector in the hot inland is *Culex annulirostris* which breeds best in shallow, warm pools of water, and reaches peak numbers depending on high local rainfall or overflows from heavy precipitation in remote head waters of the river systems. Several *Aedes* species predominate in coastal regions, where they breed at low levels throughout the colder seasons, quickly reaching peak levels with spring and early summer heat and rains that run into salt water marsh boundaries. It is thought that viruses increase cyclically in animal species by means of the mosquito species that preferentially seek them. At a critical point, a mosquito vector with a less selective appetite may then carry the virus to the human population. Other important factors include the competence of the mosquito species for transmission of the virus, and whether the virus can survive in the mosquito species alone by means of vertical (transovarial) transmission.

It is therefore clear that no all embracing guidelines can be formulated for reducing human virus infection by interrupting the infective cycle. Such a program may encompass a vast gamut of modalities, including public education through the schools and the media on mosquito avoidance, insect screening in buildings, surveillance and water control at breeding sites with mosquito trapping and virus isolation, entomological training of health surveyors, early case detection, serological studies of humans and animals, and weather and surface water surveillance by satellite. Extensive and uncontrolled insecticide spraying is discouraged, as it selects for resistant strains of mosquitoes, eliminates beneficial insects and causes other forms of environmental disruption. Larval control in identified breeding sites is preferred, preferably by biological means. Efforts have intensified as the extent of the public health problem becomes more obvious. The outcome of these measures is impossible to gauge, although local success follows the elimination of breeding sites artificially created by human activity. Each region requires approaches that consider differences in local geography, terrain, climate, demography and biology of distinctive local variations in virus vectors and reservoirs. In some countries such as New Zealand there appears to be no efficient vector of Ross River virus. Incoming aircraft are sprayed to reduce the risk of introducing new or infected insects. This route was considered a likely source of a recent major epidemic in Fiji[45].

Echoviruses and coxsackieviruses
Both of these viruses can present without other specific features and may only be recognized by an exhaustive serological survey or by direct attempts to isolate the virus from the joints, respiratory tract and gut. Echovirus 11 was isolated from a monocytic effusion in a patient who had a brief episode of monoarticular arthritis shortly after febrile diarrhea[46]. Some cases have resembled rheumatic fever and some have preceded rheumatoid arthritis. Since many cases of acute arthritis are mild or brief and laboratory results are slow to obtain, such efforts are not often undertaken.

Coxsackieviruses were first isolated in 1948 by Dalldorf and Sickles[47] in newborn mice inoculated with suspensions prepared from the feces of two patients with paralytic poliomyelitis in the village of Coxsackie in New York State. Coxsackieviruses are divided into two groups (A which has 24 immunological subtypes and B which has six), according to the types of lesions they cause in baby mice. The pathology in newborn mice is similar to that of human neonates, as both are highly susceptible to infections[48–50]. Both group A and B coxsackieviruses include important human pathogens: group A has been inculpated in herpangina[51] and fulminant myositis in infants and children. Coxsackie A16 is considered to be the cause of 'hand, foot and mouth' disease; coxsackie A9 and A23 (echo 9) infections are associated with fever, rash and meningo-encephalitis. Group B coxsackieviruses are implicated in epidemic pleurodynia[52], meningo-encephalitis, and hepatitis. Type B infections may simulate rheumatic fever by causing chronic endocarditis and potentially fatal myocarditis, and have been incriminated in postpancreatitis diabetes mellitus, and chronic disorders includ-

ing 'myalgic encephalopathy', or the chronic fatigue syndrome (Chapter 6).

Myalgia and frank myositis can occur both in coxsackie A and B infections, but frank arthritis is reported only in the latter. Coxsackie B has been associated with resolving acute arthritis, with the onset of chronic juvenile arthritis[53,54], and with erosive arthritis[55]. Infection is widespread and more common in lower socioeconomic groups, and occurs in the summer. The arthritis is benign, resolving in less than 2 weeks. Rheumatic symptoms may occur in the absence of other features. Control is the same as recommended for hepatitis A, poliomyelitis, dysentery and other gastrointestinal infections.

Pleurodynia
Epidemic coxsackie B infections characterized by severe chest and abdominal pain have been known for many years, especially in Scandinavia, where it is manifest as pleurodynia or Bornholm disease (after Bornholm Island, the Danish island in the Baltic Sea, where the first cases were recognized). A 4-day incubation period may be followed by an abrupt onset of fever and severe chest pain, often accompanied by spasms and rapid grunting respiration. The abdominal pain may be of such severity as to simulate an abdominal emergency. The illness is systemic, biphasic and may be complicated by meningoencephalitis, by cardiac involvement with myocarditis and pericarditis, or by foci of inflammation in the muscles, or in the joints. Pleurodynia is by far the commonest manifestation of coxsackie B infection, and may be an early indicator of such an epidemic; its presence should alert the medical and public health authorities of a possible outbreak in maternity wards, and acute myocarditis not only in newborn babies, but also in older children and in young adults. Myocarditis may require emergency treatment in intensive care units; some of these cardiac infections have been associated with acute myocardial infarction.

Prevention

At present, no vaccines have been developed to prevent coxsackie infections and other non-polio enteroviral disease, although such vaccines would be invaluable; in theory, formulation of a live attenuated vaccine should not be difficult. Nonetheless, current efforts should be directed to preventing exposure of pregnant women, in whose neonates the infection would be devastating.

Rickettsial infections

Diffuse pain in the limbs is one of the least obtrusive symptoms of rickettsial infections. Arthralgia, or more commonly myalgia and tenderness occur, but the rheumatic complaints are almost always overshadowed by other more severe manifestations of rickettsial infections and, understandably, receive a low priority in the patient's care.

Rickettsiae are small bacteria-like intracellular parasites of arthropods, possessing both RNA and DNA and cytochrome and thus are more closely related to bacteria than viruses. Rickettsial infections in man include the typhus group of fevers, which are classified according to their vectors as: epidemic louse-borne typhus caused by *Rickettsia prowazekii*; murine flea-borne typhus caused by *R. mooseri*; tick-borne typhus which occurs in the western hemisphere as Rocky Mountain spotted fever caused by *R. rickettsii*, in the Orient as tick typhus caused by *R. conorii*, and in Australia Queensland tick borne typhus (*R. australis)* and Q fever (*Coxiella burnetii*) occur[56].

Tick-borne typhus

Tick-borne infections are amongst the most frequent causes of acute febrile illness in many regions of the world. Tick-borne typhus[57–63] is characterized by the primary sore at the tick bite site, which begins as a raised red papule, the center of which becomes necrotic and black, comprising the classic tache noire lesion. Spread to the regional lymph nodes, which become enlarged and tender, is followed by widespread involvement of the vascular endothelium. An inflammatory reaction against these infected cells results in typhus nodes, the prototypic pathological lesion of typhus. Platelets and leukocytes, particularly mononuclear cells, adhere to the vascular surface of the infected cells, often followed by thrombosis of the affected capillary, accompanied by a perivascular infiltration of inflammatory cells, resulting in a widespread vasculitis. Typhus nodules are numerous in the skin where they result in the characteristic rash, and in the brain, where they give rise to intense headaches, delirium and stupor in severe cases. Periarticular tissues may also be involved by typhus nodules, giving rise to arthralgia and occasionally arthritis[62]. The incubation period in tick typhus is about 1 week, and in louse-borne epidemic typhus about 10 days. The onset is sudden with chills, headache, muscle pain and stiffness – especially of the neck and back, arthralgia, and fever. Fever in untreated cases of tick typhus may be intermittent, lasting 10 days or becoming remittent or continuous for up to 16 days. On the 3rd–5th day of fever, a maculopapular rash erupts, characteristically involving the palms, the soles and the face. In patients with epidemic typhus a fine maculopapular rash often with petechiae erupts about the fifth day and is prominent on the trunk more than the limbs. Arthritis is usually not a prominent feature of rickettsial diseases, although occasionally it may cause arthritis of both the large joints (e.g. knee and hip) and the small joints, especially in cases of tick typhus[62], variably accompanied by joint effusions. Timely therapy with tetracycline or chloramphenicol is usually followed by complete resolution without sequelae.

A clinical diagnosis of rickettsial infection may be confirmed by injecting a patient inoculum into guinea pigs, which develop a typical illness and antibodies that can be specifically identified in convalescence. Alternatively, the rickettsiae may be isolated in culture in embryonated hen eggs with growths after 3–5 passages in the yolk sac. *Rickettsiae* may be identified by immunofluorescent tests in skin biopsies taken from the papules of the rash. Since these procedures are only possible in specialized laboratories, the routine diagnosis depends on serological screening tests such as the Weil–Felix test in which agglutinins for *Proteus* OX19, *Proteus* OX2 and OXK are detected. A positive screening test may be followed by identification of specific rickettsial antigens by immunofluorescence, complement fixation and agglutination.

Prevention

The main preventive measures for the rickettsial diseases are directed against the arthropod vectors. The application of dichlorodiphenyl-trichloroethane (DDT) and other long-acting insecticides to the huts and houses of the community during epidemics of louse-borne typhus has resulted in the elimination of this infection from large areas of the world in which it was previously endemic. However, in some countries of Central Africa, and Central and South America, the lice have become resistant to the insecticides. There thus remains a place for vaccination[63]. Vaccines developed during World War II are highly effective and epidemic typhus, once a formidable disease, is now a relatively minor problem except in a few regions. Tick typhus, on the other hand, is endemic in vast areas of the world; it may be avoided by preventing contact with ticks, by not walking, picnicking or camping in areas where the infection is prevalent, and not allowing potentially tick-infected hosts such as cats, rats, or in particular dogs inside the rural or suburban home. Application of tick repellent to socks, stockings and the lower end of trousers which should be bound down by anklets and the lower end of shirt sleeves helps to prevent ticks from attaching. In practice, these measures are usually ignored and the possibility of suffering tick typhus is accepted

as a risk of rural life, especially since very effective treatment is available.

Vaccines, especially for protecting soldiers, and others operating in tick-infested environments, have been developed, and are of use when large numbers of susceptible army recruits and others are exposed to infection. Regular dipping of cattle in ascaricides markedly reduces the prevalence of ticks, but is a temporary measure, as the ticks soon become resistant to the ascaricides and new formulae are constantly being sought to deal with the problem. The use of insect repellents such as diethyltoluamide or dimethylphthalate, wearing of one piece suits and regular inspection of clothing for ticks is advised in infected areas. Vaccines are being developed for those at greatest risk such as laboratory workers[64].

Other typhus fevers do not produce prominent rheumatic symptoms.

Murine (endemic) typhus fever

Typhus fever, once a major scourge worldwide, is transmitted by *R. typhi*-infected fleas from rats and controlled by reducing rat populations. It does not appear to produce rheumatic symptoms. Louse-borne (epidemic) typhus is caused by *R. prowazekii* carried by human lice which are controlled by insecticides that attack the arthropod vector, e.g. lindane or DDT powder in the clothing, and by appropriate use of an already available vaccine.

Mediterranean spotted fever (African tick typhus)

This disease is caused by *R. conorii*, and frequently results in polyarthralgia, myalgia and neutrophil-rich synovial effusions, which respond quickly to treatment with doxycycline[65].

Queensland tick-borne typhus

This disease, is caused by *R. australis* and is associated with severe pain in one or two joints[66].

Q fever

This disease differs in that it is not insect-borne to man, though it is tick-borne in the enzootic state in native fauna in Australia[67] and in commercial livestock (e.g. cattle, sheep, goats) in that country, North America and Europe. Wilson and colleagues[67] did not mention any rheumatic symptoms in 13 cases of Q fever endocarditis, some of which had run a long course. Serological surveys suggest that subclinical infection may be common but one of the authors (RF) has not found any case of Q fever in the investigation of patients with acute non-specific polyarthritis who were also at occupational risk of *Coxiella burnetii* infection. A 2- to 4-week incubation period is followed by respiratory and gastrointestinal symptoms. Chest radiograph changes simulate primary atypical pneumonia. Some develop hepatitis, and endocarditis may occur[67,68]. In an extensive and detailed analysis[64], mild myalgia occurred in 47%, and joint pain in 11%, but none had signs of inflammation. In Q fever which is most commonly acquired as an occupational disease by inhalation of tick-infected dust, the vaccines which are currently under trial appear to have greatly reduced the incidence of Q fever in 'at risk' occupations, e.g. tanner and slaughter house workers, in Australia[69,70]. Those with positive skin test reactions should not be vaccinated. Laboratory workers have developed the disease which is not otherwise transmitted between humans. Milk from infected cattle should be pasteurized and inhalation risk should be reduced by minimizing exposure to infected aerosols.

REFERENCES

1. Schnitzer TJ. Viral arthritis. In Kelley WN, Harris ED, Rudd S, Sledge CB, eds., Textbook of Rheumatology. Philadelphia, WB Saunders, 1985, 2nd edn, p. 1543, 1611–1627

2. Fraser JRE. Epidemic polyarthritis and Ross River virus disease. Clin Rheum Dis. 1986; 12: 369–387

3. Silby HM, Farber R, O'Connell CJ *et al.* Acute monarticular arthritis after vaccination. Ann Intern Med. 1965; 62:347

4. Brighton SW, Simson IW. A destructive arthropathy following Chikungunya virus – a possible association. Clin Rheumatol. 1984; 3:253–258

5. Brighton SW, Pozesky OW, De La Harpe AL. Chikungunya virus infection. A retrospective study of 107 cases. S Afr Med J. 1982; 63:313–15

6. Fraser JRE, Cunningham AL, Clarris BJ, Aaskov JG, Leach R. Cytology of synovial effusions in epidemic polyarthritis. Aust NZ J Med. 1981;11:168–173

7. Sauter S, Van H, Utsinger PD. Viral arthritis. Clin Rheum Dis. 1971; 4:225–240

8. McCarty DJ, Ormiste V. Arthritis and HB Ag-positive hepatitis. Arch Intern Med. 1973; 132:264–8

9. Gocke DJ, Hsu K, Morgan C, Bombardieri S, Lockshin M, Christian CL. Association between polyarteritis and Australia antigen. Lancet. 1970; 2:1149–1153

10. Duffy J, Lodsky MD, Sharp JT, Davis JG, Person DA, Hollinger FB, Min KW. Polyarthritis, polyarteritis and hepatitis B. Medicine (Baltimore). 1976; 55:19–37

11. McMahon BJ, Steven R, Wainwright RB, Bulkow L, Lanier AP. Hepatitis B related sequelae: Prospective study of 1400 Hepatitis B surface antigen-positive Alaska native carriers. Arch Intern Med. 1990; 150:1051–1054

12. McMahon BJ, Heyward WL, Templin BW, Clement D, Lanier AP. Hepatitis B associated polyarteritis nodosa in Alaskan Eskimos: clinical and epidemiological features. Hepatology. 1989; 9: 87–101

13. Anderson MJ, Pattison JR. The human parvovirus. Arch Virol. 1984; 82:137

14. Smith CA, Woolf AD, Lenci M. Parvoviruses. Infections and arthropathies. Rheum Dis Clin North Am. 1987; 13:249–263

180

15. Reid DM, Reid TM, Brown T, Rennie JA, Eastmond CJ. Human parvovirus-associated arthritis. Lancet. 1985; 1:419–421

16. White DG, Woolf AD, Mortimer PP, Cohen BJ *et al*. Human parvovirus arthropathy. Lancet. 1985; 1:419–421

17. Cohen BJ. Buckley MM, Clewley JP, Jones VE *et al*. Human parvovirus infection in early rheumatoid arthritis in inflammatory arthritis. Ann Rheum Dis. 1986; 45:832–838

18. Shirley JA, Revill S, Cohen BJ, Buckley MM. Serological study of rubella like illnesses. J Med Virol. 1987; 21:369-379

19. Naides SJ, Scharosch LL, Foto F, Howard EJ. Rheumatologic manifestations of human parvovirus B19 infection in adults. Initial two year clinical experience. Arthritis Rheum. 1990; 33: 1297–1309

20. Goldfarb J. Parvovirus infection in children. Adv Paediatr Infect Dis. 89; 4:211–222

21. Osler W. The Principles and Practice of Medicine. 6th. edn, New York, Appleton & Co, 1906, p. 146

22. Smith CA. Petty RE, Tingle AJ. Rubella virus and arthritis. Rheum Dis Clin North Am. 1987; 13:265–274

23. Hillenbrand FKM. Rubella in a remote community. Lancet. 1956; 2:64–66

24. Brody JA, Sever JL, McAllister R, Schiff GM, Cutting R. Rubella epidemic on St Paul Island in the Pribilofs. JAMA. 1965; 191:83–87

25. McCormick JN, Duthie JJR, Gerber H, Hart H, Baker S, Marmion BP. Rheumatoid arthritis complicating rubella vaccination. Ann Rheum Dis. 1978; 37: 266–272

26. Phillips PE. Infectious agents in the pathogenesis of rheumatoid arthritis. Semin Arthritis Rheum. 1986; 16:1–10

27. Smith D, Guzowska J. Arthritis complicating rubella. Med J Aust. 1970; 1:845–847

28. Marrinan LM, Andrews J, Alsop-Shields L, Dougdale AE. Side effects of rubella immunisation in teenage girls. Med J Aust. 1990; 153: 631–632

29. Tingle AJ, Pot KH, Yong FP, Puterman ML, Hancock EJ. Kinetics of isotype specific humoral immunity in rubella vaccine associated arthropathy. Clin Immunol Immunopathol. 1989; 53:S99-106

30. Fierman AH. Varicella associated arthritis occurring before the exanthem: Case report and literature review. Clin Pediatr. 90; 29:188–190

31. Cunningham AL, Fraser JRE, Clarris BJ, Hobbs JB. A study of synovial fluid and cytology in arthritis associated with herpes zoster. Aust NZ J Med. 1979; 9:440–443

32. Devereaux MD, Hazelton RA. Acute monoarticular arthritis in association with herpes zoster. Arthritis Rheum. 1983; 26:236–237

33. Remafedi G, Muldoon RL. Acute monarticular arthritis caused by herpes simplex virus, type I. Pediatrics. 1983; 72:882-883

34. Friedman HM, Pincus T, Gilbisco P, Baker D *et al*. Acute monoarticular arthritis caused by herpes simplex and cytomegalovirus. Am J Med. 1980; 69:241–247

35. Stary A. New knowledge concerning Herpes Zoster. Z. Hautkr. 1989; 64:266–265

36. Sigal LH, Steere AC, Niederman JC. Symmetric polyarthritis associated with heterophile-negative infectious mononucleosis. Arthritis Rheum. 1983; 26:553–556

37. Panush. Adenovirus arthritis. Arthritis Rheum. 1974; 17:534–536

38. Fraser KJ, Clarris BJ, Muirden KD, Fraser JRE, Jack I. A persistent adenovirus type I infection of synovial tissue from and immuno-deficient patient with a rheumatoid-like polyarthritis. Arthritis Rheum.1985; 28:455–458

39. Maisondieu P. Etude des manifestations articulaires des orcillons. Thesis Jouve, Paris, 1924

40. Gordon SC, Lauter CB. Mumps arthritis: a review of the literature. Rev Infect Dis. 1984; 6:338–344

41. Skogh M, Espmark A. Ockelbo disease; epidemic arthritis-exanthema syndrome in Sweden caused by Sindbis-virus like agent. Lancet. 1982; 1:795–796

42. Phillips DA, Murray JR, Aaskov JG, Wiemers MA. Clinical and subclinical Barmah Forest virus infection in Queensland. Med J Aust. 1990; 152:463–466

43. Fraser JRE, Cunningham AL, Hayes, Leach R, Lunt. Rubella arthritis in adults. Isolation of virus, cytology and other aspects of the synovial reaction. Clin Exp Rheumatol. 1983; 1:287–293

44. Fraser JRE, Marshall ID. Epidemic polyarthritis (Ross River virus disease) Handbook. Common-

wealth of Australia Department of Community Services and Health, Canberra ACT

45. Marshall ID, Miles JAR, Ross River virus and epidemic Polyarthritis. Curr Topics Vector Res. 1984; 2:31–56

46. Kujala JJ, Newman JH. Isolation of echovirus type II from synovial fluid in acute monocytic arthritis. Arthritis Rheum. 1985; 28:98–99

47. Dalldorf G. The Coxsackie viruses: isolation and properties. In 2nd International Poliomyelitis Conference. Philadelphia, JB Lippincott, 1952, pp. 111–120

48. Javett SN, Heyman S, Mundel B, Pepler WJ et al. Myocarditis in the newborn infant. J Pediatr. 1956; 48:1–22

49. Montgomery J, Gear J, Prinsloo FR, Kahn M, Kirsch ZG. Myocarditis of the newborn. S Afr Med J. 1955; 29:608–612

50. Van Crefeld S, de Jager H. Myocarditis in newborns caused by Coxsackie virus. Ann Paediatr. 1956; 187:100–112

51. Robinson CR, Doan FW, Rhodes AJ. Report of an outbreak of febrile illness with pharyngeal lesions and exanthem. Toronto summer. 1957 isolation of group A Coxsackie virus. Can Med J. 1958; 79:121–134

52. Patz IM, Measroch V, Gear J. Bornholm disease, pleurodynia or epidenic myalgia. S Afr Med J. 1953; 27:397–402

53. Rahal JJ, Millan SJ, Noriega ER. Coxsackievirus and adenovirus infection. Association with acute febrile juvenile rheumatoid arthritis. JAMA. 1976; 235:2496–2501

54. Heaton DC, Moller PW. Still's disease associated with infection and haematophagocytic syndrome. Ann Rheum Dis. 1985; 44:341–344

55. Hurst NP, Martynoga AG, Nuki G, Sewell JR, Mitchell A, Hughes, GV. Coxsackie B infection and arthritis. Br Med J. 1983; 286:605

56. Gear JHS. The Rickettsial diseases of South Africa. A review of recent studies. S Afr J Clin Sci. 1954; 5:158–175

57. Gear JHS, de Meillon B, Hereditary transmission of the Rickettsiae of tick bite fever through the common dog tick *Haemaphysalis leachi.* S Afr Med J. 1941; 15:389–392

58. Gear JHS, Miller GB, Martins H, Swanpoel R *et al.* Tickbite fever in South Africa. The occurrence of severe cases on the Witwatersrand. S Afr Med J. 1983; 73:807–810

59. Gear JHS, Wagner JM, Dyssell JCG, Hutton SA, Wehde SDG,. Severe tick bite fever in young children. S Afr Med J. 1990; 77:422–424

60. Gear JHS. Tick bite fever. S Afr J Hosp Med. 1978; 4:45–49

61. Walker DH, Gear JHS. Correlation of the distribution of *Rickettsia conorii* microscopic lesions and clinical features in South African tickbite fever. Am J Trop Med Hyg. 1986; 34:361–371

62. Gear JHS. Complications of tickbite fever. A survey of fifty cases. S Afr Med J. 1939; 13:35–36

63. Gear JHS. Rickettsial vaccines. Br Med Bull. 1969; 25:171–176

64. Woodward TE. Rickettsial diseases. In Harrison's Principles of Internal Medicine. 12th edn, New York, McGraw Hill, 1991, pp. 753–763

65. Nogues X, Coll J, Gru J, Bonet M. Mediterranean spotted fever (A Rickettsial pox) and arthritis. J Rheumatol. 1989; 16:256

66. Dyer B. Personal communication re Queensland tick borne typhus (*R. australis*)

67. Wilson HG, Neilson GH, Galea EG, Stafford G, O'Brien MF. Q fever endocarditis in Queensland. Circulation. 1976; 53:680–684

68. Clark WH, Lennette EH, Railsback OC, Romer MS. Q fever in California VII; clinical features in one hundred eighty cases. Arch Intern Med. 1951; 88:155–167

69. Marmion BP, Ormsbee RA, Kyrkou M, Wright J *et al.* Vaccine prophylaxis of abbatoir-associated Q fever: eight years experience in Australian abbatoirs. Epidemiol Infect. 1990; 104:275–287

70. Shapiro RA, Siskind V, Schofield FD, Stallmen N *et al.* A randomised, controlled, double blind, crossover, clinical trial of Q fever vaccine in selected Queensland abbatoirs. Epidemiol Infect. 1990; 104:267–273

15. TROPICAL DISEASES AND ARTHRITIS – VIRAL CAUSES

James Gear

INTRODUCTION

Arthralgia and arthritis are important features of many tropical diseases. In some, they are the most prominent manifestation of the infection; in others they occur as a regular feature, while in still others the joints may be involved as an unusual complication of the infection. These conditions will be considered according to the nature of the organisms causing the disease, be they viruses, chlamydiae, rickettsiae, bacteria, fungi, spirochaetes, protozoa or helminths. Virus infections that predominate in temperate climates are described in the previous chapter and the remaining tropical infections in Chapter 16 and helminthic infections in Chapter 17.

ARTHROPOD-BORNE VIRUSES

These viruses are spread by mosquitoes and other arthropods, and have been classified according to antigenic, morphological, physical and biochemical characteristics into togaviridae, flaviviridae and bunyaviridae. There are several hundred immunologically distinct viruses in these families, causing diverse signs and symptoms, including arthralgia, arthritis and myalgia (*see* Chapter 14, Table 1). In most cases, musculoskeletal disease is transient, although infections by the chikungunya and Sindbis viruses (both members of the genus *Alphavirus* of the family *Togaviridae*), affect the joints more severely. The chikungunya virus is closely related to the o'nyong-nyong and Semliki forest viruses of tropical Africa, and the mayaro virus of South America, and more distantly related to the Sindbis virus, which in turn is related to the Ross River virus. The infections caused by the chikungunya and Sindbis viruses will be described in detail.

Chikungunya fever

The name 'chikungunya' describes a condition first seen in the Newala Province of Tanzania[1,2], which in the language of the Makonde plateau tribesmen, means 'that which bends up', referring to the bent posture assumed by the patients due to their painful stiff joints. The virus was isolated from human beings and mosquitoes during the outbreak and then was transmitted experimentally by *Aedes aegypti* mosquitoes. The strain was identified as a group A arbovirus, and subsequently classified as an alphavirus and named the CHIK virus[3]. A second outbreak occurred in the low veld of the eastern Transvaal in South Africa in early 1956[4]. Since then, the disease has been reported from most countries of tropical Africa and South East Asia.

Clinical picture

The infection is most common in rural areas that have been recently cleared of bush. Several laboratory infections have followed accidental transmission by mosquitoes. The incubation period ranges from 2 to 6 days, and is followed by an onset of pain in one or several joints, that is so abrupt and severe as to cause a person riding a bicycle to fall off the vehicle, and is generally accompanied by headache, eye pain, photophobia, sore throat, nausea, vomiting, and a fever that is typically biphasic (Figure 1).

On examination the face is flushed, with suffusion involving the open shirt area of the upper chest; the conjunctivae are markedly congested; the throat, especially the soft palate and pharynx, may be edematous and reddened; the cervical lymph glands at the angle of the jaw are enlarged and tender. In most patients no abnormal signs are detected within the chest or abdomen; in a few, the spleen is slightly enlarged and palpable. A characteristic maculopapular and erythematous eruption occurs 2–5 days after the onset of other signs, and ranges from a few scattered macules and papules to a generalized rash of the face, trunk and limbs including the palms and soles. In many cases bleeding into the papules occurs, but in Africa a fully hemorrhagic state has not been reported. Such cases have been reported in South East Asia and India, where dengue virus is a more frequent cause of the hemorrhagic state than chikungunya virus. The acute stage of the illness with fever lasts up to 10 days, but is often much shorter. The outstanding feature of chikungunya fever is the arthritis of sudden onset that develops at the beginning of illness, and persists through the febrile stage and continues into convalescence. One or several large joints, or the small joints of the hands and feet may be most affected; the painful stiffness of the joints is so severe upon awakening that the patients may express dread of the day's first movements, although the pain and stiffness lessen as the day progresses.

Some patients develop nodules adjacent to their finger joints, suggestive of rheumatoid arthritis,

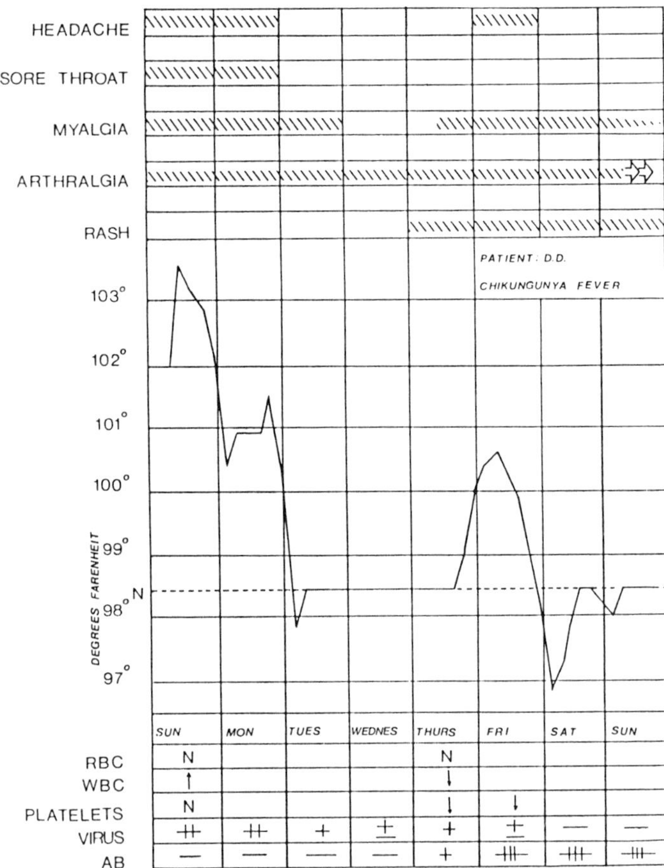

Figure 1 A typical chikungunya temperature chart

although the blood sedimentation rate is usually normal, and rheumatoid factor is usually absent. Other patients develop weakness of certain muscle groups and sensory changes suggesting local neuritis. Most patients are free from joint pain within a few weeks, while others complain of recurring painful stiffness of the small joints of the hands and feet for several months. Most patients have fully recovered within 6 months of the acute illness[5].

Pathology

Baby mice inoculated intracerebrally develop encephalitis which is fatal within a week. When inoculated subcutaneously, baby mice develop

184

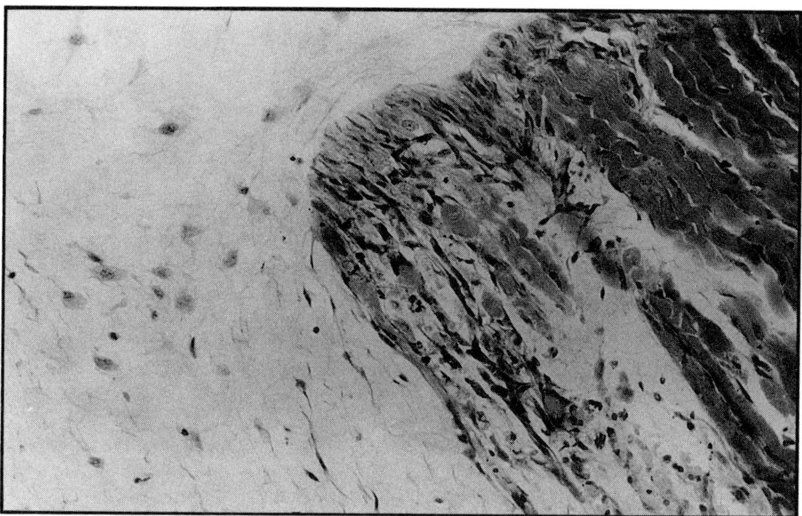

Figure 2 Acute muscle inflammation in CHIK virus infection

myositis with eosinophilic degeneration and inflammatory cell infiltration of the muscles and periarticular tissue (Figure 2). The clinical picture suggests that similar changes occur in humans.

Epidemiology

The virus has been identified in most countries of tropical Africa, and outbreaks have been described in Zambia, Zimbabwe and Zaire and serological surveys indicate that the infection occurs in Mozambique, Botswana, northern Namibia and Angola. In Asia extensive epidemics have occurred in Indonesia, the Philippines, Thailand, Vietnam and India. In South Africa, which has both tropical and temperate climates, the infection is restricted to the tropical region. Baboons and vervet monkeys circulate CHIK virus and readily infect mosquitoes. Studies on the antibody status of these primates indicate that many are infected at the time of human epidemics and they may play an important part in chikungunya's epidemiology. However, humans may also acquire the infection by intruding into a nonprimate host–vector cycle in the bush. This has not yet been elucidated. CHIK virus has often been isolated from mosquitoes frequenting the forest canopy, *Aedes africanus* and *Ae. furcifer*, both of which feed readily on baboons and vervet monkeys. *Ae. furcifer* appears to be an efficient vector of the virus and is probably the main transmitter of the infection to humans in southern Africa[6]. *Ae. aegypti* was incriminated as the vector in the first recognized epidemic of chinkungunya described in southern Tanzania. Chikungunya fever tends to occur in epidemics when conditions favor the breeding of mosquitoes and a sufficient proportion of the human population are susceptible to infection.

Prevention

The disease can be avoided by not visiting the endemic areas when outbreaks are occurring or are liable to occur. Individuals can protect themselves from mosquito bites in these areas by spraying the rooms of their houses or huts before sunset and by sleeping under mosquito nets. Patients ill with chikungunya fever should also sleep under mosquito nets to minimize the spread to mosquitoes, particularly where *Ae. aegypti* and *Ae. furcifur taylori* are prevalent and potentially serve as an initial focus of transmission. Antimos-

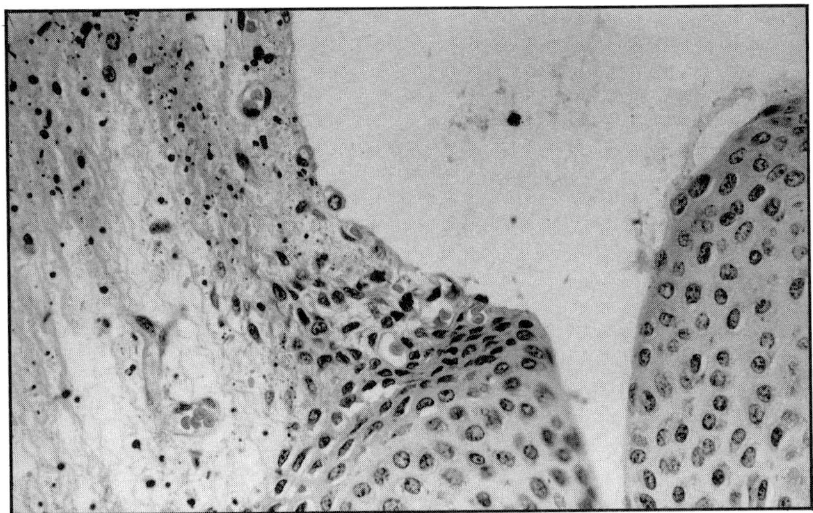

Figure 3 Acute muscle inflammation of a tendon insertion in Sindbis virus infection

quito measures are also of value in the regions where CHIK virus is endemic in preventing infection with other arboviruses, malaria and other mosquito-borne diseases.

Sindbis virus infection

Sindbis is the name of an Egyptian village near Cairo, where this virus was first isolated by Taylor and colleagues in 1952 from a trapped crow and named Sindbis virus[7], and since shown to be a not uncommon human pathogen.

Clinical picture

Studies in South Africa have clearly defined the clinical features of this infection[8]. After an incubation period of about 1 week, the patient experiences malaise, chills, fever, headache, and muscle and joint pains aggravated by movement. A characteristic rash appears on the 3rd–5th day after onset, and consists of well-demarcated red papules, often surrounded by a halo of pale skin, which often undergo vesiculation. The rash involves the face, trunk and limbs including the palms and soles, where the lesions tend to form blisters under the thicker skin. Small blisters and shallow ulcers may be seen on the mucous membranes of the mouth and throat. The fever usually lasts less than one week, but in severe cases may be more prolonged. Although slight conjunctival congestion may occur, marked conjunctivitis and swelling of the eyes are not features of Sindbis fever. In an occasional patient, the heart is involved. Myalgia, arthralgia and pain in the small joints of the hands and feet are constant symptoms; the joints are often swollen and tenderness over the insertion of tendons may be noted. The larger joints are frequently affected and become swollen and the arthritis may persist for weeks. A few patients develop neuritis with paresthesia and a pins and needles feeling, especially in the arms and hands sometimes associated with muscle weakness. Most patients recover completely within 2 weeks, but a few patients complain of fatigue and weakness for weeks, occasionally for months after the acute attack.

Pathology

There have been no reported human fatalities in Sindbis virus infection. However, Sindbis virus is pathogenic to baby mice, producing lesions which the clinical picture suggests may occur in humans. The lesions in baby mice induced by

186

virus isolated from a skin blister of a severely ill patient have been described in detail[8], and consist of necrosis of the dermal connective tissue without epidermal degeneration, accompanied by diffuse necrosis of the interstitial connective tissue of skeletal muscles and patchy eosinophilic degeneration of muscle fibers, in a background of inflammation. Of particular interest to the clinical picture seen in humans is the marked necrosis of periarticular connective tissues and capsular ligaments with involvement of the synovial membrane (Figure 3). Necrosis of smooth muscle is seen around the esophagus, gut and bladder. The cells of the brown fat undergo characteristic degeneration with nuclear pyknosis foci of myocarditis, with myocytic necrosis, may be scattered throughout the atria and ventricles, especially marked at the atrioventricular junction, and occasionally involving the valves. The extensive degeneration of the orbital muscles and connective tissue seen in newborn mice may explain the ocular pain typical of human Sindbis infection.

Diagnosis

The features of Sindbis virus infection are sufficiently characteristic to allow a diagnosis to be established on clinical grounds alone, especially when the patient has a typical rash. It is nonetheless advisable to confirm the diagnosis by the appropriate laboratory tests, since the manifestations of West Nile fever and chikungunya fever closely resemble those of Sindbis virus fever. The diagnosis may be established by isolating the virus from the blood in the early stage of disease, although in practice, this is rarely achieved; the virus has also been isolated from the blister fluid of the elements of the skin rash and from joint fluid. The Sindbis virus induces characteristic cytopathic changes in cultured vervet monkey and chick embryo cells, which display characteristic rounded eosinophilic intranuclear inclusion bodies. As the virus is rarely isolated from the blood of patients in the early acute phase, the laboratory diagnosis is based on detecting the antibodies, which appear within one week of the onset of the illness and are demonstrated by hemagglutination, hemagglutination inhibition, immunofluorescence, or by neutralization tests either in tissue culture or in baby mice.

Epidemiology

The natural history of Sindbis virus infection is somewhat complex; the virus occurs in certain common birds, in which it may reach very high titers. Studies by Jupp, McIntosh and colleagues in South Africa have implicated *Culex univittatus*, an aviophilic mosquito[9] as the primary vector of the Sindbis virus, as well as *Culex theileri*, a mosquito which feeds readily on both birds and man. Sindbis virus infection is common throughout Africa, and related viruses are prevalent in the Middle East, Europe, Asia and Australia. Epidemics of Sindbis fever tend to occur when conditions favor mosquito breeding, at which times the infection is commonly acquired in the suburbs and rural areas.

Prevention

Breeding places of mosquitoes in the vicinity of villages should be eliminated. Cleaning of huts and houses, and spraying with long-acting insecticides as practised in antimalarial campaigns greatly reduces the number of mosquitoes surviving inside dwellings. Spraying of sleeping quarters with pyrethroid insecticide will reduce further their numbers and exposure to their bites is minimized by the use of mosquito nets and repellents. Persons in open fields are well-advised to move constantly and not rest or sleep outside, although this is rarely practised. Fortunately most cases of Sindbis fever are mild, but some cases may evolve toward incapacitating arthritis.

Dengue

Dengue results from infection with a flavivirus, the dengue virus, of which four immunological serotypes, 1–4, have been identified. The infection is transmitted by *Aedes* mosquitoes, in particular under urban conditions by *Ae. aegypti.*

Clinical picture

After a 2–7-day incubation period, there is a sudden onset of high (39–40 °C) fever, accompanied by a frontal and retro-orbital headache, and back pain. The fever is often biphasic and during the second wave, the patient may have nausea and vomiting, often associated with marked anorexia, generalized lymphadenopathy and cutaneous hyperesthesia. A generalized macular erythematous rash may be seen during the first 24–28 h. Myalgia and bone pain occur soon after the onset of disease and increase in severity. On examination the patient shows conjunctival congestion, flushed face and after defervescence, a generalized morbilliform maculopapular rash erupts. At this time, the patient may develop a haemorrhagic diathesis with epistaxis and gastrointestinal bleeding, demonstrable with a tourniquet test. Some patients, especially infants and young children may develop dengue hemorrhagic fever, an often fatal condition characterized by circulatory collapse and shock, and not infrequently seen in the Philippines, Thailand, Malaya, India and, more recently, in the Caribbean islands.

Diagnosis

Chikungunya fever and dengue have many features in common, possibly because some of the epidemics described as dengue before laboratory confirmation, were actually epidemics of chikungunya fever. In the differential diagnosis, chikungunya fever is more abrupt, and the pain in the joints is sharper than dengue. Otherwise the signs and symptoms are very similar although the arthralgia with stiffness of the joints tends to persist longer in chikungunya than in dengue fever. Therefore, the confirmation of the diagnosis depends on laboratory findings.

Chikungunya virus is pathogenic to baby mice which die within 4 days of inoculation, whereas in dengue mice are relatively resistant. Serologically, the diagnosis can be clearly established, chikungunya fever is an alphavirus, whilst dengue is caused by a flavivirus. Dengue virus is not readily isolated in mice but may be isolated in mosquito cell cultures; however, reliance is usually placed on serological tests, the marked cross-reactivity with other previous flavivirus infections make the exact significance of the results of the tests difficult to interpret.

Epidemiology

Epidemics of dengue fever have occurred in most regions of the tropics, and have been particularly severe in South East Asia and the islands of the southwestern Pacific. Recently epidemics have been reported from most of the Caribbean islands, and Central America extending into the southern United States. Dengue hemorrhagic fever may occur in first infections when the virus is unusually virulent[10] or may infect children or infants who have previously had infection with another serotype of dengue virus[11].

Prevention

Preventive measures hinge on eliminating the mosquitoes responsible for transmission. The main vector, *Ae. aegypti* is essentially a domestic mosquito, breeding in man-made collections of water such as formed in water cisterns, old tins and tin cans and discarded tires. Indeed, viable eggs have been transported round the world in old tires sent from one country to another, and recently the need for proper control of this trade has become apparent. These breeding places can be eliminated by oiling or application of insecticides. Surveillance to establish the diagnosis of the first cases should be strictly applied whenever the threat of the introduction of the virus is feared. As soon as infection is detected, antimosquito measures should be intensified.

Table 1 Enteroviruses

Polioviruses types 1–3
Coxsackie A viruses types 1–25
Coxsackie B viruses types 1–6
Echoviruses types 1–72
Later isolates: Enterovirus types 34–72

ALIMENTARY TRACT VIRUS INFECTIONS

The alimentary viruses form a large group, which includes the picornaviruses, which are small RNA viruses. Those affecting humans are listed in Table 1.

Poliomyelitis

The polioviruses are well known causes of paralytic poliomyelitis, which cripples from 1 to 10% of its victims. Paralysis results from the destruction of the motor cells of the central nervous system, in particular in the anterior horn of the grey matter of the spinal cord. The illness is biphasic: the first phase or minor illness is characterized by fever, chills, sore throat, muscle and joint pains. This is followed within a week by the major illness, characterized by signs and symptoms of central nervous system involvement, including severe headache, photophobia, stiff neck, and a positive Kernig sign. Myalgia, often with tremors, develops as the temperature falls; this is followed by paralysis, involving one muscle group to complete paraplegia. Involvement of the muscles of respiration results in respiratory failure, the most frequent cause of death in polyiomyelitis. After defervescence, there is often considerable recovery of the paralysed muscles, but in many individuals, paralysis persists indefinitely, and those with respiratory paralysis may require permanent respiratory support. There is often permanent residual weakness of the limbs and joint distortion, resulting in chronic joint problems, which may be partially amenable to orthopedic surgery.

Prevention

The past efforts to limit the spread of the poliovirus by isolating patients, closing schools and places of entertainment where children congregate, and similar measures taken during the course of the epidemic were not effective. Following the discovery[12] that poliovirus would grow in tissue culture of primate cells, two highly effective vaccines were developed. The first was developed by Salk, and uses suspensions of formalin-inactivated virus[13], and consists of three injections spaced over 6 months; the other vaccine developed by Sabin, is a live attenuated oral vaccine incorporating each of the three poliovirus serotypes[14], which is administered by mouth in three doses at 3-month intervals. Mass immunization campaigns using one or other of these vaccines have been followed by a dramatic and gratifying drop in the incidence of paralytic poliomyelitis, and in North America and north west Europe have resulted in the virtual elimination of wild virus. So successful have these campaigns been that the World Health Organization and Rotary International have launched a global campaign to eliminate wild virus by supplying the vaccine to countries in need of assistance, and it is hoped that this objective will be achieved by the year 2000. In the meantime, no children should suffer from paralytic poliomyelitis provided their parents ensure that they receive the full course of immunization with either of the vaccines. Campaigns using live oral attenuated vaccine are much easier to organize than those using the injectable inactivated vaccine, given the need in the latter for sterile needles, syringes, and a semi-skilled staff to administer the vaccine. It is the duty of medical and public health authorities to ensure that every child is vaccinated, but the main responsibility rests with their parents who must be educated, not only to the existence of the poliovirus vaccine, but also to other highly effective vaccines whose use, it is hoped, will eliminate several of the common infectious diseases.

It should be noted that other enteroviruses may cause poliomyelitis-like paralysis, in particular Coxsackie A7, once described by Russian workers as poliovirus type 4[15]. Epidemics closely resembling paralytic poliomyelitis have also been reported from south east Europe and were caused by enterovirus type 71[16]. Should the threat posed by these viruses assume greater proportions it would be possible to develop vaccines to immunize against them.

Postpoliomyelitis syndrome

Recently this syndrome has attracted attention. Initially it was suggested that the increasing frequency of muscle weakness and pain occurring 30 or more years after paralytic poliomyelitis was due to reactivation of persisting viral infection. However, it is now believed that these symptoms result from years of overload of weakened muscles and of normal muscles having to carry the load, often in awkward positions. Thus, this could be classed as an overuse syndrome of the type described in Chapter 7[17,18].

REFERENCES

Arbovirus infections

Chikungunya virus

1. Robinson MC. An epidemic of virus disease in Southern Province, Tanganyika Territory in 1952–53. I. Clinical features. Trans Roy Soc Trop Med Hyg. 1955; 49:28–32
2. Lumsden WHR. An epidemic of virus disease in Southern Province, Tanganyika Territory in 1952–53. II. General description and epidemiology. Trans Roy Soc Trop Med Hyg. 1955; 49: 33–57
3. Ross RW. The Newala epidemic. III. The virus isolation, pathogenic properties and relationship to the epidemic. J Hyg. 1956; 54:177–191
4. Gear JHS, Reid FP. The occurrence of a dengue-like fever in the north-eastern Transvaal. S Afr Med J. 1957; 31:253–257
5. Brighton SW, Prozesky OW, de la Harpe AL. Chikungunya virus infection. A retrospective study of 107 cases. S Afr Med J. 1983; 63:313–315
6. McIntosh BM, Jupp PG. Attempts to transmit chikungunya virus with six species of mosquitoes. J Med Entomol. 1970; 7:615–618

Sindbis virus

7. Taylor RM, Hurlbut HS, Work TH, Kingston JR, Trothingham TE. Sindbis virus, a newly recognized arthropod transmitted virus. Am J Trop Med Hyg. 1955; 4:844–862
8. Malherbe H, Strickland Cholmley M, Jackson AL. Sindbis virus infection in man. Report of a case with recovery of virus from skin lesions. S Afr Med J 1963; 37:547–553
9. Jupp PG, McIntosh BM. Ecological studies of Sindbis and West Nile viruses in South Africa; mosquito bionomics. S Afr J Med Sci. 1967; 32:34–39

Dengue virus

10. Barnes WJS, Rosen L. Fatal hemorrhagic disease and shock associated with primary dengue infection on a Pacific Island. Am J Trop Med Hyg. 1974; 23:495–506
11. Halstead S, Rozanasuphot S, Sangukwawibba N. Original antigenic sin in dengue. Am J Trop Med Hyg. 1983; 32:154

Alimentary virus infections

Poliomyelitis

12. Enders JF, Weller TH, Robbins F. Cultivation of the Lansing strain of poliomyelitis virus on cultures of various human embryonic tissues. Science. 1949; 109:65–87
13. Salk JE. Principles of immunization as applied to poliomyelitis and influenza. Am J Public Health. 1953; 43:1384–1398
14. Sabin AB. Present position of immunization against poliomyelitis with live virus vaccines. Br Med J. 1959; 1:663–680
15. Voroshilova MK, Chumakov MP. Poliomyelitis-like properties of AB-IV Coxsackie A7 group of viruses. Progr Med Virol. 1959; 2:106–170
16. Chumakov M, Voroshilova M, Shindarov L, Lavrova I et al. Enterovirus 71 isolated from cases of epidemic poliomyelitis-like disease in Bulgaria. Arch Virol. 1979; 60:329–340
17. Peach PE. Overwork weakness with evidence of muscle damage in a patient with residual paralysis from polio. Arch Phys Med. 1990; 71:248–250
18. Jones RF. Post polio syndrome: what can we do?, Med J Aust. 1991; 155:360–361

16. TROPICAL DISEASES AND RHEUMATISM (BACTERIAL, SPIROCHETAL AND PROTOZOAL DISEASES)

James Gear

INTRODUCTION

Bacteria, fungi, spirochetes and protozoa causing rheumatic symptoms are considered in this chapter. Viruses causing rheumatic complaints were discussed in Chapters 14 and 15, and helminthic diseases in Chapter 17.

CHLAMYDIAL INFECTIONS

Chlamydiae are obligate intracellular parasites that possess both DNA and RNA, multiply by binary fission, and are more closely related to bacteria than viruses, although they were once regarded as a link between these two organisms. Chlamydiae are metabolically more rudimentary than bacteria, as they lack the ability to synthesize high-energy compounds such as adenosine triphosphate (ATP), guanosine triphosphate (GTP) and the cytochrome system.

The order chlamydiales consists of one family and one genus, containing two species, *Chlamydia trachomatis* and *Chlamydia psittaci*. *C. trachomatis* causes lymphogranuloma venereum, of which there are three serological variants or biovars, L1, L2 and L3, trachoma due to serotypes A to D, and is the most common cause of nongonococcal urethritis. Microscopically, there are two chlamydial growth forms: the elementary bodies, which are rigid spherical bodies measuring 200–300 nm in diameter and electron-dense cores of tightly packed DNA, surrounded by a trilaminar cytoplasmic membrane.

Lymphogranuloma venereum

Arthritis is a recognized complication of lymphogranuloma venereum, which is characterized by a small, often evanescent primary sore or ulcer on the genitalia followed by lymphadenitis and fever which lasts about 3 weeks. During this time the patient may develop arthritis either involving single or few joints or many joints, mainly the knees, ankles, wrists and hips. Following appropriate antibiotic therapy, the arthritis generally resolves over a period of weeks.

Sexually acquired reactive arthritis

Rheumatic complaints developing after nongonococcal urethritis have been termed 'sexually acquired reactive arthritis' (SARA) by Keat and colleagues[1], who define reactive arthritis as a sterile synovitis developing in association with a localized infection at a distant site, probably the result of toxic or immunological reactions. Most attempts to isolate chlamydia from the joints have failed or have given inconclusive findings, although high titers of chlamydial antibody have been found in the synovial fluid of many patients with SARA (*see* Chapter 18). The immunofluorescence test has also been of value in detecting antibodies in patients with SARA. Although susceptibility to *C. trachomatis* genital infection is not influenced by histocompatibility antigens, one of these, HLA-B27, is present in nearly 80% of SARA patients, and HLA-B27-positive men are approximately 100 times more likely to develop reactive arthritis than HLA-B27-negative individuals. HLA-B27-positive patients have more extra-articular lesions, a longer disease duration and a greater relapse rate than their HLA-B27-negative counterparts.

Sacroiliitis occurs in approximately 10% of patients with SARA. It is often associated with chronic prostatitis, which in turn is commonly associated with ankylosing spondylitis. In women, radiological evidence of sacroiliitis is often associated with salpingitis. More recently, Keat and co-workers examined joint fluids by the immunofluorescent monoclonal antibody technique, and found chlamydial elementary bodies in five of eight patients with SARA[2].

Psittacosis and trachoma

In neither of these other clinical presentations of chlamydial infections is arthritis a prominent feature of disease, although myalgia and muscle spasm can be pronounced in psittacosis and erythema nodosum can occur.

Diagnosis

Chlamydiae can be readily cultured from the lesions of lymphogranuloma venereum, the sputum and blood of patients with psittacosis and from eye washings from patients with trachoma, but are not readily cultured from joint fluids. However, the routine tests relied upon in lymphogranuloma, psittacosis and sexually acquired chlamydial arthritis are serological tests that detect chlamydial antibodies. There is considerable overlap of the reactions and the interpretation depends largely on the clinical manifestations.

Treatment

Chlamydial infections respond specifically to treatment with tetracycline antibiotics, the re-

sponse becoming apparent within 48 h of commencing treatment. Early antibiotic treatment of the initial chlamydial infection of the urethra may influence the outcome and prevent the occurrence of arthritis, but there is no evidence that antibiotic treatment of patients with established non-gonococcal urethritis and SARA has any influence on the development or course of arthritis.

Prevention

Like other sexually transmitted diseases, sexually acquired chlamydial arthritis may be prevented by modifying lifestyles and taking proper precautions to avoid exposure, as detailed in Chapter 18.

BACTERIAL INFECTIONS

Bacterial infections are amongst the most frequent causes of both acute (e.g. gonococcal) and chronic (e.g. tuberculous) arthritis, and many are detailed in other chapters of this monograph. In this section, the bacterial arthritides of the tropics, caused by *Mycobacterium leprae* and spirochetes, and that which occurs in both the tropics and temperate zone, *Brucella* species will be discussed in greater detail.

Leprosy

Leprosy is a chronic, contagious disease that predominantly affects the skin, mucous membranes and the peripheral nerves. It is caused by *Mycobacterium leprae*, an acid-fast bacillus that profusely proliferates within reticuloendothelial (mononuclear-phagocytic) cells, virtually packing the cytoplasm. Once widespread in Europe, leprosy is now most prevalent in developing countries in the tropics.

Clinical picture

The disease may assume one of two polar types. In tuberculoid leprosy, the patient's immune response to the infection is active or even hyperactive and the lesions are confined to the skin and peripheral nerves. The other polar form is lepromatous leprosy, in which the host is hyporeactive and there is a disseminated infection of the skin, nasal, oral and upper respiratory mucosae, peripheral nerve trunks, reticuloendothelial system, adrenal glands, testes and liver. Between these extremes are the borderline or dimorphous forms, termed borderline tuberculoid leprosy or borderline lepromatous leprosy, depending on the clinical and pathological features shared with either form. Indeterminate leprosy is characterized by poorly defined cutaneous macules with few organisms and inflamed cutaneous nerves, and may progress to any of the other, more distinct types. The invasion of the peripheral nerves results in anesthesia of the skin lesions, which in advanced cases are of glove and stocking distribution, resulting in injuries and burns to the hands and feet. This is usually followed by paralysis, foot drop, claw hand deformity, and Charcot's joints. In tuberculoid leprosy, acute reactions to the infection occur at intervals and progress to ulceration. In lepromatous leprosy, the reactions take the form of erythema nodosum leprosum, a nodular lesion causing discomfort, burning, which when pressed is painful. This lesion represents an Arthus-type reaction, is accompanied by fever, arthralgia, and lymphadenitis, and may be precipitated by intercurrent infections and drugs, especially the antileprosy sulfones.

Bone involvement is a prominent feature of leprosy, and is characterized by neurotropic atrophy of the hands and the feet, resulting in bone resorption and a gradual shortening, first of the distal, then middle and proximal phalanges. The metacarpal and carpal bones are spared. In the feet, phalanges and metatarsals are similarly resorbed, resulting in shortening of toes (Figure 1), which may remain connected to the foot by soft tissues only. Muscle paralysis may occur with ankylosis of the phalangeal, metacarpophalangeal and metatarsophalangeal joints. In lepromatous leprosy, there may also be osteitis of the long bones.

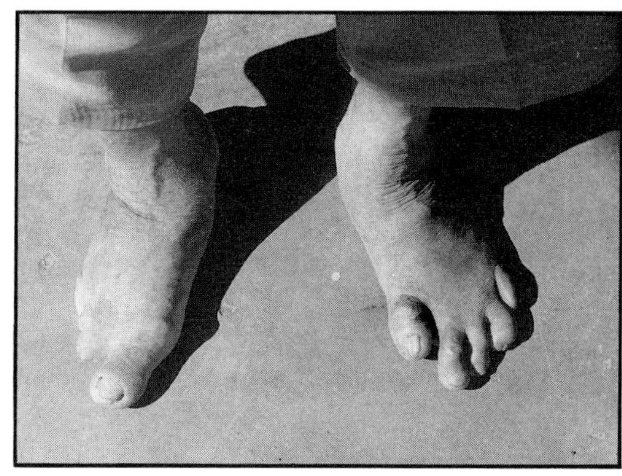

Figure 1 A case of leprosy included in the Philippines COPCORD study showing loss of toes due to sensory loss with resulting Charcot-type joint involvement

Diagnosis

The diagnosis is usually clear on clinical grounds, but early cases are often missed, and the patient may have been seen by several physicians before the diagnosis is established, often, simply because leprosy is not considered. The earliest lesions are circumscribed patches of skin that are anesthetic when tested by touching with cotton wool. At this stage, nerve thickening and tenderness may be elicited by palpating the posterior auricular nerve. Hypoesthesia of the lesion(s) may be tested by pinprick, and compared to the sensation in normal skin. Thermal sensation may also be lost and tested by using a test tube containing hot water and another ice-cold water. The diagnosis is confirmed by microscopy of clinical material, obtained by lightly incising the edge of a skin lesion with a scalpel and preparing a smear from the exudate, which is then examined for acid-fast bacilli after staining by the Ziehl–Neelsen method or by immunofluorescence.

The lepromin reaction introduced by Mitsuda in Japan is of value in differentiating the clinical

193

forms of leprosy[3]. In lepromatous leprosy, the reaction is always negative; in the borderline cases, it is usually negative but sometimes weakly positive; in the indeterminate group the reaction is variable; in tuberculoid leprosy, the Mitsuda reaction is always positive. The test antigen is prepared from homogenized lepromatous lesions and sterilized; 0.1 ml of the homogenate is injected intradermally. The reaction is interpreted at 3 weeks; a 3–5 mm in diameter nodule without ulceration, is considered a one plus (+) reaction; a greater than 5 mm nodule without ulceration, is designated as a two plus (++) reaction, and a three plus (+++) reaction is an ulcerating nodule of any size.

Treatment

Until World War II, few therapeutic options were available to patients with leprosy. In those with tuberculoid leprosy, the disease tended to burn itself out, leaving its victim severely deformed and crippled. Admission of a patient with lepromatous leprosy to a leprosy hospital meant 'abandon hope all ye who enter here'. During the War, diaminodiphenyl-sulfone (dapsone), a drug developed for the treatment of tuberculosis, was found to be highly effective in treating leprosy, and this agent has completely altered the picture of a formerly incurable disease. Since infectivity is low and quickly eliminated by treatment, the stigma of isolation is no longer necessary. Dapsone is active in all types of leprosy, and can be administered by mouth or parenterally for long periods without serious side-effects, except for mild anemia, but in patients with glucose-6-phosphate dehydrogenase deficiency (G6PDD) it may induce severe hemolysis, and the rare, but potentially fatal agranulocytosis. As resistance to dapsone has beens reported in all types of leprosy, the current treatment of choice is combined rifampicin 600 mg/day for 2 weeks, dapsone 100 mg/day indefinitely, and clofazimine 100 mg/day for 2 months, then 100 mg three times per week for 4 months. Erythema nodosum

leprosy usually responds to cortisone or prednisone 30–60 mg/day, or, if it persists, thalidomide or clofazimine are indicated.

Prevention

Prevention requires active case finding and aggressive early treatment. In areas where leprosy is endemic, case finding should be pursued actively 'by teams experienced in diagnosis. Patients detected in these surveys should be treated with sulfones, which may require years before the infection is cured. Vaccination with BCG vaccine has given equivocal results[4]. Improved living conditions in the developing countries have been accompanied by a gratifying decrease in leprosy. However, where poverty and poor living conditions are rampant, leprosy remains an important problem.

SPIROCHETAL INFECTIONS

Leptospirosis

These diseases are caused by various species of the genus *Leptospira*, and include *Leptospira interrogans* of which there are many serotypes. Leptospirosis complexes include Weil's disease caused by *L. icterohaemorrhagiae*, in which the liver bears the brunt of the infection, and *L. canicola* and *L. pomona*, both of which are often complicated by meningoencephalitis. Pretibial (or Fort Bragg) fever is due to leptospirae of the autumnalis group, and classically presents with a symmetrical macular erythematous rash over the pretibial areas on about the fourth day of disease.

Clinical picture

In general terms, leptospiral diseases are characterized by a biphasic illness; in the first stage, the patient presents with fever, marked conjunctivitis, photophobia, headache, as well as intense arthralgia, myalgia and cutaneous hyperalgesia. The second stage is characterized by signs of hepatitis, nephritis and meningoencephalitis that vary in intensity according to the different serotypes.

Diagnosis

The clinical diagnosis of leptospirosis is made on the abrupt onset of fever, its biphasic course, the marked conjunctivitis, and the characteristic pain in the back and limbs, especially in the calf muscles which are tender to palpation. The diagnosis may be confirmed in the laboratory in the first phase by isolation of the leptospirae in special culture media, in chick embryo culture or by animal inoculation of guinea pigs and hamsters. During the second phase the diagnosis is established by serological tests including micro- and macroagglutination tests, complement fixation and immunofluorescent antibody tests which give positive results after the first week of disease.

Treatment

In the early stages the infection responds to large doses of penicillin, or tetracycline.

Epidemiology

Leptospiral infections are essentially zoonoses and are common and widespread in both domestic and wild animals. Man acquires the infection from direct or indirect contact with infected animals that excrete leptospirae in their urine, often for long periods. Different animals are classically associated with different serotypes of leptospirae – *L. icterohaemorrhagae* is acquired from indirect contact with infected rats, in particular, the sewer rat *Rattus alexandrinus* or *R. norvegicus*. Common sources of infection, are the slime and water in sewers, coal mines (Britain), rivers (the Thames and others in England), canals (Netherlands), and in seaports. Outbreaks have affected fish gutters in Aberdeen and soldiers in the waterlogged trenches during World War I. *L. canicola* is acquired by contact with contaminated urine of infected dogs, especially young dogs. Some breeds of 'water' dogs, as for example spaniels, may develop chronic leptospirosis that may lead to severe terminal renal disease. *L. pomona* and

other serovar infections may be acquired by contact with pigs, cattle and other farm animals.

Prevention

Leptospirosis is often an occupational disease, most commonly infecting sewer workers, coal miners and farm workers, and may be prevented by protective clothing to prevent contamination of the skin by infected water, slime, and urine of infected animals, especially puppies that may contaminate their owners' hands with urine while being handled. Vaccines have been developed to immunize animals including cattle, pigs and dogs.

Yaws

Yaws is caused by *Treponema pertenue*, a spirochete closely related to *T. pallidum*, but is not itself a venereal disease. It is spread by direct contact with infected individuals or, as was shown in the gold mines of the Witwatersrand in South Africa, by contamination of abrasions or scratches with infected slime or water in underground workings[5]. As in syphilis, the symptoms and signs of yaws can be divided into primary, secondary and tertiary stages. The primary lesion develops in the skin after an incubation period of 1–2 months, and is a small, erythematous macule that develops into a papule or group of papules surrounded by erythema, which enlarges to several centimeters in diameter, often ulcerates, leaving a tissue-paper thin scar. If yaws is untreated, secondary lesions appear within a few weeks, which resemble the primary lesion, appearing in crops that may ulcerate and form crusts.

Many cases develop bone lesions, particularly of the long bones of the legs and forearms, and some develop multifocal dactylitis of the hands. Affected areas are tender and often edematous. Involvement of the bones of the nose may lead to a condition known as 'goundou'. Goundou are oval tumors which develop adjacent to the nose in which there is a general diffuse hyperostosis of the anterior part of the maxilla, causing the nostrils to bulge inwards, often affecting the hard palate resulting in a hideous deformity. The joints are not commonly involved, but may have increased fluid, or limited movement. In the tertiary stage, gummatous granuloma may cause skin ulceration. Gumma developing in the vicinity of large joints, especially the knees are known as juxta-articular nodules, and are painless, firm, subcutaneous tumors. Sometimes destructive lesions involve the nasal bones resulting in the condition known as 'gangosa'. Gangosa results from a spreading ulcer on the soft palate destroying the hard palate, cartilage and bones of the nose, but spread in the upper lip, leaving a gap between the nose and the tongue.

Treatment and prevention
Yaws responds to treatment with penicillin. Massive campaigns sponsored by the World Health Organization based on surveys to detect cases followed by treatment with penicillin have been highly successful in reducing the incidence of yaws in countries where it was endemic. Active surveillance, investigation of outbreaks and treatment of active cases is the appropriate control strategy for recent local resurgences in Africa[6].

BRUCELLOSIS
Brucellosis is an illness characterized in the acute stage by recurring attacks of fever with sweating, muscle and joint pains, often associated with hepato- and splenomegaly. It is caused by the gram-negative *Brucella* species, which are non-sporing coccobacilli containing three major pathogens, *B. melitensis*, an infection of goats and sheep, *B. abortus*, an infection of cattle and *B. suis*, which affects pigs. Brucella species require CO_2, produce H_2S, and grow optimally at 37 °C under aerobic conditions, taking several days before the smooth, moist, transparent, glistening 1 mm in diameter colonies are formed.

Brucella species induce abortion in animals, and abundant organisms are shed in the urine, milk and other secretions of infected animals. Man may be infected by contact with these animals or their secretions, unpasteurized milk and milk products, and tissues. It thus a disease in dairy farmers, abattoir workers, veterinary officials and laboratory workers.

Pathogenesis
Infection is followed by bacteremia, which targets the reticuloendothelial cells of the liver, spleen, lymph nodes and bone marrow. The granulomas consist of epitheloid cells, giant cells, lymphocytes and plasma cells, which are typically seen in the liver and accompanied by a marked round cell inflammation of the portal tracts. The inflammation persists in chronic infection, when local inflammation develops in various other sites, especially in the spinal column, and involves the bone, cartilage and intervertebral discs which undergo degeneration.

Clinical picture
The incubation period may vary from about 1 week to several months, and is followed by either an abrupt, typhoid fever-like onset with slight chills and fever, or may be more insidious, taking several weeks before the patient develops definite clinical signs. As the disease progresses, the patient complains of lassitude and weakness, general muscle pains, especially in the lumbar region, headache and arthralgia often associated with profuse night sweats. On examination the patient may be febrile and complain of joint swelling of the hips, knees, shoulders, ankles and wrists. After the first week of illness, the spleen becomes palpable, which may be associated with lymphadenopathy. Recurrent febrile attacks lasting from a few days to several weeks, are interspersed with afebrile periods with regression of symptoms, which may continue for months, or rarely for several years. After the acute attacks, some patients may continue to complain of symp-

196

toms without signs, and may become obsessed with persistently positive serology.

Complications
The most frequent complication of brucellosis is joint involvement. Acute inflammation with swelling of the affected joints may occur in the early stage of disease, and may be accompanied by acute suppuration, or osteomyelitis following involvement of adjacent joints. Large joints and the spine are often affected, especially the lumbar vertebrae, where bone and intervertebral discs are replaced by granulation tissue. On radiological examination, the vertebrae present a typical parrot beak appearance. Pressure on the nerve roots may cause severe radiating pain and weakness of the corresponding muscles. *B. melitensis* seems responsible for more joint affection than the other strains especially in the Middle East. Khateeb and colleagues[7] reported 96 cases of brucella arthritis from Kuwait where brucellosis is endemic (70 cases per 100 000), and found the sacroiliac joint to be involved in 26%. Other complications include meningitis, encephalitis, myelitis and neuritis, especially of the brachial plexus; respiratory complications include pneumonia and pleurisy; cardiovascular brucellosis includes subacute endocarditis, especially of the aortic valve, and recurrent thrombophlebitis; gastrointestinal brucellosis results in hepatitis and genitourinary involvement includes pyelonephritis, prostatitis, epididymitis and orchitis.

Diagnosis
The diagnosis of brucellosis is suggested on clinical grounds, and based on a history of exposure to infection by the regular consumption of raw milk and dairy products, by contact with sick animals or the carcasses of slaughtered animals or by handling of cultures in the laboratory. In the early stages of disease, the signs and symptoms most closely mimic typhoid fever. Both are often characterized by recurrent bouts of fever, splenomegaly and leukopenia. Of differential value is

an early, more complete loss of appetite, or even aversion to food, in typhoid and the occurrence of diarrhea during and after the second week of illness. Blood should be cultured with special growth media, and should be obtained during the early stages of infection, when it usually gives positive results. Multiple cultures should be taken on successive or alternate days for about a week during the fever to establish or exclude the diagnosis if the first cultures are negative. In the late stages of disease and in the chronic forms, blood cultures are often negative, and the diagnosis hinges on agglutination, complement fixation and enzyme-linked immunosorbent assay (ELISA) tests. Antibodies are usually detected during the second week of illness and thereafter may be detected for years. Although it is difficult to determine the significance of antibodies in patients complaining of vague symptoms, the persistence of high titers of antibodies suggests continued active infection.

Treatment
The therapy of choice is oral tetracycline 500 mg q.i.d. for 1 month. In patients with joints and bone involvement, streptomycin, 1 g/day for 10 days in addition to tetracycline may be necessary. Early diagnosis and early treatment is essential to avoid serious complications, such as bone and joint involvement.

Prevention
The introduction of routine pasteurization of dairy products has markedly reduced the incidence of urban brucellosis. However, it is still an important infection of those at special risk, either by occupation, e.g. farmers, veterinary surgeons and laboratory workers, or by consumption of raw milk. Some health authorities monitor dairy herds to detect and slaughter infected animals. The possibility of brucellosis should thus be considered in patients showing signs and symptoms of acute or subacute systemic infection. Appropriate and timely diagnostic labora-

Table 1 Fungi causing infections of bones and joints. (Reproduced with kind permission from Hoffman GS, Sentochnik DE. Mycobacterial and fungal infections. In Kelley *et al.*, eds., *Textbook of Rheumatology*, Philadelphia, WB Saunders, 1989, p. 1592)

Fungus	Mode of infection	Geographic distribution	Frequency of septic joint involvement
Superficial			
'maduromycoses'	fungus enters via local injury to uncovered foot	worldwide, especially in tropical climates where inhabitants do not wear shoes; rare in US	usual; soft tissue infection leading to osteomyelitis
Sporothrix schenckii	fungus enters via local injury to skin – direct implantation of plant material carrying fungus; alcoholism and myeloproliferative diseases are predisposing factors	worldwide, especially areas of high humidity; South Africa, France and Mexico are most common areas	80% of cases of systemic sporotrichosis
Candida albicans and rarely *C. stellatoidea* *C. tropicalis* *C. guilliermondi* *C. parapsilosis*	endogenous: in premature infants and other compromised hosts having malignancies, indwelling catheters, hyperalimentation, immunosuppressive therapies, multiple antibiotics; drug addicts (especially heroin)	worldwide	rare
Actinomyces israelii (anaerobic bacterium)	endogenous – host may or may not be compromised; focal cervicofacial disease or disseminated bacteremia; may follow oral trauma such as tooth extractions	worldwide	common in facial bones
Deep			
Aspergillus fumigatus	inhalation or endogenous infection in a compromised host; dissemination via respiratory tree and blood; rarely via gastrointestinal tract	worldwide	rare
Histoplasma capsulatum	inhalation; aerosol from soil rich in bird droppings (especially chickens, starlings) and bat feces	worldwide; in USA most concentrated in the Mid-West, Ohio and Mississipi River valleys	rare
H. duboisii	uncertain	Africa	about 66% with disseminated disease
Cryptococcus neoformans	inhalation, often compromised host as well as normal persons	worldwide; no regional concentration in US	5–10%
Coccidioides immitis	inhalation, especially during dry, dusty months	south-western US Central and South America especially arid dusty regions	10–20% cases with disseminated disease
Blastomyces dermatitidis	usually inhalation; very rarely inoculation into traumatized skin; most common among persons repeatedly exposed to soil. 9 males : 1 female	USA: Mississipi and River Ohio basins, middle Atlantic states, Canada, Africa, Europe, northern South America	25–50% disseminated blastomycoses cases

tory tests would facilitate prevention of the disease in others exposed to the same risk factors.

FUNGAL INFECTIONS – MYCOSES

A number of mycotic infections may be complicated by involvement of the joints and muscles. These include sporotrichosis, histoplasmosis and coccidiomycosis. The fungal diseases which can affect bones and joints are summarized in Table 1.

Sporotrichosis

Sporotrichosis is caused by the fungus *Sporothrix schenckii*; it is worldwide in distribution and cases occur sporadically, commonly affecting gardeners and others working with soil, especially after pricks from rose or other thorns. In South Africa large epidemics have affected gold miners of the Witwatersrand, involving several thousand cases[8].

Clinical picture

The sporotrichium flourishes in timber and slime of the underground workings. Human infection is usually through cuts and abrasions; a nodule develops at the site of the infection, and is followed by nodules along the tributaries of lymphatics drainage, which may undergo necrosis, forming shallow ulcers. Occasionally, the infection may involve bone and joints, with marked interference with function[9]. Rarely the infection becomes generalized and involves the lungs and other organs.

Diagnosis

The clinical picture of nodules along the course of lymphatics is so characteristic as to suggest the diagnosis. This is then confirmed by culturing the fungi on suitable media such as maltose agar where they form characteristic colonies having a characteristic morphology. Histological examination of a nodule shows microabscesses consisting of neutrophils and epithelioid cell granuloma, sometimes with typical cigar-shaped and asteroid bodies.

Treatment and prevention

Sporotrichosis responds well to prolonged treatment with potassium iodide. Ketoconazole has also been shown to be efficacious in the treatment of sporotrichosis[10]. The infection in the gold mines of the Witwatersrand was controlled by treatment of the timber with antifungal solutions.

Histoplasmosis

This condition is caused by *Histoplasma capsulatum* which is found in the soil and flourishes in pigeon and chicken droppings, and in the guano of bats in caves. The infection is widespread and has caused outbreaks of the disease especially in the eastern and central United States, in the former related to pigeon droppings, in the latter to chicken droppings, and man acquires the infection by inhaling the spores and hyphae of the fungus in the air. In South Africa, outbreaks have affected particularly speleologists and other cave visitors[11].

Clinical picture

The disease is characterized by pneumonitis with fever lasting 2 or 3 weeks; the X-ray shows a characteristic miliary pattern that may be confused with tuberculosis. Rarely, severe and potentially fatal disseminated disease develops in patients receiving immunosuppressive therapy, especially after renal transplantation. Another severe form of the disease, African histoplasmosis, has been reported from Zimbabwe, Zaire and the Sahara, which is caused by a distinct fungus, *H. duboisii*[12], and most prominently affects the skin and bones, in contrast to *H. capsulatum*, in which pulmonary lesions prevail. Involvement of the vertebrae may result in paraplegia and sometimes in death. Arthritis of the knee and wrist, and carpal tunnel syndrome have been reported but are rare[13].

Diagnosis

The diagnosis of histoplasmosis is suggested clinically by a history of exposure to potentially infected dust, as found in bat-infested caves, and may be confirmed in the laboratory by finding characteristic dimorphic fungi, obtained from the sputum. *H. capsulatum* grows readily in blood-enriched culture media, and can also be identified by the so-called exoantigen method, in which the antigens are identified by microimmunodiffusion. The presence of fungi in the air of caves can be confirmed by leaving laboratory mice or other experimental animals in cages for 24 h. After about 1 week these animals are sacrificed, the lungs examined and cultured for histoplasma. Non-pathogenic fungi are filtered out by this method. These tend to overgrow histoplasma on culture media exposed directly to cave air.

Treatment and prevention
Most cases of histoplasmosis do not require specific treatment, although progressive disease or bone involvement necessitates amphotericin B, a somewhat toxic drug whose side-effects should be closely monitored. After one attack speleologists appear to be immune to further attacks and most take no precautions; susceptible individuals exploring caves should wear protective masks with a self-contained air supply.

PROTOZOAL INFECTIONS
Chagas' disease
This is an acute, subacute, and eventually chronic condition caused by *Trypanosoma cruzi* and transmitted by reduviid bugs. This is endemic in Central and South America and may be seen in Texas. Trypanosomes are 'C' shaped organisms with a central nucleus and a large kinetoplast that are ingested by the vector whilst feeding on blood of both wild and domestic reservoir animals. They multiply in the gut, and after 3–4 weeks, are infective to man, passing from the bug's feces into the human host through cuts, abrasions and possibly the intact skin or mucous membranes.

Clinical picture
The acute form occurs in children and is charac-

terized by fever, edema of the subcutaneous tissues especially the face, local lymphadenitis, myocarditis, and occasionally involves the central nervous system. Myositis is widespread but is usually asymptomatic[14]. In adolescents and adults, Chagas' disease assumes a chronic form, the chief manifestations of which result from involvement of the heart, often leading to failure. Infection of the autonomic nervous system may result in the classic finding of esophageal and colonic dilatation, resulting in mega-esophagus and megacolon. Central nervous system involvement with meningoencephalitis, especially in infants, may result in death.

Diagnosis
The diagnosis is suggested by the clinical picture and can be confirmed by finding trypanosomes in peripheral blood smears, through diligent searching; immunofluorescent tests may detect antibodies to trypanosomal antigens. The finding of rheumatoid factor requires that rheumatoid arthritis be included in the differential diagnosis[15].

Treatment and prevention
Drug treatment, unlike that in African trypanosomiasis, is unsatisfactory, but some effect has been noted with nitrofurazone drugs and with 8-amino-quinoline. Cardiac failure requires inotropic therapy to support the cardiac muscle. Prevention depends essentially on improving living conditions, especially housing, and the elimination of the bugs by the use of DDT or other long-acting insecticides. Kirchoff[16] warns of the danger of transmitting this disease by blood transfusion, although in clinical practice this is an uncommon event.

REFERENCES
Chlamydial infections
1. Keat A, Thomas BJ, Taylor Robinson D. Chlamydial infection in the aetiology of arthritis. Br Med Bull. 1983; 39:168–174
2. Keat A, Thomas B, Dixey J, Osborn M, Sonnex

C, Taylor Robinson D. Chlamydia trachomatis and reactive arthritis, the missing link. Lancet. 1987; 1:72–74

Leprosy

3. Binford CH, Meyers WM. Leprosy. In Binford CH, Connor D, eds., Pathology of Tropical and Extraordinary Diseases. Armed Forces Institute of Pathology, Washington DC, 1976, pp. 205–225

4. Nordeen SK, Sansarricq. Immunization against leprosy – progress and prospects. Bull WHO. 1984; 62:1–6

Yaws

5. Scott CJ. Yaws special suppl. Transvaal Mine Med Off Assoc. 1933; 12:41–70

6. Perine PL. Non-venereal treponematoses: yaws, pinta and epidemic syphilis. In Harrison's Principles of Internal Medicine. 12th edn, McGraw Hill, 1991, pp. 661–663

Brucellosis

7. Khateeb MI, Araj GF, Majeed SA, Lulu AR. Brucella arthritis: a study of 98 cases in Kuwait. Ann Rheum Dis. 1990; 49:994–998

Fungal infections – mycoses
Sporotrichosis

8. Du Toit CJ. Sporotrichosis on the Witwatersrand. Proc Transvaal Mine Med Off Assoc. 1942; 22: 1–17

9. Lurie HJ. Five unusual cases of sporotrichosis from South Africa showing lesions in muscles, bones and viscera. Br J Surg. 1963; 50:585–591

10. Calhoun DL, Waskin H, White MP *et al*. Treatment of systemic sporotrichosis with ketoconazole. Rev Infect Dis. 1991; 13:47–

Histoplasmosis

11. Murray JF, Lurie HI, Kay J, Komins C, Borok R, Way M. Benign pulmonary histoplasmosis (cave disease) in South Africa. S Afr Med J. 1957; 31:245–253

12. Cockshott WP, Lucas AO. *Histoplasma duboisii*. Q J Med. 1964; 33:223–238

13. Rowe IF, Forster SM, Seifert MH *et al*. Rheumatological lesions in individuals with human immunodeficiency virus infection. Q J Med. 1989; 73:1167–1184

Chagas' disease

14. Pallis C, Lewis PD. American trypanosomiasis. In Walton J, ed., Disorders of Voluntary Muscle. Edinburgh, Churchill Livingstone, 1981

15. Harboe M. Rheumatoid factors in leprosy and parasitic diseases. Scand J Rheumatol. 1988; Suppl. 75:309–313

16. Kirchoff LV. Is *Trypanasoma cruzi* a new threat to our blood supply. Ann Intern Med. 1989; 111:773–774

17. TROPICAL DISEASES AND ARTHRITIS – HELMINTHIC INFECTIONS

James Gear

Helminthic infections may cause various forms of rheumatic complaints ranging from evanescent hypersensitivity reactions to severe damage to the joints.

FILARIAL INFECTIONS

While arthritis is not a major feature of tropical filarial diseases, the joints may become involved in the allergic reactions that commonly occur with these infections, and in their late manifestations. The filarial parasites are elongated thread worms that inhabit their host for many years, prolifically producing microfilariae that circulate in the blood or spread in the skin and subcutaneous tissues. These microfilariae are ingested by arthropod vectors, and after development, transmitted to other humans whilst the arthropod is feeding.

Bancroftian filariasis

This condition is caused by the nematode *Wuchereria bancrofti,* the adults of which are long, thread-like worms: the female is $80–100 \times 0.2–0.3$ mm and the male is about half this size. They inhabit the lymphatic channels and lymph nodes, producing abundant microfilariae that circulate in the blood with a nocturnal periodicity, a time that coincides with the peak feeding times of certain mosquito vectors, including species of the genera *Culex, Aedes* and *Anopheles.* In some south west Pacific islands, where the infection is transmitted by daytime-feeding mosquitoes, the microfilariae do not show this nocturnal peak. The presence of the adult worms in the lymphatic vessels leads to repeated inflammation, lymphangitis, lymphadenitis, fibrosis and ultimately occlusion of the vessels, which in turn leads to lymphedema, and if intense, as it commonly is, to elephantiasis, the 'classic' manifestation of filarialiasis.

Clinical picture

The manifestations of filariasis vary greatly according to the degree of involvement and the sites of obstruction. Systemic disease is manifest by fever, headache, anorexia, and intermittent lymphangitis. Local symptoms include filarial abscess, varicosities of the groin and axilliary lymphatic vessels and lymph nodes, orchitis, chyluria, chylous ascites, chylous diarrhoea, and elephantiasis of the leg, arm and scrotum, vulva and mammary glands. Arthritis and synovitis represent allergic reactions that occur during attacks of filarial fever or as a manifestation of the reaction to the presence of adult worms and microfilariae in the synovial and joint tissues. Most frequently the knee is involved, less often the ankles, the wrists and elbows and occasionally the hip and shoulder joints. Elephantiasis of the legs may seriously interfere with function of the knees and ankles. Similarly elephantiasis of the arms may restrict the movement of the elbows, wrists and fingers.

Diagnosis

The diagnosis may be confirmed by finding microfilariae in the peripheral blood smears or films, obtained both during the day, as is routine practice, as well as at hourly intervals throughout the night to detect the microfilariae. There are confirmatory skin and serological tests, but other filarial infections may interfere with the specificity of these tests.

Treatment

Single-dose therapy with ivermectin[1] is now preferred by many workers to the more traditional diethylcarbamazine (2 mg/kg, t.i.d.) per os for 3–4 weeks, both of which eliminate microfilariae from the bloodstream. The latter agent may also kill adult worms, but repeated treatments are often necessary, and may be accompanied by abscess formation and severe allergic reactions that are controlled by antihistamines and corticosteroids. Surgical removal of the elephantoid tissue of a grossly enlarged scrotum is indicated, particularly when it represents a mechanical and psychological burden to the patient. Elephantiasis of the legs may be reduced by elevating the affected limbs and pressure with elastic bandages.

Prevention

Filarial disease is prevented by eliminating as far as possible the breeding places of the mosquito vector. Long-acting insecticides may be applied to the domicile which should, if possible, have screened doors and windows, and the underbrush around the house, a favored resting place of the mosquito vector, should be cleared. The populace should sleep under mosquito nets, and possibly receive prophylactic diethylcarbamazine, a measure undertaken in Gambia (5 mg kg^{-1} day^{-1} for 5 days), which either eliminated the microfilariae or substantially reduced the parasitemia for about 1 year, after which time the number of microfilariae again increased. In other mass campaigns, a single dose of 4–6 mg/kg given once weekly for 12–24 weeks is effective in controlling *W. bancrofti* infections. The same dose given for 6–8 weeks is adequate in *Brugia malayi* infections, and is a useful prophylactic for *B. malayi* infections for those briefly visiting highly endemic regions.

Loiasis

Loiasis occurs in the equatorial rain forests of tropical Africa, involving south-east Nigeria, the Cameroon Republic, Gabon, Zaire and the Central African Republic, and is caused by the filarial worm *Loa loa*. The female measures 70 mm in length, about twice that of the male, and is transmitted by certain tabanid flies, e.g. the deer or mango fly, which breeds in densely shaded, slowly running streams. The adult filariae wander through the tissues and periodically appear beneath the skin, causing the transient subcutaneous 'Calabar' swellings. Microfilariae appear in the blood of most infected individuals, usually in greater numbers during the day, which is probably an evolutionary advantage, related to the daytime habits of their vectors. The species responsible for transmission are *Chrysops dimidiata*, *C. silicea* and *C. distinctipennis*, which ingest the microfilariae, which develop and migrate to the fly's proboscis, infecting the next human host when it feeds.

Clinical picture

Most patients with *Loa loa* have silent infections. The most common manifestations are the characteristic and locally painful swellings that first appear about 3 months after infection, and wane after several days, and then reappear for many years When these swellings appear in the vicinity of joints they may cause severe restriction of movement, and persist for weeks. The presence of the worm in the conjunctivae results in acute inflammation with edema and lacrimation.

Diagnosis

The diagnosis is suggested by the characteristic Calabar swellings and conjunctival involvement, and is confirmed by finding microfilariae in peripheral blood smears taken at midday, although the absence thereof does not exclude loiasis.

Treatment

Diethylcarbamazine is effective in eliminating microfilariae and, in some patients, in killing adult worms. Therapy should start with 1 mg/kg, increased to 4 mg/kg over the next two days and continued for 3 weeks. It may be necessary to repeat the treatment after 3 months. Allergic reactions are not uncommon and usually respond to antihistamines or corticosteroids.

Prevention

Loaisis can be avoided by not entering the rain forest or its fringes, advice which is of no value to local inhabitants. Prophylaxis with diethylcarbamazine, 200 mg b.i.d. for 3 days once a month for adults has been recommended. Flies have been successfully controlled in some areas by bush clearing and applying long-acting insecticides.

Dracontiasis

Dracontiasis is caused by Guinea worm, *Dracunculus medinensis*, which inhabits the subcutaneous tissues and may sometimes be seen subcutaneously. The adult male is rarely observed, and measures 10–30 mm × 0.4 mm; the adult female is 70–120 cm long × 0.1–0.7 cm in diameter, has a smooth, thick skin, and forms a blister when in contact with water, often around the lateral malleolus. The blister ruptures and the anterior end of the gravid female discharges larvae into the surrounding water, which are then ingested by cyclops, the intermediate host.

Clinical picture

Man acquires the infection by ingesting cyclops in drinking water, and once ingested, about 1 year passes before the developing female appears near the skin surface. Once there, its presence causes irritation and induces the patient to immerse his foot in water, whereupon the blister ruptures, discharging embryos until the worm has emptied herself. During this time the patient often experiences urticaria, or allergic reactions, vomiting and diarrhea and may suffer attacks of asthma. The ulcer may become secondarily invaded by pyogenic organisms such as staphylococci and streptococci, causing cellulitis with local pain and inflammatory edema. Arthritis and synovitis may result from the presence of the worm and its rupture in the neighborhood of joints, particularly the ankle and knee, which may develop effusions, and be followed by ankylosis with crippling limitation of movement.

Diagnosis

The diagnosis is usually obvious and typical 'rat-tail' embryos may be seen in the blister fluid. The presence of the worm is often associated with eosinophilia, and can be confirmed by intradermal and serological tests, which may be of value in cases where the worm has not made its appearance under the skin.

Treatment

The classic treatment is to gradually extract the worm after it has appeared on the surface by winding it round a stick, taking care not to break or damage it in the process. Alternatively, the worm may be extracted through surgical incisions.

Prevention

The development of the worm may be inhibited by diethylcarbamazine. The infection can easily be eliminated by eliminating the intermediate host cyclops from the water supply, which occurs naturally during periods of prolonged drought when shallow wells dry up, resulting in a marked decrease in infection. Campaigns to eliminate dracontiasis sponsored by the World Health Organization have achieved excellent results, by addressing the issue of pure water for domestic purposes.

Onchocerciasis

Onchocerciasis is caused by *Onchocerca volvulus*, a filarial nematode worm. The female worms are 30–50 cm × 0.25–0.5 mm in diameter, and have regularly spaced annular rings; male worms are 1.5–4.5 cm × 0.12–0.2 mm. The *O. volvulus* microfilaria is 220–350 × 5–10 μm, unsheathed, has a tail that tapers to a point and is free of nuclei. The nematode is transmitted by black flies of the genus *Simulium*, also known as buffalo gnats, given their hump-backed appearance. The species of flies varies in different parts of the tropics: in West Africa, in the Congo basin and the neighboring territories *S. damnosum* is the main vector; in East Africa *S. neavi* is the main vector. Several species are involved in South and Central America including *S. ochraceum* in Guatamala and Mexico, *S. metallicum* in Venezuela, and *S. amazonicum* in Brazil and Columbia. These flies typically breed in fast flowing waters such as river rapids, waterfalls and the overflow of dams. Masses of eggs are laid in the water and hatch into larvae in 2–3 weeks. The larvae of *S. damnosum* attach to vegetation and stones in the river, those of *S. neavi* to crabs. The pupae attach to aquatic weeds and the adults emerge after about 1 week, mating and feeding takes place within 24 h. Both sexes feed on plant juices but only the female flies feed on blood. The flies imbibe microfilaria with their blood meal, which then develop within the fly's thoracic muscles; the infective stage migrates to the proboscis and the infection is transmitted while the fly is feeding. *S. damnosum* tends to bite below the belt, while *S. neavi* and the simulium flies in South and Central America bite above the belt. Though the infective microfilariae may migrate some distance from their point of entry, the bite site determines to some extent the location of the nodules that subsequently develop; thus, the microfilariae are most frequent on the lower limbs and pelvic girdle in Africa and on the head, shoulders and arms in tropical America.

Pathogenesis

The infective stages develop into mature worms in the subcutaneous tissues and a fibrous capsule surrounds them, forming a nodule, often containing several females and males coiled in a mass of fibrous tissue. The female gives birth to microfilariae that migrate into the surrounding tissues and skin.

Clinical picture

Onchocerciasis is characterized by dermatitis, subcutaneous nodules and eye lesions leading, in heavy infections, to blindness (river blindness). Simulium bites are painful and often followed by transient irritation, although some of those infected develop thickened and wrinkled skin with a lichenoid appearance. The nodules first appear several months after infection, and grow slowly reaching their maximum size in 4–5 years to form rounded or ovoid masses particularly over bony prominences such as the occipital boss, the scapulae and iliac crests and periarticularly, where their presence may interfere with the free movement of the joints.

Two types of arthritis are recognized. The monoarthritic form of onchocerciasis involves large joints such as the hip, knee and elbow with nodules occurring adjacent to the affected joint. It is characterized by acute inflammation with deep pain in the joint, microfilariae in the synovial fluid, and responds well to treatment with diethylcarbamazine. The second form is a polyarthritis, possibly related to circulating immune complexes, which resembles rheumatoid arthritis and may be precipitated or exacerbated by diethylcarbamazine therapy.

Diagnosis

The diagnosis of onchocerciasis is established by finding the characteristic microfilariae within snips of affected skin or conjunctivae, which when placed in saline solution induces the migration of microfilariae from the tissues, which may be identified microscopically. Serological tests using an antigen prepared from worms are of value in surveys of the incidence of infection, although overlapping reactions occuring in those individuals harboring other filarial infections make the interpretation of results difficult. Skin tests are also useful in surveys to determine the incidence of disease. The Mazzotti test in which the patient is given a single dose of 50 mg of diethylcarbamazine should only be used if other tests are negative, as the reaction may be severe with intense pruritus, inflammation and edema of the skin, potentially severe systemic manifestations with arthralgia and aggravation of the ocular inflammation. The blood count, as in other helminthic infections, shows an eosinophilia which, in the early stages, comprises up to 70% of the granulocytes, but in long standing infections falls to lower levels; hypersensitivity reactions following treatment are associated with an increase, sometimes marked, of the eosinophilia.

Treatment
Excision of nodules interfering with movement of joints and in the vicinity of the eyes or for cosmetic reasons has been widely practised, and may help slow the progression of the lesions. Chemotherapy of onchocerciasis is remarkable for serious side-effects which are so common as to negate mass treatment campaigns, although the recent introduction of the single dose agent, ivermectin[1], may reverse this policy. The standard treatment is with diethylcarbamazine combined with Suramin. Diethylcarbamazine kills microfilariae but has little effect on the adult worms as microfilariae reappear in the vicinity within 3–12 months of their apparent elimination. The course of treatment is one tablet of 50 mg on the first day followed by two 50 mg tablets on days 2–10. This treatment may precipitate severe pruritus, fever and arthralgia and occasionally circulatory collapse within a few hours of its commencement. To lessen this hazard, a

course of corticosteroids, dexamethasone, should be given, starting with 4 mg/day 2 days before the administration of diethylcarbamazine and continued for 1 week.

Prevention
Onchocerciasis may be controlled and even eliminated by the eradication of the intermediate host, *Simulium*. As noted, these black flies breed in fast-flowing water. At one stage, soon after World War II, consideration was being given to moving the capital of the Belgian Congo (now Zaire), Leopoldville (now Kinshasa) because of the prevalence of onchocerciasis in the population. However, the application of DDT and other long-acting insecticides by aerial spraying of the Congo rapids, was highly effective. Within a few days the city was practically free from simulium and local transmission ceased and Kinshasa has remained free. A mass trial of ivermectin[2] in the control of this disease appears to have been successful.

TRICHINOSIS (TRICHINIASIS)
Trichinosis is caused by the nematode *Trichinella spiralis*, and is most common in areas where pork is consumed including east and central Europe, North America, Central and South America and in Africa. Epidemics of trichinosis may follow the consumption of raw or undercooked pork, wild bush pigs and warthogs, which contain encysted *T. spiralis*. The cysts liberate larvae which, after several months, develop in the small intestine of man, pigs, bears, rats and other carnivores into mature male and female worms, which enter the circulation and encyst in the striated muscle, where they remain viable for years.

Clinical picture
Clinical symptoms begin 10–12 days after ingesting the infected meat, and include diarrhea or constipation, abdominal pain, asthenia, weakness, fever, eosinophilia, and the highly characteristic clinical sign of subungual 'splinter'

hemorrhages. Muscle invasion is marked by myalgia, swelling of the eyelids, and in severe cases by myocarditis, nephritis, bronchopneumonia, and meningoencephalitis. While invasive disease may be associated with arthralgia, arthritis is not a prominent feature, except in chronic disease in which the patients may have rheumatoid arthritis-like symptoms.

Diagnosis
The diagnosis is suggested by the history of ingestion of raw meat followed by the characteristic high fever and muscle pains. The presence of cysts in the muscles may be confirmed by muscle biopsy examination and, when calcified, the cysts appear by X-ray examination.

Treatment and prevention
Thiabendazole is an effective larvicide in experimental animals, but its use in man is hampered by serious after-effects, which may be diminished by the use of corticosteroids. Trichinella infection may be prevented by strict supervision of abattoirs to detect infection of pork, surveillance of wild animals, and adequate cooking of pork and game meats to sterilize the cysts.

SCHISTOSOMIASIS

Schistosomiasis is a disease of man caused by parasites which have a complicated life-cycle (Figure 1), in which the adults live and lay eggs in the veins of various organs. The eggs are excreted by infected human beings, hatch in water as miracidia, which in turn infect certain species of aquatic snails, where they develop into cercariae, that are discharged into the water and infect man. Humans acquire the infection while washing, paddling and swimming in water infested with snails shedding cercariae. There are three major forms of schistosomiasis (bilharziasis) in man:

(1) Urinary schistosomiasis, characterized by hematuria and caused by *Schistosoma haema-tobium*, the larval stages of which develop in snails of *Bulinus* spp.

(2) Intestinal schistosomiasis, characterized by bloody diarrhea and mucus, caused by *S. mansoni*, the larval stages of which develop in snails of *Biomphalaria* spp.

(3) Intestinal and visceral schistosomiasis, caused by *S. japonicum*, which develops in snails of *Onchomelania* spp.

Geographical distribution
Human schistosomiasis occurs in most of Africa with the exception of the deserts, the high mountainous regions and the western half of South Africa. Both *S. haematobium* and *S. mansoni* infections occur in Malagasy, but only *S. haematobium* occurs in Mauritius, and only *S. mansoni* occurs in the western hemisphere, in the West Indies and the eastern and northern areas of South America. *S. japonicum* occurs in the Far East, in restricted areas in China, Japan and the Philippines. Small foci of *S. haematobium* infection exist in Portugal and in India, south of Bombay.

Pathogenesis and pathology
Cercariae, which are infective to man, shed their tails, penetrate the normal healthy skin, and enter the blood or lymphatic vessels, migrating via the heart and lungs to the liver. Schistosomiasis gives rise to signs and symptoms at each stage in its human cycle: at the time of first infection, there is irritation and inflammation at the penetration site, which may be quite severe in individuals sensitized by previous infections, giving rise to a transient cercarial dermatitis. Passage of schistosomules through the lungs causes coughing and occasionally blood-stained sputum. When the worms reach the portal veins they evoke the signs and symptoms of mild hepatitis, and a feeling of fullness in the right upper quadrant; in the liver, they develop in the portal veins into adult male and female worms, which mate and then migrate

208

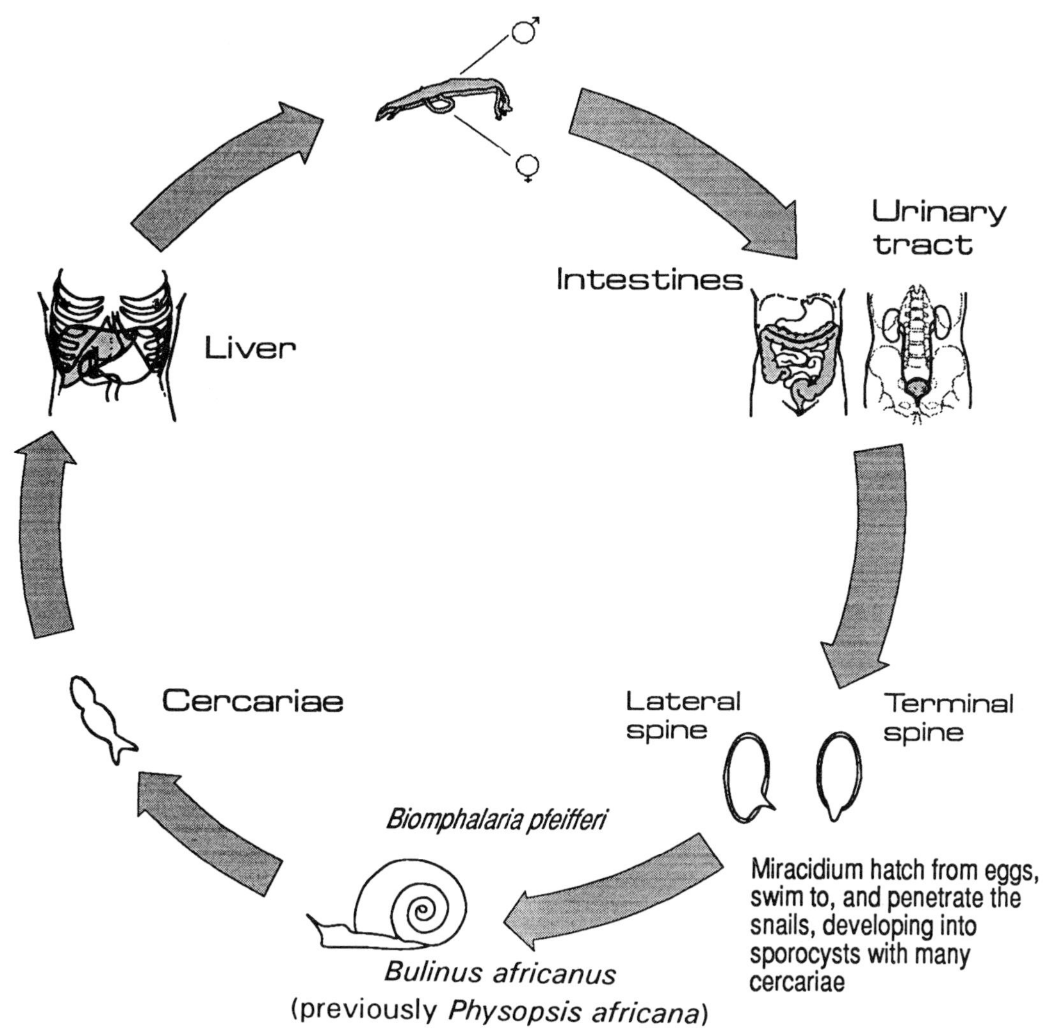

Figure 1 Life-cycle of schistosomes. The key differences between the two major forms of schistosomiasis – *Schistosoma haematobium* and *S. mansoni* is that *S. haematobium* invades the urinary tract and has an egg with a terminal spine, while *S. mansoni* infests the intestines and has an egg with a lateral spine

in pairs to the veins of the bladder or intestine, where the females lay the eggs, and live for from 10 to 30 years. Long-standing hepatic infection evokes the so-called 'pipe-stem fibrosis' of the portal tract with the development of esophageal varices which may rupture with fatal hemorrhage. The egg-laying period is the most characteristic stage of schistosomiasis. In *S. haematobium* infections, the passage of eggs is often accompanied by hematuria, first noted 10–12 weeks or longer after infection. In *S. mansoni* infections the passage of eggs is often associated with bloody diarrhea and mucus, first noted about 7 weeks after exposure. These signs and symptoms may persist in the absence of treatment for many years. Often, worms do not follow the usual and complicated itinerary through the body and deviate from their intended path, infecting other organs and tissues, causing severe complications when the central nervous system or lungs are involved.

The early stages of disease, while the schistosomules are maturing, and then as egg laying begins, are often accompanied by a serum sickness-like hypersensitivity reaction, manifest by urticaria, erythematous skin rashes, myalgia, arthralgia, and possibly swelling and tenderness of the joints. In later stages, schistosomes may be found in the tissues around the joints where tubercles may develop in the periarticular tissues, and in the synovial membranes, causing stiffness and tenderness. In a study of 96 patients from Egypt with confirmed *S. mansoni* infection, 72 suffered from polyarticular inflammatory exudative arthritis[3,4]. Three days to 2 weeks after the first symptoms of infection, these patients complained of joint pain with persistent morning stiffness lasting from 30 min to 2 h, and marked inactivity stiffness lasting up to 30 min, which resolved within 1 month of instituting schistosomiasis therapy. The arthritis affected the proximal, interphalangeal and metacarpophalangeal joints, the wrists, the knees, the ankles and the metatarsophalangeal joints. The prominence of musculoskeletal inflammation with *S. mansoni*, was an unexpected finding and a conspicuous feature of the illness; indeed in many patients it was a primary presenting complaint that prevented the patient from working. The affected joints were warm, swollen and painful. In every case, the arthritis followed the onset of the systemic illness by about a week and thereafter was one of remission and exacerbation. Eight of ten cases completely resolved within 1 month. A feature of interest was the frequency and severity of inflammation at the site of insertion of muscle through tendon or ligament into bone. Kamel and co-workers[4] describe the immunological changes in bilharzial arthropathy.

Diagnosis
The diagnosis of schistosomiasis is confirmed by finding the eggs in the excreta or in biopsy sections. Serological confirmation can be made with complement fixation, fluorescent antibody and enzyme-linked immunosorbent assay (ELISA) tests, which become positive about 3–5 weeks after exposure but are of limited value in assessing the effect of treatment since they do not revert to negative for some time after a cure has been effected.

Treatment
A number of drugs are effective schistosomacides. Praziquantel is the current drug of choice; it is effective against *S. haematobium, mansoni* and *S. japonicum*, and is administered as a single dose with minimal side-effects. Treatment of polyarticular inflammatory arthritis, with corticosteroids or non-steroidal anti-inflammatory drugs is without effect, but it may respond to antischistosomal treatment.

Control and prevention
Schistosomiasis may be controlled by breaking the parasite's life-cycle at one or more points, which is most effective when the water supply, sanitation and living conditions in endemic areas are improved, especially when accompanied by changes in human behavior. Effective prevention depends on reducing access to water containing infective snails by fencing of streams and building of bridges over them. Safe water should be provided for all domestic and recreational purposes including washing, paddling and swimming. Provision should be made for proper sanitary facilities and one of the most satisfactory latrines is that developed by the Blair Research Institute in Zimbabwe. These can be easily erected and properly maintained by the local community.

Mass treatment of the population in endemic areas has been attempted occasionally, but once cured, such individuals may again become susceptible to infection. The use of molluscicides in snail-infested water effectively controls the snails in small water bodies and irrigation schemes, at a considerable ecologic cost as these agents are also toxic to the local fish population. Education of the populace in endemic areas regarding the mode of transmission and methods of protection from infection is important. Provided proper precautions are taken, no-one should contract schistosomiasis. However human nature, especially that of young boys, usually leads to lapses which may lead to infection, even with brief immersion in snail-infected water.

MISCELLANEOUS CONDITIONS ASSOCIATED WITH ARTHRITIS AND MYOSITIS

Tropical myositis

This condition occurs sporadically in many tropical regions of Africa, affecting the native population, and rarely also expatriates. It is most common in young and middle-aged individuals, especially males, and is characterized by local swelling with edema and abscess formation in one of the muscles of limbs, most often the thighs or calves, less often the arm, chest and abdominal muscles. Usually only one abscess forms but occasionally there may be several in different muscles. The patient complains of severe local pain that may immobilize the adjacent joints, and suffers chills and rigors associated with high swinging temperatures. On examination a circumscribed, often very tender, hot and edematous swelling is present, which may resolve without discharging the pus, but may require surgical drainage.

The cause of tropical myositis is unknown, but the condition has been variously associated with *Wucheria bancrofti*, *Dipetalonema perstans*, scurvy, relapsing fever, and hookworm infection in many cases occurring on the gold mines of the Witwatersrand. The initiating factor is often hemorrhage into the muscles with the formation of a hematoma, which then becomes infected with pyogenic organisms, particularly *Staphylococcus aureus*, which has been cultured from a propor-

tion of cases, although abscesses are often bacteriologically sterile. Prevention depends on avoiding possible etiologic agents or adequately treating predisposing conditions, avoiding injury leading to hematoma and when abscesses have developed, antibiotic therapy, covering in particular the possibility of *Staph. aureus* with penicillin or tetracycline.

Mseleni joint disease

In scattered areas of the world including the tropical regions, unusual forms of joint disorders have been described, many of which may have a genetic component, while others are unclear. One such condition occurring in South Africa is commonly known as Mseleni joint disease, a strange dysplastic condition that affects a large proportion of the indigenous people living in the vicinity of the Mseleni Mission in the Ubombo district of northern KwaZulu, midway between Lake St. Lucia and Kosi Bay[5]. Lockitch, Fellingham and others found that 66.4% of the women, 25.4% of the men, 6.7% of the girls and 4.2% of the boys had osseous abnormalities of the hip, knee, elbow and wrist joints as well as in the small joints of the hands and feet. The predominant finding in young patients was epiphyseal dysplasia, and in older patients, osteoarthrosis[6]. It is suspected that genetic factors possibly resulting from long genetic isolation, play a part in the pathogenesis of this condition. Preventive measures, as in other hereditary dysplastic conditions, leave much to be desired and are directed mainly to keeping joints mobile and preventing deformities. Clearly, steps should be taken to lessen the isolation of such communities and investigations undertaken to identify its cause.

REFERENCES

1. Ottesen, EA, Vijayasakaran V, Kumaraswami V, Pillai P, Sadadandam A, Frederick S, Prabhakar R, Tripathy SP. A controlled trial of ivermectin and diethylcarbamezine in lymphatic filariasis. N Engl J Med. 1990; 322:1113–1117

2. Prod'hon J, Boussinesque M, Fobi G, Enyong P, Lafleur C, Qeillevere D. Control of onchocerciasis with Ivermectin: results of a mass campaign in northern Cameroon. Bull WHO. 1991; 69: 443–450

3. Atkin SL, Kamel M, El Hady A, El-Badawy SA, El-Fhobary A, Dick WC. Schistosomiasis and inflammatory polyarthritis. A clinical radiological and laboratory study of 96 patients infected by *S. mansoni* with particular reference to the diarthrodeal joint. Q J Med 1986; 59:479–487

5. Kamel M, Safwat E, Eltayeb S. Bilharzial arthropathy. Immunological findings. Scand J Rheumatol. 1989; 18:315–319

5. Fellingham SA, Elphinstone CD, Wittman W. Mseleni joint disease: background and prevalence. S Afr Med J. 1973; 47: 2173–2180

6. Lockitch G, Fellingham SA, Wittmann W, de Villiers PD. de Wet IS, du Toit GT. Mseleni joint disease. The pilot clinical survey. S Afr Med J. 1973; 47:2283–2293

18.   SEXUALLY TRANSMITTED DISEASES

Clifford Eastmond and Richard Wigley

INTRODUCTION

A number of sexually transmitted diseases are associated with complaints arising from the musculoskeletal system. Some complaints occur at an acute stage of infection and may be mild and transient; others may be self-limiting, but cause considerable morbidity and yet others may ultimately translate into chronic rheumatic syndromes. It is important to recognize the cause of these in order to limit the further transmission to sexual partners of these individuals. It is equally important to devise strategies of health education to prevent the transmission of sexually transmitted disease in general, and thereby the associated rheumatic syndromes.

GONOCOCCAL INFECTION[1,2]

Arthritis caused by *Neisseria gonorrhoeae* most commonly affects women under the age of 40 years. Infection by *N. gonorrhoeae* occurs most efficiently during menstruation and pregnancy, and is manifested by the typical signs of pyrexia and leukocytosis, which may be associated with polyarthralgia. In the acute phase of infection, skin lesions may be vesico-pustular with an erythematous base, or less frequently, consist of hemorrhagic bullae, and are located on the extensor surfaces of articulations. Skin lesions are thought to represent evidence of a septicemic phase, although it may not be possible to isolate bacteria from the skin lesions. Polyarthritis or monoarthritis, often accompanied by tenosynovitis, may follow the skin lesions and most commonly affect the knees and wrists, and less commonly, the ankles and small joints of the hands; bacteria can usually be isolated from the joints. When a culture specimen is taken from the joint and proves to be 'sterile', it becomes difficult to exclude the possibility of a coincidental chlamydial infection, which is a known cause of reactive arthritis and Reiter's syndrome. In suspected cases, samples should be taken in the female from the uterine cervix and in the male from the urethra, and in both, from the rectum, the oropharynx, blood and joints, *and cultured* using the appropriate (e.g. Thayer–Martin) growth media. Gram-stained slides of clinical specimens are frequently negative; indeed, 40% of slides from rectal specimens in male homosexuals are negative when infection is confirmed by other means.

Gonococcal infection, is best treated with penicillin for 14 days, if there is evidence of disseminated infection, e.g. arthritis. In cases of penicillin resistance, cefotaxime is preferred, and in the face of hypersensitivity to penicillin, co-trimoxazole is advised. Contact tracing and individual advice on prevention of further infection to affected individuals is critical in the control of gonococcal infection.

SYPHILIS[1]

Congenital syphilis

After many years of a slow decline in incidence of congenital syphilis, there has been a recent resurgence of this disease in the inner cities of certain developed nations. The most common manifestation of congenital syphilis is osteochondritis, which usually develops between the third week and third month of life, and presents with a pseudo paralysis, swelling of the limbs, which with time is associated with epiphyseal separation and fracture. Less common chondroosseous manifestations of congenital syphilis include metaphysitis, periostitis and osteoarthritis, and the quite rare dactylitis. Syphilis in pregnancy may result in spontaneous abortion, stillbirth or prematurity. It is essential to recognize syphilis in pregnant women by routine serological tests, as its recognition during early gestation and adequate treatment will prevent congenital syphilis in nearly all cases.

Childhood and adolescence
Syphilis in this age group can be acquired *in utero*, and manifest later in life as the classic Clutton's joints, which are characterized by painless swelling of the knees, usually occurring between the ages of 8 and 16 years. This must be distinguished from other forms of juvenile chronic arthritis, so that appropriate treatment can be given.

Adulthood
There are no rheumatological manifestations of primary syphilis. In secondary syphilis, hydroarthrosis similar to the Clutton's joints of children may occur with polyarthritis, tenosynovitis and periostitis. Tertiary syphilis may be associated with a number of articular diseases, e.g. periostitis principally affecting the tibia and clavicle, gummata of the synovium or periosteum and diffuse osteitis. Tabes dorsalis with lightening pains in the lower limbs may simulate arthritic pain, while neuropathic joints with gross disorganization are associated with no or minimal pain. The identification of persons with primary and secondary syphilis and their appropriate antibiotic therapy virtually eliminates the risks of tertiary syphilis. Contact tracing of cases of pri-

mary syphilis is important to ensure that such contacts are treated at an early stage, while contact tracing in the late syphilis is unlikely to prove successful.

REACTIVE ARTHRITIS
Reactive arthritis may be manifest as a sterile arthritis with or without the extra-articular features of Reiter's syndrome. Extra-articular features, particularly fever, weight loss and kerataderma blenorrhagica are usually a manifestation of more severe disease. It may also occur following infection with certain gastrointestinal pathogens. Circinate balanitis and keratoderma blenorrhagica seem to be uncommon following infection with *Salmonella*, *Campylobacter* and *Yersinia* species but are frequent with *Shigella* infection as well as the sexually acquired form of this disease.

Sexually-acquired reactive arthritis[3] (SARA) is most common in the third and fourth decades, and affects males far more frequently than females, although the condition is often underdiagnosed in females. SARA is associated with non-gonococcal urethritis, but may occur concomitantly with infection by *Neisseria gonorrheoae*. Chlamydia trachomatis accounts for 50% of cases of nongonococcal urethritis in males and is a common pathogen of the female genital tract. Some cases may be due to *Mycoplasma pneumonia* and *Ureaplasma urealyticum*. In many cases, no pathogen is identified in the genital tract. Treatment of the primary infection does not appear to influence the occurrence, duration or severity of the reactive arthritis. Urogenital symptoms usually appear 7–14 days after contact and the arthritis within 30 days. Arthritis usually follows urethritis, but may occur coincidentally or a few days prior to urethritis. One to two per cent of patients with non-gonococcal urethritis develop SARA, a finding that is partially explained by inherited susceptibility related to the presence of HLA-B27, a tissue antigen present in 70–90% of Caucasians with SARA compared with 8% in Caucasian controls. Blacks are less susceptible to reactive arthritis, which could be related to the relative absence of HLA-B27 in this racial group.

Reactive arthritis is not a totally benign syndrome and there may be long-term morbidity in a significant proportion of patients[4]. The development of subsequent ankylosing spondylitis is recognized, but it is not known whether this is a direct consequence of a previous reactive arthritis or to a common genetic susceptibility to the two diseases. SARA is a marker for the presence of sexually acquired disease, and patients with SARA should be screened not only for chlamydia infection, but other sexually transmitted disease, in particular, gonorrhea, and their sexual contacts should be identified. It is important to recognize however, the role of gastrointestinal pathogens, e.g. *Salmonella*, *Campylobacter*, *Yersinia* and *Shigella* species and that in approximately one third of patients with reactive arthritis there may be no clues either historically, bacteriologically or serologically for the pathogen[5].

LYMPHOGRANULOMA INGUINALE
This infection by *Chlamydia trachomatis* may occasionally be associated with a serum sickness-like syndrome with polyarthritis, rash, cryoglobulinemia and rheumatoid factor (*see* Chapter 16).

HIV INFECTION
The acquired immunodeficiency syndrome (AIDS) has been intimately linked to the human immunodeficiency virus (HIV)[6–9]. The impact of infection with this retrovirus, the subsequent development of AIDS and its associated morbidity and mortality is now widely recognized. Although AIDS was initially regarded as a disease of homosexuals and that of persons infected by parenteral contact with 'dirty' needles, e.g. intravenous drug abusers, or 'dirty' blood products, e.g. hemophiliacs, it is now recognized that HIV infection and its associated syndromes are,

on a global scale, more common in the heterosexual population, the so-called type II pattern of AIDS. Rheumatological complaints may be the presenting feature in HIV-infected subjects and as they contribute to the morbidity of AIDS it is important to recognize them. HIV has been isolated from joint aspirates, as well as blood products and breast milk; these infected body fluids and tissues must be handled and disposed of with the appropriate precautions.

Various rheumatological 'syndromes' have been associated with HIV infection[10–13], and can be conveniently grouped as follows:

1. Opportunistic infections
Secondary infection of joints with *Staphylococcus aureus*, *Streptococcus pneumoniae* as well as a high incidence of unusual organisms, *Cryptococcus neoformans*, *Mycobacterium haemophilum* and *Sporothrix schenckii* have been described. The microbiology laboratory should be forewarned if there is clinical suspicion of an unusual organism, so that the appropriate isolation techniques will be used.

2a. Reactive arthritis
The full triad of Reiter's syndrome occurs in HIV infection, although many patients lack the extra-articular manifestations of the triad: arthritis, conjunctivitis and urethritis.

Reactive arthritis may occur prior to, coincident with or following other features of HIV infection, and is usually severe and difficult to control. Immunosuppressive agents normally considered in the treatment of severe reactive arthritis and Reiter's syndrome should, however, be avoided in the presence of HIV infection as they may accelerate the development of the clinical AIDS and Kaposi's sarcoma. In Caucasians, AIDS-associated reactive arthritis is more common in patients with HLA-B27, an association that is not seen in Africans studied in Zimbabwe

2b. Psoriatic arthritis

Psoriasis may also occur at any time during the course of AIDS; it is often severe and usually deteriorates markedly with the onset of AIDS. Unfortunately, the most effective modalities for treating psoriasis, i.e. immunosuppressives and phototherapy, have also been associated with the clinical deterioration of AIDS.

3a. Sjögren syndrome

Although this condition when associated with AIDS is characterized by the usual features of parotid gland enlargement, xerophthalmia and xerostomia, it differs from primary Sjögren syndrome by a male predominance, the presence of massive parotid swelling and submandibular swelling and prominent extrasalivery lymphoid infiltration, an absence of arthritis, lack of anti-Ro and anti-La antibodies, and an increase in of CD8 T cells in the inflammatory infiltrate.

3b. Necrotizing vasculitis

This polyarteritis nodosa-like condition may be first manifest by peripheral sensory or sensorimotor neuropathies or mononeuritis multiplex and typical neuropathic changes occurring in association with the histological features of necrotizing vasculitis. Other vasculitic syndromes seen in AIDS include eosinophilic vasculitis, granulomatous angiitis and leukocytoclastic vasculitis, which have been described in single case reports, as have been a few cases of lymphomatoid granulomatosis.

3c. Systemic lupus erythematosus-like (SLE-like) syndrome

HIV infection and SLE share a number of clinical features including arthralgia, malar rashes, renal disease, neurological manifestations, systemic disturbance with fever, lymphadenopathy, weight loss and hematological abnormalities. Laboratory findings further demonstrate features that are common to both conditions, including the presence of antinuclear antibodies, lupus anti-coagulant and anticardiolipin antibodies, circulating immune complexes, hypergammaglobulinemia and rheumatoid factor. Two patients with pre-existing lupus had clinical improvement with the development of HIV infection and recrudescence of lupus activity with the institution of treatment with zidovudine.

3d. Polymyositis

Myalgias are common in patients with HIV infection, are usually generalized and readily respond to analgesics. A true polymyositis has been described, often appearing months to years after other clinical evidence of HIV infection. The clinical picture includes an elevation of muscle enzymes and characteristic electromyographic (EMG) changes, accompanied by the histopathological changes of inflammation, necrosis and fibrosis, which are typical of primary polymyositis. Viral-like particles have been seen in biopsy material.

Muscle atrophy of varying degrees has been reported, and in most cases, it is multifactorial and related to underlying neurological, nutritional or infectious disorders.

Myositis may occur as an uncommon side-effect of AIDS patients treated with zidovudine, which disappears upon the cessation of therapy with this drug.

4. Arthralgia and polyarthritis

Arthralgia can be a manifestation of acute HIV infection, accompanied by fever, sore throat, headache, myalgia, abdominal cramps, diarrhea and lymphadenopathy and usually resolves within 1–2 weeks. An additional syndrome characterized by severe, acute articular pain of unknown pathogenesis with painful episodes lasting from 2 to 24 h, without clinical evidence of synovitis has been described.

Recognition of the above syndromes, particularly in those who have 'high-risk' behaviors is critical

216

for identifying HIV infected individuals. Those who are infected must be counseled regarding potentially infected contacts, and in order to avoid infecting others. It is important to recognize that there are two somewhat distinct patterns of HIV infection alluded to at the beginning of this section, i.e. that of heterosexual spread seen in developing nations, which may be effectively minimized by the use of condoms. The second pattern is related to certain homosexual activities and intravenous drug abuse; it is more typical of developed nations, and may be minimized by safe sexual practices and using sterile needles and syringes to avoid the spread among drug addicts.

HEPATITIS A AND HEPATITIS B[14]

Hepatitis B may be associated with a symmetrical polyarthritis particularly affecting the hands, which may be asymmetrical, migratory or additive, and occurs in 10–30% of cases. Hepatitis B affects males and females equally, and the viral incubation periods last from 2.5 to 6 months. Prodromal manifestations include malaise, sore throat, anorexia, nausea, vomiting, chills, fever or myalgia. Clinical disease is usually several weeks in duration, but can be as short as a few days or as long as 6 months; half of the cases are associated with a purpuric rash, and in addition, there can be a low-grade fever with regional lymphadenopathy.

Hepatitis-induced polyarthritis may be due to either direct viral invasion of the synovium or can be immune complex mediated. Hepatitis B is spread through infected syringes and needles either used in medical care or by intravenous drug users, or it may be sexually transmitted. Identification of the likely mode of spread in individual cases will lead to appropriate advice on preventing further spread. Preventive strategies that are applicable to reducing the transmission of HIV, are equally true for hepatitis: drug abusers should avoid sharing needles and syringes and the number of sexual partners should be strictly limited

and condoms should be used in appropriate settings

An effective three-dose schedule[15] vaccine is available and should be offered to high-risk groups, e.g. health professionals whose contact with potentially infected persons puts them at high risk. Other workers such as police and prison service personnel are at lower risk but should nevertheless be considered for vaccination programs.

GENERAL CONTROL OF SEXUALLY TRANSMITTED DISEASE

The control of rheumatic complaints transmitted through sexual contacts hinges on sexual and other forms of transmission. The latter is particularly important where an infection may be spread through body fluids and equipment and instruments contaminated by such fluids. The precise methods of control depend upon the disease, both as regards its mode of transmission and its prevalence in a particular geographic region. Appropriate policies need to be directed to the relevant population in an appropriate manner, which will include identification of the high risk groups, the common modes of spread and cultural considerations[16].

Avoidance of exposure to infection would be the most effective way of limiting the spread of sexually transmitted disease (STD)(Figure 1(a)). However, continence outside of a monogomous relationship is likely to be an unachievable goal. The risks associated with sexual promiscuity must be made known to those at highest risk15, including teenagers and young adults, homosexuals and prostitutes, both male and female, and should be part of education on sexuality and partnerships in general. Sexually active high-risk groups are likely to require repeated re-education in the need to limit the number of sexual partners and ensure that they present themselves for voluntary STD

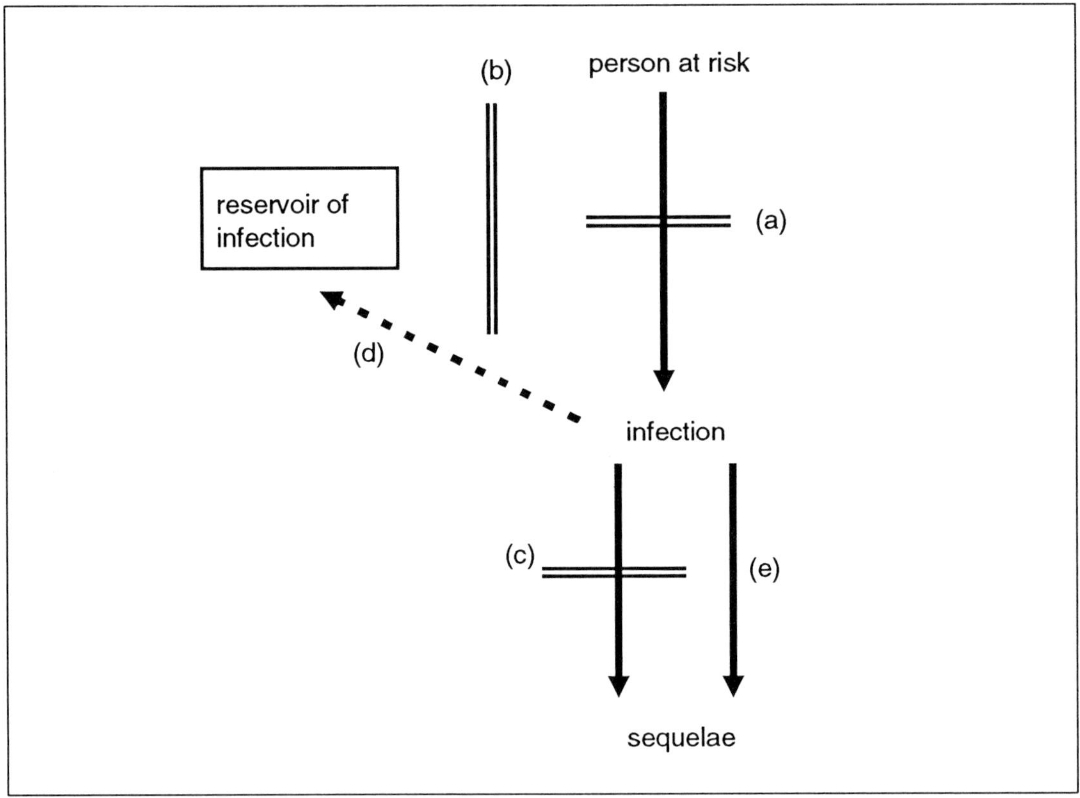

Figure 1 Sexually transmitted rheumatic diseases, preventive measures: (a) Avoidance of exposure; (b) barrier protection, e.g. condoms, and vaccination where appropriate; (c) treatment of primary infection, e.g. gonorrhea; (d) contact tracing; and (e) treatment of primary infection has no effect on sequelae

screening at regular intervals, and appropriately counselled.

The frequency of STD can be drastically reduced by the use of condoms[17] (Figure 1(b)), and the sexually active must be advised of their appropriate use, both in general education programs and the inclusion of appropriate literature. Condoms should not be reused and should be disposed of after use and tied at the end to prevent leakage; they should be put on before, and used throughout penetrative sexual, e.g. rectal, vaginal and oral intercourse. It is widely held that other forms of contraception offer no protection, including other barrier methods and spermicides.

Prompt treatment of primary infection may in the case of gonococcal and syphilitic infection prevent the rheumatic sequelae[1,2] (Figure 1(c)), but not the viral infections and reactive arthritis discussed in this chapter (Figure 1(e)). Appropriate facilities for treating these infections is essential, as is the expediency of encouraging highest risk sexually active persons to seek help early in the course of a primary infection. Contact tracing (Figure 1(d)) facilities must be available with trained staff and where appropriate, diagnostic screening and therapy should be offered to traced contacts.

It is important to recognize other routes of transmission of these 'sexual' rheumatic diseases. This is particularly the case with HIV and hepatitis B infection, where several body fluids are known to be infected and capable of transmission of disease[14,18]. Those at risk for alternative routes of transmission include intravenous drug abusers, recipients of blood products, medical personnel, medical laboratory personnel, police and prison staff. Intravenous drug abusers should not share needles and syringes, and 'needle exchange' programs need to publicly supported (Figure 1(a)). In handling blood products, clinical and laboratory personnel should adopt precautionary measures for all patients and body fluids as if they were potentially contaminated[18]. Disposable equipment should be used only once and not reused. Blood products should be manufactured and sterilized according to established protocols to eliminate risks of transmission of infection[19]. Medical staff who work in the highest risk situations should be vaccinated against hepatitis B using the three-dose schedule[15] (Figure 1(b)). HIV and hepatitis B infection probably pose the highest risk amongst this group of diseases to police and prison staff. Those most at risk of contact likely to lead to a significant risk of infection should be appropriately counselled. All measures should be taken to reduce the risk of infection. There is no vaccine available for HIV but an effective vaccine is available for hepatitis B and should be made available[15].

REFERENCES

1. Ansell BM. Infective arthritis. In Scott JT ed., Copeman's Textbook of the Rheumatic Diseases. 6th edn, Edinburgh, Churchill Livingstone, 1986
2. Goldenberg DL. Bacterial arthritis. In Kelley WN, Harris ED, Ruddy S, Sledge CB. eds., Textbook of Rheumatology. 3rd edn, Philadelphia, WB Saunders, 1989
3. Keat A. Reactive arthritis and Reiter's syndrome. In Oriel JD, Harris JRW, eds., Recent Advances In Sexually Transmitted Diseases. Edinburgh, Churchill Livingstone, 1986
4. Fox R, Calin A, Gerber RC, Gibson D. The chronicity of symptoms and disability in Reiter's syndrome. Ann Intern Med. 1979; 91: 190–193
5. Von Essen R, Nikkari S, Isomaki H. Aetiology of reactive arthritis in hospital patients in Finland. Scand J Rheumatol. 1984; Suppl. 52:61–64
6. Barré-Sinousi F et al. Isolation of a T-lymphocyte retrovirus from a patient at risk of acquired immunodeficiency syndrome (AIDS). Science. 1983; 220:868–870
7. Gallo RC et al. Frequent detection and isolation of cytopathic retrovirus (HTLV-III) from patients with AIDS and at risk for AIDS. Science. 1984; 224:500–503
8. Levy JA et al. Isolation of lymphadenopathic retroviruses from San Francisco patients with AIDS. Science. 1984; 225:840–842
9. Popovic M, Samgadharan MG, Read E, Gallo RC. Detection isolation and continuous production of cytopathic retrovirus (HTLV-III) from patients with AIDS and pre-AIDS. Science. 1984; 224:479–500
10. Davis P, Stein M, Latif A, Emmanuel J. HIV and polyarthritis. Lancet. 1988; 1:936
11. Espinoza LR, Aguilar JA, Berman A, Gutierrez F et al. Rheumatic manifestations associated with human immunodeficiency virus infection. Arthritis Rheum 1989; 32:1615–1622
12. Espinoza LR, Aguilar L, Espinoza CG, Berman A et al. HIV associated arthropathy: HIV antigen in synovial membrane. J Rheumatol. 1990; 17:1195–1201
13. Kaye B. Rheumatologic manifestations of infection with human immunodeficiency virus (HIV). Ann Intern Med. 1989; 111:158–167
14. Schnitzer TJ. Viral arthritis. In Kelley WN, Harris ED, Ruddy S, Sledge CB, eds., Textbook of Rheumatology. 3rd edn, Philadelphia, WB Saunders, 1989
15. WHO Expert Committee On Venereal Disease and Treponematoses. 6th report, 1986
16. WHO. Control Of Sexually Transmitted Disease. 1985
17. WHO. Prevention of sexual transmission of

human immunodeficiency virus. WHO AIDS Series No. 6, 1990

18. WHO. Guidelines for nursing management of people infected with human immunodeficiency virus (HIV). WHO AIDS Series No. 3, 1988

19. WHO Guidelines on sterilization and high level disinfection methods effective against human immunodeficiency virus (HIV). WHO AIDS Series No. 2, 1988

19. SPONDYLARTHROPATHIES

Sjef van der Linden and Muhammad Asim Khan

INTRODUCTION

The spondylarthropathies constitute a group of rheumatic diseases which share epidemiological, genetic and clinical features such as a familial tendency, especially in first-degree relatives, an association with the HLA-B27 antigen, and an increased prevalence of sacroiliitis. Spondylarthropathies include ankylosing spondylitis, juvenile ankylosing spondylitis, Reiter's syndrome (or reactive arthritis), psoriatic arthritis, and arthropathies that complicate inflammatory bowel diseases, i.e. Crohn's disease and ulcerative colitis. All are characterized by the absence of rheumatoid factor and other autoantibodies[1]. In 1973, it became clear that nearly all patients with ankylosing spondylitis, most patients with

Table 1 European Spondylarthropathy Study Group (ESSG) classification criteria

Inflammatory spinal pain	*or*	synovitis (asymmetrically predominantly in the legs)
	and	any of the following: positive family history psoriasis inflammatory bowel disease alternate buttock pain enthesopathy sensitivity 77% specificity 89%
	adding	sacroiliitis sensitivity 86% specificity 87%

reactive arthritis (or Reiter's syndrome), and many patients with other spondylarthropathies have in common the HLA-B27 tissue antigen.

Some patients have clinical symptoms suggestive of spondylarthropathy, but do not fit a specific spondylarthropathy pattern, and are thus labelled as 'unclassified' or 'undifferentiated'. Recently, classification criteria have been proposed for the entire group of spondylarthropathies, which encompasses the undifferentiated forms[2]. According to these criteria, a spondylarthropathy is considered to be present if a patient has either inflammatory spinal pain or synovitis (asymmetrical or predominantly in the lower limbs), and at least one of the following six items: positive family history; psoriasis; inflammatory bowel disease; alternate buttock pain; enthesopathy; sacroiliitis (Table 1). These criteria yielded 86% sensitivity and 87% specificity for all spondylarthropathies.

This chapter will focus on ankylosing spondylitis and Reiter's syndrome (or reactive arthritis).

ANKYLOSING SPONDYLITIS

Ankylosing spondylitis can be regarded as the prototypic spondylarthropathy. It is a chronic, predominantly axial arthropathy with a male predominance of 3:1, which first develops between ages 15 and 40 years of age (Figure 1), and has a prevalence of 0.1–0.2% in the Caucasian population[3].

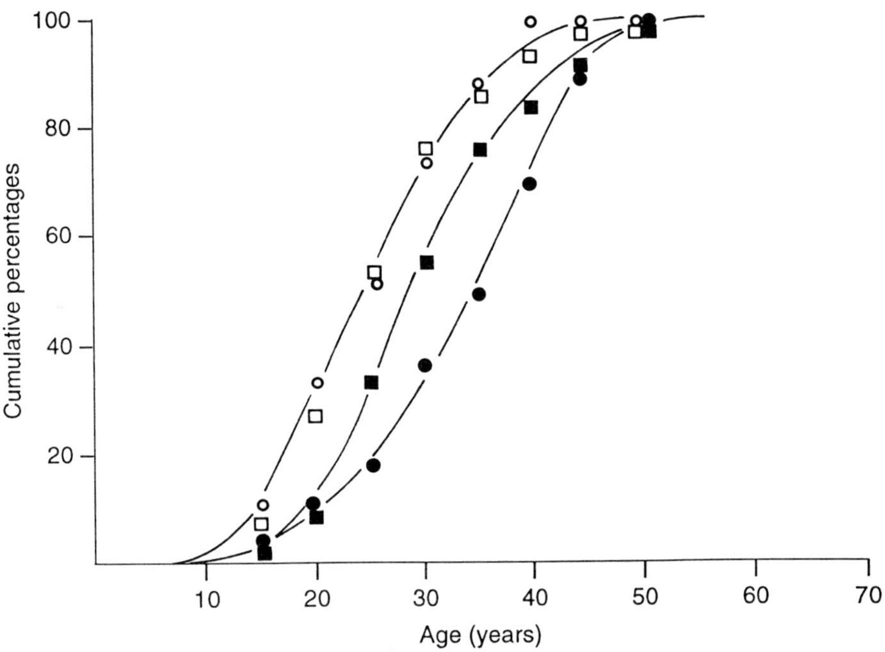

Figure 1 Age at the onset of complaints and at the time of diagnosis of ankylosing spondylitis (AS) for 135 HLA-B27 males and 30 HLA-B27 female patients. Open symbols indicate the age when complaints started, black symbols, the age at which the diagnosis was reached. Squares represent males, circles are females. Complaints started at the same age in both sexes, and the diagnosis was established later in females. By the time the patients were age 45, AS had been diagnosed in more than 92% in both sexes. (Reproduced with kind permission from reference 3)

Epidemiological and genetic aspects

The relationship between ankylosing spondylitis (AS) and HLA-B27 is by now well established. Geographic differences in the prevalence of AS might reflect differences in the distribution of the HLA-B27 antigen in different races. This antigen is present in approximately 90% of Caucasians with AS in contrast to 8% of unaffected individuals; HLA-B27 is virtually absent in African and Japanese populations. In American Blacks, owing to racial admixture with Whites, 2% possess the HLA-B27 antigen, while it is detected in only 50% of Black patients with AS. Correspondingly, American Blacks are affected far less frequently than American Whites, and the disease is rare in African Blacks and Japanese. Interestingly, healthy Indonesians of Chinese descent have a lower prevalence of HLA-B27 (4%) than native Indonesians (9%), even though AS is diagnosed more frequently in the former. In a study from Jakarta[4] 11 of 13 AS patients were of Chinese descent (nine of these 11 patients possessed HLA-B27), whereas the two AS patients of native Indonesian origin were both B27-negative. It is difficult to explain these findings on the basis of differences in access to the Indonesian health care system or by other confounding factors. Therefore, it would be of interest to survey the population for the prevalences of various B27 subtypes (*see* below) in healthy and diseased Indonesian people of Chinese and native descent.

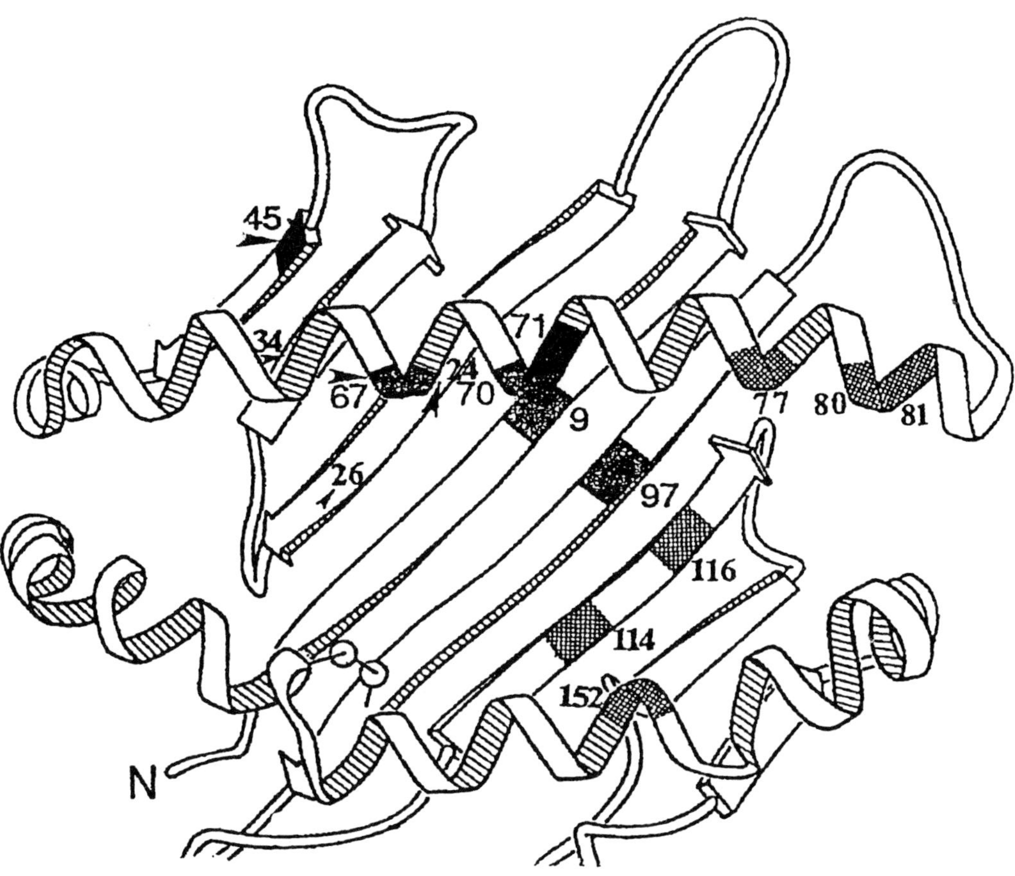

Figure 2 A ribbon diagram of the antigen-binding pocket of an HLA molecule

Currently, six subtypes of HLA-B27 are recognized by the WHO Committee on HLA nomenclature, and are designated B*2701, B*2702, B*2703, B*2704, B*2706, and B*2705, which is the major subtype of B27. B*2705 is present in 85–90% of B27-positive Whites and 45% of B27-positive Orientals. HLA-B*2701 is rare; B*2702 is present in 10% of B27-positive Whites; both are restricted to Caucasians. HLA-B*2703 is restricted to American Blacks. B*2704 is the predominant subtype in Orientals and is present in approximately 55% of Oriental B27-positive individuals, and B*2706 has so far been observed only in Orientals. A seventh subtype of B27 has been reported recently[5].

At least four of these subtypes (B*2702, B*2704, B*2705 and B*2706) have been associated with ankylosing spondylitis; these subtypes differ from each other at six amino acid residues (Figure 2) at positions 77, 80, 83, 114, 116, and 152, that are clustered on the right side of the antigen binding groove[6–8]. In contrast the amino acids that confer B27 familial specificity are located at a spatially separate site on the left side of the antigen binding groove at positions 9, 45, 67, 70, 71 and 97[7,8]. There is great interest in the '45-pocket', which is situated below the α-helix of the α_1 domain with Gly_{45} at its base surrounded by Thr_{24}, Gly_{26}, Val_{34}, and Cys_{67}[7,8]. These residues are highly diverse among HLA-B molecules, but show sequence similarity or 'homology' in the B27 subtypes. The combination of Thr_{24}, Glu_{45} and Cys_{67} is specific to B27 among HLA class-I molecules of known structure and confers uniqueness to the '45-pocket', which may act as a 'cul-de-sac' for the side chains of the putative antigenic peptides, and play a pivotal role in setting off the arthritogenic trigger.

HLA-B*2703 may not be associated with ankylosing spondylitis. This may account for the rarity of the disease in Blacks and the lower relative risk for ankylosing spondylitis in HLA-B27-positive Blacks[9]. It is interesting that B*2703 differs from the most common Caucasian subtype B*2705 by a substitution of histidine for tyrosine at position 59 of the α_1 domain[8,10]. T-lymphocytes that respond to the common B27, B*2705 and B*2702 in cytotoxicity assays do not recognize B*2703[9], a finding that more strongly supports the 'arthritogenic peptide' model of HLA-B27 disease pathogenesis than the 'altered-self' and 'molecular mimicry' models[9]. The arthritogenic peptide model invokes a central role for cytotoxic lymphocytes reactive with a B27-specific oligopeptide, possibly derived from a foreign pathogen[7,11]. If it could be established that B*2703 is not associated with susceptibility to AS, then position 59, which is in the vicinity of the '45-pocket', becomes extremely interesting in the pathogenesis of AS. The tyrosine to histidine mutation in B*2703 is the first recorded polymorphism of a HLA-class I molecule at position 59; the tyrosine residue is normally conserved in humans and other homologous species[10].

In addition to HLA-B27, at least one other B-locus antigen has been associated with an increased susceptibility to ankylosing spondylitis. HLA-Bw60 (or B40 when the Bw60, 61 split of B40 was not typed for) was shown to be increased among B27-positive AS patients in each of five independent data sets[12]. The 655 patients included in this study were representative of AS cases from The Netherlands ($n = 37$), Canada ($n = 150$), Switzerland ($n = 297$), Norway ($n = 75$), and the United States ($n = 96$), and demonstrated that the susceptibility to AS in B27-positive individuals was increased threefold when Bw60 was also present. The increase in Bw60 (B40) was statistically significant in four of the five data sets studied, and the overall significance was $p < 0.00001$. The distribution of HLA-A alleles on the B27-bearing haplotypes was not significantly different from that in normal controls, while the distribution of HLA-A alleles on Bw60-bearing haplotypes was significantly different from the general population. It is not yet clear whether among B27-positive individuals, Bw60 itself or a locus that is in linkage disequilibrium with Bw60, predisposes to ankylosing spondylitis. Bw60 was not increased in B27-negative patients with AS[12].

It should be stressed that a *positive family history* for AS is a very strong risk factor for the disease. About 20–25% of first-degree relatives of HLA-B27-positive patients also develop AS in contrast to 1–2% of B27-positive Caucasians in the general population[3]. There appear, however to be regional differences; For example, for HLA-B27-positive Nords native to northern Norway a risk of 6.7% was calculated. It is presently unknown whether these differences are due to differences in study designs, selection bias(es), or reflect actual differences, for example in the distribution of HLA-B27 subtypes.

Pathogenesis

An altered host response to an environmental factor in genetically susceptible individuals appears to be the most plausible basis for the pathogenesis of AS and related diseases, although HLA-B27's modus operandi is as yet unknown. Any hypothesis that explains an association between B27 and AS must accommodate the following findings: not all individuals with B27 develop the disease; the presence of B27, even in the homozygous form, is insufficient to cause the disease; and a small percentage of patients with ankylosing spondylitis do not possess HLA-B27[13]. Two major theories have been advanced to explain the association between B27 and AS: one states that HLA-B27 itself is unimportant, but its coding allele is in strong linkage disequilibrium with another (as yet unidentified) gene that predisposes to the development of the disease, which may act by modifying the immune response. The second postulated pathogenic mechanism holds that the B27 antigen itself plays a functional role in AS pathogenesis, and the B27 molecule may act as a receptor for a microbial or other environmental factor, or may mimic an antigen in the environment capable of triggering the disease.

In view of the well-recognized association of Reiter's syndrome (also known as reactive arthritis) with enteric bacterial infection, many workers have looked for similar microbiological associations in AS[7] especially *Klebsiella* which has been studied extensively. Raised levels of IgA antibody to *Klebsiella* have been found in spondylitic sera but there was no correlation with disease activity[14]. Other workers have found normal or low levels of antibody to a variety of gram-negative bacteria, including *Klebsiella*. A number of studies, primarily by two groups of investigators, have also suggested a possible role for certain *Klebsiella* strains in triggering AS[15,16]. Because of the inability of other investigators to independently confirm these findings, a possible role for *Klebsiella* in triggering ankylosing spondylitis remains controversial[17].

Schwimmbeck and colleagues renewed interest in *Klebsiella* when they demonstrated a short sequence homology between B27 and a *Klebsiella pneumoniae* protein, nitrogenase reductase[18]. It is, however, unlikely that this enzyme plays a role in AS, as it is used for nitrogen fixation and the gene is expressed only when the bacteria are in nitrogen-free media, a highly unlikely environment in the human host. Moreover, the observed sequence similarity was only with the major B27 subtype, although other B27 subtypes also confer a similar increased susceptibility to AS. Other investigators have failed to confirm the presence of antibodies in the sera of AS patients and Reiter's syndrome directed against a synthetic peptide based on the short sequence homology between B27 and nitrogenase reductase.

Although some form of gastrointestinal infection may be important in the etiology of AS, the significance of serological cross-reactivity between a determinant on the HLA-B27 molecule and enteric bacteria is open to discussion. Antigenic cross-reactivity between gut bacteria and human cell surface antigens appears to be a commonplace phenomenon, exemplified by the sharing of ABO blood group antigens between human erythrocytes and *Escherichia coli*. It is possible that cross-reactivity between HLA-B27 and bacterial antigens may occur, but lacks pathogenic significance[14].

At present, the divide among unique major histocompatiblity complex-related determinants at the cell surface and the characteristic clinical features of AS remains largely unbridged, although knowledge is expanding rapidly. Indeed the detailed three dimensional X-ray crystallographic structure has now been reported[19], and reveals electron density compatible with a 9-amino-acid long bound peptide in the binding groove of the B27 molecule. It appears that the side chain of the second residue of the bound peptide extends into the '45-pocket'. This observation and the increasing evidence for bacterial triggering in many forms of spondylarthropathies, further enhance our understanding of how B27 may tie into its function. The propensity of the antigen binding groove of B27 to bind arthritogenic oligopeptides may explain the increased susceptibility of B27 individuals to AS and related spondylarthropathies[11]. Knowledge of HLA-B27's structure, and the occurrence of spontaneous inflammatory disease with striking resemblance to spondylarthropathies in B27 transgenic rats, would enable investigators to find the antigenic structure recognized by cytotoxic T cells and the oligopeptides that preferentially bind to B27 molecules[20,21]. This, then, might in turn lead to identification of an arthritogenic trigger for AS and related spondylarthropathies in genetically susceptible individuals. Such progress in our understanding of the pathogenesis would, hopefully, provide tools for the primary prevention of this disease as well as for other spondylarthropathies.

REITER'S SYNDROME AND REACTIVE ARTHRITIS
Epidemiological and genetic aspects
The typical features of Reiter's syndrome (or reactive arthritis) are asymmetrical oligoarthritis predominantly of the lower limbs, affecting, in particular the knees, ankles, and metatarsophalangeal joints, although back pain or upper limb involvement also may also occur. Between 60 and 80% of Caucasians with Reiter's syndrome or reactive arthritis are HLA-B27-positive. Extra-articular manifestations of Reiter's syndrome include conjunctivitis, uveitis, urethritis, cervicitis, circinate balanitis, stomatitis, and keratitis blenorrhagica. The spectrum of this disease has been broadened considerably and 'incomplete' forms of Reiter's syndrome are now much more common than those that fulfil the criteria of the classic triad of arthritis, conjunctivitis, and urethritis[22]. The term 'B27-associated reactive arthritis' has been used in recent years to refer to spondylarthropathies following enteric or urogenital infections, and the disease spectrum includes the clinical picture of typical Reiter's syndrome.

The arthritogenic organisms that are generally included in the list of organisms that may give rise to Reiter's syndrome or reactive arthritis include *Salmonella* species, *Yersinia* species, e.g. *Y. enterocolitica*, *Campylobacter* species, and *Chlamydia trachomatis*. Recent findings suggest that *Borrelia burgdorferi*, which causes Lyme disease (Chapter 13) may join human immunodeficiency virus (HIV) on the growing list of infectious agents that must be considered for a patient with reactive arthritis[23–27]. Reiter's syndrome, psoriasis, and psoriatic arthritis occupy an intriguing place in the spectrum of spondylarthropathies; some HIV-infected patients have developed severe psoriasis (with or without psoriatic arthritis) and/or Reiter's syndrome, usually at the onset of the development of acquired immunodeficiency syndrome (AIDS) or AIDS-related complex (ARC). Indeed, since the first reports of Reiter's syndrome and psoriasis in HIV-infected persons, it has become clear that several rheumatoid factor-negative syndromes occur in the presence of HIV infection[28].

Pathogenesis
Despite many attempts, no viable organisms have been successfully cultured from the joints in these patients, although the presence of *Chlamydia*, *Salmonella*, and *Yersinia* antigens in the synovial white blood cells of synovial tissue has now been observed in some patients with reactive arthritis. Recent findings suggest that in genetically predisposed individuals, an arthritogenic immune response giving rise to Reiter's syndrome might be triggered by persisting infectious agents independent of their antigenic specificities[23–27]. According to Inman, the working hypothesis for the pathogenesis of Reiter's syndrome and reactive arthritis maybe formulated as follows:

(1) Reiter's syndrome often follows genitourinary or gastrointestinal tract infections;

(2) Certain microorganisms can cause a sterile synovitis;

(3) Reiter's syndrome is due to an aberrant host immune response to the pathogen[29]; and

(4) The disease occurs primarily in HLA-B27-positive persons.

PREVENTION

The primary prevention of Reiter's syndrome and reactive arthritis would require prevention of urogenital infections and AIDS as detailed in Chapter 18, and the control of gastrointestinal infections in general. Hand washing and fly (vector) control are indicated. Travellers to developing countries should rigorously avoid bowel infections, by boiling water, or treating it with chlorine, eating only hot cooked food and should personally peel fruit. Vaccines are available only for typhoid and paratyphoid infection. Relatives of those with spondylarthropathy or those known to be HLA-B27-positive individuals are at greater risk of developing these forms of arthritis, and they should be especially careful to avoid these infections. Routine tissue typing is neither currently feasible nor cost-effective.

There is as yet no firm evidence that early antibiotic treatment of *Salmonella, Yersinia enterocolitica, Campylobacter jejuni,* or *Chlamydia trachomatis* infections would prevent the development or improve the prognosis of reactive arthritis. There are as yet no clear options for the primary prevention of AS; more research is desperately needed to provide tools for the primary prevention of this as well as for the other spondylarthropathies.

REFERENCES

1. Arnett FC. Seronegative spondylarthropathies. Bull Rheum Dis. 1987; 37:1–12
2. European Spondylarthropathy Study Group: Preliminary criteria for the classification of spondylarthropathy. Arthritis Rheum. 1991; 34: 1218–1227
3. Van der Linden SM, Valkenburg HA, de Jongh BM, Cats A. The risk of developing ankylosing spondylitis in HLA-B27-positive individuals: a comparison of relatives of AS patients with the general population. Arthritis Rheum. 1984; 27: 241–249
4. Nasution AR, Adiwirawan M *et al*. J Rheumatol. 1993; in press
5. Lopez de Castro JA, Bragardo R, Lauzurica P *et al*. Structure and immune recognition of HLA-B27 antigens. Scand J Rheumatol. 1990; 87 (Suppl.):51–69
6. Taurog JD. Immunology, genetics, and animal models of the spondyloarthropathies. Curr Opin Rheumatol. 1990; 2(4):586–591
7. Benjamin R, Parham P. Guilt by association: HLA-B27 and ankylosing spondylitis. Immunol Today. 1990; 11:137–142
8. Lopez de Castro JA, Bragardo R, Lauzurica P *et al*. Structure and immune recognition of HLA-B27 antigens. Scand J Rheumatol. 1990; 87 (Suppl.):21–31
9. Hill AVS, Allsopp CEM, Kwiatkowski D, Anstey NM, *et al*: HLA class I typing by PCR: HLA-B27 and an African B27 subtype. Lancet. 1991; 337:640–642
10. Breur-Vriesendorp BS, Vingerhoed J, Kuipjers KC *et al*. Effect of Tyr-to His point mutation at position 59 in the α_1 helix of the HLA-B27 class-I molecule on allospecific and virus specific cytotoxic T-lymphocyte recognition. Scand J Rheumatol. 1990; 87 (Suppl.): 36–43
11. Benjamin RJ, Madrigal JA, Parham P. Peptide binding to empty HLA B27 molecules of viable human cells. Nature (Lond). 1991; 351:74–77
12. Robinson WP, van der Linden SM, Khan MA, Rentsch HU *et al*. HLA-Bw60 increases susceptibility to ankylosing spondylitis in HLA-B27+ patients. Arthritis Rheum. 1989; 32:1135–1141
13. Khan MA, van der Linden SM. Ankylosing spondylitis: clinical aspects. Spine: State Art Rev. 1990; 4:529–551
14. Keat A. Is spondylitis caused by *Klebsiella*? Immunol Today. 1986; 7:144–149
15. Ebringer A. The relationship between *Klebsiella* infection and ankylosing spondylitis. Baillière's Clin Rheumatol. 1989; 3:321–338
16. Geczy AF, van Leeuwen A, van Rood JJ *et al*. Blind confirmation in Leiden of Geczy factor on

the cells of Dutch patients with ankylosing spondylitis. Hum Immunol. 1986; 17:239–245

17. Terasaki PI, Yu DTY. Regarding the ankylosing spondylitis/*Klebsiella*/HLA-B27 problem. Arthritis Rheum 1987; 30:353–354

18. Schwimmbeck PL, Yu DTY, Oldstone MBA. Auto antibodies to HLA-B27 in the sera of HLA-B27 patients with ankylosing spondylitis and Reiter's syndrome: molecular mimicry with *Klebsiella pneumoniae* as potential mechanism of autoimmune disease. J Exp Med. 1987; 166:173–181

19. Khan MA. An overview of clinical spectrum and heterogeneity of spondyloarthropathies. Rheum Dis Clin North Am. 1992; 18:1–10

20. Hammer RE, Maika SD, Richardson JA *et al.* Spontaneous inflammatory disease in transgenic rats expressing HLA-B27 and human B2m: an animal model of HLA B27 associated human disorders. Cell. 1990; 63:1099–1112

21. Tsomides TJ, Eisen HN. Antigenic structures recognised by cytotoxic T lymphocytes. J Biol Chem. 1991; 266:3357–3360

22. Khan MA, van der Linden SM. A wider spectrum of spondyloarthropathies. Semin Arthritis Rheum. 1990; 20:107–113

23. Arnett FC. The Lyme spirochaete: another cause of Reiter's syndrome? Arthritis Rheum. 1989; 32:1182–1184

24. Weyand CM, Goroncy JJ. Immune responses to *Borrelia burgdorferi* in patients with reactive arthritis. Arthritis Rheum. 1989; 32:1057–1064

25. Rowe IF, Keat ACS. Human immunodeficiency virus infection and the rheumatologist. Ann Rheum Dis. 1989;48:89–91

26. Espinoza LR, Aguilar JL, Berman A *et al.* Rheumatic manifestations associated with human immunodeficiency virus infection. Arthritis Rheum. 1989; 32:1615–1622

27. Khan MA, van der Linden SM. Ankylosing spondylitis and other spondyloarthropathies. Rheum Dis Clin North Am. 1990; 16:551–579

28. Keat A. Reiter's syndrome and associated arthritides. Rheum Dis Clin North Am. 1991; 17:25–42

29. Inman RD. Reiter's syndrome and reactive arthritis. Spine: State Art Rev. 1990; 4:627–636

20. THE PRIMARY PREVENTION OF RHEUMATOID ARTHRITIS

Alan J. Silman

INTRODUCTION

Rheumatoid arthritis (RA) is the most prevalent of the inflammatory joint diseases. Its public health impact is substantial given the disease's prolonged duration, the large size of the population that it affects and the degree of disability that the disease causes. Indeed, in a population survey of causes of disability in those under the age of 65, RA figured most prominently[1]. RA is a clinically heterogeneous disease that overlaps considerably with many of the disorders considered in this text. This clinical heterogeneity in part reflects an etiological heterogeneity and thus attempts at finding causes by studying random samples of RA cases are likely to be subject to this 'noise'. Nor is there a single, clinical, radiological or serological feature that can be used reliably to diagnose the disease. Thus, classification into disease-negative and disease-positive individuals is based on satisfying a number of arbitrary criteria in the absence of an alternative diagnosis[2] (Table 1). It is perhaps not surprising that against this background there has been little progress in identifying causes for RA. The Scientific Advisory Committee to the Empire Rheumatism Council reported on a major case-control study of etiological factors in RA[3], and their conclusion of 40 years ago is still sadly applicable: 'At the present time it is both honest and wise to admit our ignorance of the etiological factors causing rheumatoid arthritis'. In this review such clues as do exist will be discussed having first considered those aspects of the epidemiology of RA that point to possible areas requiring further investigation.

EPIDEMIOLOGICAL ASPECTS OF RHEUMATOID ARTHRITIS

The descriptive epidemiology of RA is unhelpful in posing environmental hypotheses of etiology. Firstly, there is the lack of clues from investigating RA's geographical distribution, and in contrast to the other major chronic diseases, there is surprisingly little variation in the prevalence of RA in different populations[4]. Nonetheless, dissenting reports have appeared, such as those which compared rural and urban Bantu populations in South Africa. The urbanized groups had the same prevalence as the European population[5], whereas the rural groups had a very low rate[6]. Within a population, cases of rheumatoid arthritis in general do not tend to cluster either in time or place, characteristics which, when present, would suggest an environmental cause such as an infection.

Two aspects of the epidemiology of RA are of interest. Firstly, RA is a disease that largely affects females, in particular premenopausal women[7] (Figure 1). This female excess is unexplained but there are a number of other intriguing observations to suggest a role for gynecological/endocrinological factors. The disease remits during pregnancy and relapses or indeed may be precipitated by the postpartum period[8–10]. The pregnancy history of women who subsequently

Table 1 The 1987 revised criteria for the classification of rheumatoid arthritis (traditional format)*

Criterion	Short title	Definition
1	morning stiffness	morning stiffness in and around the joints, lasting at least 1 hour before maximal improvement. At least three joints
2	arthritis of three or more joint areas	areas simultaneously have had soft tissue swelling of fluid (not bony overgrowth alone) observed by a physician. The 14 possible areas are right or left PIP, MCP, wrist, elbow, knee, ankle and MTP joints
3	arthritis of hand joints	at least one area swollen (as defined in 2) in a wrist, MCP or PIP joint
4	symmetric arthritis	simultaneous involvement of the same joint areas (as defined in 2) on both sides of the body (bilateral involvement of PIPs, MCPs or MTPs is acceptable without absolute symmetry)
5	rheumatoid nodules	subcutaneous nodules, over bony prominences, or extensor in juxtaarticular regions, observed by a physician
6	serum rheumatoid factor	demonstration of abnormal amounts of serum rheumatoid factor by any method for which the result has been positive in < 5% of normal subjects
7	radiographic changes	radiographic changes typical of rheumatoid arthritis on posteroanterior hand and wrist radiographs, which must include erosions of unequivocal bony decalcification localized in or most marked adjacent to the involved joints (osteoarthritis changes alone do not qualify)

*For classification purposes, a patient shall be said to have rheumatoid arthritis if he/she has satisfied at least four of these seven criteria. Criteria 1–4 must have been present for at least 6 weeks. Patients with two clinical diagnoses are not excluded. Designation as classic, definite, or probable rheumatoid arthritis is not to be made.
Alternative classification based on fulfilling the following subsets:
(i)   Criteria 1 and 3   (iv)   Criteria 4 and 6
(ii)   Criteria 1 and 6   (v)   Criteria 3 and 6
(iii) Criteria 1 and 7
Criteria 3 for this classification excludes PIP.
(Reproduced with kind permission from reference 2)

develop RA may be abnormal (*see* below) with an increased rate of subfertility and fetal loss prior to the onset of RA. There is also the suggestion in some studies of an earlier age at menopause[11] in women who develop RA. These observations have led to a considerable number of studies on the role of exogenous sex hormones in the prevention of RA and these studies are reviewed in detail below.

A second aspect of RA is also of interest. For unknown reasons, RA appears to be declining in incidence, an epidemiological finding for which there is a considerable unanimity in the available results[7,12–14]. An example of such data drawn from the number of new cases presenting to general practitioners in the UK is shown in Figure 2. One possible explanation is that RA may be due to an as yet unproven infectious cause, and like any other epidemic disease, should decline over time and ultimately disappear[15]. The possible role for specific infectious agents is also discussed in detail below.

One of the most persuasive arguments for a possible environmental cause to RA is the rela-

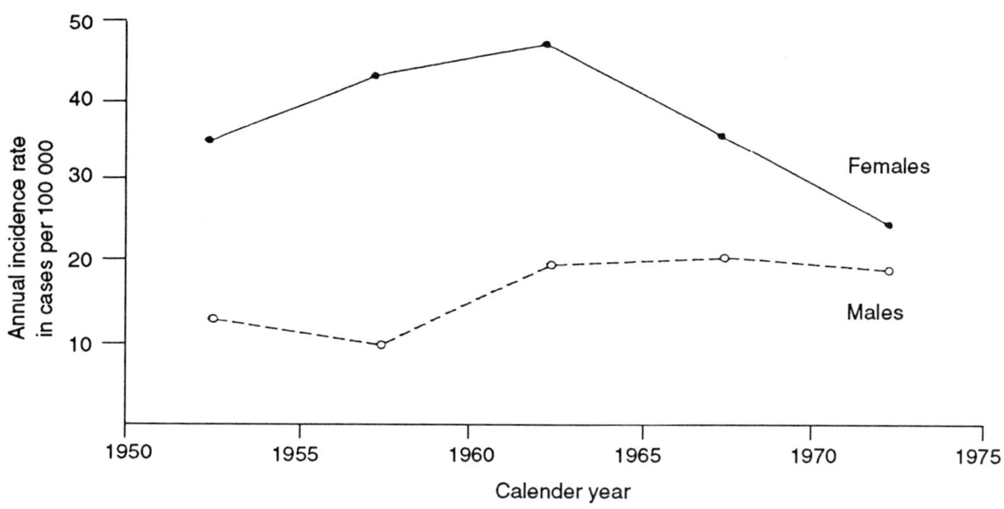

Figure 1 Incidence of rheumatoid arthritis by age in males and females. (Reproduced with kind permission from reference 7)

tively low (between 12 and 30%) concordance rate in monozygotic twins[16–17]. The variation in concordance in the different studies may in part be explained by the selection of probands: hospital ascertained probands are more likely to be concordant for RA with their co-twin than community ascertained probands[18]. The twin data, which show greater monozygotic than dizygotic concordance, are often interpreted as proving a genetic contribution to the disease, while such data suggest an environmental cause. The presumed increased concordance in monozygotic twins might actually reflect a greater shared environment in such twins. It is indeed the anecdotal experience of this reviewer during the course of a major twin survey that monozygotic twins are more likely to live in the same area and share the same occupation than same-sex dizygotic twins. Much of the etiological enquiry in RA has concentrated on heredity, particularly following the recognition of an association between the HLA class II antigen DR4 and RA[19]. In non-European populations, associations with other class II markers in the DR region have been found and linked to an epitope in the third hypervariable region of the $DR\beta_1$ chain[20]. This observation is

of limited utility given that the shared epitope is also present in 50% of normal individuals against a population frequency of RA of 0.8%[21]; this association is uncommon in RA cases identified from population screening surveys, and this putative genetic linkage may be associated with disease severity rather than susceptibility[22]. Thus, despite these immunogenetic and molecular biological advances, the role for environmental factors seems sound.

This review will concentrate on three areas of interest of potential for primary prevention, addressing possible roles for (a) an infectious agent, particularly a virus, (b) pregnancy and hormones, and (c) occupation and related exposures.

INFECTIOUS CAUSES
General considerations
The most likely etiological model for RA, based on its immunopathological appearance, is an infection, possibly viral, occurring in a genetically susceptible host. The occurrence of an inflammatory polyarthritis after some viral infections, such as rubella is well described; but the overwhelming majority of these postviral arthritides remit

231

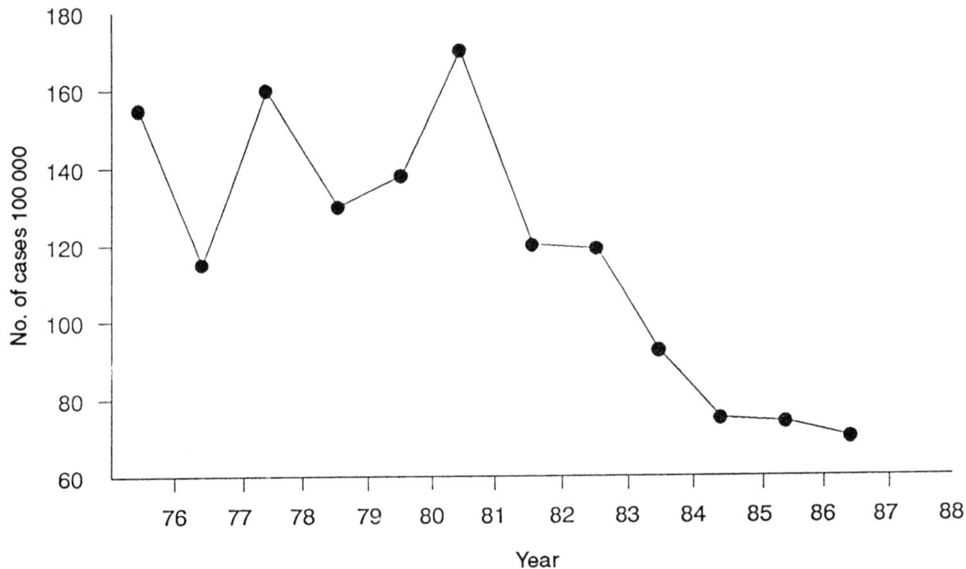

Figure 2 Trends in crude new episode incidence in patients attending general practice in UK 1976–1987. (Reproduced with kind permission from reference 13)

relatively rapidly and do not proceed to a chronic destructive phase. The identification of possible agents in RA has been the target of considerable study, which has met with only limited success.

The identification of *Borrelia burgdorferi* as the spirochete responsible for Lyme disease[23], a regional infection of late summer[24], serves as a reminder that infectious agents may be responsible for rheumatic diseases, which justifies the efforts of those seeking a similar cause for the more endemic, albeit clinically distinct, rheumatoid arthritis.

Clinical evidence based on prospective studies of asymptomatic individuals positive for rheumatoid factors[25,26] suggests that this family of antibodies may precede the clinical onset of RA by years. Thus exposure to any relevant infection might have occurred years prior to clinical presentation, making retrospective studies very difficult to interpret. Given this conundrum, a potentially useful epidemiologic tool is a birth cohort study, which examines a group of subjects sharing a common period of birth. The rationale for such a study is that the period of birth might influence a person's chances of exposure to specific infections early in life, and differences in the subsequent incidence of RA among birth cohorts might emerge, as many infectious diseases occur in relatively short lived epidemics. There does appear to be a birth cohort effect in regard to rheumatoid factor positivity both in the general population[27] and in patients with RA[12] although there are no data on any such influences on RA itself. This could be compared to a recent study on juvenile arthritis suggesting a clustering of births around 1963, a year which coincided with an epidemic of a particular strain of influenza[28]. Such data are of some interest but are widely open to contrasting interpretations.

Other circumstantial support for an infective etiology came from the observation, 10 years ago, of an increased risk of tonsillectomy and appendicectomy for the development of RA[29] with the suggestion that such surgery reduced host-defence mechanisms. Despite further evidence supporting this association[30], other studies failed to corroborate these data[31–33], and moreover, criticism was raised in the methodology used in the first study[34]. Detailed investigation of etiological factors within family clusters provides little to suggest an infectious cause. This applies to both affected sibling pairs[35,36] and spouse couples[37], where there was a considerable median delay between the onset of disease in both the affected members. Investigation of disease discordant, but HLA-identical, sibling pairs showed no evidence of differences in exposure to a long list of possible infectious agents[38]. Nonetheless, it is relevant to consider available data from studies of a number of specific agents.

Human parvovirus

This agent stimulated recent wide interest after it was associated with a post-infectious arthritis[39]. The acute form of this arthritis was reported to be clinically similar to RA, and demonstrated transient rheumatoid factor positivity. The first of two reports from the UK regarding this association was a retrospective study in which 19 of 153 patients with early synovitis, possibly RA, had evidence of parvovirus infection[40]. The second was a prospective study which described the occurrence of joint problems in 17 patients following an outbreak of parvovirus[41]. Neither study had appropriate control groups and there were no patients with persistent arthritis. An analysis of possible HLA associations[42] of the patients in the retrospective series[40] showed that the DR4-positive rate was similar to that found in rheumatoid arthritis. Parvoviral infection is, however, very common in the community especially with increasing age, and evidence of infection is a poor predictor of the subsequent development of RA. A final twist in the parvovirus story is the report of isolation of a serologically distinct parvovirus, RA-1 from the synovium of patients with RA[43]. Further studies showed that isolates from cultured synovial cells from these patients reacted with antisera to RA-1 in six of 11 patients with RA but in none of the six controls. There are little data however on the basic epidemiology of this virus.

Epstein–Barr virus

The most widely studied agent that may be etiologically linked to RA is the Epstein–Barr virus (EBV), which first evoked interest in this regard after a report in 1975[44] identified EBV antibodies in the sera of RA patients. Subsequent seroepidemiological studies comparing the frequency of antibodies to various EBV antigens in RA patients and controls have confirmed the high titers of antibodies against the viral capsid antigen (VCA), early antigen (EA), EB nuclear antigen (EBNA) and nuclear antigen (RANA) in RA patients[45–48]; EBV can, moreover, *in vitro* induce B lymphocytes to produce rheumatoid factor. However, not all studies have been positive[49] and the differences from the control population have not always been either biologically or statistically significant. A broad conclusion from such studies would be that there is probably no difference in rates of EB infection between RA and normal individuals, but that the former group either has a more active infection or perhaps an altered regulation of their immune response.

Epidemiologically, EBV is worthy of study for several reasons. First, the geographical distribution of infectious mononucleosis, an EB-induced condition, and RA are similar. Second, the former is apparently unknown in countries with a reportedly low prevalence of RA[50]. The explanation for these observations in the face of the geographical ubiquity of EBV infection is the effect of age. In low prevalence RA countries, infection with EBV is virtually universal by the age of 3 years and the infection is clinically silent, while in high RA prevalence countries, infection occurs at a later age and is more likely to be clinically apparent as in the case of infectious mononucleosis. The major problem in linking EBV infection to RA is the lack of clinical evidence that EBV is arthritogenic unlike, for example rubella, hepatitis and mumps[51].

Other infectious agents

A large number of other potential RA-inducing infectious agents have been proposed including *Proteus* species, *Mycobacterium tuberculosis* and others, and the recent recent emergence of AIDS has fostered interest in retroviruses. There are similarities between RA and the arthritis induced by lentiviruses in animals, for example caprine arthritis encephalitis in goats, although a link between retroviral infection in RA is, at best, tenuous[52–54]. There are good *Mycoplasma*-induced animal models of RA, and the chronicity and severity of mycoplasma infections in humans have been related to genetic factors[55]. Clinical and epidemiological studies in humans have, however, failed to link mycoplasma to RA, although a recent report demonstrated the isolation of mycoplasma antigens from the synovial fluid of six patients with RA[56]. It is also likely that the response to mycobacterial antigen is enhanced in HLA-DR4-positive individuals[57].

In summary, both clinically and epidemiologically, RA does not behave as an infectious disease, although the abnormality resulting in the persistence of an immune response may not require the continued presence of microbial antigen(s). The conventional application of Koch's postulates in linking a putative microbial agent to disease causation is likely to be too restrictive in revealing possible agents for RA, given the nature and time course of the disorder. A reasonable conclusion is that a viral cause for RA may exist, but that it is unlikely that a single agent is responsible even within well circumscribed populations. Given the other difficulties mentioned above, the scope for identifying causes from epidemiological methods seems remote.

SEX HORMONES AND PREGNANCY

There has been much interest in a possible role for sex hormones in the etiology of RA, which has been the subject of a recent review[58].

Oral contraceptive pill

The hypothesis that oral contraceptives (OC) are protective against the development of RA, arose from a prospective study of 23 000 female OC users in the UK[59]. This study was primarily designed to evaluate the overall safety of OCs, and it was observed that current OC use halved the risk of RA, although subsequent follow-up analysis of the same cohort of women showed that this protection was not sustained[60]. At least 13 other studies on a possible association between RA and OC use have been reported, the results of which are summarized in Table 2. There is a considerable disparity in the results between studies and an attempt has been made to resolve this by undertaking statistical meta-analysis (overview) of the various studies[61,62] and the results of this are shown in Figure 3. In brief, the overall conclusion is that OC use probably delays the clinical development of RA, by masking its signs until the use of OCs has ceased. The differences in the conclusions reached by these studies can be explained, if this masking or protective effect is more common in random cases of RA than in those identified in hospital settings and hence the protection may be against severity of disease.

Postmenopausal hormone therapy

A major problem of the oral contraceptive hypothesis is that their use is largely confined to women under age 40 years, which is a decade younger than the peak age of onset of RA. It is therefore reasonable to consider the possible role for non-contraceptive hormones that are being increasingly used to reduce menopausal symptoms and prevent osteoporosis. There have been at least three formal studies; the first was a case–control study[63] showing a halving in RA risk in

Table 2 Studies of the possible protective effect of oral contraceptive use against the development of rheumatoid arthritis

Author	Year	Study design	Relative risk for ever use (95% confidence interval*)	
Wingrave	1978	prospective	0.68	(0.45–1.03)
Allebeck	1982	case–control	0.70	(0.40–1.24)
Vandenbroucke	1982	case–control	0.42	(0.27–0.65)
Linos	1983	case–control	1.7	(0.8–3.5)
del Junco	1985	case–control	1.1	(0.7–1.7)
Vandenbroucke	1986	case–control	0.57	(0.32–1.00)
Vessey	1987	prospective	1.12	(0.79–1.79)
Darwish	1987	case–control	1.29	(0.64–2.58)
Koepsell	1989	case–control	0.27[1]	(0.06–0.97)
Hernandez-Avila	1990	prospective	1.0	(0.6–1.4)
Moskowitz	1990	case–control	2.0[1]	(0.97–4.2)
Spector	1990	case–control	0.56[2]	(0.29–1.12)
			0.60[3]	(0.30–1.17)
Hazes	1990	case–control	0.39	(0.24–0.63)
Hazes	1990	case–control	0.37[4]	(0.11–1.24)

*Odds ratios for case–control studies; [1]current oral contraceptive use; [2]osteoarthritis controls; [3]population controls; [4]sister controls

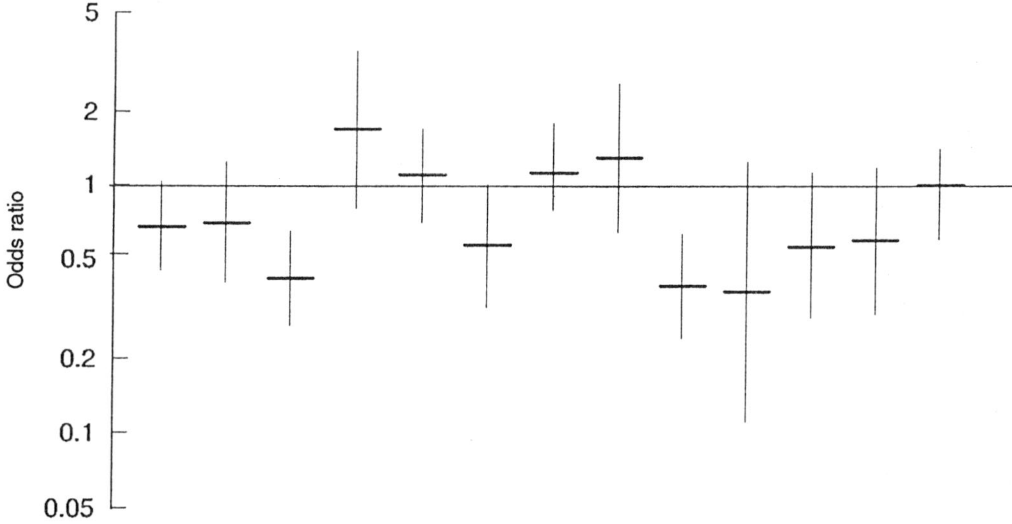

Figure 3 Overview of results of observation studies of oral contraceptive use and rheumatoid arthritis (results expressed as odds ratios (relative risks) with 95% confidence intervals. (Reproduced with kind permission from reference 62)

those receiving this form of hormonal therapy. Another case–control study[64] and a retrospective cohort study[65] showed no such protection, and thus, the contradictory findings in these studies militates against a role of post menopausal hormone therapy in the pathogenesis of RA.

Pregnancy and nulliparity
In addressing the sex difference in the incidence of RA, the question is raised of whether pregnancy is protective or a risk factor for RA, taking into account potentially confounding factors such as marriage, and whether single women are at increased risk. Further, given the well-described immunological background of RA, this question becomes all the more interesting. In particular, if fetal loss is considered to be (at least in part) an immunological response, does fetal loss predispose to RA? This possibility[66] is based on similar observations in other autoimmune disorders[67]. As with other aspects of the pathogenesis of RA considered in this review, there are inconsistencies in the results obtained. Nonetheless, currently available data suggests that nulliparous women are at an increased risk for RA with the more recent studies providing the strongest evidence[68–70]. It is unknown whether this actually reflects some preclinical effect of RA on reproductive function or whether pregnancy itself is protective, as it appears to be in breast cancer. This does not appear to be the case and thus the relationship between RA and parity is far from simple. This might also reflect an increase in fetal loss particularly in the early weeks of pregnancy and thus, for the reasons stated above, it might be expected that women with RA would have an increased rate of either spontaneous abortion (loss prior to 28 weeks) or stillbirth. Here again, the results are conflicting. Kay and Bach's data from the 1960s[72] showed no increased fetal loss but there was an increased fetal loss in the subgroup of patients who had rheumatoid factors, which would beg the question of whether these factors might, as is the case of the

antiphospholipid (or anticardiolipin) antibody syndrome play a role in the fetal loss. Two subsequent studies showed an increase in both spontaneous abortions[73] and stillbirths[74], although more recent studies have failed to confirm these observations[69,75] (Table 3).

Occupation and related exposures
Despite studies suggesting that the risk for RA is inversely related to income and occupational status[76,77], most reports show no relationship with occupational class[78–81]. Specific occupational hazards were studied following the report of an increased incidence of RA in miners with massive pulmonary fibrosis in South Wales[82]. A subsequent formal epidemiological analysis did not confirm this association in coal miners. An association between RA and silicosis was reported in Italian pyrite miners, but the study was uncontrolled and most of the cases detected were 'probable' rather than definite RA[83]. A more recent study of 1026 granite workers, who had worked in the industry between 1940 and 1971 and followed to 1981 showed that the incidence of RA was 1.7/1000 compared to a general population risk of 0.25, yielding a relative risk of 5. Most of the affected miners however did not have silicosis[84]. It has been suggested that those working in outdoor industries such as fishing have a high risk[85]. Other occupational data are scanty or anecdotal in nature (Table 3).

Diet
The role of nutrition in the pathogenesis of RA is somewhat problematic, and has been and has been recently reviewed in detail[86]. Most work on the relation between diet and RA has concentrated on its effects on modifying the course of the disease. Although such effects, if real, may be relevant to disease causation, these data must be interpreted with caution. Patients often regard diet as an environmental factor of import, perhaps because it is under their own control. Data sug-

Table 3 Results of case–control studies of fetal loss prior to onset of rheumatoid arthritis

Study (first author)	Cases (N)	Controls (N)	Odds ratios (95% confidence limits) Spontaneous abortion		Still birth	
Kay (1965)	111[a]	111	0.7	(0.4–1.4)	0.7	(0.2–2.7)
Kaplan (1986)	89	113	1.8	(1.2–2.7)	not tested	
Silman (1988)	40	67	1.2	(0.9–2.9)	12.4	(1.6–91.1)
Spector (1990)	260	296[b]	0.4	(0.3–0.7)	1.0	(0.4–2.6)
		267[c]	0.9	(0.5–1.6)	1.8	(0.5–6.9)
Hazes (1991)	135	378	0.7	(0.5–1.1)	not tested	

[a]Postmenopausal onset; [b]osteoarthritis controls; [c]general population

gesting a causative role of diet are however scanty. Retrospective studies suffer from the possible long latency period prior to clinical expression of the disease and hence the difficulty in recalling premorbid dietary intake. Prospective studies would require large sample sizes and a long follow-up period and in the absence of a specific hypothesis cannot be justified on the current evidence.

Trace elements

RA has been linked both to increased serum copper[86] and copper deficiency[88]; there is also an ample body of folklore attached to the use of copper bracelets in preventing rheumatic complaints, making it difficult to separate fact from fancy. Serum selenium is also low in RA[89] and although this could be a result of disease activity, it might be of etiological importance[90]. Evidence linking zinc deficiency to the pathogenesis of RA is also weak.

PREVENTION

Though so many avenues have been explored no realistic prospect of prevention of rheumatoid arthritis is available. Being a woman and of reproductive age are the only risk factors established so that hormonal intervention would seem

the only possible intervention, but that would be unacceptable unless reproduction is not possible or undesired. So, further progress with etiological studies will have to be made before prevention of this formidable disease is feasible.

REFERENCES

1. Martin J, Meltzer H, Elliot D. The prevalence of disability in adults. OPCS surveys of disability in Great Britain. Report 1, London HMSO, 1988
2. Arnett FC, Edworthy SM, Bloch DA *et al.* The American Rheumatism Association. 1987 Revised Criteria for the Classification of Rheumatoid Arthritis. Arthritis Rheum. 1988; 31:315–324
3. Lewis-Fanning E. Report of enquiry into the aetiological factors associated with rheumatoid arthritis. Ann Rheum Dis. 1950; 9:1–94
4. Spector TD. Rheumatoid arthritis. Rheum Dis Clin North Am. 1990; 16:513–537
5. Solomon L, Robin G, Valkenburg HA. Rheumatoid arthritis in an urban South African negro population. Ann Rheum Dis. 1975; 34:128–135
6. Beighton P, Solomon L, Valkenburg HA. Rheumatoid arthritis in a rural South African negro population. Ann Rheum Dis. 1975; 34:136–141
7. Linos A, Worthington JW, O'Fallon M *et al.* The epidemiology of rheumatoid arthritis in Rochester, Minnesota: a study of incidence, prevalence and mortality. Am J Epidemiol. 1980; 111:87–98
8. Hench PS. The ameliorating effect of pregnancy on chronic atrophic (infectious rheumatoid) arth-

ritis, fibrositis and intermittent hydrarthritis. Mayo Clin Proc. 1938; 13:161–167

9. Persellin RH. The effect of pregnancy on rheumatoid arthritis. Bull Rheum Dis. 1977; 27:9226

10. Silman AJ, Kay A, Brennan P. Timing of pregnancy in relation to the onset of rheumatoid arthritis. Arthritis Rheum. (in press)

11. Del Junco DJ, Annegers JF, Coulam CB, Luthra HS. The relationship between rheumatoid arthritis and reproductive function. Br J Rheumatol. 1989; 28: Suppl. 1:33

12. Silman AJ, Davies P, Currey HLF, Evans SJW. Is rheumatoid arthritis becoming less severe?. J Chronic Dis. 1983; 36:12:891–897

13. Silman AJ. Has the incidence of rheumatoid arthritis declined in the United Kingdom? Br J Rheumatol. 1987; 27:77–78

14. Hochberg M. Changes in the incidence and prevalence of rheumatoid arthritis in England and Wales – 1970–1982. Semin Arthritis Rheum. 1990; 19:294–302

15. Buchanan WW, Murdoch RM. Hypothesis that rheumatoid arthritis will disappear. J Rheum. 1979; 6: 324–329

16. Lawrence JS, Ball J. Genetic studies on rheumatoid arthritis. Ann Rheum Dis. 1958; 17:160–168

17. Aho K, Koskenvuo M, Tuominen J, Kaprio J. Occurrence of rheumatoid arthritis in a nationwide series of twins. J Rheum. 1986; 13:899–902

18. Silman AJ, Ollier WER, Hayton RM, Holligan S, Smith IL. Twin concordance rates for rheumatoid arthritis: preliminary results of a nationwide study (Abstr). Br J Rheumatol. 1989; 28: Suppl 2:95

19. Stastny P. Association of the B cell alloantigen DRw4 with rheumatoid arthritis. N Engl J Med. 1978; 298:869–871

20. Gregersen PK, Silver J, Winchester RJ. The shared epitope hypothesis. An approach to understanding the molecular genetics of susceptibility to rheumatoid arthritis. Arthritis Rheum. 1987; 30:1205–1213

21. Hazes JMW, Silman AJ. Review of UK data on the rheumatic diseases – rheumatoid arthritis. Br J Rheumatol. 1990; 29:310–312

22. De Jongh BM, Van Romunde LKJ, Valkenburg HA, De Lange GG. Epidemiological study of HLA and GM in rheumatoid arthritis and related symptoms in an open Dutch population. Ann Rheum Dis. 1984; 43:613–619

23. Steere AC, Grodzicki RL, Kornblatt AN, Craft JE, Barbour AG. The spirochetal etiology of Lyme disease. N Engl J Med. 1983; 308:733–739

24. Steere AC, Malawista SE, Snydman DR, Shope RE *et al.* Lyme arthritis – an epidemic of oligoarticular arthritis in children and adults in three Connecticut communities. Arthritis Rheum. 1977; 20:7–37

25. Aho K, Palosuo T, Raunio V, Puska P, Aromaa A, Salonen JT. When does rheumatoid disease start? Arthritis Rheum. 1985; 28:485–489

26. Aho K, Heliovaara M, Maatela J, Tuomi T, Palosuo T. Rheumatoid factors antedating clinical rheumatoid arthritis. J Rheum. 1991; 18: 1202–1284

27. Lawrence JS. Rheumatism in Populations. London, Heinemann, 1977

28. Pritchard MH, Matthews N, Munro J. Antibodies to influenza in a cluster of children with juvenile chronic arthritis. Br J Rheumatol. 1988; 27:176–180

29. Gottlieb NL, Page WF, Appelrouth DJ, Palmer R, Kiem IM. Antecedent tonsillectomy and appendectomy in rheumatoid arthritis. J Rheumatol. 1979; 6:316–323

30. Fernandez-Madrid F, Reed AH, Karvonen RL *et al.* Influence of antecedent lymphoid surgery on the odds of acquiring rheumatoid arthritis. J Rheumatol. 1985; 12:43–48

31. Wolfe F, Young DY. Rheumatoid arthritis and antecedent tonsillectomy. J Rheumatol. 1983; 10:309–312

32. Patel SB, Eastmond CJ. Preceding tonsillectomy and appendicectomy in rheumatoid and degenerative arthritis. J Rheumatol. 1983; 10:313–315

33. Linos AD, O'Fallon WM, Worthington JW, Kurland LT. The effect on tonsillectomy and appendectomy on the development. J Rheumatol. 1986; 13:707–709

34. Bombardier C. Some pitfalls of the case-control approach to investigation of rheumatoid disease. J Rheumatol. 1979; 6:247–250

35. Silman AJ, Ollier WER, Currey HLF. Failure to find disease similarity in sibling pairs with rheumatoid arthritis. Ann Rheum Dis. 1987; 46: 135–138

36. Sanders PA, Grennan DM. Age and year of onset differences in siblings with rheumatoid arthritis. Br J Rheumatol. 1990; 29:128–130

37. Schweiger F, Bell DA, Little AH. Coexistence of rheumatoid arthritis in married couples: a search. J Rheum. 1981; 8:416–422

38. Walker DJ, Griffiths ID, Madeley D. Autoantibodies and antibodies to microorganisms in rheumatoid arthritis: comparison of histocompatible siblings. J Rheumatol. 1987; 14: 426–428

39. Anderson MJ, Higgins PG, Davis LR et al. Experimental parvoviral infection in humans. J Infect Dis. 1985; 152:257–265

40. White DG, Mortimer PP, Blake DR, Woolf AD, Cohen BJ, Bacon PA. Human parvovirus arthropathy. Lancet. 1985; 419–421

41. Reid DM, Reid TMS, Brown T, Rennie JAN. Human parvovirus-associated arthritis: a clinical and laboratory description. Lancet. 1985; 422–425

42. Klouda PT, Corbin SA, Bradley BA et al. HLA and acute arthritis following human parvovirus infection. Tissue Antigens. 1986; 28:318–319

43. Simpson RW, McGinty L, Simon L et al. Association of parvoviruses with rheumatoid arthritis in humans. Science. 1984; 223:1425–1428

44. Alspaugh MA, Tan EM. Antibodies to cellular antigens in Sjögren's syndrome. J Clin Invest. 1975; 55:1067–73

45. Alspaugh MA, Henle G, Lennette ET, Henle W. Elevated levels of antibodies to Epstein–Barr virus antigens in sera and synovial fluids of patients with rheumatoid arthritis. J Clin Invest. 1981; 67:1134–1140

46. Catalano MA, Carson DA, Slovin SF, Richman DD, Vaughan H. Antibodies to Epstein–Barr virus-determined antigens in normal subjects and in patients with seropositive rheumatoid arthritis. Proc Natl Acad Sci. 1979; 76:5825–5828

47. Ferrell PB, Aitcheson CT, Pearson GR, Tan EM. Seroepidemiological study of relationships between Epstein–Barr virus and rheumatoid arthritis. J Clin Invest. 1981; 67:681–687

48. Ng KC, Perry JD, Brown KA, Holborrow EJ. Anti-RANA antibody is a marker of seronegative and seropositive rheumatoid arthritis. Lancet. 1980; 1:447–449

49. Venables PJW, Ross MGR, Charles PJ et al. A seroepidemiological study of cytomegalovirus and Epstein–Barr virus in rheumatoid arthritis and sicca syndrome. Ann Rheum Dis. 1985; 44: 742–746

50. Aho K, Raunio V. EB-Virus and rheumatoid arthritis: new insights into their interrelation. Med Biol. 1982; 60:49–52

51. Depper JM, Zvaifler NJ. Epstein–Barr virus – its relationship to the pathogenesis of rheumatoid arthritis. Arthritis Rheum. 1981; 24:755–761

52. Pelton BK, North M, Palmer RG, Hylton W, Smith-Burchnell CS. A search for retrovirus infection in systemic lupus erythematosus and rheumatoid arthritis. Ann Rheum Dis. 1988; 47:206–209

53. Panayi G, Dalgleish AG. Retroviruses in rheumatoid arthritis. Ann Rheum Dis. 1986; 45:439

54. Galeazzi M, Tuzi T, Amici C, Benedetto A. Rheumatoid arthritis and helper T cell lymphotropic retroviruses. Arthritis Rheum. 1986; 29:1533–34

55. Cassell GH, Davis JK, Lindsey JR, Cole BC, Hartley MW. Mycoplasma-induced arthritis. Israel J Med Sci. 1981; 17:608–615

56. Clark HW, Cokervann MR, Vailey JS et al. Detection of mycoplasmal antigens in immune complexes from rheumatoid arthritis synovial fluids. Ann Allergy. 1988; 60:394–98

57. Ottenhoff THM, Torres P, Terencio de Las Aguas J, Fernandez R. Evidence for an HLA-DR4-associated immune-response gene for *Mycobacterium tuberculosis*. Lancet. 1986; 310–313

58. Silman AJ, Vandenbroucke JP. Female sex hormones and rheumatoid arthritis. Br J Rheumatol. 1989; 28: Suppl. 1:1–73

59. Wingrave SJ. Reduction in incidence of rheumatoid arthritis associated with oral contraceptives. Lancet. 1978; 569–571

60. Hannaford PC, Kay CR, Hirsch S. Oral contraceptives and rheumatoid arthritis: new data from the RCGP OC study. Ann Rheum Dis. 1990; 49: 744–746

61. Hernandez Avila M et al. Exogenous sex hormones and the risk of rheumatoid arthritis. Arthritis Rheum. 1990; 33:947–953

62. Spector TD, Hochberg MC. The protective effect of the OC pill on RA. J Clin Epidemiol. 1990; 43:1221–1230

63. Vandenbroucke JP, Witteman JCM, Valkenburg HA, Boersma JW. Noncontraceptive hormones and rheumatoid arthritis in premenopausal and postmenopausal women. JAMA. 1986; 255:1299–1303

64. Carette S, Marcoux S, Gingras S. Postmenopausal hormones and the incidence of rheumatoid arthritis. J Rheumatol. 1989; 16:911–913

65. Spector TD, Brennan P, Harris P, Studd JWW, Silman AJ. Does estrogen replacement therapy protect against rheumatoid arthritis? J Rheumatol. 1991; 18:1473–1476

66. Silman AJ. Is pregnancy a risk factor for rheumatoid arthritis? Ann Rheum Dis. 1986; 45:1031–34

67. Beral V, Roman E, Colwell R. Poor reproductive outcome in insulin dependent diabetic women associated with later development or other endocrine disorders to the mothers. Lancet. 1984; 1:4–7

68. Spector TD, Silman AJ. Is poor pregnancy outcome a risk factor in rheumatoid arthritis? Ann Rheum Dis. 1990; 49:12–14

69. Hazes JMW, Dijkman BAC, Vandenbroucke JP, de Vries RRP, Cats A. Pregnancy and the risk of developing rheumatoid arthritis. Arthritis Rheum. 1990; 33:1770–1775

70. Del Junco DL, Annegers JF, Coulam CB, Luth HS. The relationaship between rheumatoid arthritis and reproductive function. Br J Rheumatol, 1986; 28: Suppl. 1, 33

71. Koepsell T, Dugowson C, Voigt L, Bley L, Nelson JL et al. Preliminary findings from case-control studies of risk of rheumatoid arthritis in relation to oral contraceptive use. Br J Rheumatol. 1989; 28:41

72. Kay A, Bach F. Subfertility before and after the development of rheumatoid arthritis in women. Ann Rheum Dis. 1965; 24:169–173

73. Kaplan D. Fetal wastage in patients with rheumatoid arthritis. J Rheumatol. 1986; 13:875–877

74. Silman AJ, Roman E, Beral V, Brown A. Adverse reproductive outcomes in women who subsequently develop rheumatoid arthritis. Ann Rheum Dis. 1988; 47:979–981

75. Spector TD, Silman AJ. Is poor pregnancy outcome a risk factor in rheumatoid arthritis? Ann Rheum Dis. 1990; 49:12–14

76. King SH, Cobb S. Psychosocial factors in the epidemiology of rheumatoid arthritis. J Chronic Dis. 1958; 7:466–475

77. Engel A. Rheumatoid arthritis in US adults. 1960–62. In Bennett PH, Wood PHN, eds., Population Studies of the Rheumatic Diseases, 1968

78. Lawrence JS. The epidemiology and genetics of rheumatoid arthritis. Population studies and genetics. Rheumatology (Basel). 1969; 2:1–36

79. Kato H, Duff IF, Russell WJ, Uda Y et al. Rheumatoid arthritis and gout in Hiroshima and Nagasaki, Japan. A prevalence and incidence study. J Chronic Dis. 1971; 23:659–679

80. Marcolongo R, Spaziani L. Analisi computerizzata su alcuni fattori condizionanti la preval. Reumatismo. 1971; 23:185–210

81. Jacob DL, Robinson H, Masi AT. A controlled home interview study of factors associated with early rheumatoid arthritis. Am J Public Health. 1972; 1532–1537

82. Miall WE, Caplan A, Cochrane AL, Kilpatrick GS. An epidemiological study of rheumatoid arthritis associated with characteristic X-ray appearances in coal workers. Br Med J. 1953; 4:1231–1236

83. Franzinelli A, Marcolongo R. Epidemiologia dell'artrite, reumatoide e del fattore reumatoide. Reumatismo. 1971; 23:222–235

84. Klockars M, Koskela RS, Jarvinen E et al. Silica exposure and rheumatoid arthritis: a follow up study of g. Br Med J 1987; 294:997–1000

85. Hellgren L. Prevalence of rheumatoid arthritis in occupational groups. Acta Rheum Scand. 1970; 16:106–113

86. Buchanan HM, Preston SJ, Brooks PM, Buchanan WW. Occasional review. Is diet important in rheumatoid arthritis? Br J Rheumatol. 1991; 30:125–134

87. Scudder PR, Al-Timimi D, McMurray W, White AG, Zoob BC, Dormandy TL. Serum copper and related variables in rheumatoid arthritis. Ann Rheum Dis. 1978; 37:67–70

88. Rainsford KD. Environmental metal ion perturbations, especially as they affect copper status, are factors in the etiology of arthritis conditions: an hypothesis. In Sorenson JRJ, ed., Inflammatory Disease and Copper. Clifton: Humana Press, 1982; 137–142

89. Mottonen T, Hannonen P, Seppala O, Alfthan G, Oka M. Glutathione and selenium in rheumatoid arthritis. Clin Rheum 1984; 3:195–200

90. Peretz A, Neve J, Vertongen F, Famaey JP, Molle L. Selenium status in relation to clinical variables and corticosteroid treatment in rheumatoid arthritis. J Rheumatol. 1987; 14:1104–1107

21. CONNECTIVE TISSUE DISEASES

Marc C. Hochberg and Richard Wigley

SYSTEMIC LUPUS ERYTHEMATOSUS
Systemic lupus erythematosus (SLE) is a multisystem connective tissue disease characterized by a plethora of immunological abnormalities including loss of self tolerance, polyclonal B-lymphocyte activation and the production of autoantibodies to a variety of cellular constituents. Although cutaneous lupus was described as early as the thirteenth century, systemic involvement was not appreciated until the latter part of the nineteenth century when Kaposi described the occurrence of fever, arthritis, lymphadenitis, pleuropneumonia, anemia and mental disturbance in patients with cutaneous lupus[1]. The clinical features of SLE are now well described and include, in descending order of frequency, cutaneous and mucous membrane involvement, arthritis, pleurisy and/or pericarditis, renal involvement, central nervous system involvement, Raynaud's phenomenon and peripheral vasculitis. Constitutional symptoms including malaise, fever and weight loss are common. Laboratory abnormalities include anemia, which may on occasion be hemolytic, leukopenia, thrombocytopenia and the presence of autoantibodies including antinuclear antibodies and antibodies to native deoxyribonucleic acid, extractable nuclear antigens such as nuclear ribonucleoprotein, and phospholipids, including cardiolipin. The diagnosis of SLE is based on clinical and historical evidence of multisystem disease and confirmed by laboratory tests, most often the presence of antinuclear antibodies. For purposes of epidemiological studies, the 1982 American

Table 1 Revised criteria for the diagnosis of systemic lupus erythematosus (from the American College of Rheumatology, 1982). (Modified with kind permission from reference 2)

1.	Malar rash
2.	Discoid rash
3.	Photosensitivity
4.	Oral ulcers
5.	Non-erosive arthritis
6.	Pleuritis or pericarditis
7.	Renal disorder
8.	Seizures or psychosis
9.	Hematological disordery
10.	Immunological disorder
11.	Positive test for antinuclear antibodies

Table 2 Prevalence of systemic lupus erythematosus by country

Country (Ref)	Cases per 100 000
United States	
Rochester[7]	40
San Francisco[6]	51
Sweden[10]	39
England/Wales[15]	12
New Zealand[13]	15
Finland[11]	28
Japan[17]	21
China[16]	40

College of Rheumatology's 'Revised criteria' for SLE should be used for case definition[2] (*see* Table 1). The presence of four or more of the 11 items boasts a sensitivity and specificity of 96%. Although alternative classification schema have been suggested [3], a recent analysis suggests that the 1982 revised criteria are more accurate, especially in African–American patients[4].

Prevalence

Lupus erythematosus is considered to be a rare disease in Caucasian populations as it has overall prevalence of less than 80 in 100 000[5]. Studies to estimate the prevalence of SLE have been performed worldwide in the United States[6–8], Sweden[9,10], Finland[11], Iceland[12], New Zealand[13,14], England and Wales[15], China[16] and Japan[17]; in general, overall prevalence ranges from 12 to 51 cases per 100 000 for both sexes combined (Table 2). Prevalence is greater in females than males in all racial groups studied; in Caucasians, the prevalence in females aged 18 years and older approaches 100 cases per 100 000[6,10]. Prevalence is greater in African–American than Caucasians in both sexes, and in African–American females, the prevalence is as high as 400 per 100 000[6]. Prevalence has also been reported to be higher in various Polynesians than in Caucasians, particularly in the State of Hawaii[18,19] and New Zealand[14] (Figure 1). The results of a population survey conducted in China under the auspices of the International League Against Rheumatism and the World Health Organization are pending (four cases of SLE were found among 12 000 adults in North and South China). The above data have been reviewed extensively elsewhere[20].

Incidence

The incidence rate is nearly five cases per 100 000 per year in Caucasian females aged 18 years and above[7,10,21], and exceeds ten cases per 100 000 per year in African–American females of the same age[21].

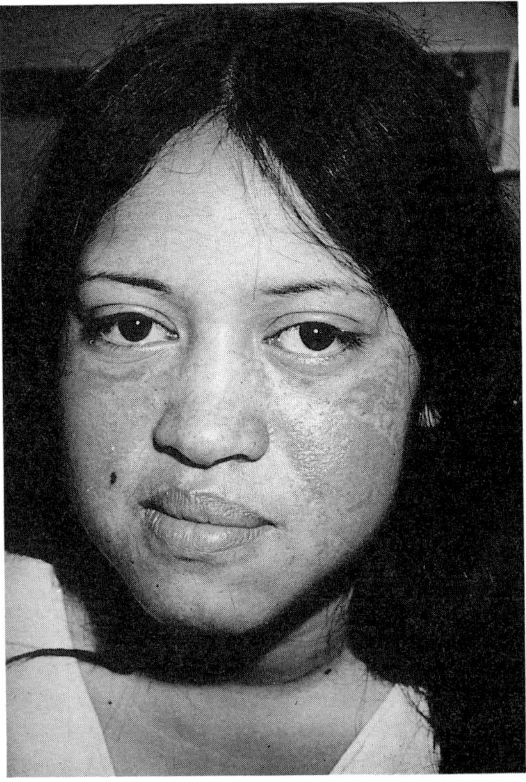

Figure 1 A Maori girl with a light-sensitive eruption. Maoris are thought to be affected more frequently with this disease than Caucasians

Etiological factors

Epidemiological studies have focused on three broad areas of potential risk: endocrine–metabolic, genetic and environmental. The strongest risk factor for SLE is female gender, and about 90% of patients in most series are women. Studies in murine models of SLE have demonstrated that treatment with androgens prevents, and estrogens accelerates, the development of renal disease and mortality of SLE. Despite these experimental data, there is no evidence that use of oral contraceptives is a risk factor for developing SLE[20].

Table 3 Pharmaceuticals associated with drug-induced lupus

Procainamide
Hydralazine
Isoniazid
Methyldopa
Quinidine
Chlorpromazine
Diphenylhydantoin
Carbamazepine
D-Penicillamine
β-Blockers

Genetic factors are known to be important in the development of SLE[20,22], and SLE demonstrates familial aggregation and a greater concordance in monozygotic than in dizygotic twins. Studies of the mode of inheritance support a polygenic model with a contribution of an autosomal dominant 'autoimmune' gene and modification of expression of the phenotype by gender. Several HLA Class II gene products, including HLA-DR2 and DR3, and the presence of the null phenotype of complement protein C4A [C4AQO] due to gene deletion are also associated with the presence of SLE.

Finally, non-infectious environmental factors also appear to be associated with SLE[20]. The most prominent example of such an association is that displayed by pharmaceutical agents, some of which may cause so-called drug-induced lupus: agents definitely associated with this syndrome are listed in Table 3[23]. The diagnosis of drug-induced lupus requires demonstration of a temporal association between drug administration and development of symptoms and signs of SLE which remit on discontinuation of the agent. In addition, several chemicals such as hydrazine, found in mushrooms, tobacco and tobacco smoke, and tartrazine (a food colorant, also known as FD&C yellow number 5) have been implicated in cases of SLE and lupus-like syndromes[24]. Finally, in a case–control study conducted in the south east United States, the use of hair dyes was associated with the development of SLE with an odds ratio of 7.1[25]. In this study, use of hair permanent solutions, hair spray and working as a beautician were also more common in cases than controls but did not reach statistical significance.

An increased sensitivity to ultraviolet light is inferred from the photosensitivity of malar rash seen in SLE[26]. Baer and Harber[27] found that radiation in the 285 to 315 nm range produced abnormal cutaneous reactions and exacerbation of systemic disease. Epstein and colleagues[28] were able to produce skin lesions with rays shorter than 320 nm only in those with a light sensitive rash. More recently, light sensitivity was found to be a common feature of SLE and all subtypes of cutaneous LE[29].

Primary prevention

Few opportunities exist for primary prevention of SLE as modifiable risk factors (except as above noted), have not been identified. High-risk groups, include non-Caucasian females, especially those with a positive family history, i.e. SLE in a first-degree relative, should be cautioned regarding the use of hair dyes and, possibly, other hair treatments. Avoidance of sunlight and the use of protective ultraviolet blocking cream would appear to have a secondary protective effect in those with light sensitivity but may not have significant primary protective value. Secondary prevention of manifestations of SLE, such as renal insufficiency, and primary prevention of complications of SLE, such as coronary atherosclerosis, are not discussed here as they have been recently reviewed elsewhere[30].

MYOSITIS

Primary polymyositis and dermatomyositis by definition have no identified cause, which by

Table 4 Average incidence and prevalence of systemic sclerosis per million population.(Reproduced with kind permission from reference 39)

Author	Study population	Period	Incidence/prevalence	
Medsger	Tennessee	1947–1952	0.6	4
		1953–1958	1.5	7
		1958–1962	4.1	21
		1963–1968	4.5	28
Wigley	New Zealand	1950–1973	2.3	45
Michet	Minnesota	1950–1979	10	253
Bosmansky	USSR	1961–1969	7	—
Medsger	US veterans	1963–1972	10	—
Eason	New Zealand	1970–1979	6.3	—
Asboe–Hansen	Denmark	1977–1979	—	126
Haustein	Leipzig, Germany	1980–1981	—	20
			—	100
Silman	England	1980–1985	3.7	31
Steen	Pennsylvania	1963–1972	9.6	—
		1973–1982	19.1	—

extension negates any means of primary prevention. In adults Barnes and co-workers found that malignant tumors are 5–11 times more common in dermatomyositis than in controls[31] so that in theory, prevention of the former might also prevent the latter, although this is unlikely to be a profitable preventive approach.

Myositis may occur as part of rheumatoid arthritis, systemic lupus erythematosus or systemic sclerosis. Drug-induced myopathies have been reviewed in detail[32], and are best controlled by avoiding or closely monitoring the use of these drugs, as discussed under iatrogenic disorders in Chapter 26. Other poisons and natural toxins that may damage muscle are discussed in Chapter 22. Preventable causes of myositis include alcohol[32], lovastatin[33], epsilon amino caproic acid[34], heroin, clofibrate[35], fenfluramine, phencyclidine and penicillamine[36]. Zidovudine, recently introduced for the treatment of HIV infection, has been reported to cause a polymyositis-like syndrome[37].

SYSTEMIC SCLEROSIS

This condition has been divided into a primary or idiopathic form and a secondary form which appears to be caused by controllable environmental factors. Systemic sclerosis may also be divided into clinical forms, including limited scleroderma, generalized scleroderma and scleroderma localized to the skin, also known as morphea. Masi[38] and more recently Steen[39] have reviewed the clinical epidemiology of systemic sclerosis (Table 4). Steen concluded that the apparent increased prevalence of systemic sclerosis may be explained by improved survival rates through effective control of the severe hypertension that was once the most common cause of death (and presumably continues to be in developing countries). Allowing for methodological variation and the general difficulty of estimating incidence from clinical samples, the reported studies do not show clear geographical differences from which general risk factors might be inferred. Maricq and colleagues[40] have since published a population based study of 6998 adults in South Carolina, and estimated a prevalence of between 670 and 2650 per million. Although this is much higher than that described in the clinic based studies, Silman[41] noted that only two cases satisfying the ARA criteria were found, so that very large samples would need to be studied in order to establish prevalence with greater confidence: still greater populations would need to be studied in order to establish incidence. Nonetheless, such data support expectations that many of the less severe cases will not be discovered in clinic-based studies. An increased frequency reported in young black women[39] raises the possibility of environmental or hormonal causes. Maricq and colleagues[42] have reviewed the evidence for clustering of cases of this disease. Silman has found a possible risk factor in pet ownership[43].

Occupational causes of systemic sclerosis

Occupational exposure to a number of chemicals is associated with systemic sclerosis and Raynaud's phenomenon providing an opportunity for prevention for a small proportion of cases.

Vinyl chloride

Workers who are exposed to vinyl chloride fumes in the production of polyvinyl chloride[44] may develop Raynaud's phenomenon and sclerodactyly-acro-osteolysis and pulmonary fibrosis typical of systemic sclerosis, but may also have other skin lesions, parasesthesia and liver involvement not expected in systemic sclerosis. Predisposition to this toxic effect has been related to HLA-DR5 in severe disease and to A1-B8-DR3 and C4AQO in mild disease[44]. Organic solvents such as benzene, toluene, xylene and to trichlorethylene, napthhexane and meta phenyldiamine rarely cause a systemic sclerosis like disease[39].

Silica

Silica dust exposure has been estimated to increase the risk of developing systemic sclerosis in East Germany by a factor of 110[45]. Sluis-Cremer and co-workers noted a 20-fold increase of this condition in a case–control study of South African gold miners[46]; they found in miners that systemic sclerosis was related to cumulative life time exposure to silica but was unrelated to silicosis as defined by chest radiograph(s). They reviewed evidence of possible disturbances induced by silica, and concluded that different mechanisms are involved in silica's induction of systemic sclerosis and pulmonary silicosis. They also noted six cases of SLE associated with silica.

Silicone

Silicone breast implants may also be associated with systemic sclerosis-like disease and other autoimmune type conditions described collectively as human adjuvant diseases[47]. Improvement has been reported to follow removal of the prosthesis in about half the cases. Francisco and co-workers[48] have described a case in which systemic sclerosis completely remitted following removal of the silicone implant (Chapter 27). Recent data from a multicenter case–control study, however, failed to demonstrate a difference in the frequency of antecedent augmentation mammoplasty in patients with systemic sclerosis compared with population-based controls[49].

Bleomycin causes Raynaud's phenomenon but not the full picture of systemic sclerosis[50].

Eosinophilia myalgia syndrome may simulate systemic sclerosis in some respects but has been attributed to taking excess L-tryptophan so is described in Chapter 27.

Prevention

Preventive measures are currently available only for the above noted secondary forms of systemic sclerosis, most of which occur in specific occupational settings and account for a small fraction of the cases of systemic sclerosis. The control of silica dust in mines and in grinding is detailed in texts on occupational medicine[51].

ARTERITIS (VASCULITIS)

Arteritis is found on histological examination of tissue from a wide range of disorders. Where the arteritis is regarded as part of other clinical entities, e.g. SLE and rheumatoid arthritis, it will not be included in this discussion, as the control of these, so far as is feasible, will be that of the underlying disease. In this section, only well-defined clinical entities apparently based on vasculitis will be discussed. Since the cause of most of these vasculitides, is as yet unknown, the options for prevention are limited so these complaints will not be considered in detail.

POLYARTERITIS NODOSA

This disease was described by Kussmaul and Maier[52] as a disease in which there was generalized vasculitis of medium-sized arteries with a tendency to aneurysm formation with frequent renal involvement and a characteristic mononeuritis multiplex. This disease is rare and difficult to diagnose, so that prevalence and incidence statistics are of limited value. Incidence per million has been estimated at nine in Olmsted county USA[53], 4.6 in England[54] and 2.7 in New Zealand[55], and men are affected about twice as often as women. Andrews and colleagues[56] studied cases of polyarteritis nodosa and Wegener's granulomatosis selected for renal involvement, and found that the incidence of both diseases had risen from 1.5 to 6.1 since 1987 when the anti-neutrophil cytoplasmic antibody test (ANCA)[57] was introduced. They concluded that the more recently diagnosed cases were less severe, and that it was probable that the new test had enabled the diagnosis of less severe disease rather than that there had been an actual increase in prevalence.

An association with polyarteritis nodosa and hepatitis B was described by Gocke[58], and subsequently, in 10–30% of cases, with immune complexes, which suggests a role of these complexes in this form of vasculitis. In an Alaskan Eskimo population with endemic hepatitis B, polyarteritis nodosa was found in 77 per million[59]. Of 1400 hepatitis B surface carrying native Alaskans, none had polyarteritis nodosa but 20 developed carcinoma, 14 developed chronic active hepatitis and 8 cirrhosis. It would thus appear that the individual risk of developing polyarteritis nodosa in hepatitis B virus carriers is very low. Other viral infections have been reported in association with polyarteritis nodosa, including hepatitis A[60], cytomegalovirus[61], HIV[62], parvovirus[63], and T cell leukemia virus 1[64]. A virally-induced arteritis occurs in horses and a similar disease occurs in mice and many other species[65].

At best, therefore the only possibility of preventing polyarteritis nodosa, if indeed there is a relationship thereto, is by controlling viral infections, in particular hepatitis B, which is widespread particularly in developing countries with high carrier rates. Avoidance of needle and venereal transmission is important but a safe effective genetically engineered vaccine is now available. Hepatitis A is controlled by food and water hygiene; a prophylactic serum is available particularly for susceptible travelers moving into an endemic area.

WEGENER'S GRANULOMATOSIS

Wegener's granulomatosis[66] is a similar rare entity in which vasculitis mainly affects the upper and lower respiratory tract and renal vessels but may be widespread. As with polyarteritis, the ANCA antibody is positive in the majority of cases so the opportunity now arises for diagnosis at an earlier phase when possible risk factors such as virus infections may be detectable so allowing possible control measures.

CHURG–STRAUSS SYNDROME

This is also a rare condition in which asthma and eosinophilia are associated with a systemic vasculitis and the majority have allergic rhinitis[67].

Table 5 Diagnostic criteria for polymyalgia rheumatica

Major criteria
Age > 50 years
Bilateral pain for at least one month involving
  two of the following: neck, shoulder girdle and
  hip girdle associated with morning stiffness and
  gelling.
ESR greater than 40 mm/h
Exclusion of other diseases except GCA

Lesser criteria
Caucasian race
Evidence for a systemic illness
No primary muscle disease
No infection
Clinical synovitis
Clinical response prednisone < 16 mg daily

ESR, erythrocyte sedimentation rate

There appear to be no established risk factors that would enable preventive measures for this syndrome.

HENOCH–SCHÖNLEIN PURPURA

This vasculitic form of purpura is not uncommon, and occurs in 13.4 per 100 000 annually in Belfast[68]. It is more common in boys and is uncommon in adults. This condition has been attributed to infectious agents such as streptococci, drugs, foods, environmental chemicals and insect bites. The agricultural chemical tetramethylthiuram disulfide has been implicated[69]. However there are no established risk factors to enable prevention and the same is true of the following disorders though geographical and ethnic differences may eventually provide clues to control measures.

POLYMYALGIA RHEUMATICA AND GIANT CELL ARTERITIS

These conditions overlap to such an extent that they are usually considered to be variations on a single disease pattern[70]. Diagnostic criteria for polymyalgia rheumatica are shown in Table 5[71].

Table 6 Incidence per 100 000 of giant cell arteritis

Site, period studied	Cases	Incidence rate
Minnesota, 1950–1985	94	17.0
Israel, 1969–78	46	0.49
Scotland, 1964–1977	136	4.2
Tennessee, 1971–1980	26	1.58
Sweden, 1973–1979	74	16.8
France, 1975–1985	110	9.4
Italy, 1981–1985	28	8.8
Denmark, 1982	46	23.3

The incidence of giant cell arteritis by country is summarized in Table 6[72].

One author (RW) and his colleagues, though well aware of this syndrome from publications from the UK and two neighboring districts, were unable to find a single case of polymyalgia rheumatica in the Palmerston North Health District before 1980. The only two cases suspected of having this complaint developed florid rheumatoid arthritis. Since 1980 the number of cases diagnosed has been similar to that expected in other communities. In Italy Cimmino and co-workers[73] observed that more cases of polymyalgia rheumatica occurred in summer whereas matched rheumatoid arthritis cases did not show this pattern suggesting a temperature or sunlight risk factor. Similar patterns emerging from further time–space–season cluster studies may disclose evidence for a transmissible agent and hopefully a means of prevention. Several studies have shown an association with DR4 and polymyalgia rheumatica and temporal arteritis[74,75].

TAKAYASU, KAWASAKI AND BEHÇET'S DISEASES

There are no effective measures for preventing Takayasu's arteritis[76], Kawasaki syndrome or Behçet's disease, given the lack of understanding of the pathogenesis of these diseases. All appear to be more prevalent in Japan and possibly in north China, and thus heredity may play a role in these complaints; since renal arteritis is a common cause of renovascular hypertension in China[77], and each of these complaints have clinical forms of vasculitis, it is possible that investigation of environmental factors in this region may eventually yield a means of control.

ERYTHEMA NODOSUM

Erythema nodosum is not a disease *a sui generis*, but rather a lesion that may herald a number of preventable disorders[78], including tuberculosis, leprosy, psittacosis, coccidiodomycosis, histoplasmosis, North American blastomycosis, lymphogranuloma venereum, cat scratch disease, streptococcal, yersinia infections. It has also been associated with the use of oral contraceptive hormones, and other drugs including sulphonamides, bromides and iodides, Apparent joint involvement in erythema nodosum may in fact result from a tender skin nodule (panniculitis) occurring over a joint. The Stevens Johnson syndrome may follow the use of sulphonamides[79].

ALLERGY

Though is has been postulated that allergy to foreign substances as opposed to autoallergy (autoimmunity) is an important cause of arthritis, well documented cases of such an event involving exogenous antigens are uncommon. Golding[80] has described eight cases in which arthritis was associated with atopy. Three had type I immediate allergy and three had urticarial arthralgia in which urticaria and joint pain occurred simultaneously. Three had evidence of food allergy. Allergy to drugs such as penicillin may cause serum sickness type reactions with urticaria, angioedema[81] or generalized skin erythema with transient inflammatory arthritis clearing with withdrawal of the drug. When serum was commonly used for tetanus, serum sickness was common and this included an acute polyarthritis. Rarely, major disease with systemic vasculitis

and renal involvement with hematuria occurs. Anaphylaxis followed by serum sickness has been reported after maintenance antigen injection for allergy[82] but no allergen was identified in three.

Panush and co-workers[83] described a patient with rheumatoid arthritis in whom ingestion of certain foods was followed by arthritic pains that decreased on fasting. Panush also found that 30% of rheumatoid arthritis cases alleged that their arthritis was related to food. On double-blind food challenges to 15 of these, subjective and objective rheumatic symptoms occurred in three patients on challenge to milk, shrimp and nitrates. Panush concluded that not more than 5% of arthritics are immunologically sensitive to food. Martin and colleagues[84] found that 11 of 69 cases of rheumatoid arthritis improved on elimination of food allergens. As such clinics are likely to have a bias towards the collection of such cases the population prevalence may be much lower but if confirmed this work would suggest that prevention is possible for a small proportion of arthritis cases.

HYPERSENSITIVITY ANGIITIS

Myalgia and arthritis may occur in the so-called leukocytoclastic vasculitis[85], in which small arteries and veins are diffusely involved, which contrasts to polyarteritis nodosa that affects larger vessels in a segmental and patchy manner. Serum sickness type reactions to drugs and possibly to viruses, bacteria and parasites and antibiotics particularly the penicillins have been implicated. Recent reports involve naproxen[86], streptokinase[87,88], terbutaline sulfate[89] and phenytoin; the latter producing rhabdomyolysis[90]. This syndrome has also followed immunization with human diploid cell rabies vaccine[91]. Lohr[92] has reviewed the rheumatic manifestations associated with drug abuse, which include septic spondylitis, arthritis, alcoholic myopathy, rhabdomyolysis, fibrous myopathy, vasculitis, hypertrophic pulmonary osteoarthropathy, in addition to subacute bacterial endocarditis, and hepatitis B infection.

Eosinophilic fasciitis and toxic oil syndrome are discussed in Chapter 25.

PREVENTION OF ALLERGY

Clearly prevention depends on an awareness of these causes and protection of susceptible individuals from the causative agent. This is difficult in practice since only a small proportion of the community will be susceptible to any one antigen. A history of allergies should be routinely recorded on all medical records. These patients' medical records must be labelled in such a way that attending medical staff are immediately aware of the risk even in an unconscious patient. Wearing engraved metal wrist bands or neck pendants ensures adequate warning even in emergencies such as road accidents. Full labeling of all medication is also important. Subjects known to be allergic should be fully informed of this, and if there is any doubt, small test doses should be used initially if an alternative cannot be used.

REFERENCES

1. Hochberg MC. History of lupus erythematosus. Md Med J. 1991; 40:871–873
2. Tan EM, Cohen AS, Fries JF *et al*. The 1982 revised criteria for the classification of systemic lupus erythematosus. Arthritis Rheum. 1982; 25:1271–1277
3. Edworthy SM, Zatarain E, McShane DJ *et al*. Analysis of the 1982 lupus criteria data set by recursive partitioning methodology: new insights into the relative merit of individual criteria. J Rheumatol. 1988; 15:1493–1498
4. Perez-Gutthann S, Petri M, Hochberg MC. Comparison of different methods of classifying patients with systemic lupus erythematosus. J Rheumatol. 1991; 18:1176–1179
5. Safavi KH, Heyse SP, Hochberg MC. Estimating the incidence and prevalence of rare rheumatic diseases: a review of methodology and available data sources. J Rheumatol. 1990; 17:990–993
6. Fessel WJ. Systemic lupus erythematosus in the community: incidence, prevalence, outcome and first symptoms; the high prevalence in black women. Arch Intern Med. 1974; 134:1027–1035
7. Michet CJ, McKenna CH, Elveback LR *et al*. Epidemiology of systemic lupus erythematosus and other connective tissue disease in Rochester, Minnesota, 1950 through 1979. Mayo Clin Proc. 1985; 60:105–113
8. Siegel M, Lee SL. The epidemiology of systemic lupus erythematosus. Semin Arthritis Rheum. 1973; 3:1–54
9. Leonhardt T. Family studies of systemic lupus erythematosus. Acta Med Scand. 1964; 416 (Suppl.):1–156
10. Nived O, Sturfeldt G, Wollheim F. Systemic lupus erythematosus in an adult population in Southern Sweden: incidence, prevalence and validity of ARA revised classification criteria. Br J Rheumatol. 1985; 24:147–154
11. Helve T. Prevalence and mortality rates of systemic lupus erythematosus and causes of death in SLE patients in Finland. Scand J Rheumatol. 1985; 14:43–46
12. Teitsson I, Thorsteinsson J. Systemic lupus erythematosus in Iceland. Iceland Med J. 1978; 64:116
13. Meddings J, Grennan DM. The prevalence of systemic lupus erythematosus in Dunedin. NZ Med J. 1980; 91:205–206
14. Hart HH, Grigor RR, Caughey DE. Ethnic difference in the prevalence of systemic lupus erythematosus. Ann Rheum Dis. 1983; 42:529–532
15. Hochberg MC. Prevalence of systemic lupus erythematosus in England and Wales, 1981–2. Ann Rheum Dis. 1987; 46:664–666
16. Zhang N C. Rheumatic diseases in China. J Rheumatol. 1983; 10 (Suppl. 10):41–45
17. Nakae K, Furusawa F, Kasukawa R *et al*. A nation-wide epidemiological survey on diffuse collagen diseases: estimation of prevalence rate in Japan. In Kasukawa R, Sharp GC, eds., Mixed Connective Tissue Disease and Anti-nuclear Antibodies. Amsterdam, Elsevier Science Publishers, 1987, pp. 9–20
18. Serdula MK, Rhoads GG. Frequency of systemic lupus erythematosus in different ethnic groups in Hawaii. Arthritis Rheum. 1979; 22:328–333

19. Catalano MA, Hoffmeier M. Frequency of systemic lupus erythematosus among the ethnic groups of Hawaii. Arthritis Rheum. 1989; 32 (Suppl.4): 530 (Abstr.)

20. Hochberg MC. Systemic lupus erythematosus. Rheum Dis Clin North Am. 1990; 16:617–639

21. Hochberg MC. The incidence of systemic lupus erythematosus in Baltimore, Maryland, 1970–1077. Arthritis Rheum 1985; 28:80–86

22. Hochberg MC. Genetic epidemiology of systemic lupus erythematosus. In Proceedings of the Second International Conference on Systemic Lupus Erythematosus, Tokyo, 1989, pp. 9–13

23. Hess EV, Mongey AB. Drug-related lupus. Bull Rheum Dis. 1991; 40(4):1–8

24. Reidenberg MM. Aromatic amines and the pathogenesis of lupus erythematosus. Am J Med. 1983; 75:1037–1042

25. Freni-Titulaer LWJ, Kelley DB, Grow AG et al. Connective tissue disease in Southeastern Georgia: a case–control study of etiologic factors. Am J Epidemiol. 1989; 130:404–409

26. Shulman LE, Harvey AM. Systemic lupus erythematosus. In Hollander and McCarty, eds., Arthritis and Allied Conditions. Lea and Feabiger, 1976, p. 875

27. Baer RL, Harber LC. Photobiology of lupus erythematosus. Arch Dermatol. 1965; 92: 124–128

28. Epstein JH, Tuffanelli DL, Dubois EL. Light sensitivity and lupus erythematosus. Arch Dermatol. 1965; 91:483–485

29. Beutner EH, Blaszczyk M, Jablonska S et al. Studies on criteria of the European Academy of Dermatology and Venereology for classification of cutaneous lupus erythematosus. I. Selection of clinical groups and study factors. Int J Dermatol. 1991; 30:411–417

30. Hochberg MC. Epidemiology of systemic lupus erythematosus. In Hahn BH, Wallace D, eds., Dubois Lupus Erythematosus. 4th edn, Philadelphia, WB Saunders, 1992 (in press)

31. Barnes BE, Dermatomyositis and malignancy. Ann Intern Med. 1976; 84:68–76

32. Zuckner J. Drug-induced myopathies. Semin Arthritis Rheum. 1990; 19:259–268

33. East C, Alivizatos PA, Grundy SM et al. Rhabdomyolysis in patients receiving lovastatin after cardiac transplantation. N Engl J Med. 1988; 318:47–48

34. Randall J, Taylor K. Epsilon-aminocaproic acid myopathy. Aust NZ Med J. 1990; 20:851

35. Langer T, Levy RI. Acute muscular syndrome associated with administration of Clofibrate. N Engl J Med. 1968; 279:856–858

36. Dawkins RL, Zilko PJ, Carrano J et al. Immunobiology of D-penicillamine. J Rheumatol. 1981 Suppl. 8:56–61

37. Bessen LJ, Greene JB, Louie E, et al. Severe polymositis like syndrome associated with zidovudine therapy of AIDS and ARC. N Engl J Med. 1988; 318:708

38. Masi AT. Clinical-epidemiological perspective of systemic sclerosis. (scleroderma). In Jayson MIV, Black CM, eds., Systemic Sclerosis (Scleroderma). New York, John Wiley, 1988, pp. 7–31

39. Steen VD. Systemic sclerosis. Rheum Dis North Am. 1990; 16:641–654

40. Maricq HR, Weinrich MC, Keil JE, Smith EA, Harper FE, Nussbaum AI, LeRoy EC, McGregor AR, Diat F, Rosl EJ. Prevalence of scleroderma spectrum disorders in the general population of South Carolina. Arthritis Rheum. 1989; 32: 998–1006

41. Silman A, Symmons D. Comment on article by Maricq et al. Arthritis Rheum. 1989; 33:1062

42. Maricq HR. Geographic clustering of scleroderma. Br J Rheumatol. 1990; 29:241–244

43. Silman AJ. Pet ownership: a possible risk factor for scleroderma. Br J Rheumatol. 1990:29:494

44. Black CM, Pereira S, McWhirter A. et al. Genetic susceptibility to syndrome in symptomatic and asymptomatic workers exposed to vinyl chloride. J Rheumatol. 1986; 13:1059–1062

45. Haustein UF, Ziegler V, Environmentally induced systemic sclerosis-like disorders. Int J Dermatol. 1985; 24:147–151

46. Sluis-Cremer GK, Hessel PA, Nizdo EH, Churchill AR, Zeiss EA. Silica, silicosis and progressive systemic sclerosis. Br J Indust Med. 1985; 42:838–843

47. Kumagai Y, Shiokawa Y, Medsger TA Jr. et al. Clinical spectrum of connective disease after cosmetic surgery: Observations on eighteen patients and a review of the Japanese literature. Arthritis Rheum. 1984; 27:1–12

48. Francisco J, Gutierrez FJ, Espinoza LR. Progressive systemic sclerosis complicated by severe hypertension: Reversal after implant removal. Am J Med. 1990; 89:390–392

49 Wigley F, Miller R, Hochberg MC, Steer V. Augmentation mammoplasty in patients with systemic sclerosis: Data from the Baltimore Scleroderma Research Center and Pittsburgh Scleroderma Data Bank. Arthritis Rheum. 1992: 3S (Suppl 9); S46

50. Finch WR, Rodnan GP, Buckingham RB, Prince RK, Winkelstein A. Bleomycin induced scleroderma. J Rheumatol. 1980; 7:651–659

51. Dalton S, Hazelman BL. In Raffle PAB, ed., Hunter's Diseases of Occupations. London, 1987; pp. 649–653

52. Kussmaul A, Maier R. Ueber ein bisher nicht bescreibene eigenthumliche Artieren-krankung, die mit Morbus Brightii und rapid fort screitender allgemeiner Muskellahmung einher geht. Deutch Arch Klin Med. 1866; 1:484

53. Kurland MT, Chuang TY, Hunder GH, Epidemiology of the Rheumatic Diseases. New York, Gower Publishing, 1984

54. Scott DGI, Bacon PA, Elliott PJ. et al. Systemic vasculitis in a district general hospital. 1972–1980; Clinical and laboratory features, classification and prognosis of 80 cases. Q J Med. 1982; 203:292–311

55. Wigley R, Borman B. Medical geography and the aetiology of the rare connective tissue diseases in New Zealand. Soc Sci Med. 1980; 14D:175–183

56. Andrews M, Edmunds M, Campbell A, Walls J, Feehally J. Systemic vasculitis in the 1980s – is there and increasing incidence of Wegener's granulomatosis and microscopic polyartertis. J R Coll Physicians London. 1990; 24:284–288

57. Davies DJ, Moran JE, Niall JF, Ryan GB. Segmental necrosing glomerulitis with antineutrophil antibody: possible arbovirus aetiology? Br Med J. 1982; 285:606

58. Gocke DJ, Hsu K, Morgan C, Bombardieri S, Lockshin M, Christian CL. Association between polyarteritis and Australia antigen. Lancet. 1970; 1:1148–1153

59. McMahon BJ, Alberts SR, Wainwright RB, Bulkow L, Lanier AP. Hepatitis B related sequelae. Prospective study of 1400 surface antigen-positive Alaska native carriers. Arch Intern Med. 1990; 150:1051–1054

60. Inman R, Hodge M, Johnston MEA *et al.* Arthritis vasculitis and cryoglobulinemia associated with relapsing hepatitis A virus infection. Ann Intern Med. 1986; 105:700–703

61. Curtis JL, Egbert BM. Cutaneous cytomegalovirus vasculitis: An unusual clinical presentation of a common opportunistic pathogen. Hum Pathol. 1982; 13:1138–1141

62. Calabrese LH, Estes M, Yen-Lieberman B *et al.* Systemic vasculitis in association with human immunodeficiency virus infection. Arthritis Rheum. 1989; 32:569–576

63. Li Loong TC, Coyle PV, Anderson MJ *et al.* Human serum parvovirus associated vasculitis. Postgrad Med J. 62:493–494

64. Haynes BF, Miller SE, Parker TJ, Moore JO *et al.* Identification of human T cell leukemia virus in a Japanese patient with adult T cell leukemia and cutaneous lymphomatous vasculitis. Proc Natl Acad Sci USA. 1983, 80:2054–2058

65. Wigley RD, Craig AS, Williamson KI, Couchman KG. Spontaneous arteritis and glomerulitis in mice. A comparison of light and electronmicroscopic renal changes in PN/n, NZB/Bl, 101/MAC mice. Lab Invest. 1975; 33:8–15

66. Conn DL. Vasculitic syndromes. Rheum Dis Clin N Am. Philadelphia, WB Saunders, 1990

67. Guillevin L, Du LTH, Godeau P, Jais P, Wechsler B. Clinical findings and prognosis of polyarteritis nodosa and Churg–Strauss syndrome: a study of 165 patients. Br J Rheumatol. 1988; 27:258–264

68. Stewart M, Savage JM, Bell B, McCord B. Long term renal prognosis of Henoch–Schönlein purpura in an unselected childhood population. Eur J Paediatr. 1988; 147:113–115

69. Duell PB, Morton WE. Henoch–Schönlein purpura following thiram exposure. Arch Intern Med. 1987; 147:778–779

70. Paulley JW. Giant cell (temporal) arteritis-polymyalgia rheumatica: A critical review. Recent Prog Med. 1990; 81:176–183

71. Cohen MC, Ginsburg WW. Polymyalgia rheumatica. Rheum Dis Clin North Am. 1990; 16: 325–339

72. Machado EBV, Michet CJ, Ballard DJ, Hunder GG, Beard CM, Chu C, O'Fallon MW. Trends in incidence and clinical presentation of temporal arteritis in Olmsted county, Minnesota. Arthritis Rheum. 1988; 31:745–749

73. Cimmino MA, Caporali R, Montecucco CM, Rovida S, Baratelli E, Broggini M. A seasonal pattern in the onset of polymyalgia rheumatica. Ann Rheum Dis. 1990; 49:521–523

74. Sakkas LI, PLoqueman N, Panayi GS, Myles AB, Welsh KI. Immunogenics of polymyalgia rheumatica. Br J Rheumatol. 1990; 29:331–334

75. Cid MC, Ercilla G, Vilaseca J, Sanmarti R, Villalta J, Ingelmo M, Marquez A. Polymyalgia rheumatica. A syndrome associated with HLA DR4 antigen. Arthritis Rheum. 1988; 31:678–682

76. Hall S, Buchbinder. Takayasu's arteritis. Rheum Clin N Am. 1990; 16:411–422

77. Liu LS, Huang SW. Renovascular hypertension in China-report of 200 cases. J Hum Hypertens. 1990 4:133–134

78. Blomgren SE. Erythema nodosum. Semin Arthritis Rheum. 1974; 4:1–24

79. Chan HL, Stern RS, Arndt KA, Langlois J, Jick SS, Walker AM. The incidence of erythema multiforme, Stevens–Johnson syndrome and toxic epidermal necrolysis. A population-based study with particular reference reactions caused by drugs among outpatients. Arch Dermatol. 1990; 126:43–47

80. Golding DN. Is there an allergic synovitis? J R Soc Med. 1990; 83:312–314

81. Chopra R, Roberts J, Warrington RJ. Severe delayed onset hypersensitivity reactions to amoxycillin in children. Can Med Assoc J. 1989; 140:921–923

82. Umetsu DT, Hahn JS, Perez-Atayde AR, Geha RS. Serum sickness triggered by anaphylaxis A complication of immmunotherapy. J Allergy Clin Immunol. 1985; 76:713–718

83. Panush RS. Food allergy and arthritis. Proceedings of the XVII ILAR Congress of Rheumatology, Rio de Janiero, p. 631

84. Martin AFJ, Van de Laar Van de Korst JK. Rheumatoid arthritis influenced by elimination of food allergens. XVII ILAR Congress, Rio de Janiero, 1989, Abstract F217

85. Zeek PM. Periarteritis nodosa and other forms of necrotizing angiitis. N Engl Med J. 1953; 248: 764–772

86. Singhal PC, Faulkner M, Venkatesan J, Molho L. Hypersensitivity angiitis associated with naproxen. Ann Allergy. 1989; 63:107–109

87. Ong AC, Handler CE, Walker JM. Hypersensitivity vasculitis complicating intravenous streptokinase therapy. Int J Cardiol. 1988; 21:71–73

88. Manoharan A, Ramsay D, Davis S, Lvoff R. Hypersensitivity vasculitis associated with streptokinase. Aust NZ J Med. 1986; 16:815–816

89. Enat R, Katz R, Munichoir M, Pollack S. Hypersensitivity vasculitis induced by terbutaline sulfate. Ann Allergy. 1988; 61:275–276

90. Engel JN, Mellul VG, Goodman DB. Phenytoin hypersensitivity: A severe case of rhabdomyolysis. Am J Med. 1986; 81:928–930

91. Warrington RJ, Martens CJ, Rubin M, Rurtherford WJ, Aoki FY. Immunologic studies in subjects with a serum sickness-like illness after immunisation with human diploid cell rabies vaccine. J Allergy Clin Immunol. 1987; 79:605–610

92. Lohr KM. Rheumatic manifestations of diseases associated with substance abuse. Semin Arthritis Rheum. 1987; 17:90–111

22. CHEMICAL AND PHYSICAL CAUSES OF RHEUMATIC PROBLEMS

Richard Wigley

INTRODUCTION

Rheumatic complaints secondary to chemicals or physical agents, i.e. non-infectious or environmental are of therapeutic, industrial or accidental origin. These complaints are, by their very origin, preventable, and are discussed in this section. Rheumatic conditions related to therapeutic drugs are discussed in Chapter 26; those related to diet, in Chapter 25 and those related to allergy, in Chapter 21.

CHEMICAL CAUSES OF RHEUMATIC PROBLEMS

Rheumatic symptoms due to chemicals are rare, and often confined to particular regions or occupations. Awareness of the potential role these agents play in the pathogenesis of rheumatic complaints would enable early intervention and speed the recognition of possible new syndromes, which might result from the development of new chemicals or the use of old chemical agents in new industries.

Fluoride

Fluorosis, which can cause periarticular calcification and stiffening of joints, especially of the spine, is discussed in more detail under diet. Fluorides are used in the manufacture of pesticides and aluminum products, in smelting nickel, copper and gold and in glass works. Skeletal fluorosis due to occupational exposure to fluorides is reviewed by Nemeth[1]; serum fluorine levels in 353 aluminum metallurgy workers exposed to fluoride for 10–18 years were found to be six-fold higher than recommended limits; minor osteosclerosis was found in twelve, and one person suffered from fluorosis of moderate intensity. For those who are occupationally exposed, the maximum recommended air levels of fluoride are $2\,mg/m^3$; radiographs should be taken after 5 years exposure, and those demonstrating changes should be removed from the environment. Urinary levels reflect the fluorine intake from all sources including water, diet and fluorinated drugs, and urinary fluoride levels above 8 mg/l allow a definitive diagnosis of fluorosis (*see also* Chapter 25).

Other metals associated with rheumatic complaints

Lead

Saturnine gout resulting from lead intoxication is detailed in Chapter 23, and may produce a painful neuropathy.

Iron

Iron overload may result from injections of iron or multiple blood transfusions for anemia[2,3], from cheap wine containing excessive iron and in those genetically predisposed to iron retention in the form of hemochromatosis. Iron overload may cause chondrocalcinosis and pseudogout (*see* Chapter 23).

Calcium

Pseudogout and chondrocalcinosis may also result from an excessive intake of calcium and/or vitamin D (*see* Chapter 23).

Cadmium

Cadmium was thought to cause muscular weakness in Japan from renal osteomalacia, but this syndrome is now considered to have been to coincidental calcium deficiency (*see* Chapter 25).

Aluminum

Aluminum has been implicated (as has, to a lesser degree, iron) in the arthropathy of renal dialysis[4], which may be related to deposition of amyloid β-microglobulin. Although this is only a problem in a small specialized field, this phenomenon may prove instructive in preventing other forms of arthritis.

OTHER ENVIRONMENTAL TOXINS AND/OR CLINICAL CONDITIONS

Vinyl chloride

Vinyl chloride can cause acro-osteolysis, a systemic sclerosis like syndrome, arthritis, and a Raynaud's phenomenon that is not reversible on withdrawal of the agent. The United States National Institute of Occupational Safety and Health (NIOSH) recommends limiting exposure to three parts per million over 1 year[5]. Perchlorethylene and trichlorethylene used in dry cleaning have also been considered to cause similar problems[6].

Silicone

An adjuvant-type illness accompanied by symptoms of systemic sclerosis has been reported in women with silicone mammoplasty implants or inserts silicone joint implants may cause a foreign body type synovitis[7,8] (*see* Chapter 27).

Pulmonary osteoarthropathy

Hypertrophic pulmonary osteoarthropathy is a painful periostitis affecting one or more bones, including the tibia, fibula, radius and ulna that may signal various intoxications or malignancy, and may occur in asbestosis with mesothelioma, berylliosis, arsenic poisoning, silicosis, aluminum dust inhalation, smoking and lung cancer[9].

Neuropathy

A vast palette of toxic chemicals and drugs can simulate rheumatic symptoms by inducing neuropathies, and these must be appropriately ruled out. Prevention requires that these substances, e.g. arsenic, beryllium and aluminum dust, be monitored in industry, in the food and in the air.

RHEUMATIC DISORDERS DUE TO PHYSICAL AGENTS

In this section the rheumatic effects of high and low environmental pressures, vibration, burns, electrical and radiation injuries are considered; direct trauma to the joints are discussed in Chapters 4 and 5. As with chemical agents, physical causes of rheumatic symptoms are rare but equally preventable, and thus should not be forgotten when investigating any new or unfamiliar rheumatic complaints.

The 'bends' (dysbaric osteonecrosis)

Osteonecrosis occurred in the Japanese pearl divers who traditionally did not use diving equipment (Moon Sik Han. Bends in Japanese and Korean pearl divers. Personal communication). The 'bends' occur in 17% of those working in compressed air environments, and in 4.2% of professional divers, despite current careful decompression guidelines[10] (scuba divers are also at risk but they rarely go to the depths required of professional divers), and is usually accompanied by a history of decompression sickness. The bone lesions, which may occur months or years after exposure to the high pressure environment, are bilateral, and affect the large bones of the extremities. Joint involvement leads to secondary osteoarthritis, and considerable disability. Regular X-ray followed by bone scan monitoring of divers is necessary. Decompression time is related to the depth and the duration of exposure[11]. It is particularly noteworthy that the risk of decompression disease is increased by flying after diving, as the pressure in airliners is equivalent to that at 2000 meters[5], and those who take diving vacations should be warned about this possibility.

Vibration

Kakosy reviewed vibration injuries[12], and divided vibrating machines into those causing:

(1) Hand and arm vibrations, e.g. pneumatic tools, grinders, power saws and shoe pounding machines;

(2) Whole body vibration, e.g. in vehicles and from floor vibration from sheet iron presses, turbines and similar equipment; and

(3) Both hand and body vibration, e.g. concrete preparing machines and vehicles such as trucks, self-propelled power machines and earth moving equipment.

Vibration of the hand and arm has long been known to cause Raynaud's phenomenon. Vibration induced white finger has been renamed 'hand–arm vibration syndrome'[13]. Vascular and neurological complications occur independently so that a two-tier grading system has been introduced:

First tier: Vascular
(1) Blanching of finger tips without disability;

(2) Symptoms lying between 1 and 3;

(3) Blanching to the finger base with a loss of fine motor skills and work time; and

(4) Loss of finger tip tissue due to arterial occlusion.

Second tier: Neurogenic
(1) Episodic numbness without tingling;

(2) Numbness; reduced sensory perception; and

(3) Numbness; reduced tactile discrimination and manipulative dexterity.

Additional cold provocation and neural conduction studies are also indicated. James and colleagues studied 118 subjects with neurological symptoms, and found that the mean period from the time of prolonged exposure to vibration, and the development of symptoms was 13 years, and these symptoms more often affected domestic activities than work[14]. Vibration may contribute to carpal tunnel syndrome, osteoarthritis and spinal disk disease.

Carpal tunnel symptoms

The carpal tunnel syndrome (*see* Chapter 8), occurs in as many as 26% of forestry chain saw operators in Finland compared with white fingers in 5%[15] and polyneuropathy in 4%, and it is thought that the carpal tunnel swelling is reversible. In a case reference study, Wieslander found that the carpal tunnel syndrome was significantly associated with the use of hand-held tool vibration and with repetitive wrist movements but not with work producing a heavy load on the wrist[16]. Avascular necrosis of carpal bones was reported in a higher proportion of chain saw operators and miners than in controls, and necrosis of the lunate bone leads to the workers retirement due to permanent disability[12]. Environmental noise may have an additive effect to vibration in causing white finger[17].

Prevention of vibration

This is essential as response to treatment is poor. If avoidance of vibration is not possible, plastic or polystyrene handles reduce vibration by 50% in the 300–500 Hz range for chain saws and 95% for pneumatic hammers. As cold contributes to vibration injury, heated handles have been used. Polystyrene foam lined gloves reduce high frequency vibration and protect against cold. Pyykko has reported a fall in vibration injuries due to improved tool design and reduction in exposure to vibration[18].

Whole-body vibration can be reduced by installing vibration free bases under machinery, improving vehicle suspension, truck and tractor seats and using thick rubber shoe soles. Degenerative changes in the lumbar spine are more frequent than is expected for age in those exposed to whole-body vibration[12]. Kelsey[19] found the risk of herniated lumbar disc is nearly three-fold greater in those spending half their working time driving than in non-drivers, a finding that applies to airline pilots[20] and tractor drivers[21].

An increased risk for vibration injuries is present in women, older persons, those with an asthenic body type and previous cold sensitivity[12]. Taylor[13] deplores the delay in instituting the international standards organization recommendations for longitudinal and transverse whole body vibration. Prevention requires improved design of machinery and tools to reduce vibration, and need for vibration standards in machines known to cause injuries has been accepted since 1911. When redesign is not possible, automation may remove the risk or the worker may be insulated from the source of the vibration for example, by wearing thick gloves while handling vibrating tools or using vibration absorbing seats in vehicles and machinery. The British Standards Institution has now established vibration limits (BS 6842, 1987)[3]. Regular medical checks

should be made and all should be informed of the risk and need to attend regularly for examination.

Ultrasound and ultrasonics

There is little evidence that normal clinical use of therapeutic ultrasound causes bone or joint damage, although it was suspected of causing transient increase in sciatic pain in two patients[22].

Electrical injuries

Electric shocks may cause peripheral fractures, vertebral compression or cervical disc degeneration which may be followed by prolonged pain and disability[23]. Skin burns may lead to contractures that limit joint movement, and fractures may result from spasmodic muscle contraction. In children, bone growth may be arrested from necrosis of epiphyses. The prevention of such injuries is implicit in the extensive legislation in most countries, and will not be considered further here.

Burns

Kolar[22] found disuse osteoporosis in 70% of 1740 with third degree burns and 17% had reflex sympathetic dystrophy. Most (80%) of these were from combined crush injuries and burns from hot rollers. Myositis ossificans occurred in two patients who eventually died. These injuries can be prevented by fitting guards on machines that automatically release the rollers.

Cold

Trench foot, paddy foot and immersion foot result from inactivity and exposure to damp cold. Cold pulseless and numb hands or feet later swell with discoloration and blister over many weeks with eventual recovery, which may accompanied by temporary limitation of joint movement[23]. Frostbite follows exposure to cold air usually at temperatures less than 13 °C: vessels are damaged, resulting in thrombosis and potentially, gangrene and tissue loss. X-rays shows osteoporosis, osteolysis, destructive arthritis and periostitis, and the extremity may require amputation[23]. Cartilage is susceptible to cold injury, and von Tempsky in 1931 found joint damage in 40% of subjects who had been occupationally exposed to cold temperatures for 20 or more years; in younger age groups, necrosis of epiphyseal cartilage may lead to growth defects[24].

It is generally believed that workers in meat freezing rooms have more rheumatic pain than those working at normal temperatures, although this has not been well studied. Working in polar regions has always presented formidable risks of cold injury and outer space poses even greater risks of extreme cold, although sophisticated protective clothing has been developed to prevent this problem. Such work is liable to cause overuse syndromes. If this results from sustained muscle tension (Chapter 7) it would be expected that the shivering in response to cold would increase such symptoms, which would provide a possible explanation of the higher prevalence of general rheumatic pain in north as compared with south China (Chapter 3). All forms of cold injury are preventable by adequate protective clothing and minimizing exposure times to severe cold. Automation may also be necessary to prevent cold injuries.

Aeronautical problems

Vertebral fractures occur in 6–25% of ejections from aircraft, and may lead to chronic disability[25]. In early designs of the ejection equipment, impact of the head on the canopy was responsible for the injury, but the rate of neck injury has been reduced by jettisoning the canopy first. Less dramatic is the back pain of aeroplane and helicopter pilots, which is attributed to prolonged sitting and vibration as with tractor, truck and bus drivers. Lytic spondylolisthesis is an occupational hazard of helicopter pilots[19]. Reduction in this problem has been achieved by using amortized equipment for the surface of the pilot's seat[25]. Scoliosis, Klippel–Feil syndrome

Table 1 Grades of radiation injury

1. Demineralization without symptoms
2. Hypertrophic bone atrophy with pain and fractures which may heal
3. Bone necrosis; fractures do not heal
4. Malignancy, usually osteogenic sarcoma

and Scheuermann's disease increase susceptibility to aviation injury, thus in these occupations, pre-employment X-rays should be taken to rule out these conditions. Improved seat design and periodic mobility and exercises are required for prevention of back problems in pilots. Astronauts rapidly develop disuse osteoporosis, which may be accompanied by irreversible muscle atrophy if the muscles are not regularly exercised[25]. In the absence of gravity, intervertebral discs swell leading to an increase in height and sometimes back pain (Nachemson A. Disc swelling in astronauts. Personal communication).

Radiation injury

Joint injury may follow the use of therapeutic ionizing radiation for various malignancies, causing either direct bone and joint injury and/or indirect injury by impairing circulation through obliterative vascular disease. This does not appear to be a problem with supervoltage radiation[23]. Four grades of severity of radiation changes of the bone are recognized (Table 1).

Kolar[22] found arthritis in one of 100 physicians occupationally exposed to X-rays over more than 25 years. Workers who had been heavily exposed to radium and luminescent paints during the 1920s had a 50-fold greater incidence in osteogenic sarcoma than the normal population. Radium ingestion, thorium, uranium, plutonium, yttrium, strontium all potentially affect bones and joints. Bone-seeking isotopes[23] are taken up in an irregular pattern so that calculation of exposure limits is difficult, but present control measures appear to be adequate. Radiation joint damage was not reported in a study of arthritis in survivors of the Hiroshima atomic bomb[26].

Thorn arthritis

Arthritis following penetration of joints by thorns is rare, judging from the paucity of reports in the literature. Box thorns produce local granulomatous arthritis from penetration of joints in Britain[27]. Phoenix Palm thorns cause this condition in California[28] and the author has seen a case of knee arthritis in New Zealand. Hawkins[29] reported a case of rheumatoid arthritis that followed thorn dermatitis. Ormerod and co-workers[30] reported a case in which a plant thorn was located in the same sites as that of psoriatic arthritis. Periostitis has been attributed to thorn penetration[31] and arthritis[32]. Awareness of the risk to joints from thorns and the use of protective gloves by gardeners should reduce the risk of such accidents.

CONCLUSIONS

Prevention of the many disorders listed in this chapter, clearly hinges on avoiding the causative factor. There are numerous combinations of rheumatic syndromes and causes, but each one is rare, except in some high risk occupations. The purpose of bringing this information under one heading is to provide a quick reference to possible associations for use in daily practice and to raise the general level awareness of these risks and the possibility of recognizing new causes. Proving that an agent causes the symptoms may be difficult and compensation awards may be made for legal expediency, even in the absence of scientifically valid data. Preventive measures, if easily applied, may also be advisable where causation is not clearly established.

REFERENCES

1. Nemeth L, Zsogon E. Occupational skeletal fluorosis. Clin Rheumatol. 1989; 3:81–98
2. Abbott DF, Gresham GA. Arthropathy in transfusional siderosis. Br Med J. 1972; 1:418–419
3. Sella EJ, Goodman AH. Arthropathy secondary to transfusion hemochromatosis. J Bone Joint Surg. 1973; 55A:1077–1081
4. Netter P, Kessler M, Gaucher A, Bannwarth B. Does aluminum have a pathogenic role in dialysis associated arthropathy? Ann Rheum Dis. 1990; 49:573–575
5. Howard P. In Harrington, ed., Recent Advances in Occupational Health. No 3. Edinburgh, Churchill Livingstone, 1987, p. 13–14
6. Straniero NR, Furst DE. Environmentally-induced systemic sclerosis-like illness. Clin Rheumatol. 1989; 3:63–79
7. Christie AJ. Silicone synovitis. Semin Arthritis Rheum. 1989; 19:166–171
8. Seleznick MJ, Martinez-Osuna P, Espinoza P, Vasey FB. Is silicone associated with connective tissue disease. J Med Assoc. 1991; 78:85–87
9. Hypertrophic pulmonary osteoarthropathy. In Seaton *et al.*, eds., Crofton and Douglas, Respiratory Diseases. Oxford, Blackwell Scientific Publications, 1989, pp. 115 & 827
10. Davidson JK. Dysbaric disorders: aseptic bone necrosis in tunnel workers and divers. Clin Rheumatol. 1989; 3:1–23
11. Amako T, Kawashima N, Torisu T, Hayashi K. Semin Arthritis Rheum. 1974; 4:151–190
12. Kakosy T. Vibration disease. Clin Rheumatol. 1989; 3:25–50
13. Taylor W. Hand–arm vibration syndrome: a new clinical classification and an updated British standard guide for hand transmitted vibration. Br J Indust Med. 1988; 45:281–282
14. James CA, Aw TC, Harrington JM, Trethhowan WN. A review of 132 consecutive patients referred for assessment of vibration white finger. J Soc Occup Med. 1989; 39:61–64
15. Farkkila M, Pyykko I, Aatola A *et al.* Forrestry workers exposed to vibration: A neurological study. Br J Indust Med. 1988; 45:188–192
16. Wieslander G, Norback D, Goethe CJ, Juhlin L. Carpal tunnel syndrome and exposure to vibration, repetitive wrist movements and heavy manual work: a case referent study. Br J Indust Med. 1989; 46:43–47
17. Miyakita T, Miura H, Futatsuka M. An experimental study of the physiological effects of chain saw operation. Br J Indust Med. 1987; 44: 41–46

18. Pyykko I. Clinical aspects of the hand–arm vibration syndrome. Can J Work Environ Health. 1986; Spec No.12/4:439–447

19. Kelsey JL, Hardy RJ. Driving of motor vehicles as a risk factor for acute herniated intervertebral disc. Am J Epidemiol. 1975; 102:63–75

20 Wilder DG, Woodworth BB, Prymover JW. Vibration and the spine. Spine. 1982; 7:243–254

21. Auquier L, Siaud JR, Le Parc LE, Lasne E. Resultat d'une nouvelle enquete controlée sur le rachis des tractoristes. Rev Rheum. 1983; 50:421–426

22. Gnatz SM. Increased radicular pain due to therapeutic ultrasound applied to the back. Arch Phys Med Rehabil. 1989; 70:493–494

23. Kolar J. Locomotor consequences of electrical and radiation injuries, burns and freezings. Clin Rheumatol. 1989; 3:99–110

24. Carrera FG, Kozin F, Flaherty L, McCarthy DJ. Radiographic changes in the hands following childhood frostbite injury. Skeletal Radiol. 1981; 6:33–37

25. Remes P. Locomotor problems of supersonic aviation and astronautics. Clin Rheumatol. 1989; 3:111–120

26. Kato H, Duff I, Russell WJ, Yutaka U *et al.* Rheumatoid arthritis and gout in Hiroshima and Nagasaki, Japan. J Chronic Dis. 1971; 23:659–679

27. Kelly JJ. Black thorn inflammation. J Bone Joint Surg. 1966; 48B:474–477

28. Sugarman M, Stobie DF, Quismorio FP *et al.* Plant thorn synovitis. Arthritis Rheum. 1977; 20:1125–1128

29. Hawkins SJ, Blake DR, Doherty M, Hall ND. Rheumatoid arthritis developing after plant thorn synovitis. Br Med J. 1982; 285:1620

30. Ormerod AD, White MI, Eastmond CJ, Chesney RB. Plant thorn synovitis occurring in a child with psoriatic arthritis. Br J Rheumatol. 1984; 23:296–297

31. Rosenfeld R, Spigelblatt L, Chicoine R, Laverdiere M. Thorn induced periostitis associated with *Enterobacter agglomerans* infection. Can Med Assoc J. 1978; 119:925–928

32. Barton LL, Saied KR. Thorn-induced arthitis. J Paediatr. 1978; 93:322–323

23.   METABOLIC CAUSES OF ARTHRITIS

Bryan Emmerson and Richard Wigley

GOUT
Bryan Emmerson

INTRODUCTION

The diagnosis of gout requires either the demonstration of urate crystals (monosodium urate-monohydrate or MSUM) within the synovial fluid of an affected joint, or the combination of hyperuricemia with a classical pattern of recurrent acute monarticular arthritis of considerable severity and sudden onset, which completely remits between attacks[1].

RELATIONSHIP OF GOUT TO HYPERURICEMIA

Acute gout is an inflammatory response to the formation of needle-shaped urate crystals[2]. The formation of these crystals depends on several factors of which only some are well defined. These include:

Supersaturation of urate

The solubility of urate will vary with the composition of the fluid in which it is dissolved, and is dependent upon the pH, ionic strength and the presence or absence of other compounds in the solution; as an example, urate is more soluble in plasma than water[3].

Temperature

The solubility of urate in a solution falls with temperature; it has been suggested that the tendency for gout to affect peripheral joints may relate to the lower temperature of these joints[4].

Presence or absence of inhibitors of crystallization

Many proteins and proteoglycans can affect the tendency to crystal formation from a urate solution, acting either to maintain solubility or inhibit crystallization.

Despite this, urate crystal formation does not invariably induce an inflammatory response, and the extent of such a response is probably dependent upon the protein coating of the crystals[5], with gammaglobulin coating inducing a greater inflammatory response than albumin. These factors determine the different predispositions to urate crystal formation and an inflammatory response thereto in the different body sites. Thus the factors inducing the classical gouty toe (acute gout of the first metatarsophalangeal joint) may be distinct from those inducing a microtophus in the kidney[6]. Similarly, local factors, particularly pH, can determine whether urate precipitates as acicular crystals of MSUM or whether, at a lower pH, it precipitates as amorphous crystals of uric acid.

EPIDEMIOLOGY OF HYPERURICEMIA

Hyperuricemia is defined as a serum urate concentration exceeding 0.42 mmol/l (7 mg/dl) in males or 0.36 mmol/l (6 mg/dl) in females[7]. This is more a pragmatic than a physicochemical definition, as there is overlap between serum urate concentrations in normal subjects and in patients with gout. Between 5 and 10% of normal males (without gout) have serum urate concentrations >0.42 mmol/l, but it is uncommon for patients with gout to have serum urate concentrations below this arbitrary cut-off point; moreover the frequency of gout increases exponentially as the serum urate concentration rises beyond this value so that it is twice as great at a serum urate concentration of 0.54 mmol/l as at a serum urate of 0.42 mmol/l. Serum urate levels rise in males at puberty, and the mean value remains approximately 0.6 mmol/l (1 mg/dl) greater in men than women until middle age when, usually after the menopause, the mean value for females rises to nearly male levels[8]. Thus the mean serum urate levels in females is usually lower than that of males of similar age, which in part accounts for the greater prevalence of gout in men. After menopause, the frequency of gout in women approaches that of men.

CAUSES OF GOUT

The major prerequisite for the development of gout appears to be hyperuricemia of sufficient intensity, which is present for an adequate time period. As hyperuricemia becomes more common in the community from various acquired causes, it has been suggested that gout may develop in any individual with sufficiently high levels of uricemia. The risk of an acute attack of gout in a person with a serum urate of 0.6 mmol/l (10 mg/dl) is estimated to be about one in 20 per annum[9]; this

would mean that five out of every 100 patients with this degree of hyperuricemia would develop an acute attack of gout in any one year, and some of these subjects who do not develop acute gout for 18 or 19 years, might develop it by the twentieth year. Nonetheless, it is difficult to predict if and when acute gouty arthritis will occur in an individual with persistent hyperuricemia, and it is difficult to predict the risk of developing gout at a particular time from knowledge of the serum urate levels. This highlights the gap in our understanding of the factors that precipitate acute gout in any individual at a particular time, and is an issue that begs further study.

'GOUTY DIATHESIS'

While genetic factors are clearly important in the development of hyperuricemia, there is no clear evidence that heredity plays a major role in precipitating acute gouty arthritis in a hyperuricemic individual. The most important factor in developing acute gouty arthritis is the severity and duration of the hyperuricemia and there is no need to postulate, as have some workers, the existence of an inherited 'gouty diathesis', which has been alleged to predispose an individual to gout. The term gouty diathesis then, may have outlived its conceptual utility and would be better forgotten.

PREVENTION

The main approach to preventing gout lies in correction or prevention of hyperuricemia. Accordingly, the causes of hyperuricemia will be considered in detail and those with a genetic component will be separated from those with an environmental component, which have the greatest potential for manipulation. If modification of life-style factors cannot be achieved, a range of drug treatments is available to reduce hyperuricemia and thereby reduce the risk of gout. The risk of developing acute gout can also be reduced at any given serum urate concentration by administering a low dose of colchicine (0.5 mg b.i.d.)[10]. Prophylactic administration of colchicine reduces the frequency of acute gout in individuals who are hyperuricemic, or whose serum urate levels have been reduced to normal by drugs or life-style modification, or who suffer from fluctuations in the serum urate due to various factors. Once the serum urate has remained normal for a year or more, the risk of acute gout becomes small and prophylactic colchicine is no longer needed. The dose given should not exceed 0.5 mg/day in individuals with even minor degrees of renal dysfunction. This will include many patients over 60 years of age. Higher doses of colchicine have been associated with an increased risk of the development of myopathy.

CAUSES OF HYPERURICEMIA

Hyperuricemia results from an imbalance between urate production and urate excretion. Nucleoprotein degradation into purine nucleotides is the principal mechanism of urate production within the body. Excretion of urate occurs mainly by the kidney where two-thirds of the urate produced is usually excreted, with the remainder being eliminated into the alimentary tract as a constituent of alimentary secretions. An increase in urate production can be balanced by an increase in excretion of urate without there being any resultant hyperuricemia. Likewise, impaired urate excretion need not be followed by hyperuricemia provided urate production is reduced in proportion. Accordingly, when considering the causes of hyperuricemia in an individual patient, it is vital to consider those factors which promote an increase in urate production and those which can modify or reduce urate elimination. In each patient, more than one of these factors is likely to operate at any one time, so that hyperuricemia in a patient is often multifactorial[11]. Frequently, some factors are operating to increase urate production and others to reduce urate elimination simultaneously.

An increase in urate production can have either a genetic or an acquired cause.

Overproduction of urates
Inherited overproduction of urate
The major cause of genetic overproduction is a deficiency of activity of hypoxanthine guanine phosphoribosyl transferase (HGPRT), an enzyme without which there is defective control of purine synthesis, and an excessive *de novo* production of purines[12]. A similar result may also be seen with the rarer mutation of the enzyme phosphoribosyl-pyrophosphate (PRPP) synthetase. Severe HGPRT deficiency results in the Lesch–Nyhan syndrome, which is almost invariably accompanied by neurological features including choreoathetosis, self-mutilation and mental impairment. Identification of HGPRT deficiency in a family can lead to the early diagnosis of urate overproduction in affected individuals, which can allow appropriate management to prevent the development of hyperuricemia, gout and renal disease, or form the rationale for *in utero* diagnosis.

Acquired overproduction of urate
Increased marrow activity Since most nucleoprotein turnover occurs in the bone marrow, increased bone marrow activity from any cause can lead to increased production of purines and urate. Thus, acquired overproduction of urate can occur in myeloproliferative disorders, in primary and secondary polycythemia and during treatment of these by irradiation or cytotoxic agents. Infectious mononucleosis may also be associated with increased urate production.

High purine content of diet A high purine intake causes an increase in the serum urate concentration in any individual, the extent of which depends on the amount of purine consumed and on the ability to eliminate urate. A high consumption of nucleoproteins, particularly in the form of meat, or yeasts or plants high in nuclear material produces a purine load which the body will catabolize according to its capacity. Affluence is often associated with hyperuricemia, especially since foods high in purines and nucleoprotein tend to be costly.

Increased ATP degradation This can occur with alcohol consumption, fructose ingestion, exercise and a range of other diseases associated with tissue hypoxia[13]. Fructose requires phosphorylation, which dephosphorylates ATP, and leads to AMP production in excess of that which can be re-utilized and which, therefore, is degraded to inosine and hypoxanthine initially, and subsequently to uric acid[14]. The metabolism of ethanol increases urate production by a similar mechanism. Vigorous exercise may also contribute to an increase in urate production in a similar fashion. Of these factors, alcohol is the most important because it tends to be most widely and heavily consumed; moreover, its consumption is often associated with obesity and hyperlipidemia.

Increased body weight Epidemiologically, hyperuricemia is associated with an increased body weight and particularly with increased body mass index. The particular component of body weight causing the increase in urate production in such subjects is not finally defined because in some it relates to muscle mass but in others the increase in urate production is reversible with weight loss and it seems to relate to fat stores[15,16].

Hypertriglyceridemia This is associated with hyperuricemia, probably due to an increase in urate production. However, the precise mechanism is not yet well defined, as there is conflicting evidence whether the association is primary between hypertriglyceridemia and gout or secondary to the associated obesity and alcohol consumption[17,18].

Hyperuricemia due to decreased renal excretion of urate
Inherited defects in urate excretion
Genetic factors that affect renal handling of urate, although clearly known to exist, are not well defined. Support for genetic factors is provided by a greater similarity in urate clearances in identical twins than is seen in non-identical twins[19]. The urate clearance in normal subjects ranges from 5 to 14 ml/min, so that a normal individual with a urate clearance of 14 ml/min would intrinsically have a greater facility for renal elimination of urate than an individual with a clearance of 5 ml/min. This variation in urate excretion is normal and not the result of intrinsic renal disease; it appears to be limited to urate handling and is not associated with any other defect in renal function.

Acquired causes of reduced renal urate excretion
Chronic renal disease Most chronic renal disease, whether reversible or irreversible, is associated with a reduced urate excretion[20]. Although urate excreted per nephron may rise, the absolute excretion of urate in the urine falls as creatinine clearance falls. In chronic renal disease, there is also evidence for increased urate elimination by extra-renal routes, so that the serum urate does not rise to the same extent as other non-protein nitrogen compounds. Some forms of chronic renal disease, e.g. chronic lead nephropathy, polycystic disease of the kidneys, and several other varieties of chronic tubulointerstitial disease, including medullary cystic disease and several familial nephropathies, are associated with sub-optimal renal elimination of urate and a disproportionate degree of hyperuricemia for the level of the glomerular dysfunction[21].

Plasma volume contraction A reduction in circulating volume of any etiology is associated with increased tubular reabsorption of urate and hyperuricemia[22]. Likewise, any suboptimal urine flow (e.g. flow rates of less than 1 ml/min) is associated with hyperuricemia.

Hypertension Hypertension, particularly essential hypertension, is associated with altered renal hemodynamics, altered renal handling of urate and frequently with hyperuricemia.

Drugs and metabolites The most important drugs causing hyperuricemia are oral diuretics[20], especially the thiazides. All oral diuretics (except those that primarily retain potassium) can cause significant and persistent hyperuricemia by blocking urate excretion. Similarly, a reduced renal excretion of urate can occur with low dose aspirin and low doses of some uricosuric agents. Lactic acidosis of any cause will reduce renal excretion of urate, as will the presence of ketone bodies. This occurs because of the presence of these metabolites within the tubular fluid interfering with tubular handling of urate.

A number of systemic diseases are also associated with hyperuricemia, such as myxedema, hyperparathyroidism, respiratory acidosis, acute myocardial infarction, toxemia of pregnancy and psoriasis[20], and in each, the dominant factor would operate through an effect upon genetic or acquired components of either an increase in urate production or a reduction in urate excretion.

In summary, many factors may affect either the production or elimination of urate, and in an individual with hyperuricemia, multiple factors are likely to act simultaneously. A person from a culture with a traditionally low consumption of dietary purines may have a normal serum urate despite a low–normal urate clearance and a normal glomerular filtration rate. However, when such an individual is exposed to a high purine diet, alcohol on a regular basis, or becomes obese from ready access to high calorie food, hyperuricemia may result because the kidneys do not have the ability to respond by increasing urate elimination. In contrast, another individual with a higher–normal urate clearance may well remain normo-uricemic despite similar purine consumption, as this can be compensated for by an increased capacity for urate elimination. Many of

these factors can be defined from the history of a patient with hyperuricemia or can be seen by the effect of dietary purine restriction on the serum urate concentration of such a patient[23].

PREVENTION OF HYPERURICEMIA

Hyperuricemia results from the interplay of intrinsic or genetic factors with a wide variety of extrinsic or acquired factors. Hyperuricemia secondary to increased urate production can be corrected, by controlling the consumption of alcohol and foods high in purines, and correcting obesity and hyperlipidemia , assuming the absence of the myeloproliferative disorders (which lead to secondary overproduction of urate). Hyperuricemia secondary to reduced renal excretion of urate can be best controlled if a reversible cause for the renal insufficiency can be found, or if the patient is taking therapeutic agents, such as the oral diuretics, which reduce renal excretion of urate. Likewise, the control of ketosis or lactic acidosis can lead to an improved elimination of urate. In this regard, a urine flow rate of greater than 1 ml/min facilitates renal excretion of urate. Thus, identification of factors contributing to hyperuricemia and correction thereof leads to correction of hyperuricemia, and thereby to the prevention of gouty arthritis.

Various population studies have identified several environmental factors contributing to hyperuricemia. While it is difficult to compare different populations, the available data suggests than increased purine-rich food and beer consumption in certain regions of Europe has resulted in an increasing mean serum urate concentration in the population and a higher prevalence of gout[24]. These concepts are supported by a low prevalence of gout in indigenous Pacific populations, as long as they consume their traditional diet; when they change to a more opulent (western) diet, and consume alcohol, hyperuricemia and an increased prevalence of gout ensue. Much of the hyperuricemia and gout in these populations is explained by a combination of a low renal capacity to eliminate urate (although this capacity would have been sufficient for their normal diet), upon which is added a purine load through adoption of a western diet and alcohol consumption[25,26]. Nonetheless, Darmawan found a relatively high prevalence of gout in villagers in central Java living on a subsistence diet (*see* Chapter 3), the mechanism for which has not yet been defined. Figure 1 demonstrates gross tophaceous gout in such a patient.

An appreciation of the factors contributing to hyperuricemia provides a basis for understanding the differences in the degree of hyperuricemia and the incidence of gout both among different populations and in one population at different times. Many population studies have tabulated the range of serum urate concentrations and the prevalence of gout. While each study has provided important data, few address the important issue of differing susceptibilities to hyperuricemia and gout in differing populations. Analysis of populations migrating to countries with a different life-style, environment and dietary pattern has contributed appreciably to our understanding of environmental factors capable of modifying the serum urate, particularly in those with an inherited low–normal urate clearance. The only intervention that can correct a low urate excretion is the maintenance of a good urinary flow. Environmental manipulations aimed at minimizing hyperuricemia include reducing the consumption of alcohol, purines and total calories and maintenance of an ideal body weight[23].

It is appropriate to review the history of gout over the centuries. Hippocrates recognized the greater prevalence of gout in males, and that gout in females tended to occur only after the menopause[27]. Illustrations of the eighteenth century, as depicted by such social satirists as Hogarth clearly recorded

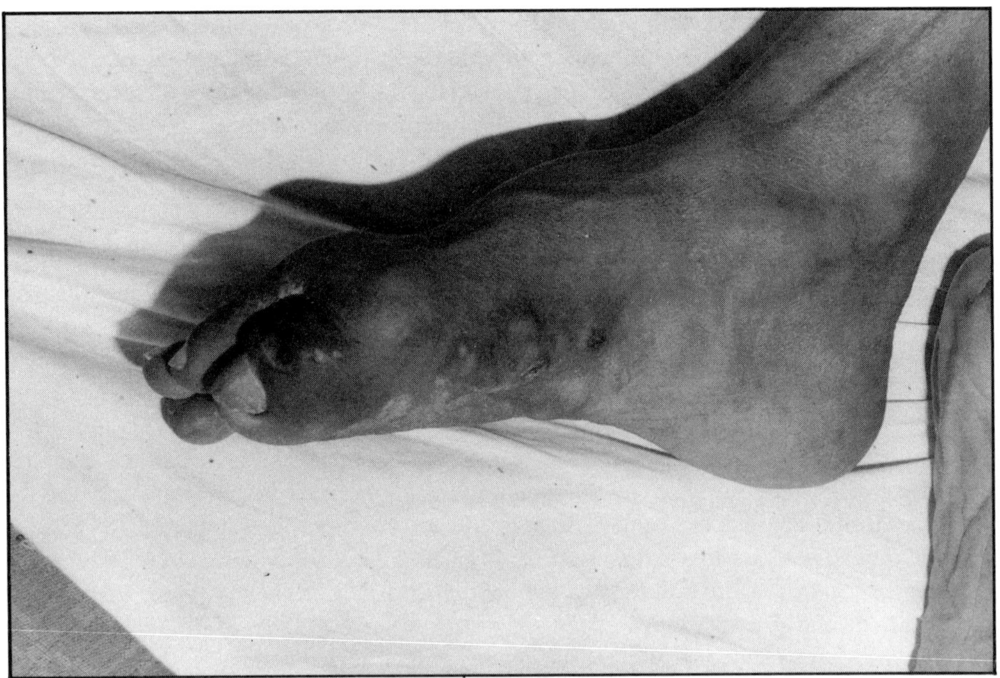

Figure 1 Gross tophaceous disabling gout

the belief that gout was associated with obesity and the consumption of large amounts of alcohol, food, flesh[28]. Evan Garrod[29] in 1859 wrote that 'There is no truth in medicine better established than that the use of fermented or alcoholic liquors is the most powerful of the predisposing causes of gout'. All of the early writings on gout are consistent with our current understanding of the interaction between these environmental factors and the renal elimination of urate. Many of the current community health programs designed to correct hyperlipidemia, obesity, the risk of coronary artery disease, and minimize the prevalence of diabetes in populations, also reduce the tendency to hyperuricemia and gout. Accordingly, gout in such populations can be looked upon as only one of the effects of affluence, and usually one which contributes to morbidity much more than to mortality.

Prevention of hyperuricemia and gout in populations should therefore devote special attention towards:

(1) Maintenance of a high urine volume, at least exceeding 1 ml/min throughout the day;

(2) Reduction in alcohol consumption, preferably to minimal levels plus moderation of dietary purine consumption;

(3) Restoration of body weight to an optimum, with correction of hypertriglyceridemia; even a modest reduction in weight can have a beneficial effect upon hyperuricemia; and

(4) Avoidance whenever possible of drugs that retain urate, such as the oral diuretics, and replacement by alternative treatment.

Such measures should result in a reduction in hyperuricemia and gout in the population. Individuals with persistent hyperuricemia and gout may require appropriate therapeutic agents, such as uricosuric drugs in those with a solitary defect in renal urate excretion, or allopurinol in those with an intrinsic overproduction of urate and/or increased consumption of purines and alcohol. Early diagnosis of renal disease and correction where possible is desirable, together with the early treatment of hypertension to prevent renal vascular disease. The use of the urate-retaining diuretics should be minimized. Knowledge of intrinsic overproduction of urate would be useful in HGPRT deficiency, since this would allow early diagnosis and the adoption of measures including allopurinol to minimize the complication of hyperuricemia, gout and renal disease.

REFERENCES

1. Wallace SL, Robinson H, Masi AT, Decker JL *et al*. Preliminary criteria for the classification of the acute arthritis of gout. Arthritis Rheum. 1977; 20:895–900
2. McCarty DJ, Hollander JL. Identification of urate crystals in gouty synovial fluid. Ann Intern Med. 1961; 54:452–460
3. Kippen I, Kleinenberg JR, Weinberger A, Wilcox WR. Factors affecting urate solubility *in vitro*. Ann Rheum Dis. 1974; 33:313–317
4. Simkin PA. The pathogenesis of podagra. Ann Intern Med. 1977; 86:230–233
5. Terkeltaub RA, Dyer CA, Martin J, Cortiss LK. Apolipoprotein (apo)E inhibits the capacity of monosodium urate crystals to stimulate neutrophils. J Clin Invest. 1991; 87:20–26
6. Emmerson BT, Row PG. The pathogenesis of the gouty kidney. Kidney Int. 1975; 8:65–71
7. Brøchner-Mortensen K, Cobb S, Rose BS. Report of subcommittee on criteria for the diagnosis of gout in surveys. In Kellgren JH, Jeffrey MR, Ball S, eds., The Epidemiology of Chronic Rheumatism, Vol I. Oxford, Blackwell Scientific Publications, 1963, pp. 295–297
8. Mikkelsen WM, Dodge HJ, Valkenburg H. The distribution of serum uric acid values in a population unselected as to gout or hyperuricemia. Am J Med. 1965; 39:242–251
9. Campion EW, Glynn RJ, Delabry LO. Asymptomatic hyperuricemia; risks and consequences in the normative ageing study. Am J Med. 1987; 82:421–426

10. Yu TF. The efficacy of colchicine prophylaxis in articular gout – a reappraisal after 70 years. Semin Arthritis Rheum. 1982; 12:256–264

11. Emmerson BT. Hyperuricaemia and gout in clinical practice. Sydney, ADIS Health Science Press, 1983

12. Kelley WN, Rosenbloom FM, Henderson JF, Seegmiller JE. A specific enzyme defect in gout associated with over-production of uric acid. Proc Natl Acad Sci. 1967; 57:1735–1739

13. Faller J, Fox IH. Ethanol-induced hyperuricemia; evidence for increased urate production by activation of adenine nucleotide turnover. N Engl J Med. 1982; 307:1598–1602

14. Fox IH. Metabolic basis for disorders of purine necleotide degradation. Metabolism. 1981; 30:616–634

15. Emmerson BT. Alteration of urate metabolism by weight reduction. Aust NZ J Med. 1973; 3:4 10–412

16. Yamashita S, Matsuzawa Y, Tokunaga K et al. Studies of the impaired metabolism of uric acid in obese subjects: marked reduction of renal urate excretion and its improvement by a low-calorie diet. Int J Obesity. 1986; 10:255–264

17. Feldman EB, Wallace SL. Hypertriglyceridemia in gout. Circulation. 1964; 29:508–513

18. Matsubara K, Matsuzawa Y, Jiao S, Takama T et al. Relationship between hypertriglyceridermia and uric acid production in primary gout. Metabolism. 1989; 38(7):698–701

19. Emmerson BT, Nagel SL, Duffy, Martin NG. Genetic control of the renal clearance of urate: a study of twins. Ann Rheum Dis. 1992; 51: 375–377

20. Emmerson BT. Abnormal urate excretion associated with renal and systemic disorders, drugs and toxins. In Kelley WN, Weiner IM, eds., Uric Acid. Berlin, Springer–Verlag, 1978, pp. 287–315

21. Emmerson BT. Gout and renal disease. In: Massry SG, Glassock RJ, eds., Textbook of Nephrology. 2nd edn, Baltimore, Williams and Wilkins, 1988, pp. 756–760

22. Steele TH. Evidence for altered renal urate reabsorption during changes in volume of the extracellular fluid. J Lab Clin Med. 1969; 74:288–299

23. Emmerson BT. Identification of the causes of persistent hyperuricaemia. Lancet. 1991; 337: 1461–1463

24. Gresser U, Gathof B. Epidemiology of hyperuricemia. In Gresser U, Zöllner N, eds., Urate Deposition in Man and its Clinical Consequences. Berlin, Springer–Verlag, 1991, pp. 82–96

25. Prior IAM. Epidemiology of rheumatic disorders in the Pacific with particular emphasis on hyperuricemia and gout. Semin Arthritis Rheum. 1981; 11:213–229

26. Prior IAM, Welby TJ, Østbye T, Salmond CE, Stokes YM. Migration and gout: the Tokelau Island migrant study. Br Med J. 1987; 295:457–480

27. Hippocrates. The genuine works of Hippocrates. Translated from the Greek with a preliminary discourse and annotations by F Adams. New York, Wood, 1886

28. Rodnan GP. A gallery of gout. Arthritis Rheum. 1961; 4:27–45; ibid, 4:176–194

29. Garrod AB. The Nature and Treatment of Gout and Rheumatic Gout. London, Walton and Maberley, 1859

OTHER METABOLIC AND ENDOCRINE CAUSES OF RHEUMATIC DISEASE
Richard Wigley

CHONDROCALCINOSIS AND PSEUDOGOUT

Calcium pyrophosphate (CPPD) deposition (chondrocalcinosis) in joint cartilage is a widespread age-related phenomenon that often occurs in the absence of any joint symptoms[1]. In 50 patients with pseudogout[2], 15 women and 35 women with an average age of 71 years, attacks in 10 were induced by mild trauma, long walks, knee arthroplasty or injection of crystalline glucocorticoid. Of these 25 had fever, five, confusion, and 14 were initially misdiagnosed as having septic arthritis. More than one joint was affected in 21 cases. Acquired and spontaneous chondrocalcinosis increase with age and may facilitate the onset of osteoarthritis, and there is evidence that osteoarthritis causes chondrocalcinosis. In an autopsy study[3] of 130 asymptomatic knees, calcification was found in 27, and these were more commonly associated with severe destructive changes. In another study of surgical material, it was not possible to determine whether the association of calcinosis with osteoarthritis was cause or effect[4].

In the Framingham study[5], osteoarthritis of the knee and chondrocalcinosis both increase with age, and those with chondrocalcinosis have a relative risk of 1.52 for the development of osteoarthritis. In another study with an average follow-up of 8 years, secondary chondrocalcinosis developed in five of 31 cases with osteoarthritis of the knee[6].

There is a definite association of pseudogout with hyperparathyroidism. Of 531 surgical cases of hyperparathyroidism, eight of 20 patients with intermittent attacks of arthritis were diagnosed as having pseudogout because of these attacks[7]. In another 12 patients, pseudogout occurred after successful parathyroidectomy, coinciding with the lowest serum calcium levels. This suggests that a fall in calcium may lead to shedding of crystals into the joint[8] and that a high serum calcium level may lead to chondrocalcinosis. Thus any measures preventing hypercalcemia, including hyperparathyroidism, excessive vitamin D from high fish oil intake, vitamin supplements, possibly combined with high food and water calcium content would be expected to have primary preventive value. A possible role of ethnic susceptibility to chondrocalcinosis has not been formally studied, but it was noted in a few individuals in population samples in China.

HEMOCHROMATOSIS

In 25 cases of hemochromatosis with arthritis[9], 14 had inflammatory arthritis, mostly in the hands and knees, and five had chondrocalcinosis. In hereditary hemochromatosis[10], arthritis was not found to be an early predictor of this condition, and chondrocalcinosis appears to be a late manifestation of hemochromatosis-arthropathy.

Other hereditary causes of chondrocalcinosis predisposing to pseudogout and premature osteoarthritis[1] which do not present an opportunity for primary intervention, include hypophosphatasia, Bartter's syndrome, Wilson's disease, hypomagnesemia and possibly ochronosis.

Apart from the general problem of minimizing joint injury, the only possibility for primary prevention at present would seem to be by identifying and treating hyperparathyroidism and hemochromatosis as early as possible and reducing calcium and iron intake where appropriate.

AMYLOID ARTHROPATHY

Primary amyloidosis is a rare cause of rheumatic symptoms. In the Mayo Clinic, where rarities are collected, of 229 cases, half were associated with myeloma[11]. Carpal tunnel syndrome often accounts for the rheumatic symptoms of amyloidosis. Amyloid may involve periarticular structures leading to a mistaken diagnosis of rheumatoid arthritis, although secondary amyloid arthritis may occur in severe rheumatoid arthritis. Amyloidosis secondary to chronic infections offers the only opportunity for prevention by controlling infections as in bronchiectasis, osteomyelitis, leprosy and tuberculosis. Amyloidosis is a rare complication in countries where these infections are prevented or treated by antibiotics. It is unclear how secondary amyloidosis causes symptomatic joint involvement or whether better control of rheumatoid, psoriatic arthritis or ankylosing spondylitis would reduce the frequency of amyloidosis. The author has only once diagnosed amyloidosis in rheumatoid arthritis in 30 years of practice in New Zealand.

HYPERLIPOPROTEINEMIAS

The hyperlipoproteinemias are classified in Table 1. Rheumatic complaints may occur in all except types I and III.

Type II hyperlipidemia has been associated with a migratory polyarthritis[12], which is more severe in homozygotes than in heterozygotes, with attacks of pain recurring from two to 12 times per year. Achilles tendinitis was reported in 14 patients from nine kindreds[13]. In a study of 69 cases of type IIa hyperlipidemia, joint pain was found in 48% of cases and 26% of controls. The pain was more frequent in the feet and ankles than in controls but is unrelated to local effects of xanthomata and there was no evidence of inflammatory arthritis.

Table 1 Types of hyperlipidemia and possible rheumatic complications

---

Primary hyperlipidemias

Type I	xanthomata of skin
Type II	xanthomata, migratory polyarthritis, tendinitis
Type III	xanthomata of palms
Type IV	xanthomata, arthralgia arthritis, hyperuricemia, gout
Type V	xanthomata, hyperuricemia, gout

Secondary hyperlipidemias

diabetes
alcoholism
oral contraceptives

Type III hyperlipidemia Xanthomata in the palms occur but no rheumatic symptoms are reported.

Type IV hyperlipidemia In 1975, 12 cases with carbohydrate-induced hyperglyceridemia[14] were described with mild persistent bilateral oligoarticular inflammatory arthritis of large and small joints. Metaphyseal and epiphyseal bone cysts were found in five subjects. This syndrome did not fit the American College of Rheumatology criteria for gout or rheumatoid arthritis and was considered a separate syndrome. Restriction of dietary carbohydrate and alcohol reduced symptoms in four cases. The authors suggested that this relationship is causal. In a lipid clinic[15] eight men with type IV had recurrent attacks of gout. There was a transient polyarthritis in three subjects which may have been related to the lipid disorder.

Type V hyperlipidemia Typical gout occurs in this syndrome.

Secondary hyperlipoproteinuria Hyperlipidemia due to biliary cirrhosis has been reported to cause infiltration of foam cells and xanthoma tendinosum in joint tissue with joint symptoms[16].

Alcohol and estrogens increase lipids in those with genetic predisposition.

Prevention

As discussed above, type II[17], and presumably also type IV[18], hyperlipidemias increase the risks of serious heart disease and strokes, as well as the accompanying rheumatic symptoms. Both can be controlled by dietary intervention and or drugs. Routine surveillance of serum lipids in rheumatic patients would facilitate early treatment and the detection of more significant pathology, enabling preventive intervention in susceptible family members. Control of hyperlipidemia due to diabetes, and alcoholism depends on control of those complaints; those receiving exogenous estrogens should have serial testing of blood lipid levels.

ENDOCRINE CAUSES OF RHEUMATIC DISEASES

Primary prevention of rheumatic complaints secondary to endocrinopathies requires control of the underlying disease itself. This is possible for hypothyroidism due to iodine deficiency and to treatment with radioactive iodine. A need for secondary prevention also arises in managing acromegaly; other relevant associations are listed in Table 2.

Prevention of non-insulin-dependent diabetes mellitus (NIDDM) would appear to be an attainable goal, since there is a lower rate of NIDDM in non-migrant Tokelau Islanders than in migrant Tokelauans living in New Zealand[19] on a more affluent diet. Weight control is obviously desirable in preventing both diabetes and osteoarthritis, whether or not the diabetes itself contributes to the arthritis. Moern and Hybbinette[20] found that diabetics receiving insulin for more than 10 years, or those with diabetic retinopathy, had an increased risk of developing chronic shoulder complaints. Two-thirds of those with shoulder pain had one or several hand syndromes described in diabetics and half of these had bilateral

Table 2 Relationship between potentially preventable endocrine disorders and rheumatic disease

Diabetes mellitus[21,22]
    neuropathic joints in diabetic neuritis
    osteoarthritis
    association with DISH (disseminated
      idiopathic skeletal hyperostosis)
    diabetic hand syndrome
    dupuytrens contracture
    frozen shoulder (capsulitis)
    calcific bursitis
    reflex sympathetic dystrophy
Thyroid disease
    myxedema; carpal tunnel syndrome
    thyrotoxic myopathy
    thyroid arthropachy
Acromegaly
    osteoarthritis; hyperparathyroidism
    primary (pseudogout q.v.)
    secondary to renal failure
Menopause and amenorrhea
    osteoporosis (Chapter 24)

shoulder involvement. Limited joint mobility, trigger finger and Duypuytren's contracture have been included in under the diabetic hand syndrome[21,22]. Data from this nationwide interview study in Sweden suggested that diabetic individuals younger than 54 years tended to have more rheumatic disorders than age-matched non-diabetics. Half of the diabetic persons granted disability pensions reported chronic rheumatic symptoms at various sites. Among the disability pensioners reporting rheumatic symptoms, this was considered the main diagnosis for granting a disability pension in 25% of the cases.

There is also scope for prevention in osteoporosis due to the menopause and amenorrhea if these are regarded as hormone deficiency states (Chapter 24). Routine checking of blood lipids before and after initiating oral contraceptives would identify those at risk of developing hyperlipidemia in response to estrogens.

PAGET'S DISEASE

This disease is not strictly a metabolic disorder, although there is a localized and sometimes diffuse disorder of bone growth and breakdown increasing in frequency with age. The subject has been recently reviewed by Freeman[23], and Yates[24]. There is ultrastructural evidence of a viral cause of Paget's disease, with paramyxovirus, measles, and respiratory syncytial viruses each having been postulated to cause a form of slow virus infection leading to this disease, possibly providing preventive strategies in the future[25,26]. Because Paget's disease has also been associated with canine distemper virus, an association with earlier or present pet ownership has been sought. O'Driscoll and colleagues in northwest England[31] and Holdaway and co-workers[32] in New Zealand found an association but Siris and colleagues[33] were not able to confirm this in the USA. Canine distemper virus RNA has been demonstrated in Paget's disease but not in controls[34]. In Spain an association was shown with the use of bovine meat without sanitary control[35].

Epidemiology

Radiological surveys suggest that it is less prevalent in India, Japan, Middle East and Scandinavia than in USA, UK and Australia. In Madrid[27], 6.4% of those over 40 years were found to have the disease and this is thought to represent a very high prevalence. In a geriatric study in the USA, Blacks were as often affected as Whites[28]. In South Africa[29] a rate similar to that reported in Europe (2.5%) was found in Whites and 1.3% in Blacks over 55 years of age. In Nigeria, Paget's[30] is rare but it is seen in Sierra Leone.

Treatment

Although editronate, calcitonin and cytotoxic agents are effective in treating Paget's disease, primary prevention is presently beyond reach. If it is indeed due to measles, distemper virus or it is a prion disease, then control of these infections would reduce the incidence of Paget's disease, bearing in mind that decades might pass before the impact of such measures would be reflected by a reduction in the incidence of this disease.

Other bone diseases such as rickets, scurvy and osteoporosis which may cause bone and joint pain are discussed in Chapters 24 and 25.

REFERENCES

1. Doherty M, Dieppe P. Clinical aspects of pyrophosphate dihydrate crystal deposition. Rheum Dis Clin North Am. 1988; 14:395–414

2. Masuda I, Ishikawa K. Clinical features of pseudogout attack. A survey of 50 cases. Clin Orthop. 1988; 6:173–181

3. Mitrovic DR, Stankovic A, Iriarte-Borda O, Uzan M, Quintero M, Miravet L, Kuntz D. The prevalence of chondrocalcinosis in the human knee joint: an autopsy study. J Rheumatol. 1988; 15:633–641

4. Sokoloff L, Varma AA. Chondrocalcinosis in surgically resected specimens. Arthritis Rheum. 1988; 31:750–756

5. Felson DT, Anderson JJ, Naimark A, Kannel W, Meenan RF. The prevalence of chondrocalcinosis in the elderly and its association with knee osteoarthritis: The Framingham study. J Rheumatol. 1989; 19:1241–1245

6. Massardo L, Watt I, Cushnaghan J, Dieppe P. Osteoarthritis of the knee joint. Ann Rheum Dis. 1989; 48:893–897

7. Geelhoed GW, Kelly TR. Pseudogout as a clue and complication in primary hyperparathyroidism. Surgery. 1989; 106:1036–1041

8. Yashiro T, Hara H, Ito K, Tanaka R et al. Pseudogout associated with primary hyperparathyroidism: management in the immediate postoperative period for prevention of pseudogout. Endocrinol Jpn. 1988; 38:617–624

9. Huaux JP, Geubel A, Koch MC, Malghem J et al. The arthritis of hemochromatosis, a review of 25 cases with special reference to chondrocalcinosis, and a comparison with patients with primary hyperparathyroidism. Clin Rheumatol. 1986; 5:317–324

10. Mathews JL, Williams HJ. Arthritis in hereditary hemochromatosis. Arthritis Rheum. 1987; 30: 1137–1141

11. Kyle RA, Greip PR. Amyloidosis (AL) – clinical and laboratory features in 229 cases. Mayo Clin Proc. 1983; 58:665–683

12. Khachadurian AK. Migratory polyarthritis in familial hypercholesterolemia. Type II hyperlipoproteinemia. Arthritis Rheum. 1968; 11:385–393

13. Glueck CJ, Levy RI, Frederickson DS. Acute tendonitis: a presenting symptom of familial hyperlipoproteinemia. JAMA. 1968; 206:2895–2897

14. Buckingham RB, Bole GG, Bassett DR. Polyarthritis associated with type IV hyperlipoproteinemia. Arch Intern Med. 1975; 135:286–290

15. Struthers GR, Scott DL, Bacon PA, Walton KW. Musculoskeletal disorders in patients with hyperlipidemia. Ann Rheum Dis. 1983; 42:519–523

16. Mills PR, Rooney PJ, Watkinson G, MasSween RNM. Hypercholesterolemic arthropathy in primary biliary cirrhosis. Ann Rheum Dis. 1978; 37:179–180

17. Rooney PJ. Atheroma, arthritis and all that. J Rheumatol. 1989; 16:5–7

18. Wysenbeek AJ, Shani E, Biegel Y. Musculoskeletal manifestations in patients with hypercholesterolemia. J Rheumatol. 1989; 16:643–645

19. Ostbye T, Welby TJ, Prior IA, Salmond CE, Stokes YM. Type 2 (non-insulin dependent) diabetes mellitus, migration and westernization: the Tokelau migrant study. Diabetologia. 1989; 32:585–590

20. Moern Hybbinette I. The painful diabetic shoulder. Relationship between diabetes, rheumatic symptoms and disability pensioning. Thesis, University of Lund. 1987

21. Forgacs SS. Diabetes mellitus and rheumatic disease. Clin Rheum Dis. 1986; 12:729–753

22. McGuire JL. Arthropathies associated with endocrine disorders. In Kelley *et al.* ed., Textbook of Rheumatology, 3rd edn, Philadelphia, WB Saunders, 1989, pp. 1648–1664

23. Freeman DA. Paget's disease of bone. Am J Med Sci. 1988; 295:144–158

24. Yates AJ. Paget's disease of bone. Baillières Clin Endocrinol Metab. 1988; 2:267–285

25. Basle MF, Rebel A, Fournier JG, Russell WC, Malkani K. On the trail of myxoviruses in Paget's disease of bone. 1987; 217:9–15

26. Mills BG, Singer FR. Critical of viral antigen data in Paget's disease of bone. Clin Orthop. 1989; 217:16–25

27. Piga M, Lopez-Abente G, Vadillo GA, Ibanez AE, Gonzales-Lanza M. Features of Paget's disease of bone in a new high-prevalence focus. Med Clin (Barc). 1990; 95:169–174

28. Polednak AP. Rates of Paget's disease of bone among hospital discharges, by age and sex. J Am Geriatr Soc. 1987; 35:550–553

29. Guyer PB, Chamberlain AT. Paget's disease of bone in South Africa. Clin Radiol. 1988; 39:51–52

30. Dahniya MH. Paget's disease of bone in Africans. Br J Radiol. 1987; 60:113–116

31. O'Driscoll JB, Buckler HM, Jeacock J, Anderson DC. Dogs, distemper and osteitis deformans: a further epidemiological study. Bone Mineral. 1990; 11:209–216

32. Holdaway IM, Ibbertson HK, Wattie D, Scragg R, Graham P. Previous pet ownership and Paget's disease. Bone Mineral. 1990; 8:53–58

33. Siris ES, Kelsey JL, Flaster E, Parker S. Paget's disease of bone and previous pet ownership in the United States: dogs exonerated. Int J Epidemiol. 1990; 19:455–458

34. Gordon MT, Anderson DC, Sharpe PT. Canine distemper virus localised in bone cells of patients with Paget's disease. Bone. 1991; 12:195–201

35. Piga AM, Lopez-Abente G, Ibanez AE, Vadillo AG, Lanza MG, Jodra VM. Risk factors for Paget's disease: a new hypothesis. Int J Epidemiol. 1988; 17:198–201

24. INVOLUTIONAL OSTEOPOROSIS

Erik Allander

INTRODUCTION

This chapter deals with involutional osteoporosis. Drug-induced osteoporosis is discussed in Chapter 26 and sport-induced osteoporosis in Chapter 5.

Osteoporosis is both 'sitting on and falling between the stools' of the major fields, rheumatology, endocrinology and orthopedic surgery. One thing is, however, clear that over the last decades several possibilities for the prevention of osteoporosis have been focused on.

The major stimulus for primary prevention of osteoporosis is not the condition as such, but its consequences, the fractures[1]. The rate of fractures increases with increasing bone loss[2]. The major manifestation of osteoporosis in terms of social impact and economic consequences is hip fracture[3], a major health problem[4].

In a WHO report 1988[5] it was stated that more information was needed on the socioeconomic importance of fractures as well as how much disability they cause. There are also some indications that the number of hip fractures, though increasing sharply by increasing age are exceeding this very sharp age tendency[6]. Many good reviews of osteoporosis, its diagnosis, treatment and prevention have been published, e.g. by Dequeker and Geusens[7]. The reader is referred to this for details.

Prevention of osteoporosis (Figures 1 and 2) is sometimes strongly advocated as by Ford[8]:

In spite of obstacles inherent in the present system of health care financing in the United States, we also must move in this direction if we are to apply actively all of what we know now about the prevention and treatment of hip fracture. If we can accomplish this, then at last the elderly will be able to reduce their apprehension about the likelihood of breaking a hip.

There are also financial profits to be made in prevention of osteoporosis[9]. In the US there has been a 30-fold increase in the number of offices, clinics, and hospitals offering screening examination for bone mineral density. In the same paper the pros and cons for screening are discussed. Their conclusion was negative with regard to screening because of economic restrictions, also because a better case can be made for mammography in the prevention of breast cancer.

The pattern of prevention of fractures has two main directions. The *first* includes various attempts at increasing bone mass and thereby acting indirectly in creating a more trauma-resistant skeleton. The *second* is how to influence the circumstances leading to falls, which in turn can be divided into internal (individual) and external (environmental) factors.

275

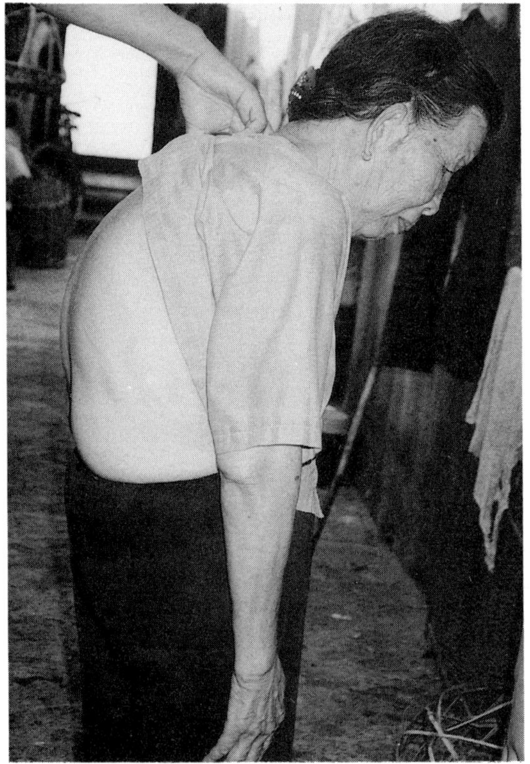

Figure 1 The rounded kyphos secondary to osteoporosis seen in a rural community in south east China

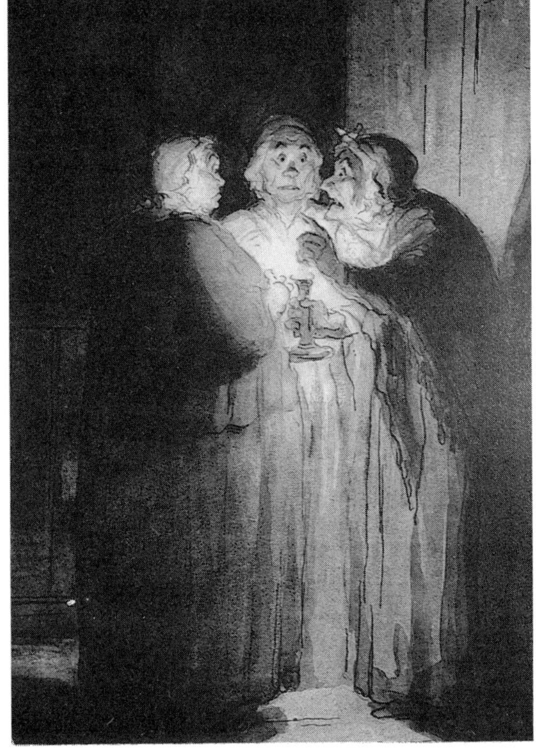

Figure 2 This picture of *The Three Gossips* by Honore Daumier in 1878 reminds us that osteoporosis and obesity were health problems in the nineteenth century. The thin old lady has a more pronounced kyphos than the obese one as one would expect from current research. (Reproduced with kind permission from Daumier by Roger Passeron, Phaidon Press Ltd.)

WHAT SHOULD BE PREVENTED?
Definition of osteoporosis

The prevention of fractures is the main target of preventive activities for osteoporosis but this is intimately related to the definition and grading of osteoporosis.

Within the framework of prevention, involutional osteopenia should be separated from postmenopausal osteoporosis, in spite of an overlap[10]. Osteoporosis has also been classified as *disease*, but could also be regarded as a disorder when not causing symptoms.

Osteoporosis can appear principally by two mechanisms; a *fast rate* of bone mineral loss from a normal level or a *normal loss* of bone from a lower level. Thus the means of reducing osteoporosis might also differ.

Bone mineral density is a major factor in the determination of the risk of fracture[11–13]. Genetic factors operate in osteoporosis also. The difference in

276

bone mineral density between monozygotic twins was small and definitely less than between dizygotic[14]. The proneness to osteoporosis might also be influenced genetically as in alcoholism or smoking. The process of bone remodeling in osteoporosis has been used as a basis for this. It has been shown, 1989, by de Vernejoul[15] that it was, however, not possible to use results from bone morphometry to distinguish subgroups among osteoporotic women.

The methods of measurement of bone density for screening are radiogrammetry, photodensitometry, single photon absorbiometry, quantitative computerized tomography, dual photon absorbiometry (DPA) and dual energy X-ray absorbiometry (DEXA). The latter two (DPA and DEXA) are presently regarded as the best methods[16]. Conventional radiography is generally not acceptable as insufficient information about bone mineral content is provided.

It should be noted, however, that the correlation between different measurement sites, spine, forearm, hip and femoral shaft for bone mineral density (BMD) does not show the same rate of decline with age. Bone loss is not homogeneous. Trabecular and cortical bone are probably independently modulated[17].

The peak bone mass concept[18] is frequently used and is certainly important in understanding and interpreting the efficiency of any preventive activities taken or proposed.

A procedure that has become more and more applied is to use the results from a single-measurement bone mineral density to predict the risk of a future fracture for an individual. This has been advocated in several publications by Christiansen and others[19]. Several screening procedures have been proposed to identify persons at risk for a fracture by using various methods to establish bone density.

Christiansen has argued strongly for the identification of the 'fast bone loser'[20].

Fracture epidemiology
It was estimated in 1969 that up to 70% of fractures in persons aged 45 or older are attributable to osteoporosis[2]. It has been estimated in the USA that about one-quarter of all women over the age of 60 had spinal compression fracture and about 15% of women sustained hip fractures in their life time[3].

There are certainly other limb fractures that could also be prevented. The fracture pattern of wrist fracture (Colle's fracture) is quite different from the pattern of hip fractures. The peak is earlier and the increase in old age is much less than for hip fractures.

For vertebral compression fractures, the pattern is more complicated. The epidemiology is not quite clear, but the studies are ongoing, e.g. a major survey in Europe (EVOS)[21]. Measurement of vertebral osteoporosis is more difficult technically and conceptually more complicated. It usually progresses gradually in contrast to the yes/no condition for limb fractures.

A recent comprehensive overview on key issues in the epidemiology of osteoporosis can be found in reference 22. Some key recommendations on the epidemiological study of hip fractures can be found in the WHO report[5].

Although the prevention of osteoporosis relates very much to females it should certainly also be mentioned that males suffer osteoporotic fractures although to a much lesser extent that females.

Screening
In a review[23] Cummings and Black discuss whether perimenopausal women should be screened for osteoporosis. Their conclusion was that although the mortality and morbidity caused

by hip fracture would warrant routine screening, measurement of bone mass is of uncertain value in assessing risks for hip fracture. In their opinion serial measurements of bone mass to estimate women's rate of bone loss are relatively imprecise and increases the cost of screening and have at best a limited role in screening women to assess risk of osteoporotic fractures.

Routine screening to detect low bone mineral content is not yet recommended[16]. The 1984 National Institutes of Health consensus development conference on osteoporosis came up with the same conclusion: presently no test could be recommended to identify persons with mild osteoporosis[24].

The WHO consultation on osteoporosis 1988[5] came to the conclusion on screening that the application of currently available techniques for identifying patients at risk at the menopause should be further researched together with estimates of cost effectiveness and possible methods of implementation, in addition to studies under way in Europe, United States, and Australia.

OSTEOPOROSIS AND THE CONCEPTUAL STRUCTURE OF PREVENTION

Much of the efforts on prevention is based upon the assumption that a high or at least improved bone mass implies that the number of fractures are reduced. Although studies provide results in this direction, that assumption is, however, not yet sufficiently proven.

The pattern of prevention of vertebral osteoporosis deals not only with reduction of the pain that may or may not arise from fractures, but also with the secondary effects on cardiovascular and pulmonary function imposed by the kyphotic back.

To clarify the concept of prevention, especially primary prevention, in osteoporosis the reader is referred to Figure 3.

First some general comments. To the left is the disease process for a specific disease that starts from individuals with 'no symptoms', but with 'positive heredity' to the presence of clinical signs and/or positive tests. By means of bone density measurements or otherwise a group can be identified that might be positively influenced, at least in part by certain specified measures by postponing the risk for fractures, or by stopping or reducing the osteoporotic process, even completely blocking or alternatively reversing it.

The distinction between 'in part' and 'completely' stopping osteoporosis and fractures is not conceptually clear. As indicated lower down the disease or, in the case of hip fracture, the morbid condition is easy to trace but it could neither be postponed, nor partly influenced. The only possibility of avoiding a fracture is to avoid it completely. The conceptual difference is between a *disease*, the start of which can not be exactly defined, and a *fracture* that can be linked to an exact moment of time. For sake of simplicity, I have considered the possibility of 'partial fractures' or *silent* fractures as in the case of vertebral compression fractures.

Other lines of *secondary* prevention refer to late effects after a hip fracture, that is to eliminate, postpone, or partly reduce these complications, but could also be looked upon as a complete elimination of these effects after an 'ideal' fracture. For instance good physical condition before fracture might reduce the severity of complications and thereby also reduce the mortality.

The WHO's purpose with introducing the concept of 'underlying cause of death' in 1948, was to identify the most appropriate point at which 'to cut the chain of events or institute the cure', in order to

278

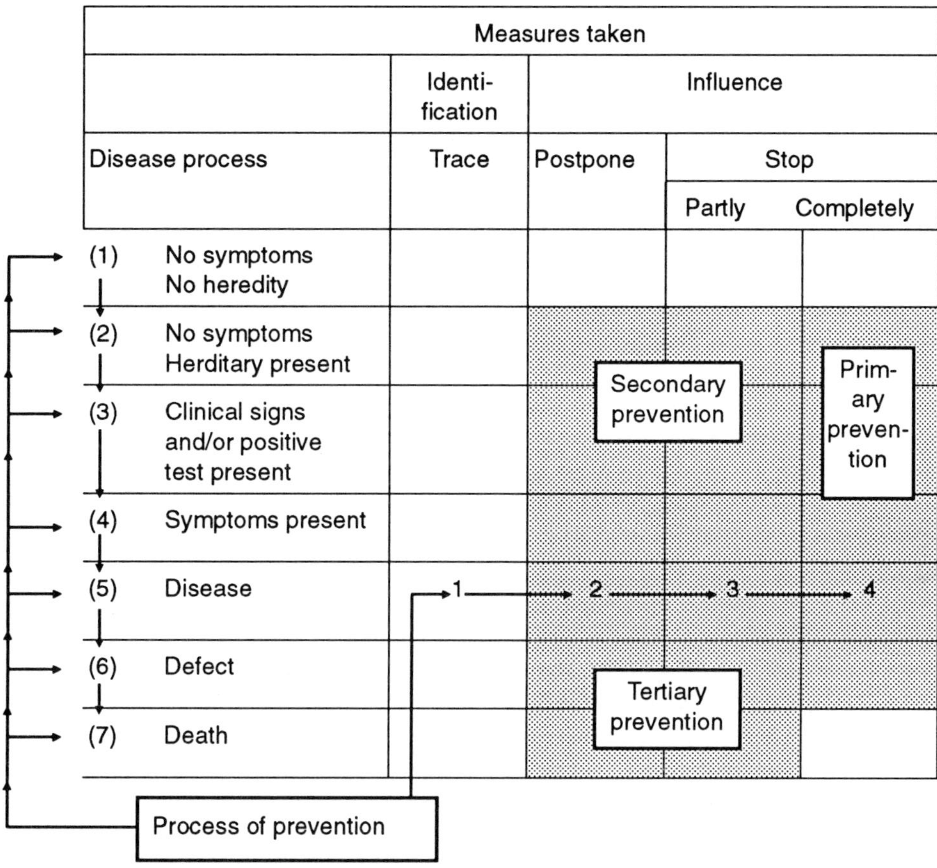

Figure 3 Structure and prevention. Prevention implies actions serving to avert a transition from one condition with fewer or less severe manifestations to another condition with more or severe manifestations

prevent untimely death[25]. The interpretation of 'prevention' in this context has been discussed and the appropriateness of the current WHO cause-of-death registration principles for this purpose has been seriously put in question[26-28].

It is not only osteoporosis as such that should be prevented, but also the mortality rate for elderly patients after fracture of hip[29]. In a 2-year follow-up of 241 USA patients the mortality rate after the fracture was 21.6% for the total group with 8% for the low risk group and 49.4% for the high risk group. The standard mortality ratio was six times higher in the high risk group than in the general population. It has been pointed out that the purposes and criteria for attributing death to osteoporosis or to other causes related to hip fractures needs to be carefully considered when interpreting mortality data. The problem of establishing the cause of death in cases of hip fracture has been thoroughly analyzed in a recent study[26].

Eleven percent of the injury deaths in the United States in an elderly population results from falls[30]. Persons with mental disorders including senile dementia constitute a high risk group for hip fractures[37]. The prevention of senile dementia or confusion states is therefore a part of the prevention of fractures as also is multipharmacy. When an individual takes six or more drugs daily the relative risk of fracture is 2.68[30].

The 'condition' or 'disease' osteoporosis identified on the vertical line (Figure 3) may or may not produce symptoms. If preventive measures are taken and are successful an individual could be moved from one category *with* symptom to one *without* although osteoporosis may still be present. That could be regarded secondary prevention.

The vertical line of prevention also presupposes one or several causal mechanisms. A question in that context is the classification if a preventive action moves him from a condition *with* symptoms to one *without*, this could be some action that results in a measurable increase in bone mass.

In summary, with these few examples I wanted to point out that the classification pattern for prevention of osteoporosis *and* fractures is not completely clear. The causal relationships in osteoporosis are never unifactorial, but always multifactorial, parallel and/or sequential. To clarify the logical pattern for primary prevention more work remains to be done.

THINGS TO BE DONE

Exercise

Some studies suggest a reduced incidence of hip fractures among persons who have regular exercise[32,33]. and further prospective studies were recommended. The rate of bone loss is reduced by exercise[34].

Although age and bone mass serve as predictors of fracture this association is gradually reduced by increasing age[35]. It has been shown that young men engaged in regular and vigorous exercise have a bone mineral content greater than controls[36,37]. The WHO recommendations concluded that bone loss created by immobilization

could be reversed by weight bearing activity and that this was valid for the elderly[5].

The effect of physical exercise in the prevention of osteoporosis has been studied by Dilsen and colleagues[38]. An exercise period resulted in a 4.76% *increase* of bone mineral content (BMC) as opposed to 2.7% *decrease* in a control group. In Sweden a combined effort with increased physical exercise, reduced smoking and increased calcium intake is reducing the speed of bone loss in older persons[39]. Further studies are needed to establish how much this combination increased bone mass *and* improved physical fitness are the result of physical activity and also what this means in reduction of fracture rates and, if so, do such fractures lead to fewer complications than average.

Nutrition

It has been shown that women with low weight and low body mass index (BMI) loose bone at a greater rate than heavy women[20]. A study from the US showed that the BMI increased over a 20-year period for both white and black women at all levels of income and education[40]. Though this would be expected to reduce the number of hip fractures, the rate actually rises over the 20-year period. The reduction of one risk must be outweighed by the increase of another, perhaps a decreasing lower level of physical exercise. Failing eyesight with the use of bifocal lenses, making the ground less visible, would also contribute.

Calcium

Good nutrition is believed to be associated both with a sufficient peak bone mass as well as a reduced fracture rate. Figures concerning milk intake during childhood are not convincing. It seems possible that a higher calcium intake results in higher bone mineral density, only when a higher level of physical activity is maintained[41,42]. A 14-year study showing that there was an inverse association between dietary calcium and the subsequent risk of hip fracture supported the hypothesis that increased dietary calcium intake protects against hip fracture. However, the need for calcium intake has been much discussed[43].

In one study it was found that only 2–4% gain in bone mass resulted from a combination of a high calcium intake and physical activity[44]. It is not clear whether the reverse hypothesis is true – that low physical activity and a low calcium means a higher fracture risk.

Calcium alone can probably not prevent bone loss. The nutritional importance of calcium intake was stated to be unclear in the WHO report[5]. 'It was recognized that there is still much uncertainty concerning the nutritional requirements for calcium and other nutrition, not only at different stages of skeletal development, but also across cultural and racial boundaries.' As opposed to estrogen, calcium intake seem to be effective only in the presence of other factors, such as physical activity.

In Heaney's position paper[45], for the WHO consultation 1988[5], 17 cross-sectional studies on calcium intake were reviewed. Eleven showed a positive correlation between current calcium intake and bone mass; six showed no effect and no study showed a negative correlation. Of ten controlled intervention studies, eight showed a slowing down of age-related bone loss at high calcium intakes and only two studies failed to show any such effect. Four studies of the association between early life calcium intake and perimenopausal bone mass found it to be positive.

It has been proposed that 1000 mg/day should be a minimum intake, and that less that 500 mg/day will be clearly insufficient[46]. Dietary calcium of 800 mg/day has been recommended for adults and 1200 mg/day for adolescents and pregnant or lactating women[47,48]. Some studies have suggested that a reduced calcium intake means an increased risk for bone mineral loss and postmenopausal osteoporosis. It remains unclear whether postmenopausal osteoporosis is reduced or stopped by calcium supplementation[10,49,50].

In a review[51], calcium carbonate was recommended to be the main calcium supplement given because it was inexpensive, but this should be combined with low intensity exercise. The practical recommendation was brisk walking for 1 h three times a week. Vitamin D supplementation was recommended only for those patients who do not get an adequate dietary intake or sunlight exposure.

Fluoride

As fluoride increases bone mass it has been tried in the prevention of osteoporotic fractures. Fluoride did not reduce the fracture rate in a 4-year prospective clinical trial in 202 postmenopausal women with osteoporosis and other studies have also been negative[50,52,53]. That means that the quality of bone is also a factor to consider in prevention, not just only bone mass[54] as fluoride intake increases bone fragility[53]. Bone mineral density increased in the predominantly cancellous lumbar spine, the femoral neck, and trochanter sites, but it decreased by 4% in the predominatly cortical bone of the shaft of the radius. The number of new vertebral fractures was similar in both groups but the number of new non-vertebral fractures in the fluoride group in this controlled trial was significantly increased in the group receiving fluoride.

Estrogens

More than 20 years ago the bone-sparing action of estrogen was observed by Meema and Meema[55]. The reduction of fracture rates was shown by a study in 1979 by Nachtigall[56] and by Lindsay[57] in 1976. In a 10-year study in which Lindsay measured midshaft radius density the loss of bone was 0.22% per year of bone mineral content in the treated group whereas the placebo group lost 0.95% per year, that is a 4.5-fold increase[58].

A reduction of 50% in vertebral crush fractures with estrogen treatment was shown by Ettinger and colleagues, 1985[59]. The effect of estrogens on bone formation and prevention of osteoporosis and fracture has been studied in much detail[60].

All estrogens maintain bone mass. Estrogen diminished bone resorption and bone turnover, decreased serum calcium and decreased serum phosphate concentration. It has been shown that a 1 mg dose of 17β-estradiol kept the BMC constant but with 2 mg the gain was 0.8% and 1.5% after 12 months[61]. The combination of estrogen and progestogen has been studied by many authors and several methods have been shown to protect bone mass.

In a larger study on a population-based cohort of 23 246 the greatest protective effect with a relative risk of 0.47 was found for trochanteric fracture in women receiving potent estrogen, who were under 60 years of age at cohort entry[62].

From the Framingham study it was possible to show that estrogen replacement was effective in preventing hip fracture in spite of the long-term selection processes that have taken place in that study. Estrogen effects were compared after controlling for age, age at menopause, metropolitan relative weight, smoking and alcohol consumption. The authors, however, have some reservations and did state that they were unable to determine the ideal duration of exposure to estrogen[63].

Theoretically, if it is possible to postpone the onset of osteoporosis 5–6 years it would reduce the occurrence of hip fracture by 50%[60]. Estrogen use does mean an increased risk for endoetrial carcinoma, but this can be to some extent reduced by giving simultaneous progesterone[64].

There is at present insufficient evidence to recommend the routine prescription of prophylactic estrogen therapy to all women[16], but estrogen therapy is recommended for postmenopausal women who are at particular risk of developing osteoporosis. Estrogen is not recommended for all women as the risk of osteoporosis is low in the general population despite the increasing risk of hip fracture. The risk of breast and endometrial cancer must be taken into consideration. The ideal duration of estrogen treatment is not known. The proven reduction in the incidence of cardiovascular disease is an additional advantage of estrogen therapy[65].

Calcitonin

Calcitonin has been shown to increase bone mass and probably also to lead to a reduction in fractures[66]. Information on the effect on osteoporosis is rapidly growing.

Editronate

In a multicenter study with a rather complex design 220 women who had from one to four vertebral compression fractures were treated with phosphate, editronate or placebo, in cycles that were repeated eight times. The rate of new vertebral fractures was reduced by half in the editronate (diphosphonate)-treated patients as compared with patients who did not receive etitronate. The treatment effect was greatest in the subgroup of patients with the lowest spinal bone mineral density at baseline[67].

THINGS TO AVOID

Alcohol, tobacco, coffee

Excess use of alcohol constitutes a risk through not only creating osteoporosis by inhibiting bone formation as such, but also by increasing the risk of injury. For moderate use of alcohol the data are inconclusive. A high intake of coffee and alcohol, creates a higher risk[5]. The mode of action of caffeine might be through inhibition of the formation of new bone and/or an increase in urinary calcium loss.

It has been found that the risk of hip and forearm fracture is elevated in thin women and in those who smoked cigarettes, particularly among non-users of estrogen[68]. Smoking as a risk factor could be primary or as a part of the smoking package, smokers being thinner, having earlier menopause, and a higher estrogen metabolism.

WHO has no definite recommendation to reduce smoking and drinking specifically for osteoporosis because there are other better reasons against smoking and excess alcohol[5,69]. Further, to prove a graded effect on osteoporosis of moderate use of alcohol, tobacco, and coffee is methodologically difficult.

Falls

As indicated in the introduction and in Chapter 4, falls are a major problem for the elderly population[70].

In a study of falls and subjective health rating in a sample for 3494 Israelis over 65 years of age, the 1-year incidence for 1985 was estimated to be 23–24% for those over 65[71]. Falls at the same level constitute 75% of all falls[72].

In a study of hip fractures it was found that the consumption of benzodiazepines was not significantly different in cases and controls, but that the hip fracture patients had a higher incidence of stroke, an odds ratio of 3.5 and among social risk factors an odds ratio 1.5[73].

In a review on risk factors for hip fracture it is underlined that the prevention of falls is also likely to be an important protective measure in the elderly[31]. Each year almost one-third of patients 65 or older fall. Two per cent of all elderly persons who seek medical advice do this because of falls[3]. A number of drugs have been suspected to create imbalance, and dizziness[73].

In another study it was concluded that muscle strength and bone density were important factors in determining the risk of fracture in women between 45 and 70 years of age. The authors proposed that muscular action may absorb much of the energy of the fall, so protecting the bones. This was, however, not found for the older cases in the group[74].

CONCLUSIONS

In 1990 Cummings and co-workers tried to estimate the size of the hip fracture problem in the USA. They claimed that the universal use of estrogen therapy by postmenopausal white women may slow down but not prevent the rise in hip fractures, therefore new effective and widely applicable strategies to prevent hip fractures are urgently needed[75].

The timing and the sequence of preventive measure taken is important. From several studies it is known that peak bone mass, that is the maximum bone mass before menopause, is critical for determining the rate of development of osteoporosis. The peak bone mass is in turn dependent on conditions during childhood and early adulthood, such as the amount of physical exercise, calcium intake and nutritional status including vitamin D supplementation. In essence this means that the most extended time lag between preventive action taken and the positive effect on such prevention could be 70–80 years. So far this stepwise approach to prevention and its results has not yet been sufficiently quantified. Thus, the development of fracture prediction modes for osteoporosis prevention is very important to elucidate the real long-term outcome on a population level of preventive measures[76].

Recommendations for prevention

In the present state of knowledge an adequate calcium intake and exercise level combined with avoidance of smoking, alcohol and falls can be confidently recommended in prevention for all. Hormone therapy with cyclical estrogen and progestogen is recommended only for those at particular risk.

REFERENCES

1. Christiansen C, Riis BJ. The silent epidemic. Postmenopausal osteoporosis. A handbook for the medical profession. National Osteoporosis Society and the European Foundation for Osteoporosis and Bone Disease. 1990 87–89172–28–0

2. Iskrant AP, Smith RW Jr. Osteoporosis in women 45 and over related to subsequent fractures. Public Health Rep. 1969; 84:338

3. Cummings SR, Kelsey JL, Nevitt C *et al.* Epidemiology of osteoporosis and osteoporotic fractures. Epidemiol Rev. 1985; 7:178–208

4. McIlwain HH, Bruce DF, Silverfield JC, Burnette MC. Osteoporosis. Prevention, Management, Treatment. New York, Chicester, Brisbane, Toronto, Singapore, John Wiley, 1988

5. World Health Organization. Report of the Joint WHO/EOPF/NIAMS (NIH) Consultation on Oosteoporosis. Geneva, 13–15 July, 1988, NCD/OND/OSTEO/88.1

6. Johnell O, Nilsson B, Obrant K *et al.* Age and sex pattern of hip fracture changes in 30 years. Acta Orthop. Scand. 1984; 55:290–292

7. Dequeker J, Geusens P. Treatment of established osteoporosis and rehabilitation: current practice and possibilities. Maturitas. 1990; 12:1–36

8. Ford AB. Reducing the threat of hip fracture. Am J Public Health. 1989; 79:269–70

9. Hall FM, Davis MA, Baran DT. Bone mineral screening for osteoporosis. N Engl J Med. 1987; 316:212–214

10. Resnick MM, Greenspan SL. 'Senile' osteoporosis reconsidered. JAMA. 1989; 261:1025–1029

11. Cooper C, Barker DJP, Morris J *et al.* Osteoporosis, falls and age in fracture of the proximal femur. Br Med J. 1987; 295:13–5

12. Jensen GF, Christiansen C, Boesen J *et al.* Relationship between bone mineral content and frequency of postmenopausal fractures. Acta Med Scand. 1983; 213:61–63

13. Smith DM, Khairi MRA, Johnston CC. The loss of bone mineral and its relationship to the risk of fracture. J Clin Invest. 1978; 36:311–318

14. Smith DM, Nance WE, Kang KW *et al.* Genetic factors in determining bone mass. J Clin Invest. 1973; 52:2800–2808

15. de Vernejoul MC. Bone remodelling in osteoporosis. Clin Rheumatol. 1989; 8: Suppl. 2, 13–15

16. Wahner HW. Measurements of bone mass and bone density. Endocrinol Metab Clin North Am, 1989; 18:995–1012

17. Thomsen K, Gotfredsen A, Christiansen C. Is postmenopausal bone loss an age-related phenomenon? Calcif Tissue Int. 1986; 39:123–127

18. Burckhardt P, Michel C. The peak bone mass concept. Clin Rheumatol. 1989; 8: Suppl. 2, 16–21

19. Christiansen C, Riis BJ. New methods of identifying 'at risk' patients for osteoporosis. Clin Rheumatol. 1989; 8: Suppl. 2, 52–5

20. Christiansen C, Riis BJ, Rodbro P. Prediction of rapid bone loss in postmenopausal women. Lancet. 1987; 1:1105–7

21. Silman A. The EVOS project. To be published.

22. Allander E. The epidemiology of osteoporosis. A selective overview. Clin Rheumatol. 1989; 8: Suppl. 2, 9–12

23. Cummings SR, Black D. Should perimenopausal women be screened for osteoporosis? Ann Intern Med. 1986; 104:817–23

24. National Institutes of Health. Consensus conference: osteoporosis. JAMA, 1984; 252:799–802

25. World Health Organization. Manual of the International Statistical Classification of Diseases, Injuries, and Causes of Death. Sixth revision. Vol. 1. Geneva, WHO, 1948

26. Lindahl BIB. On weighting causes of death. An analysis of purposes and criteria of selection. In Brandstrom A, Tedebrand L-G, eds., Society, Health and Population During the Demographic Transition. Stockholm, Almqvist and Wiksell International, 1988 pp 131–156

27. Lindahl BIB. The development of population research on causes of death: growth of knowledge or accumulation of data? In ten Have HAMJ, Kimsma GK, Spicker SF, eds., The Growth of

Medical Knowledge. Dordrecht, Kluwer Academic Publishers, 1990, pp 103–119

28. Lindahl BIB, Glattre E, Lahti R *et al.* The WHO principles for registering causes of death: suggestions for improvement. J Clin Epidemiol. 1990; 43:467–74

29. White BL, Fisher WD, Laurin CA. Rate of mortality for elderly patients after fracture of the hip in the 1980's. J Bone Joint Surg. 1987; 69A: 1335–1339

30. Fos PJ, McLin CL. The risk of falling in the elderly: a subjective approach. Med Decision Making. 1990; 10:195–200

31. Kelsey JL. Risk factors for hip fracture. N Engl J Med. 1987; 316 (7):404–406

32. Chalmers J, Ho KC. Geographic variations in senile osteoporosis: the association of physical activity. J. Bone Joint Surg. 1970; 52:667–75

33. Paganini-Hill A, Ross RK, Gerkins JR *et al.* Menopausal estrogen therapy and hip fractures. Ann Intern Med. 1981; 95:28–31

34. Fisher M (ed.), Exercise counselling. In Guide to Clinical Preventive Services. An Assessment of 169 Interventions. Report of the US Preventive Services Task Force. Baltimore, Hong Kong, London, Sydney, Williams and Wilkins, Chap. 49, 1989

35. Hui SL, Slemeda CW, Johnstone CC Jr. Age and bone mass as predictors of fracture in a prospective study. J Clin Invest. 1988; 81:1804–1809

36. Block JE, Genant HK, Black D. Greater vertebral bone mineral mass in exercising young men. West J Med. 1986; 145:39–42

37. Dalen N, Olsson KE. Bone mineral content and physical activity. Acta Orthop Scand. 1974; 45:170–4

38. Dilsen G, Berker C, Oral A *et al.* The role of physical exercise in prevention and management of osteoporosis. Clin. Rheumatol. 1989; 8: Suppl. 2, 70–5

39. Mellstrom D, Rundgren A. Benskorhet kan motverkas med okad motion, minskad rokning och okat kalciumintag. Lakartidningen. 1983; 80:2048–2050

40. Flegal KM, Harlan WR, Landis JR. Secular trends in body mass index and skinfold thickness with socioeconomic factors in young adult women. Am J Clin Nutr. 1988; 48:535–43

41. Kanders B, Dempster DW, Lindsay R. Interaction of calcium nutrition and physical activity on bone mass in young women. J Bone Minerol. Res. 1988; 3:145–9

42. Picard D, Ste-Marie LG, Carrier L *et al.* Influence of calcium intake during early adulthood on bone mineral content in premenopausal women. In Cohn DV, Martin TJ, Meunier PJ, eds., Calcium Reg Bone Metab.: Basic and Clin. Aspects, Vol. 9, pp. 128–32. Elsevier, 1987

43. Holbrook TL, Barrett-Connor E, Wingard DL. Dietary calcium and risk of hip fracture: 14-year prospective population study. Lancet. 1988; 2:1046–9

44. Mazess RB, Barden H, Towsley M *et al.* Bone mineral density of the spine and radius in normal young women. J Bone Minerol Res. 1986; 1 (Abstr): p.118

45. Heaney RP. Nutrition and bone health. A position paper prepared for a WHO consultation on osteoporosis, 13–15 July, 1988

46. Fisher M (ed.). Nutrition. In Guide to Clinical Preventive Services. An Assessment of 169 Interventions. Report of the US Preventive Services Task Force. Baltimore, Williams and Wilkins, Chap. 50, 1989

47. National Center for Health Statistics. In Carroll MD, Abraham S, Dresser CM, eds., Dietary Intake Source Data: United States, 1976–80. Vital and Health Statistics, Series 11, No. 231. Washington, DC, Government Printing Office, 1983. (Publication No. DHHS (PHS) 83–1681)

48. National Research Council, Food and Nutrition Board. Recommended Dietary Allowances, 9th revised edn. Committee on Dietary Allowances. Washington, DC, National Academy of Sciences, 1980

49. Nordin BEC, Horsman A, Crilly RG *et al.* Treatment of spinal osteoporosis in postmenopausal women. Br Med J. 1980; 280:451–454

50. Riggs BL, Seeman E, Hodgson SF *et al.* Effect of the fluoride/calcium regimen on vertebral fracture occurrence in postmenopausal women: comparison with conventional therapy. N Engl J Med. 1982; 306:446–450

51. Trachtenbarg DE. Treatment of osteoporosis. What is the role of calcium? Postgrad Med Osteoporosis. 1990; 87:263–270

52. Hodsman AB, Drost DJ. The response of vertebral bone mineral density during the treatment of osteoporosis with sodium fluoride. J Clin Endocrinol Metabol. 1989; 69:932–8

53. Riggs BL, Hodgson SF, O'Fallon WN *et al.* Effect of fluoride treatment on the fracture rate in postmenopausal women with osteoporosis. N Engl J Med. 1990; 322:802–809

54. Lindsay R. Fluoride and bone – quantity versus quality. N Engl J Med. 1990; 322:845–6

55. Meema HE, Meema S. Prevention of postmenopausal osteoporosis by hormone treatment of the menopause. Can Med Assoc J. 1968; 99:248–251

56. Nachtigall LE, Nachtiall RH, Nachtigall RD *et al.* Estrogen replacement therapy I: a 10-year prospective study in the relationship to osteoporosis. Obstet Gynecol. 1979; 53:277–81

57. Lindsay R, Hart DM, Aitken JM *et al.* Long-term prevention of postmenopausal osteoporosis by oestrogen. Lancet. 1976; 1:1038–41

58. Lindsay R, Hart DM, Forrest C *et al.* Prevention of spinal osteoporosis in oophorectomised women. Lancet. 1980; 2:1151–4

59 Ettinger B. Genant HK, Cann CE. Long-term estrogen replacement therapy prevents bone loss and fractures. Ann Intern Med. 1985; 102:319–324

60. Nagant de Deuxchaisnes C, Devogelaer J-P. Endocrinological status of postmenopausal osteoporosis. Clin Rheum Dis. 1986; 12:559–635

61. Christiansen C, Christensen MS, Larsen NE *et al.* Pathophysiological mechanisms of estrogen effect on metabolism. Dose-response relationships in early postmenopausal women. J. Clin. Endocrinol Metabol. 1982; 55:1124–30

62. Naessen T, Persson I, Adami H-O *et al.* Hormone replacement therapy and the risk for first hip fracture. A prospective, population-based cohort study. Ann Intern Med. 1990; 113:95–103

63. Kiel DP, Felson DT, Anderson JJ *et al.* Hip fracture and the use of estrogens in postmenopausal women. N Engl J Med. 1987; 317:1169–1174

64. MacDonald PC, Edman CD, Hemsell DL *et al.* Effect of obesity on conversion of plasma androstenedione to estrone in postmenopausal women with and without endometrial cancer. Am J Obstet Gynecol. 1978; 130:448–455

65. Fisher M (ed.). Estrogen prophylaxis. In Guide to Clinical Preventive Services. An Assessment of 169 Interventions. Report of the US Preventive Services Task Force. Baltimore, Williams and Wilkins, Chap. 59, 1989

66. Gennari C. Salmon calcitonin (Miacalcic) nasal spray in prevention and treatment of osteoporosis. Clin Rheumatol. 1989; 8: Suppl. 2, 61–5

67. Watts NB, Harris ST, Genant HK *et al.* Intermittent cyclical editrodronate treatment of postmenopausal osteoporosis. N Engl J Med. 1990; 323:73–79

68. Williams AR, Weiss NS, Ure Cl *et al.* Effect of weight, smoking, and estrogen use on the risk of hip and forearm fractures in postmenopausal women. Obstet Gynecol. 1982; 60:695–699

69. World Health Organization. WHO consultation on an integrated programme for community health in noncommunicable diseases. Report of a meeting, Geneva, 16–18 December, 1985. NCD/IP/86.1

70. Stevens A, Mulrow C. Drugs affecting postural stability and other risk factors in the hip fracture epidemic – case-control study. Community Med. 1989; 11:27–34

71. Cwickel J, Kaplan G, Barell V. Falls and subjective health rating among the elderly: evidence from two Israeli samples. Soc Sci Med. 1990; 31:485–90

72. Hedlund R, Ahlbom A, Lindgren U. Hip fracture incidence in Stockholm. 1972–1981. Acta Orthop Scand. 1985; 57:30–4

73. Ray WA, Griffin MR, Schaffner W *et al.* Psychotropic drug use and the risk of hip fracture. N Engl J Med. 1987; 316:363–369

74. Eriksson SAV, Lindgren JU. Outcome of falls in women: Endogenous factors associated with fracture. Age Aging. 1989; 18:303–8

75. Cummings SR, Rubin SM, Black D. The future of hip fractures in the United States. Numbers, costs and potential effects of postmenopausal estrogen. Clin Orthop Rel Res. 1990; 252:163–6

76. Ross PD, Wasnich RD, Davis JW. Fracture prediction models for osteoporosis prevention. Bone. 1990; 11:327–331

286

25. DIET AND RHEUMATIC DISEASES

Richard Wigley

INTRODUCTION

The relationship of diet to rheumatic problems may be summarized by five key questions, which are not mutually exclusive and may operate together:

(1) Does diet cause rheumatism and if so, is this due to allergy or biochemical effects?

(2) Can diet cure or prevent rheumatism?

(3) Is dietary modification for rheumatic complaints merely another medium for faith healing?

(4) Does obesity aggravate rheumatic complaints or does enforced inactivity from the rheumatism cause the increase in weight?

(5) Do dietary deficiencies cause neuropathies that simulate rheumatic disease?

In addition to these complexities, there are the difficulties inherent in controlled studies on diet, an emotive susceptibility of the subjects in the study (which may be exploited by purveyors of alleged health foods), and the intangible impact of the news media. The result is that firm conclusions on the relation of diet to diseases which are often marked by non-specific signs and symptoms (as are the rheumatic diseases), are difficult to reach. The less controversial and less common issues will be dealt with first, beginning with rheumatic symptoms possibly arising from excess or deficit of vitamins and essential nutrients. At the end of this section, the ever-present problem of alternative or fringe diets and medicines will be discussed.

HYPERVITAMINOSIS A

Diffuse bone pain and radiologic evidence of periosteal neo-osteogenesis can result from excessive vitamin A intake, which may occur in Eskimos consuming large quantities of polar bear liver or may be iatrogenic from taking Vitamin A or other retinols[1], used in treating severe acne[2]. Retinol has also been recommended for the treatment of rheumatoid arthritis[3], although there is little beyond anecdotal data to support this suggestion, and it should be withdrawn if bone pain arises. The radiographic changes seen in hypervitaminosis A simulate those of Forrestier's disease (disseminated idiopathic hyperostosis, DISH), a condition that has been associated with high blood retinol levels, as well as diabetes mellitus[3,4]. Tendon and ligament calcification have also been described[5]. Prevention requires a reduced vitamin A intake, which may be difficult in a population that traditionally consumes bear and fish liver, both of which are high in vitamin A.

CALCIUM AND VITAMIN D

A high calcium and/or vitamin D intake can result in pseudogout from calcium pyrophosphate crystal deposition in joints (*see* Chapter 23). A low intake of either or both results in bone pain and deformity from rickets in children and osteomalacia in adults, causing bone pain and deformity with partial (Milkman's) fractures. Such long-term deformities in turn may induce degenerative arthritis later in life. In developed countries this more likely to be due to malabsorption states as in the post gastrectomy syndrome.

VITAMIN B

In Indonesia, it is sometimes difficult to separate rheumatic symptoms from those of peripheral neuropathy due to endemic thiamine (vitamin B_1) deficiency[6]. Despite the epoch-making discovery made a century ago by Eijkman[7] that this disease results from removing (polishing) the thiamine-rich husks of rice, white (polished) rice continues to be a main stable food. The opportunity for prevention is clear but established customs are not easily broken, and require adequate nutritional education. Riboflavin (vitamin B_2) and pyridoxine (vitamin B_6) deficiencies may cause neuropathy also, often on a background of alcoholism. Vitamin B_{12} deficiency may cause pain, paresthesiae and discomfort from peripheral neuropathy, thereby simulating rheumatic complaints. Usually this deficiency is most often due to gastric atrophy, in which there is an absence of intrinsic factor, but also occurs in those on strict vegan diets, which are devoid of any form of animal protein. Vitamin B_{12} deficiency is rare in India, despite a complete vegans diet in some areas as the potable water in India contains sufficient bacteria to synthesize the vitamin. Ironically, attempts to lower the bacterial content in the water to control infectious disease may result in vitamin B_{12} deficiency (personal communication, L. Bieder).

VITAMIN C

Severe scurvy can lead to subperiosteal hematomas or hemarthrosis. Prevention by using limes on British ships in the eighteenth century led to the identification of ascorbic acid in fresh fruit and uncooked vegetables (light cooking of green vegetables and potatoes conserves ascorbic acid). In developed countries, scurvy is now confined to various neglected groups, e.g. the elderly, and alcoholics, and is not uncommon in migrant laborers in South Africa, who have a high alcohol intake, which may be accompanied by thickening of the subcutaneous tissues around the ankles simulating scleroderma (personal communication, Anthony Gear).

KASHIN–BECK DISEASE

This bone and joint disease was described in the Lake Baikal area of Siberia by Kashin and Beck last century, and occurs in Helionjiang province in northeast China extending across to southwest China (Figure 1). Kashin–Beck disease causes irregular, defective epiphyseal growth of the long bones particularly at the hands, feet and knees, which may be observed radiologically. The typical swelling of the knees has evoked the local name of 'big joint disease'. Although the joint cartilage is generally preserved, interference with growth results in premature degenerative arthritis. A toxin, from the fungus *Fusaria* which infects wheat and maize but is not found on rice has been etiologically linked to the disease[8]. An alcohol, threitol, has been isolated from affected grain but not from rice or from wheat or maize from non-endemic areas. In an exhaustive series of epidemiological and interventional studies, Yang Jian Bo and colleagues linked consumption of contaminated grain to Kashin–Beck disease, and prevention hinges on changing from wheat to rice production. It had been suggested that the growth of *Fusaria* species might be facilitated by selenium deficiency which occurs in a similar but not identical band across China (Figure 2) Kashin–Beck disease does not occur in the selenium-deficient area in southwest China. This is an area where Keshan disease occurs. Rice is the staple diet in that region and rice may concentrate selenium better than wheat or maize (Figures 1 and 2).

SELENIUM DEFICIENCY

Selenium is a strong antioxidant similar in action to vitamin E (see below). Keshan disease occurs in the selenium deficient area of northeastern China, and consists of a juvenile cardiomyopathy responding to vitamin C in the acute form, and preventable by selenium supplements. Kashin–Beck disease has been claimed to respond to selenium tablets, but not to selenium added to salt[9]. Several patients on prolonged total parenteral nutrition suffering from muscle tenderness of thighs and inability to walk responded to selenium[10,11].

Selenium is deficient in the soil in southern New Zealand; selenium drenches are given to sheep in this area to prevent 'white muscle disease', in which the sheep become progressively weaker and at postmortem examination, have extremely pale musculature. From this, selenium has acquired a certain (and completely unproven) mystique as a therapy for rheumatic complaints. Any claims for symptomatic relief from selenium 'therapy' are likely to be a non-specific placebo response, and as confirmatory evidence there is no relation of selenium levels to rheumatic symptoms[12], and treatment trials have proved negative for muscle complaints[13] and osteoarthritis[14]. Thus the evidence that selenium deficiency is a significant cause of rheumatic symptoms is minimal. Thompson[13] has recently reviewed the consequences of low selenium levels and found no relationship to human rheumatic disease in New Zealand.

VITAMIN E

Like selenium, vitamin E is a potent antioxidant, so that to a certain extent, one can replace the other. Large doses of vitamin E have been promoted by purveyors of 'natural health foods' as beneficial for most of the agonies of human existence, from sexual dysfunction to rheumatic complaints, although evidence indicates that it only promotes the health of rodents. Any modifi-

cation of rheumatic pain is probably due to a placebo effect[15]. In a different context[16] omission of this vitamin from the diet of PN/n inbred mice with a systemic lupus erythematosus-like disease and hypertension brought the blood pressure to normal. The pressure rose again when pure α-tocopherol was added to the diet, possibly due to the vitamin's stabilizing effect on the cell membrane, making arachidonic acid less available for the prostaglandin pathway, thereby lowering the blood pressure and so having a pharmacological effect not unlike that of non-steroidal anti-inflammatory drugs. Vitamin E is regarded as relatively innocuous even in large doses, but the effect on mouse blood pressure raises the possibility of similar undesired effects in man. Despite these unanswered questions, no further work appears to have been done in this area.

ESSENTIAL FATTY ACIDS

Of all the dietary hypotheses, the one that seems to be the most promising is that which proposes that the polyunsaturated fatty acids, eicosapentanoic, docosahexanoic, linolenic or linoleic acids taken in large quantity, may ameliorate rheumatic pain. Eicosapentanoic acid diverts the prostaglandin pathway, suppressing proinflammatory prostaglandin production, an effect that is similar to that of the prostaglandin blocking non-steroidal anti-inflammatory drugs or NSAIDs[18]. A beneficial effect on the development of renal lesions in NZB/NZW mice with SLE[17] encouraged trials of this oil in rheumatoid arthritis. The results were equivocal in three controlled trials[18–20] but the non-steroidal anti-inflammatory (NSAID) prostaglandin blocking drugs had not been stopped. In one trial[19] when NSAIDs were withdrawn, the oil group did not deteriorate whereas the control group did. The presumption is that the effect is equivalent to the effect of these drugs but not additive. Considering that the large amount of oil taken caused some gastric disturbance, the practical use of fish or fish oil may be

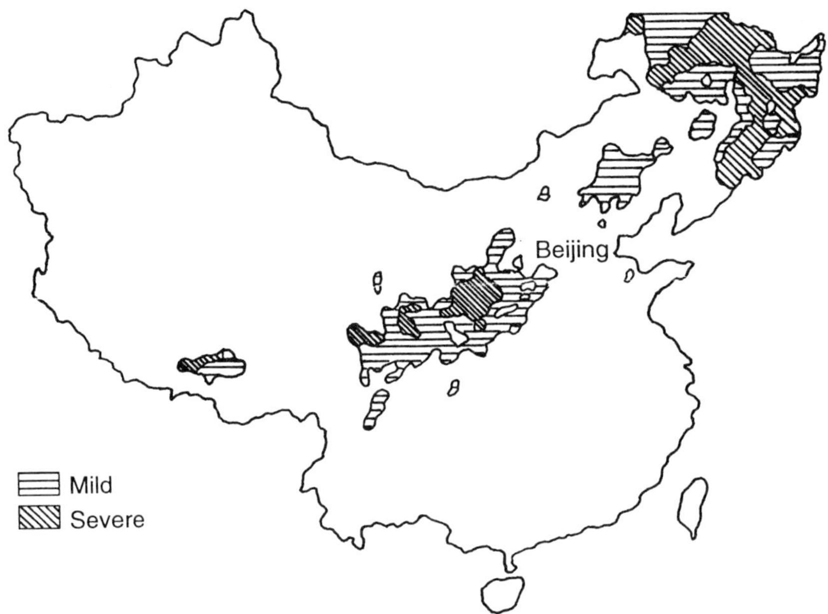

Figure 1 This map shows the distribution of Kashin–Beck Disease in China. (Modified with kind permission from Tan J, Zhu W, Li R *et al*. Geographic distribution of Kashin–Beck disease. (From China and the Relation of Ecological Chemico-geography to its Occurrence. Institute of Geography, Academica Sinica, Beijing, China))

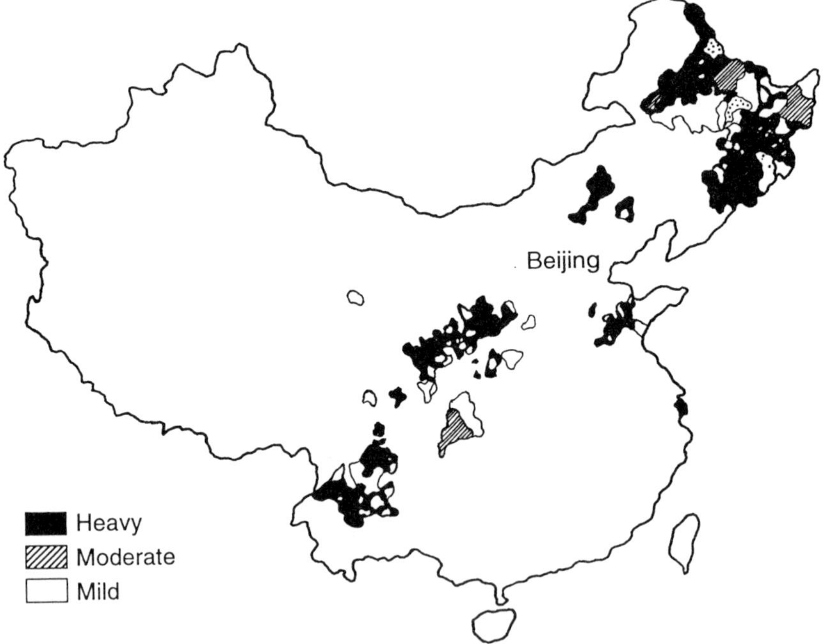

Figure 2 The distribution of selenium deficiency and Keshan disease in China. (Modified with kind permission from Guanqi Y, Wang S, Ruihua Z, Shuzhuang S. Am J Clin Nutr. 1983; 37:872–881)

limited. Moreover, large quantities of fish or fish oil must be consumed to provide the necessary oil and oily fish is not very palatable.

Kremer compared fish oil with olive oil dietary supplementation[20]. The improvement in the fish oil groups was not significantly greater than in the olive oil group, although drop-outs from the latter group were significantly higher. NSAID therapy was continued in this study possibly obscuring a pharmacological effect of the oil. It is possible that life-long high fish oil intake may have prophylactic value in rheumatic disease, and epidemiological data suggests that musculoskeletal pains are lower with a high fish diet. Since these oils are also said to have prophylactic value for atheroma there is an added incentive to investigate this further. In a population survey of rheumatic disease in Taiwan, Chou[21] quantified the fish consumption in the diet and found a negative association with rheumatic pain in those with high fish consumption. In similar surveys in mainland China[22,23] higher rates for rheumatic symptoms and in particular knee pain were found in the Beijing region than in the Shantou region of the warmer Quantung province, where fish and eels are consumed in greater quantities. The possibility that the fish oil content of the diet has a protective effect for all rheumatic pain could be studied further by taking samples of blood for eicosapentanoic acid estimation. Clearly there are other variables to consider such as climate to explain this difference (*see* Chapter 3). As discussed above, there is a possibility of inducing symptoms from an excess of vitamins A and D.

Against the fish oil hypothesis is the experience of the Tokelauans who subsisted largely on fish and coconut in their tropical atoll, but did not suffer more rheumatic symptoms after moving to New Zealand except for gout which increased as did weight[24]. Eskimos from Greenland, who have a high fish oil diet, were reported to have a low prevalence of rheumatoid arthritis but the sample size was small[25], and thus a possible relationship is not established. Another Eskimo study from Canada showed a higher prevalence of rheumatoid arthritis, although their fish consumption was not quantified[26]. Coastal urban Javans had more rheumatic symptoms than rural Javans[6].

A book written 30 years ago by a laboratory technician, *Common Sense in Arthritis*, which continues to be popular among the lay public, promotes the use of cod liver oil, based on the theory that sore joints need this oil. Despite the fact that (a) oil is degraded in the stomach and (b) the joint lubricant is not an oil but a proteoglycan, the author may yet prove to be right, though for the wrong reasons. The amounts used by his followers were probably insufficient to affect prostaglandin production. A non-medical fashion for taking green lipped mussels for rheumatism in New Zealand faded when this proved no better than placebo[27]. The mussels are now used as food which is more appropriate. A Californian Chinese, Dr Dong, having recovered from rheumatoid arthritis upon changing to a Chinese diet high in rice, extrapolated his experience to all arthritides, enthusiastically promoting his rice diet as a therapy for rheumatic disease, thereby achieving worldwide popularity. Although rheumatoid arthritis is no less common in Shantou than Beijing, there were less subjective complaints of pain of all categories than those in the north where the diet is wheat-based[22,23]. So this theory cannot be ignored in further epidemiological research. In the Malaysian COPCORD study of an inland rural area where fish would not be readily available[28] Chinese originally from Fukien in southeastern China had less rheumatic complaints than Malays or Tamil Indians raising the possibility of a genetic factor.

Evening primrose oil containing a high proportion of homo-gamma-linolenic acid, is also under trial in animal models of arthritis and rheumatoid arthritis[29]. The oil in toxic oil syndrome is discussed in Chapter 21. The arthritic symptoms that may arise from hyperlipoproteinemias and their relation to diet are detailed in Chapter 23.

In conclusion, much further work has to be done to define the role of essential fatty acids, wheat, rice and other dietary factors, if any, in the primary prevention of rheumatism. Climate and other possible risk factors should be studied. The pattern appearing in the Asian Pacific area should provoke further work to interrelate these variables with various rheumatic syndromes.

CADMIUM

This toxic metal ion once contaminated crops in Japan, and was once to cause severe bone pain from osteomalacia, the so-called 'itai-itai' or 'ouch-ouch' disease, in which there was proteinuria and high cadmium in the rice and water pollution with this element from a mine. It is now believed that deficiency of calcium and vitamin D were responsible[30] for the symptoms.

Vitamin and trace element deficiencies are rare in Caucasian populations unless there is malabsorption, renal disease, alcoholism or milk intolerance. Sprue causes malabsorption in the tropics. Clearly, deficiency of vitamins is preventable by dietary modification where sufficient food is available or prescription of vitamins is affordable.

ALLERGY

Sensitivity to food allergens as a cause of inflammatory arthritis remains controversial, except when it constitutes part of allergic vasculitis or serum sickness as discussed in Chapter 21. Some determined allergists progressively remove various items from the diet to try to identify a causative allergen, and may claim success in this regard, although causation is proven in only a few cases[31]. As discussed below, apparent success

can be due to non-specific effects. Reproducing symptoms by challenge is claimed as proof but even if the challenge is double blinded, the improvement could in fact result from spontaneous regression. There are also potential harmful side-effects from dietary deficiency. Because milk is often implicated in 'food allergies', calcium deficiency may persist for years in susceptible children who, at least theoretically, could develop rickets. Gluten sensitivity though an established cause of malabsorption does not cause arthritis but may cause neuropathy from vitamin deficiency related to malabsorption.

FLUORIDE

Fluorosis is endemic in the Pubjab, Madras, parts of North America, China (Figure 3), South Africa, Japan and Europe. More than 4 mg/day is considered to be an adequate daily requirement. Excessive fluoride intake affects the dental enamel in the first 2 years of life and permanently discolors the teeth at water levels of 2.4/4 ppm[32]. Muscle weakness, stiffness, spasm and pain have been reported to occur before florid fluorosis develops. This consists of calcification in the spinal ligaments and ligamentum flavum, causing spinal stenosis and nerve root pain and signs[33]. Teotia and Teotia[34] describe arthralgia, difficulty closing the fingers and ankylosis of the hips, knees and elbows as well as the spine. These symptoms occur in children often with coxa vara, with knee and chest deformities, especially if there is associated calcium deficiency. Anteroposterior narrowing of the spinal canal leads to stenosis with root signs and pain from narrowing of root foramina. Fusion of the vertebrae may simulate ankylosing spondylitis. As fluorine is present in food and particularly in tea, the blood and urine should be examined for fluoride in addition to drinking water. A simple and inexpensive screening of an entire community can be performed by measuring the fluoride in pooled urine samples. This averages those who may be deficient and those who are ingesting dietary

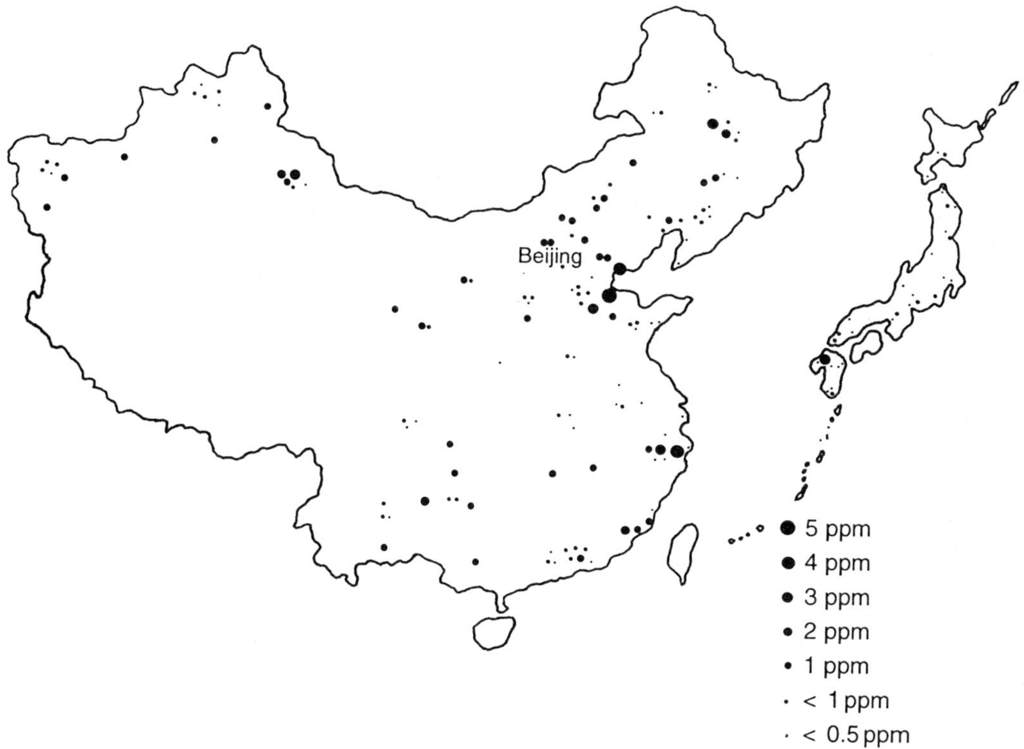

Figure 3 This map shows the water fluoride content of various water supplies in China. (Modified with kind permission from Liu M, Sun RY, Zhang JH *et al*. Elimination of excess fluoride in potable water with coacervation by electrophoresis using an aluminum anode. Fluoride. 1987; 20:54–63)

supplements of this ion. Fluoride is included in many modern drugs, such as corticosteroids.

Susheela[33] advises care in use of fluoride in the prevention of dental caries and notes that fluorosis may complicate the therapeutic use of fluoride in treating osteoporosis. Where fluoride is added to water supplies to prevent caries, levels fall short of that needed to produce fluorosis but a possible positive relationship between water fluoridation levels and hip fracture rate has been reported from Britain and the USA[35] with levels from zero to 1 mg/l but further work is needed to control the effect of other variables. Medication for osteoporosis with 75 mg/day of sodium fluoride which is greatly in excess of the recom-

mended intake of 1 mg/day, resulted in a greater frequency of fractures than in untreated controls (*see* Chapter 24)

Primary prevention of fluorosis is essential as treatment is not effective. Lowering the fluoride intake can at best arrest progression of bone disease. Activated alumina has been used to reduce fluoride in water. Ming and colleagues[36] have developed a method using electrolysis with an aluminium anode, which also removes bacteria. Serpentine (meta-silicate of magnesium) has also been used to remove fluorine from water[37]. Teotia[38] found that by putting down deeper wells, water with less fluorine could be obtained. In Sinjiang and Inner Mongolia in

China, water supplies have been successfully changed to achieve lower fluorine levels[39]. Filtering through burned bone is the cheapest and most practicable method.

OBESITY

Obesity is widely considered to be a risk factor for osteoarthritis of hip and knees (*see* Chapter 10), gout and overuse syndromes. In advanced arthritis enforced inactivity can lead to further weight gain. Though weight control is not definitively proven to have primary preventive effect on osteoarthrosis, it is highly desirable for many other reasons, in particular as a cardioprotective measure.

IRON

Iron overload may result from the high iron content of cheap wine, high red meat intake, iron-containing medication or injections, and cause chondrocalcinosis and pseudogout as described in Chapter 23. This may also occur in hemochromatosis, a hereditary condition, the expression of which may be facilitated by exogenous factors, e.g. transfusions[40] or as above noted, dietary indiscretions. This is illustrated by a father and son with hemochromatosis. The father, a butcher, presented with knee pain due to chondrocalcinosis (Figure 4), and was treated by venesection for some years, which arrested his disease. Venesection was discontinued when he developed iron deficiency anemia from the therapeutic leechings, and as a result of his decreased access to inexpensive red meat upon retirement. The son later presented with diabetes mellitus and cirrhosis of the liver but no arthritis. Low serum iron in rheumatoid is usually due to failure of utilization. Though piridoxine, histidine and zinc may also be low and copper and ceruloplasmin may be raised in rheumatoid arthritis, these changes are thought to reflect inflammatory activity and have no dietary or causal significance in this disease[41].

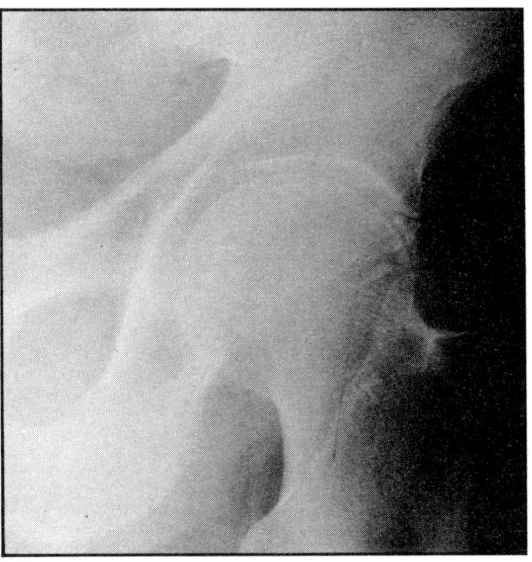

Figure 4 depiction of chondrocalcinosis

L-TRYPTOPHAN AND THE TOXIC OIL SYNDROME

Use of this amino acid, available over the counter as a mild sedative, was recently associated with the eosinophilia myalgia syndrome which may simulate scleroderma and other connective tissue diseases[42–44]. By February 1990, 1305 cases had been reported in the USA. Following withdrawal of a particular formulation of this amino acid the condition has essentially disappeared. Whether this was due to L-tryptophan itself or a contaminant introduced during manufacture or a breakdown product in a particular batch from one manufacturer is not yet clear[45].

Previously in 1981, a clinical complex with certain similar features appeared in epidemic form in Spain and was attributed to the use of rapeseed cooking oil denatured with aniline, a toxic contaminant. The toxic oil syndrome resulted in more than 20000 reported cases and over 300 deaths[46,47], and was characterized by myalgia, scleroderma-like skin changes, nerve damage, joint contractures and the sicca syndrome.

294

LAY BELIEFS

The claims of laymen, pseudoprofessionals and professionals who uncritically believe that rheumatism can be prevented or cured by an enormous variety of seemingly illogical maneuvres are very difficult to assess. The promoters of these agents may not be aware of the remarkable healing power of nature, but may assume the credit for the results of her labors. For instance 95% of back pains will settle with the passage of time (a good result; even better than a placebo). This can be explained since most rheumatic symptoms are cyclical. Help will be sought when symptoms are at their worst so the trend will be back to the previous condition (the reversion to the mean phenomenon). In addition to this time effect, boosted by belief of the treater and the treated in efficacy (faith-healing), increases this effect at least for mood and pain problems. The healer's belief in his/her own powers increases since, usually, only his successful cases report back so that the power of his suggestion increases. The author has discussed this phenomenon in detail[48].

It could be argued that this is a harmless, or even partly helpful, phenomenon, which might free the physician to spend his time more effectively on the more seriously ill. Unfortunately many of these patients do have major complaints needing a therapy that is more effective than a placebo. If the public can be educated regarding these false therapeutic gods, the outlook for most rheumatic complaints is indeed good, and the optimism that reassurance brings is more lasting than a continuous search for a promised cure. Education in stress and pain coping is of use, as suggested above, for the overuse syndromes in Chapter 7, and may be taught by faith-healing groups. Others[49] view faith-healing, especially if associated with religion, to be advantageous. This may well satisfy basic needs for direction, communication and support. The qualified doctor, as father figure, consciously or otherwise, dispenses faith-

healing in any interaction with patients, though he may not feel comfortable with this thought. Despite all this, many will put their hopes for a panacea in diet.

A serious objection to 'alternative' medicines is the tendency for its pedlars to claim that their particular nostrum will prevent rheumatic disease. This may mean that proven preventive methods are neglected and that the public may expend large amounts on supporting a profitable industry to their own ultimate disadvantage. As shown in this section, some alleged health food supplements can actually induce rheumatic symptoms, i.e. excessive iron, calcium and vitamins A and D. Public education is necessary for prevention of these problems.

PREVENTION

In general, what *needs* to be done in the primary prevention of dietary disorders is clear. What *can* be done must be planned according to the resources of the affected population. Public education must be tailored to local needs, traditional dietary patterns and budgetary limitations. For further reading on this difficult subject the reader is referred to the monograph on nutrition and rheumatic diseases edited by Panush[50].

REFERENCES

1. Cuny JF, Schmultz JL, Terver MN, Aussedat R, Cointin M, Weber M, Beurey J. Effets rheumatologiques de l'etretinate. Ann Dermatol Venereol. 1989; 116:95–102
2. Peck GL, Olsen TG, Yoder FW, Strauss JS *et al.* Prolonged remissions of cystic and conglobate acne with 13-cis-retinoic acid. N Engl J Med. 1979; 300:329
3. Mezes M, Bartosiewicz G, Nemeth J. Comparative investigations on vitamin A level of plasma in some rheumatic diseases. Clin Rheumatol. 1986; 5:221–224
4. Lussier A, Menard H, Myhal D, Gagne M *et al.* DISH, diabetes and retinol metabolism: the physiopathologic core. PANLAR Congress Guadalajara 1990, Abstr. 287

5. Digiovanna JJ, Helfgott RK, Gerber LH. Extraspinal tendon and ligament calcification associated with long-term therapy with etretinate. N Engl J Med. 1986; 315:1177–1182

6. Darmawan J. Rheumatic conditions in the northern part of central Java. Doctoral thesis. Erasmus University, Holland. 1988

7. Eijkman. Beriberi. Quoted in Goodman and Gilman, New York, MacMillan, 1966, p. 1653

8. Yang J. Kaschin–Beck disease: study of cause and intervention measures. Report to WHO, 1989

9. Combs GK, Combs SB. The role of selenium in nutrition. Academic Press, 1986, pp. 367–371

10. Van Rij A, Thomson CD, McKenzie JM, Robinson MF. Selenium deficiency in total parenteral nutrition. Am J Clin Nutr. 1979; 32:2076–2085

11. Kien Cl, Ganther HE. Manifestations of chronic selenium deficiency in a child receiving total parenteral nutrition. Am J Clin Nutr. 1983; 37:319

12. Robinson MF, Stewart RDH, Thompson CD, Snow PG, Aquires IHW. Effect of daily supplements of selenium on patients with muscular complaints in Otago and Canterbury. N Z Med J. 1981; 93:289–292

13. Thompson CD. Clinical consequences and assessment of low selenium status. N Z Med J. 1991; 104:376–377

14. Hill J, Bird HA. Failure of selenium to improve osteoarthritis. Br J Rheumatol. 1990; 29:211–213

15. Langley GB, Sheppeard H, Wigley RD. Placebo therapy in Rheumatoid arthritis. Clin Exp Rheumatol. 1983; 1:17–21

16. Wigley RD, Vlieg M. α-tocopherol and blood pressure in PN/n mice. Aust J Exp Biol Med. 1978; 56:631–637

17. Sperling RI. The effects of fish oil fatty acids on inflammatory mediator generation. Proc. ILAR Congress. Rio de Janeiro, 1989, pp. 632–634

18. Cleland LG, French JK, Betts WH, Murphy GA, Elliott MJ. Clinical and biochemical effects of dietary fish oil supplements in rheumatoid arthritis. J Rheumatol. 1988; 15:1471–1475

19. Kremer JM, Jubiz W, Michalek A, Rynes RI et al. Fish oil fatty acid supplementation in active rheumatoid arthritis. Ann Intern Med. 1987; 106: 497–503

20. Kremer JM, Lawrence DA, Jubiz W, DiGiacomo R et al. Dietary fish oil and olive oil supplementation in patients with rheumatoid arthritis. Arthritis Rheum. 1990; 33:810–820

21. Chou CT, Pai L, Chang DM, Lee CF, Liang MH, Schumacher RH. The epidemiologic studies of rheumatic diseases in Taiwan. ILAR 17th congress, Rio de Janeiro, 1989, Abstr. p. 418

22. Wigley RD, Zhang NC, Zeng CQ, Duff I, Bennett P. ILAR study of rheumatic disease in China III. APLAR Bull. 1989. 7:51–55

23. Wigley RD, Zhang NC, Duff I, Bennett P. ILAR study of rheumatic disease in China IV. APLAR Bull. 1989; 7:72–75

24. Wigley RD, Prior IAM, Salmond C, Stanley D, Pinfold B. Rheumatic complaints in Tokelau: II. A comparison of migrants in New Zealand and non-migrants. The Tokelau island migrant study. Rheumatol Int. 1987; 7:61–65

25. Oen K, Postl B, Chalmers IM et al. Rheumatic diseases in an Inuit population. Arthritis Rheum. 1986; 29:65–74

26. Boyer GS, Lanier AP, Tempin DW. Prevalence rates of spondyloarhtropathies. Rheumatoid arthritis, and other rheumatic disorders in an Alaskan Eskimo population. J Rheumatol. 1988; 15:678–683

27. Huskisson EC, Scott J, Bryans R. Seatone is ineffective in rheumatoid arthritis. Br Med J. 1981; 282:1358–1359

28. Veerapen K, Wigley RD, Valkenburg HA. The Malaysian COPCORD study. 1989 (unpublished data)

29. Buchanan HM, Preston SJ, Brooks PM, Buchanan WW. Is diet important in rheumatoid arthritis. Br J Rheumatol. 1991; 30:125–134

30. McCallum TI. Cadmium poisoning. In Raffle et al., eds., Hunter's Diseases of Occupations. London, Hodder and Stoughton, 1987, pp. 257–259

31. Panush RS. Possible role of food sensitivity in arthritis. Ann Allergy. 1988; 61:31–35

32. Kaminsky LS, Mahoney MC, Leach J, Melius O, Miller MJ. Fluoride benefits and risks of exposure. Crit Rev Oral Biol Med. 1990; 1:261–281

33. Susheela AK. Elements in Health and Disease. India, Said Hamdard University Press, 1987, pp. 225–230

34. Teotia SPS, Teotia M. Endemic skeletal fluorosis. Clinical and etiological variants. Fluoride. 1988; 21:39–44

35. Cooper C, Wickham CAC, Barker DJR. Water fluoridation and hip fracture. JAMA. 1991; 266:513–514

36. Ming L, Sun RY, Zhang JH, Bina Y, Wei L, Liu P, Kei CF. Elimination of excess fluoride in potable water with coacervation by electrolysis using an aluminium anode. Fluoride 1987; 20: 54–62

37. Marathamutu M, Reddy JV. A native index of defluoridation by serpentine. Fluoride. 1987; 20: 64–67

38. Teotia SPS, Teotia DP, Singh DP, Rathour RS, Singh CV, Tomar NPS Nath M, Singh NP. Endemic fluorosis: change to deeper bore holes as a practical community-acceptable approach to its eradication. Fluoride 198?; ??: 48–52

39. Editorial. Environmental fluoride problems in China. Fluoride. 21:164–165.

40. Abbott DF, Gresham GA. Arthropathy in transfusional siderosis. Br Med J. 1972; 1:418–419

41. Espiranza B, Robinson DR, Nutrition and rheumatic diseases. In Kelly *et al.*, eds., Textbook of Rheumatology. Philadelphia, WB Saunders, 1989. pp. 560–561

42. Shulman L. The eosinophilia-myalgia syndrome associated with ingestion of L-tryptophane. Arthritis Rheum. 1990; 33:913–917

43. Kaufman LD, Seidman RJ, Gruber GL. l-Tryptophane associated eosinophilic perimyositis, neuritis, and fasciitis. A clinicopathologic and laboratory study of 25 patients. Medicine. 1990; 187–199

44. Martin R, Duffy J. PANLAR Congress, Guadalajara. 1990 Abstracts 49, 50

45. Love LA, Rader LJ, Crofford LJ, Page SW *et al.* L-tryptophane and 1,1′-ethyldibene-bis(tryptophane). A contaminant in eisinophilia myalgia syndrome case-associated l-TRP; cause myofascial thickening and pancreatic fibrosis in Lewis rats. Am Coll Rheumatol. 55th Congress Proc. 1991; Abstr. b201; Ps131.

46. Escribano PM, Atauri MJ, Sanchez MAG. Persistence of respiratory abnormalities four years after onset of toxic oil syndrome. Chest. 1991; 100:336–33

47. Kilbourne EM, La Paz MP, Borda IA, Ruiz-navarro MD, Ohilen RM, Falk H. Toxic oil syndrome: a clinical and epidemiologic summary, including comparisons with the eosinophilia myalgia syndrome. J Am Coll Cardiol. 1991; 18:711–717

48. Wigley RW. Placebo and time therapy: can they be used in rehabilitation and research? 1987; 1:47–52

49. Glik DC. Symbolic, ritual and social dynamics of spiritual healing. Soc Sci Med. 1988; 27:1197–1206

50. Panush RS. Nutrition and rheumatic diseases. Rheum Clin North Am. 1991; 17:254–272

26. DRUG-INDUCED RHEUMATIC PROBLEMS (IATROGENIC DRUGS AND DRUGS OF ABUSE)

Patrick J. Rooney and W. Watson Buchanan

Medicine is a collection of uncertain prescriptions which kill the poor, and succeed sometimes with the rich; and the results of which, collectively taken, are more fatal than useful to mankind. Speak to me no more about these fine things; I am not a man for drugs.

Napoleon Bonaparte

INTRODUCTION

It is a platitude, but nevertheless a truth, that modern medicaments are double-edged weapons, often offering dramatic benefit to the patient, but also at times causing iatrogenic illness. Antirheumatic drugs are no exception and, indeed, cause a considerable morbidity in themselves, and also not an insignificant mortality. Adverse drug reactions are generally easily recognized when they affect organs other than the musculoskeletal system, e.g. the gastrointestinal tract, but are more difficult to detect when they impact on a system well known for producing vague symptoms in the face of inflammation. This problem forms the basis for the present review.

CORTICOSTEROIDS

One of the major causes of morbidity and mortality among patients with rheumatic disease is long-term corticosteroid therapy[1,2], which causes global osteoporosis, affecting trabecular bone more than cortical bone[3], and all parts of the skeleton[4–8]. There is a direct relationship between the duration and total dose of corticosteroids[9], but age, years since the menopause, and duration and severity of arthritis also contribute[6–8]. Osteoporosis also occurs with intermittent corticosteroid regimens, and apparently no less than with continuous therapy. Corticosteroids cause increased bone resorption[10] and generally inhibit, while low doses enhance certain anabolic processes, such as collagen and protein synthesis of osteocytes[11]. Receptors for corticosteroids have also been demonstrated on osteocytes[12]. Corticosteroids also have effects on absorption of calcium from the gastrointestinal tract, on vitamin D metabolism, on the renal excretion of calcium and phosphorus, and on sex hormones, parathormone, prostaglandins and others. Nonetheless, the precise role, if any, that each of these effects plays on the pathogenesis of osteoporosis is unknown[13].

Osteoporosis is clinically silent until bone failure occurs. The axial skeleton appears to be more prone to fractures, but the entire skeleton is vulnerable. Certain races appear to be more susceptible to fractures, for example, fair-haired, light-skinned Caucasians in contrast to Africans. This may to a large extent reflect a greater pre-existing bone mass in the latter. Bone mass decreases with age, especially in females, so that elderly women receiving corticosteroid therapy are especially prone to fractures. Skin atrophy with bruising, seen in both the elderly and patients receiving corticosteroid therapy, has been found to correlate with spinal osteoporosis[14].

The diagnosis of osteoporosis is generally made by radiography, and may be appreciated in radiographs of the hip joint, and by other techniques (*see* Chapter 24). In the long bones, the secondary trabeculae are resorbed, the primary weight-bearing trabeculae are accentuated and the bone cortex is attenuated. In the vertebral bodies resorption of the secondary trabeculae results in apparent increased density of the cortical end plates, which may become biconcave due to central weakening, giving rise to the so-called 'codfish' or 'fish mouth' appearance. The apparent increased density of the vertebral end-plates is often referred to as 'penciling'. The relative retention of the vertical trabeculae, which are subject to greatest stress, gives rise to a vertical streaking effect, imparting an appearance that has been fancifully likened to the handiwork of an amateur painter. These become especially apparent in the vertebral body, and indeed may be the earliest radiological sign. Eventually, the vertebrae collapse in a wedge-shaped fashion, and the vertebral bodies may become sclerosed due to compression of bone. It is not possible to differentiate a wedge-shaped vertebral fracture from a secondary tumor unless other features elsewhere allow this distinction. Microfractures may also occur in osteoporotic bones and cause pain, but these cannot be identified with plain radiographs.

Cortical changes in the long bones may be most apparent in the metacarpals and phalanges, and are characterized by small scalloped defects and a decreased density of the peripheral portion of the cortex. In acute osteoporosis of adults, a 'spotty' form may be apparent which is characterized by small, sphenoid, lucencies within the carpal or tarsal bones and the ends of the metacarpals and metatarsals. These changes are related to the blood supply, which in the peripheral portion of the adult bone cortex is received from the periosteum. In late adolescence, a lamellated cortex is often present, especially in the bones of the feet, but also, to a lesser extent in the hands. In young patients, linear translucent bands may appear in the metaphyses, due to residual hypervascular blood supply of the epiphyseal plate during growth.

It has been suggested that patients receiving corticosteroid therapy should be routinely screened for osteoporosis[15], using sensitive techniques[16], e.g. dual energy X-ray absorptiometry[17], or dual photon absorbiometry. However, the only known method of preventing corticosteroid-induced osteoporosis is to discontinue corticosteroid therapy. Estrogens may reduce the rate of development of osteoporosis in postmenopausal females[18], but do not prevent it. There is no evidence that any of the currently recommended methods of treatment such as calcium and vitamin D supplements, estrogen therapy, fluoride or physical exercise can prevent the disease in corticosteroid treated patients[15]. In contrast, Reid and colleagues[19] have suggested that low-dose oral corticosteroid therapy may prevent the development of osteoporosis in patients with rheumatoid arthritis due to improvement in mobility.

Osteonecrosis

Corticosteroid therapy is frequently cited in textbooks as one of the most common causes of osteonecrosis (Figure 1). However, it is not clear whether the osteonecrosis is related to vascular occlusion, as it appears to be in systemic lupus erythematosus, fat embolism, or as many believe, the final result of osteochondral fractures, which cause bone collapse and resultant joint disorganization. Whatever the pathogenesis, the lesion is most commonly seen in the hip and knee. Prevention is only possible by avoiding corticosteroid therapy, the adverse effects of which are ameliorated by the smallest possible dose for the patients'

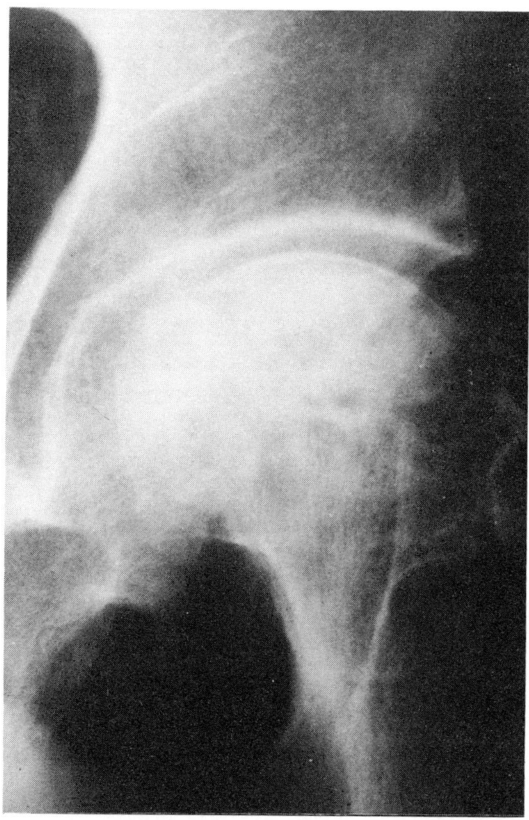

Figure 1 Necrosis of the femoral head in a man with severe systemic lupus erythematosus who had been treated with moderate doses of prednisone for more than 10 years. Both hips and both ankles were affected

particular needs[20]. Bone scintigraphy is the best method of diagnosis in the early stages, and reduction in radionuclide uptake may precede any change on conventional radiographs[21]. In early stages, core decompression is recommended[22], which relieves intraosseous pressure and creates a channel through which bone can regrow[23]. The latter may be promoted by insertion of a cortical bone graft. When joint destruction ensues patients usually require a replacement arthroplasty[24].

Myopathy

Muscle weakness and wasting are common in rheumatic disease and make a diagnosis of ster-oid myopathy difficult, especially as muscle enzyme levels remain normal. Corticosteroids, especially 9α-fluoro-corticosteroids are a known cause of myopathy, an insidious and relatively painless condition that most commonly affects the shoulder and pelvic girdle muscles. Usually the myopathy occurs with high-dose therapy, e.g. 40 mg prednisone/day or equivalent[25], may occur after intravenous pulse therapy[26], and is related in part to the hypokalemia induced by corticosteroids. Muscle biopsy in corticosteroid myopathy usually shows atrophy of type 2B fibers, although the electromyographic results are usually normal[27]. Prevention requires avoidance of corticosteroid therapy if possible, especially with halogenated compounds, and alternate day therapy. Other drugs may also cause muscle weakness, especially D-penicillamine and chloroquine, or antacids by phosphorous depletion.

Intra-articular corticosteroids

Intra-articular injection of corticosteroids is widely employed both for rheumatoid arthritis and osteoarthritis, and osteonecrosis may occur after repeated injections, especially in weight-bearing joints. Hollander and co-workers[28] reported such damage in 79 joints in 62 patients in a total of 23 500 injections in 8000 patients. The etiology of this osteonecrosis is uncertain, and is likely to be neuropathic[29], although a direct toxic effect on cartilage cannot be excluded[30]. Joint sepsis as a result of intra-articular corticosteroid injections is an extremely rare[31] event that could be reduced further by rapid skin sterilization (i.e. preparation of the skin with cetrimide in surgical spirit) and the exclusive use of disposable, factory-sterilized needles and syringes, single-dose vials or ampoules and scrupulous no-touch technique. Tendon and ligamentous rupture may also occur, but is not uncommon with tendon sheath and ligament injections[32].

The commonest cause of joint pathology following intra-articular injection is crystal-induced synovitis[33]. Some subjects develop skin flushing between 24 and 48 hours following injection of triamcinalone or betamethasone preparations. This effect was reproduced by injection of the pure preservative. This rarely occurs after injection of methyl prednisone which contains a different preservative. (Personal communication, Ed.)

MISCELLANEOUS DRUGS

Five patients have been described who developed severe polyarthritis while being treated with cimetidine for duodenal ulcer[34]. The arthritis disappeared when the drug was discontinued, and reappeared when it was restarted in two of the patients. The authors postulated that histamine H_2 blockade in joints might decrease the vascular clearance of inflammatory mediators. Whatever the pathogenesis, the incidence of this complication is very low. Quinidine-induced polyarthritis was reported by Kertes and Hunt[35]. This resolved on discontinuing the drug and reappeared on rechallenge. β-Blocking drugs have been implicated in arthritic symptoms[36–38]; amphotericin B has been reported to cause both muscle and joint pain[39]; it is uncertain whether levamisole may cause polyarthritis since the reported cases had also been diagnosed of Crohn's disease and Behçet's disease, where arthritis is a feature of the primary disease[40–42]. Muscle aches and pains may be induced by medications affecting fluids and electrolytes, e.g. magnesium deficiency may result from excessive purgation causing muscle pains and cramps[43,44]. The shoulder–hand syndrome has long been attributed to barbiturates, especially phenobarbitone[45–47] and to isoniazid[48], but no controlled studies have been performed to prove an association. Serum sickness type reactions to drugs is frequently associated with a severe polyarthritis[49].

DISEASE-MODIFYING DRUGS

The so-called disease-modifying or remission-inducing drugs may cause rheumatic symptoms and signs.

D-Penicillamine

This agent may cause a variety of musculoskeletal complaints, including polymyositis[50–53], dermatomyositis[54–56] or a myasthenia gravis-like syndrome (see below), each of which may be accompanied by acetylcholine antibodies[57] A systemic lupus erythematosus (SLE)-like syndrome may also occur in D-penicillamine-treated patients[65], and is often associated with high titers of anti-DNA antibody, unlike other forms of drug-induced SLE. Scleroderma has also been reported following D-penicillamine therapy[66]. The only distinction between D-penicillamine-induced and spontaneous polymyositis and dermatomyositis is that the disease subsides on cessation of therapy in the former[59]. Recurrence may occur with resumption of therapy[59] and with subsequent exposure to ampicillin[51], perhaps because of molecular structural similarities between these two drugs. The pathogenesis of D-penicillamine-induced polymyositis and dermatomyositis is unclear[58], although its ability to induce antinuclear[59], antistriational[60], and acetylcholine receptor antibodies, implies that an immunological mechanism is at play. Extractable nuclear autoantibodies are not found in D-penicillamine polymyositis and dermatomyositis[61], as in idiopathic disease[62]. Anti-DNA antibodies have also been described in iatrogenic polymyositis and dermatomyositis, but without clinical evidence of SLE[63]. An association with HLA-B18, -B35 and -DR4 haplotypes have been reported in the iatrogenic disease; B8 and DR3 haplotypes are increased in the idiopathic forms of the disease[59,64]. Thus, although there may be a genetic predisposition to these diseases in patients treated with D-penicillamine, this is not strong enough to deny an individual patient the benefit of D-penicillamine therapy. D-penicillamine can induce a number of different autoantibodies[67] and affect T lymphocytes[68–70], but it is not clear whether these play any role in causation.

The pathogenesis of D-penicillamine-induced myasthenia gravis is probably immune-mediated in a similar manner to the spontaneous disease. Acetylcholine receptor (AChR) antibodies usually decline when D-penicillamine is discontinued, and as clinical improvement occurs. The antibody probably blocks transmission by combining with the post-synaptic AChR. A high incidence of other autoimmune diseases, including SLE, thyroiditis and immune complex nephritis, in D-penicillamine induced myasthenia gravis supports an immunological mechanism. Thymoma has not been reported in D-penicillamine induced myasthenia gravis. HLA antigens have not been studied in a sufficient number of patients with iatrogenic myasthenia gravis to determine whether there might be a genetic basis, as has been shown for spontaneous myasthenia gravis. Although D-penicillamine induced myasthenia gravis is rare, it is important to recognize as it is reversible; if not, it may be fatal. The clinical features of iatrogenic myasthenia gravis are identical to those of the spontaneous disease, and thus must be differentiated from neuromyotonia secondary to D-penicillamine therapy[71]. An Ehler–Danlos-like syndrome has been reported in a newborn baby possibly related to D-penicillamine treatment during the mother's pregnancy[72]. Unusual creaking of the joints in patients with rheumatoid arthritis treated with D-penicillamine has been reported[73].

Crysotherapy

Transient arthralgia and joint swelling have been reported 6–24 h after injection of gold, and since it was only been reported with gold sodium thiomalate[74], it may be caused by the particulate nature of this compound.

Antimalarial drugs

Myopathy, neuromyopathy and myasthenia gravis have been reported following the use of antimalarial drugs[75–77], and appear to most prominently affect the granular type I muscle fibers[78]. In general, myopathy is related to the dose[78] and duration of therapy[79]. Estes and colleagues[80] have admirably summarized the electrophysiological and histological features of antimalarial drug-induced neurotoxicity.

Cytotoxic drugs

Patients treated with single-agent drugs or combination chemotherapy may develop aseptic bone necrosis, especially of the femoral head[81–84]. This complication usually occurs after 3–6 weeks of therapy, but occasionally sooner[84]. Ansell and co-workers[85] reported a patient with psoriatic arthritis treated with methotrexate who developed bone infarcts. Children with acute lymphatic leukemia treated with long-term oral methotrexate may develop severe osteoporosis, especially of the lower limbs, which may result in fractures and be associated with a thick dense zone of calcification close to the epiphysis[86–88]. The cause of this methotrexate osteopathy has been attributed to increased resorption of bone[88]. Extensive nodule formation has been described during methotrexate therapy for rheumatoid arthritis[89]; since methotrexate is used only in the most severe cases, the effects of drugs may be confused with the underlying disease process. Cytotoxic therapy may result in hyperuricemia and acute gouty arthritis[90]. Acute gout has been reported, especially with cyclosporin A and if the patient is also receiving diuretics[91–93]. Acute myopathy has also been ascribed to cyclosporine[94]. Myopathy, possibly due to azathioprine, was described in two patients[95]. Lipid storage myopathy has been reported in a patient treated with azathioprine. This fully recovered with L-carnitine therapy[96].

RAYNAUD'S PHENOMENON

Raynaud's phenomenon was first described in 1862, and is most commonly induced by exposure to low temperatures. Classically, it consists of episodic digital ischemia provoked by cold or emotion, and is manifest by pallor due to vasospasm, followed by cyanosis due to deoxygenation of venous blood, and rubor due to reactive hyperemia on return of blood flow[97]. It affects 5–10% of the population in temperate climates, and may on occasion be so severe as to cause digital ulceration and gangrene[98]. The full triphasic color change is no longer considered to be essential for diagnosis[97]. There are, in fact, no internationally agreed diagnostic criteria[99] other than the subdivision into a primary or idiopathic form, and form that is secondary to etiologies listed in Table 1[100]. Hormonal changes during the normal menstrual cycle[101] and smoking[102] can increase the severity of an attack.

The commonest occupational cause of Raynaud's phenomenon is vibration disease[103]. The pathogenesis of vibration-induced Raynaud's phenomenon remains obscure[104]. The most popular hypothesis is hyperactivity of the sympathetic nervous system, since vasoconstriction has been abolished by proximal nerve blockade[105]. Some workers believe that the primary lesion is in the vessel wall[106,107], while others have invoked rheological changes in the blood[108]. Whatever the pathogenesis, prevention is the only therapy[109]. Reversal of vibration-induced Raynaud's phenomenon can only be achieved in the very early stages[110]. If occupational vibration cannot be avoided, it can be mitigated by installing antivibration devices in the handles of tools and by installation of vibration-free bases under machinery[103]. Polystyrene foam-layered gloves also can help reduce high frequency vibration and protect against cold[103]. There are no international guidelines regarding pre-employment medical standards to prevent vibration-induced Raynaud's phenomenon[103] (*see* Chapter 22).

The toxic oil syndrome due to ingestion of cooking oil from plastic containers in Spain resulted in scleroderma-like changes in the limbs, which may be accompanied by Raynaud's phenome-

non[111,112]. Acro-osteolysis may subsequently develop[113,114]. The exact substance present in the cooking oil responsible for the syndrome has not been identified[112], but a recent epidemic of eosinophilic myalgia syndrome attributable to tryptophan ingestion[115] has led to suggestions that the toxic oil syndrome was an early manifestation of this disorder[116–118]. Eosinophilic myalgia syndrome consists of a protean collection of clinical features and may present to many different clinical specialists. It affects all ages but has a very striking female preponderance[119,120] and an even more striking predilection for white Caucasians. Eosinophilia myalgia syndrome generally develops over several weeks with intense disabling muscle pain and fatigue. There is often a low-grade fever with cough, shortness of breath and a pulmonary infiltrate. A maculopapular or urticarial rash occurs in most patients and some tightening of the skin of the limbs suggestive of eosinophilic fasciitis[119]. Although true arthritis is rare, joint contractures of elbows and knees is common. There is anemia, and a striking eosinophilia but immunoglobulins and serum antibody profiles are usually normal. Almost all patients had been ingesting L-tryptophan, although discontinuation of this agent allowed only a slow recovery of the syndrome. Steroids are only of limited therapeutic value[115,116,121].

Vinyl chloride is used in the plastics industry and may cause Raynaud's phenomenon as well as acro-osteolysis of the fingers, finger clubbing and scleroderma-like skin changes[122,123]. Capillary microscopy has demonstrated dilated capillary loops in the nail fold similar to those in scleroderma[124], and angiography has demonstrated obstructions and tortuosity of digital arteries[125]. Prevention, i.e. controlling exposure to the vinyl chloride monomer, is the only means of avoiding the illness[112].

Raynaud's phenomenon has also been described in workers exposed to certain solvents, such as

Table 1 Secondary causes of Raynaud's phenomenon. (Reproduced with kind permission from Dr France Joyal and the Editor of 'Diagnosis'

Occupational
pianist's or typist's vasospasm
vibration tool users, e.g. chain saw or pneumatic drill operators
exposure to vinyl chloride, and solvents such as perchlorethylene and trichloroethylene, and silica

Traumatic and neurogenic
frostbite
thoracic outlet and shoulder-hand syndrome
carpal tunnel syndrome
paralysis and peripheral neuropathy
disorders of arterial supply
atheromatous obliterans
arteriovenous shunt, brachial aneurysm
Takayasu's disease
thromboangiitis obliterans

Connective tissue disease
progressive systemic sclerosis, systemic lupus erythematosus, and dermatomyositis
Sjögren's syndrome
primary pulmonary hypertension

Blood disorders
cold hemagglutination
cryoglobulinemia
polycythemia
paraproteinemia
macroglobulinemia

Iatrogenic
ergotamine
β-blockers (with no intrinsic sympathomimetic activity)
bromocriptine
bleomycin, *cis*-platinum, vinblastine; nicotine resin complex
pseudoephedrine

perchlorethylene and trichloroethylene. These workers subsequently developed scleroderma-like illnesses[112]. In contrast, workers exposed to certain epoxy-resins develop sclerodermatous induration of the skin, but not Raynaud's phenomenon[112]. Exposure to silica has been reported to cause progressive systemic sclerosis and Raynaud's phenomena[125]. Although exposure to silica is less well established in progressive systemic sclerosis than pneumoconiosis, it would seem prudent to control worker exposure by the use of masks and ventilation[112]. Silastic breast implants may induce Raynaud's phenomenon and scleroderma[126]. Improvement does not occur after mastectomy, and drug therapy has proved disappointing[127]. Augmentation mammoplasty is used widely in Japan. The complications which arise indicate that this operation is unlikely to be approved for cosmetic purposes but may still be permitted following mastectomy.

Vasospasm of the digital vessels leading to gangrene occurred in ergot poisoning due to eating rye or wheat bread infected with the parasitic fungus, *Claviceps purpurea*. Today, ergotism may result from excessive and prolonged medicinal use of ergotamine for migraine. Other drugs which may cause digital vasospasm and Raynaud's phenomenon include: β-blockers (with no intrinsic sympathomimetic activity), bromocriptine, bleomycin, *cis*-platinum, vinblastine, nicotine resin complex, and pseudoephidrine[100] (*see* Chapter 21).

TOBACCO SMOKING

Smoking may induce bronchogenic carcinoma. About 10% of these carcinomas may be complicated by the clinical features of hypertrophic osteoarthropathy[128,129], which usually regresses with removal of the lung tumor or even following thoracotomy[129]. Other complications are common in males with rheumatoid arthritis, and may be associated with smoking. Smokers with rheumatoid arthritis being treated with injectable gold therapy have a sixfold greater amount of gold within erythrocytes than similar patients who do not smoke[129]; this is attributed to the increased concentrations of cyanide and thiocyanate in the blood of smokers, which complex with the gold and enter the red blood cells[129]. The significance of this pharmacokinetic effect remains, as yet, obscure. Smoking reduces the erythrocyte sedimentation rate in patients with rheumatoid arthritis, but again the clinical significance is not known[130]. Patients with arthritic diseases, such as ankylosing spondylitis, and connective tissue disorders, such as progressive systemic sclerosis, who are prone to respiratory complications are well advised to stop smoking. Patients with Raynaud's phenomenon frequently notice benefit on stopping smoking.

Clinical data suggest that cigarette smoking may be linked to osteoarthritis of the spine[131–133], although this may merely reflect anxiety associated with low back pain[134]. Epidemiological evidence that cigarette smoking is associated with osteoporosis continues to mount[135], and this association may be related to an earlier menopause[136], lower body weight ('the slender smoker') or to chronic lung disease and systemic acidosis. Everson and colleagues[137] have shown that even passive smoking may be associated with early menopause. Cigarette smoking also has a direct effect on the hepatic biotransformation of estrogens. As a result of increased hepatic 2-hydroxylation of estradiol, 2-hydroxyestrogens are formed, which have less effect on bone[138] either directly or by competition with estradiol at estrogen binding sites[139]. Other effects of nicotinic alkaloids on estrogen biotransformation have been described, and may affect bone metabolism[140–142]. Calcium absorption is inversely related to the amount of cigarette smoking[143]. Not only is cigarette smoking a factor in

postmenopausal bone loss in the spine[135], but also in the bones of the upper and lower limbs[144,145]. Smoking is of particular importance in leading to hip and wrist fractures, especially in thin women[146,147], even when receiving estrogens[148]. Obesity protects against hip and wrist fractures, and can overcome the effects of smoking[148].

DRUG-INDUCED SYSTEMIC LUPUS ERYTHEMATOSUS

A lupus-like syndrome[149] may be caused by a wide range of drugs, in particular hydralazine, and procainamide which is the most potent[150]. With 100-mg daily doses of hydralazine some 15% of patients will develop antinuclear antibodies, and some 5–10% SLE: in contrast, some 50–100% of patients receiving 1.25 g procainamide daily doses can be expected to develop antinuclear antibodies, and some 25%, SLE[151]. Antinuclear antibodies develop in 15–80% of patients with tuberculosis treated with isoniazid, but the development of SLE is extremely rare[152].

Whether anticonvulsants cause drug-induced SLE is uncertain. Most workers believe that the disease was exacerbated rather than caused by the drug, especially as the disease often persists for years[153]. Antinuclear antibodies, including antibodies to denatured DNA frequently occur in patients receiving chlorpromazine, but these patients do not usually develop SLE[154,155]. Likewise, patients treated with methyldopa develop antinuclear antibodies[156] in addition to positive Coombs tests[157] and hemolytic anemia[158], but not SLE. Another drug evoking positive antinuclear antibody tests without clinical disease is chlorthalidone[156].

Of the numerous other drugs which have been implicated to cause drug-induced SLE, such as the sulfonamides and penicillin and oral contraceptives, most authorities believe that they have merely caused an exacerbation of pre-existing disease[159–161].

Drug-induced SLE differs in a number of respects from the disease arising *de novo*: The illness ceases when the drug is stopped[162], and there is a higher incidence of pleuro-pericardial involvement than in idiopathic SLE, although this may be because most of the patients are elderly[163,164]. Involvement of the central nervous system and kidneys is rare in drug-induced SLE; anemia and leukopenia are less common[153,160] The sex ratio is the same in iatrogenic lupus, but blacks appear to be rarely affected[160], and although the disease is usually mild, fulminant SLE may develop with renal involvement[153,165]. The immune profile of drug-induced lupus also differs from spontaneous SLE: although antibodies to denatured DNA are found not infrequently[166], antibodies to native DNA and to Sm antigen are rarely present[167,168]; low complement levels are unusual in iatrogenic SLE. (Additional references to drug-induced SLE are included[169–176].)

HYPERURICEMIA AND GOUT

Oral diuretics are the most commonly used drugs to cause hyperuricemia and acute gouty arthritis, and approximately two-thirds of those treated with oral diuretics, such as thiazides, furosemide and ethacrynic acid, develop hyperuricemia[177–180], although this is of modest degree, 0.04 mmol/l (0.7 mg/dl)[181], even after prolonged therapy[182]. Hyperuricemia is particularly common in patients with hypertension treated with oral diuretics[183], but is also common in untreated hypertension[184,] acute gouty arthritis, however, is rare[180,185]. The mode of action of oral diuretics is complex, but probably is due to extracellular volume depletion, leading to increased renal tubular reabsorption of uric acid, with a consequent reduced filtered load of uric acid[186–188]. Perhaps of greater importance than acute gouty arthritis is the potential risk, especially in elderly patients with reduced renal function, of further kidney impairment secondary to hyperuricemia[189]. Paradoxically, in very high doses, urate excretion is enhanced by chlorothiazide[190], and perhaps by other oral diuretics, as with salicylates, probenecid, phenylbutazone and sulfinpyrazone.

Acute gouty attacks should be treated like other cases of primary or secondary gout. Unless there is excessive hyperuricemia, renal calculi, progressive renal failure, or recurrent attacks of gouty arthritis, treatment with uricosuric agents and allopurinol is not necessary.

Salicylates[191] and other drugs such as chlorothiazide[190], pyrazinamide[192], and probenecid, phenylbutazone and sulfinpyrazone, have a biphasic effect on renal urate excretion, causing a reduced uric acid excretion in low dosage and an increase in excretion at high doses. The critical factor, at least for salicylate, is the concentration of free drug in the tubular urine, so that alkalinization which promotes the renal excretion of salicylate also increases renal urate excretion. Salicylates at plasma concentrations exceeding 50 µg/ml diminish the uricosuric effect of probenecid[193] and sulfinpyrazone[194]. Neither acetaminophen nor ibuprofen have this effect[195]. Nicotinic acid and the antituberculous drug, ethambutol, may also cause hyperuricemia by reduction of renal urate excretion.

Saturnine gout has been recognized since ancient times, and lead poisoning, associated with alcoholism, may have contributed significantly to the decline of the Roman Empire[196]. Lead poisoning affects those who drink 'moonshine' whiskey (which is distilled in copper tubing, using lead solder) in America[197], and as a result of lead paint in Australia[198] and in the urban US population[199], and leaded petroleum in Spain[200]. Renal failure in lead poisoning has been reported in 6–50% of patients[200,201], and is generally implicated as the cause of hyperuricemia. Patients who present with gout and renal failure should always be tested for lead poisoning[202–205]. Increased serum lead concentrations have been reported in patients with primary gout in Glasgow, Scotland, who otherwise showed no evidence of lead toxicity[206]. The significance of this observation is obscure. Graziano and Blum[207] have recently found that wines and spirits stored in crystal decanters for a long time contain lead at concentrations up to 21530 µg/l which may partly explain why the rich are more commonly affected by gouty arthritis.

Alcohol has long been associated with gout. Habitual intake of alcohol and serum urate concentrations show a strong correlation[208–210], and acute ingestion or intravenous infusion of alcohol results in hyperuricemia[211]. Patients who suffer from gout consume more alcohol than normal subjects[209,210,212]. Hyperlacticacidemia has traditionally been the explanation why alcohol causes hyperuricemia[213], as it appears to also do in fasting[212,213], exercise[214], toxemia of pregnancy and labor[215], glycogen storage disease[216] and chronic beryllium poisoning[217]. However, Faller and Fox[218] showed convincing evidence that alcohol also increased urate production by activation of adenine nucleotide turnover. The effect of alcohol on osteoporosis is discussed in Chapter 24.

CONCLUSIONS

The prevention of these undesirable side-effects of drug treatment requires constant vigilance by the prescriber.

Recommendations include:

(1) Avoid using drugs with major side-effects when simpler measures are available or if there is a safer, equally effective alternative. For instance, the use of hydralazine in hypertension or procainamide for arrhythmias is no longer justified, given the plethora of viable alternatives.

(2) Monitor the blood for early warnings of side-effects, for instance urate levels for those taking diuretics.

(3) Patients should be informed of warning symptoms to watch for. This should preferably be in writing, as people forget quickly. For some drugs such as corticosteroids, cards should be carried with details of dosage at all times, or an engraved bracelet or pendant (Medicalert) should be worn.

(4) Catalogues distributed by the drug firms to all doctors and pharmacies, regularly updated with detail on side-effects, are of great value in developed countries. Abbreviated versions appropriate to the shorter list of drugs available in developing countries are desirable but not likely to be available.

(5) Finally, physicians have to keep constantly in mind that a patient's symptoms may result from medicaments.

Primum non nocere

REFERENCES

1. Lee P, McCusker S, Allison A *et al*. Adverse reactions in patients with rheumatic diseases: retrospective analysis of causes of admissions and outpatient attendance in a specialist centre. Ann Rheum Dis. 1973; 32:565–573
2. Brooks PM, Stephens WH, Stephens MEB, Buchanan WW. How safe are anti-rheumatic drugs? A study of possible iatrogenic deaths in patients with rheumatoid arthritis. Health Bull (SHHD). 1975; 33:108–111
3. Dempster DW, Arlott MA, Herndon CH. Mean wall thickness and formation periods of trabecular bone pockets in corticosteroid-induced osteoporosis. Calcif Tissue Int. 1983; 35:410–417
4. Kennedy AC, Smith DA, Anderson JA, Buchanan WW. Osteoporosis in rheumatoid arthritis: its natural history and statistical prediction. Rheumatologie (Paris). 1974; 4:441–445

5. Kennedy AC, Smith DA, Buchanan WW, Anderson JB, Samuels BB, Jasani MK. Osteoporosis in rheumatoid arthritis. Rheumatologie (Paris). 1974; 4:25–35

6. Kennedy AC, Smith DA, Anton HC, Buchanan WW. Generalised and localised bone loss in patients with rheumatoid arthritis. Scand J Rheumatol. 1975; 4:209–215

7. Kennedy AC, Smith DA, Buchanan WW, Anderson JB, Jasani MK. Bone loss in patients with rheumatoid arthritis. Scand J Rheumatol. 1975; 4:73–79

8. Kennedy AC, Smith DA, Grey G, Jasani MK, Buchanan WW. Osteoporosis in patients with rheumatoid arthritis. Ann Rheum Dis. 1975; 34:542–543

9. Shubin H. Long term administration of corticosteroids in pulmonary disease. Dis Chest. 1965; 48:287–290

10. Reid IR. Steroid osteoporosis. Calcif Tissue Int. 1989; 45:63–67

11. Dietrich JW, Canalis EM, Maina DM, Raisz LG. Effects of glucocorticoids on fetal rate bone collagen synthesis in vitro. Endocrinology. 1979; 104:715–721

12. Feldman D, Dziak R, Koehler R, Stern P. Cytoplasmic glucocorticoid binding proteins in bone cells. Endocrinology. 1975; 96:29–36

13. Gennari C, Civitelli R. Glucocorticoid-induced osteoporosis. Clin Rheum Dis. 1986; 12:637–654

14. McConkey M, Fraser GM, Bligh AS. Osteoporosis and purpura in rheumatoid arthritis: prevalence and relation to treatment with corticosteroids. Q J Med. 1962; 1:419–427

15. Gennari C. Glucocorticosteroids and bone. In Peck WA, ed., Bone and Mineral Research, Vol. 3. Amsterdam, Elsevier, 1985, pp. 213–231

16. Huth EJ. Radiologic methods to evaluate bone mineral content. Ann Intern Med. 1984; 100:908–11

17. Sartoris DJ, Resnick D. Dual-energy radiographic absorptiometry for bone densitometry: current status and perspective. Am J Radiol. 1989; 152:241–247

18. Lindsay R, Hart DM, Aitken JM, MacDonald EB, Anderson JB, Clarke AC. Long-term prevention of postmenopausal osteoporosis by oestrogen. Lancet. 1976; 1:1038–1041

19. Reid DM, Kennedy NSJ, Smith MA, Tothill P, Nuki G. Total body calcium in rheumatoid arthritis: effects of disease activity and corticosteroid treatment. Br Med J. 1982; 285:330–332

20. Solomon L. Mechanisms of idiopathic osteonecrosis. Orthop Clin North Am. 1985; 16:267–282

21. Bonnarens F, Hernandez A, D'Ambrosia R. Bone scintigraphic changes in osteonecrosis of the femoral head. Orthop Clin North Am. 1985; 16:697–703

22. Zizic TM, Hungerford DS, Stevens MB. Ischemic bone necrosis in systemic lupus erythematosus. Part 1: The early diagnosis of ischemic necrosis of bone. Medicine. 1980; 59:134–142

23. Springfield DS, Enneking WJ. Surgery for aseptic necrosis of the femoral head. Clin Orthop. 1978; 130:175–185

24. Kenzora JE. Treatment of idiopathic osteonecrosis: the current philosophy and rationale. Orthop Clin North Am. 1985; 16:717–725

25. Bowyer SL, LaMothe MP, Hollister JR. Steroid myopathy: incidence and detection in a population with asthma. J Allergy Clin Immunol. 1985; 76:234–242

26. Knox AJ, Mascie-Taylor BH, Muers MF. Acute hydrocortisone myopathy in acute severe asthma. Thorax. 1986; 41:411–412

27. Askari A, Vignos PJ, Moskowitz RW. Steroid myopathy in connective tissue disease. Am J Med. 1976; 61:485–492

28. Hollander JL, Jessor RA, Brown EM. Intrasynovial corticosteroid therapy: a decade of use. Bull Rheum Dis. 1961; 11:239–240

29. Laroche M, Arlet J, Mazieres B. Osteonecrosis of the femoral and humeral heads after intra articular corticosteroid injections. J Rheumatol. 1990; 17:549–551

30. Behrens F, Shepard N, Mitchell N. Metabolic recovery of articular cartilage after intra articular injections of glucocorticoid. J Bone Joint Surg. 1976; 58A:1157–1160

31. Hollander JL. Intrasynovial corticosteroid therapy in arthritis. Md Med J. 1969; 19:62–66

32. Sweetman R. Corticosteroid arthropathy and tendon rupture. J Bone Joint Surg. 1969; 51B:397–8

33. McCarty DJ, Hogan JM. Inflammatory reaction after intra-synovial injection of microcrystalline adrenocorticosteroid esters. Arthritis Rheum. 1964; 7:359–367

34. Khong TK, Rooney PJ. Arthritis associated with cimetidine. Lancet (Letter). 1980; 2:1380

35. Kertes P, Hunt D. Polyarthritis complicating quinidine treatment. Br Med J. 1982; 284: 1373–1374

36. Fraser DM, Irvine NA. Joint effusions and practolol. Lancet (Letter). 1976; 1:89

37. Kaplan R, Robinson CA, Scavulli JF, Vaughan JH. Propranolol and the treatment of rheumatoid arthritis. Arthritis Rheum. 1980; 23:253–255

38. Savola J. Arthropathy induced by beta blockade. Br Med J. 1983; 287:1256–1257

39. Hart DF. Drug-induced arthritis and arthralgia. Drugs. 1984; 28:347–354

40. Segal AW, Pugh SF, Levi AJ, Loewi G. Levamisole induced arthritis in Crohn's disease. Br Med J. 1977; 2:555

41. Sigidin JA, Bunchuk NV. Neurological complication of levamisole. Lancet (Letter). 1977; 2:980

42. Siklos P. Levamisole induced arthritis. Br Med J. 1977; 2:773

43. Davies DM. Drug induced aches and pains. Adverse Drug React Bull. 1971; 30:88–90

44. Hart FD. Drug induced arthritis. Curr Med Res Opin. 1974; 2:505–509

45. Maillard G, Renard G. Un nouveau traitement de l'epilepsie. Presse Med. 1925; 33:315–317

46. Maillard G, Thomazi P. Douleurs provoquees par certains derives barbituriques au cours du traitement de l'epilepsie. Presse Med. 1931; 39:851–852

47. Van der Korst JK, Colenbrander H, Cato A. Phenobarbital and the shoulder–hand syndrome. Ann Rheum Dis. 1966; 25:553–555

48. Good AE, Green RA, Zarafontenis CJD. Rheumatic symptoms during tuberculous therapy. Ann Intern Med. 1965; 63:800–807

49. Bethel GH. Severe arthritis with carbimazole. Br J Clin Pract. 1979; 33:294

50. Atcheson SG, Ward JR. Ptosis and weakness after start of D-penicillamine therapy. Ann Intern Med. 1978; 89:939–940

51. Ostensen M, Husby G, Arrli J. Polymyositis with acute myolysis in a patient with rheumatoid arthritis treated with penicillamine and ampicillin. Arthritis Rheum (Letter) 1980; 23:375–377

52. Brousson A, Pélissier J, Lepeu G et al. Polymyosite induite par la D-penicillamine. Rev Rhum. 1981; 48:267–271

53. Takahashi K, Ogita T, Okudaira H et al. D-Penicillamine-induced polymyositis in patients with rheumatoid arthritis. Arthritis Rheum. 1986; 29:560–564

54. Fernandez L, Swinton DR, Hamilton EBD. Dermatomyositis complicating penicillamine treatment. Ann Rheum Dis. 1977; 36:94–95

55. Wojnarorowska F. Dermatomyositis induced by penicillamine. J Roy Soc Med. 1980; 73:884–880

56. Swartz M, Silver RM. D-penicillamine induced polymyositis in juvenile chronic arthritis: reports of a case. J Rheumatol. 1984; 11:251–252

57. Dawkins RL, Christiansen FT, Garlepp MJ. Autoantibodies and HLA antigens in ocular, generalized and penicillamine-induced myasthenia gravis. Ann NY Academy Sci. 1981; 377: 372–384

58. Medsger TA, Dawson WN, Masi AT. The epidemiology of polymyositis. Am J Med. 1970; 48:715–723

59. Carroll GJ, Will RK, Peter JB, Garlepp J, Dawkins RL. Penicillamine induced polymyositis and dermatomyositis. J Rheumatol. 1987; 14:995–1001

60. Carrano JA, Swanson NR, Dawkins RL. An enzyme linked immunosorbent assay for anti-striational antibodies associated with myasthenia gravis and thymoma. Comparison with indirect immunofluorescence. J Immunol Methods. 1983; 13:301–14

61. Nishikai M, Reichlin M. Heterogeneity of precipitating antibodies in polymyositis and dermatomyositis. Characterization of the Jo-I antibody system. Arthritis Rheum. 1980; 23:881–888

62. Leddy JP, Grigs RC, Klemperer MR. Hereditary complement (C2) deficiency with dermatomyositis. Am J Med. 1975; 58:83–91

63. Takahasni K, Ogita T, Okuraida H, Yoshinoya S, Yoshizawa H, Myamoto T. D-penicillamine induced polymyositis in patients with rheumatoid arthritis. Arthritis Rheum. 1986; 29:560–564

64. Garlepp MI, Dawkins RL, Christiansen FT. HLA antigens and acetylcholine receptor antibodies in penicillamine induced myasthenia gravis. Br Med J. 1983; 286:338–340

65. Delamere JP, Jobson S, Mackintosh IP, Wells L, Walton KW. Penicillamine induced/myasthenia in rheumatoid arthritis: its clinical and genetic features. Ann Rheum Dis. 1983; 42:500–504

66. Liddle BJ. Development of morphea in rheumatoid arthritis treated with penicillamine. Ann Rheum Dis. 1989; 48:963–964

67. Kolarz G, Maida EM. Acetylcholin-Rezeptorantikorper unter D-Penicillamintherapie. Z Rheumatol. 1986; 45:118–121

68. Lipsky PE, Ziff M. Inhibition of human helper T cell function in vitro by D-penicillamine and CuSO4. J Clin Invest. 1980; 65: 1069–1076

69. Morimoto C, Reinherz EL, Borel Y, Schossman SF. Direct demonstration of the human suppressor inducer subset by anti-T cell antibodies. J Immunol. 1983; 130:157–161

70. Morimoto C, Letvin NL, Distaso JA, Aldrich WR, Schlossman SF The isolation and characterization of the human suppressor inducer T cell subset. J Immunol. 1985; 134:1508–1515

71. Reeback J, Benton S, Swach M. Penicillamine-induced neuromyotonia. Br Med J. 1979; 1:1464–1465

72. Mjolnerod OK, Dommerud SA, Rasmussen K, Gjeruldsen ST. Congenital connective tissue defect probably due to D-penicillamine treatment in pregnancy. Lancet. 1971; 1:673–675

73. Sturrock RD, Brooks PM. Penicillamine and creaking joints. (Letter to Ed.) Br Med J. 1974; 3:575

74. Gordon OA. Gold compound. In Kelley et al., eds., Textbook of Rheumatology. Philadelphia, WB Saunders, 1989, pp. 804–823

75. Schumm F, Wietholter H, Fateh-Moghadam A. Myasthenie-Syndrom unter Chloroquin-Therapie. Dtsch Med Wochenschr. 1981; 106:1745–7

76. Sghirlanzoni A, Mantegazza R, Mora M et al. Chloroquine myopathy and myasthenia-like syndrome. Muscle Nerve. 1988; 2:114–119

77. Rynes RI. Antimalarial drugs. In Kelley et al., eds., Textbook of Rheumatology. Philadelphia, WB Saunders, 1989, pp. 792–803

78. Hughes JT, Esiri M, Oxbury JM et al. Chloroquine myopathy. Q J Med. 1971; 40:85–93

79. Ebringer A, Collwille P. Chloroquine neuropathy associated with keratopathy and retinopathy. Br Med J. 1967; 1:219–220

80. Estes ML, Ewing-Wilson O, Chou SM et al. Chloroquine neurotoxicity. Clinical and pathologic perspective. Am J Med. 1987; 82:447–455

81. Ihde DC, DeVita VT. Osteonecrosis of the femoral head in patients with lymphoma treated with intermittent combination chemotherapy. Cancer. 1975; 36:1585–1588

82. Obrist R, Hartmann D, Obrecht JP. Osteonecrosis after chemotherapy. Lancet (Letter). 1978; 1:1316

83. Harper PG, Trash C, Souhami RL. Avascular necrosis of bone caused by combination chemotherapy without corticosteroids. Br Med J. 1984; 288:267–268

84. Marymont JV, Kaufmann EE. Osteonecrosis of bone associated with combination chemotherapy without corticosteroids. Clin Orthop. 1986; 204:150–153

85. Ansell G, Evans S, Jackson CT, Lewis-Jones S. Cytotoxic drugs for neoplastic disease (Letter). Br Med J. 1983; 287:762

86. Ragab AH, Frech RS, Vietti TJ. Osteoporotic fractures secondary to methotrexate therapy of acute leukemia in remission. Cancer. 1970; 25:580–585

87. Nesbit M, Kriwit W, Heyn R, Sharp H. Acute and chronic effects of methotrexate on hepatitis pulmonary and skeletal system. Cancer. 1976; 37:1048–1054

88. Schwartz AM, Leonidas JC. Methotrexate osteopathy. Skeletal Radiol. 1984; 11:13–16

89. Segal R, Caspi D, Tischler M, Fishel B, Yaron M. Accelerated nodulosis and vasculitis during methotrexate therapy for rheumatoid arthritis. Arthritis Rheum. 1988; 31:1182–1185

90. Martin JH, Gordon M, Wallace R. Methotrexate in psoriasis. Arch Derm. 1967; 96:431–433

91. Kahl LE, Thompson ME, Griffith BP. Gout in the heart transplant recipient: physiologic puzzle and therapeutic challenge. Am J Med. 1989; 87: 289–93

92. Lin HY, Rocher LL, McQuillan MA, Schmaltz S, Palella TD, Fox IH. Cyclosporine-induced hyperuricemia and gout. N Engl J Med. 1989; 321:287–292

93. Noordzij TG, Leunissen KML, VanHooff JP. Cyclosporine-induced hyperuricemia and gout (reply). N Engl J Med. 1990; 322:3335

94. Noppen M, Velkeniers B, Diercks R et al. Cyclosporine and myopathy. Ann Intern Med. 1987; 107:945–946

95. Clayton R. Azathioprine in psoriasis. (Letter) Br Med J. 1974; 1:443

96. Lossner J, Huhn HJ, Lehmann J, Ziegan J. Secondary muscular carnitine deficiency following immunosuppressive treatment. Psychiatr Neurol Med Psychol (Leipzig). 1989; 41:614–620

97. Belch JJF. The phenomenon, syndrome and disease of Maurice Raynaud. Br J Rheumatol. 1990; 29:162–165

98. Porter JM, Rivers SP, Anderson CJ, Baur GM. Evaluation and management of patients with Raynaud's syndrome. Am J Surg. 1981; 142:183–189

99. Maricq HR. Raynaud's phenomenon and microvascular abnormalities in scleroderma (systemic sclerosis). In Jayson MIV, Black, CM eds., Systemic Sclerosis: Scleroderma. Chichester, John Wiley, 1988, pp. 151–166

100. Joyal F. Workup for Raynaud's phenomenon. Diagnosis. 1988; 169–175

101. Lafferty K, De Trafford JC, Potter C, Robert VC, Cotton LT. Reflex vascular responses in the finger to contralateral thermal stimuli during the normal menstrual cycle: a hormonal basis to Raynaud's phenomenon? Clin Sci. 1985; 68:10–15

102. Goodfield MJD, Hume A, Rowell NR. The acute effects of cigarette smoking and non-smoking subjects with and without Raynaud's phenomenon. Br J Rheumatol. 1990; 29: 89–91

103. Kakosy T. Vibration disease. Baillière's Clin Rheumatol. 1989; 3:25–50

104. Behrens V, Taylor W, Wilcox T et al. Vibration syndrome in chipping and grinding workers. Epidemiol J Occup Med. 1984; 26:756–788

105. Olsen N, Petring OU. Vibration elicited vasoconstriction reflex in Raynaud's phenomenon. Br J Indust Med. 1988; 45:413–419

106. Gemme G, Pyykko I, Starck J et al. Circulatory reaction to heat and cold in vibration-induced white finger with and without sympathetic blockade. Scand J Work Environ Health. 1986; 12 (Special Issue No. 4):371–377

107. Freedman RR, Subharwal SC, Desai N, Wenig P, Mayes M. Increased α-adrenergic responsiveness in idiopathic Raynaud's disease. Arthritis Rheum. 1989; 32:61–65

108. Okada A, Arizumi M, Fujinaga N. Diagnosis of vibration syndrome by blood viscosity. In Brammer AJ, Taylor W eds., Vibration Effects on the Hand and Arm in Industry. New York, John Wiley, 1982, pp. 67–70

109. Thulesius O. Vascular spasm in the hands and vibration trauma – prevention is the only therapy. Lalkartidningen. 1985; 82:2873–2877

110. Cohen SR, Bilinski DL, McNutt NS. Vibration syndrome. Arch Dermatol. 1985; 121:1544–1547

111. Tabuenca JM. Toxic-allergic syndrome caused by ingestion of rapeseed oil denatured with aniline. Lancet. 1981; 2:567–568

112. Straniero NR, Furst DE. Environmentally-induced systemic sclerosis-like illness. Baillière's Clin Rheumatol. 1989; 3: 63–79

113. Alonso-Ruiz A, Zea-Mendoza AC, Gonzalez-Lanza M et al. Digital tuft alterations in toxic oil syndrome. Lancet. 1983; 2:520–521

114. Mateo IM, Izquierdo M, Fernandez-Dapica MP et al. Toxic epidemic syndrome: musculoskeletal manifestations. J Rheumatol. 1984; 11:333–338

115. Roubenoff R, Cote T, Watson R, Levin ML, Hochberg MC. Eosinophilia-myalgia syndrome due to L-Tryptophan ingestion: report of four cases and review of the Maryland experience. Arthritis Rheum. 1990; 33: 930–938

116. Bulpitt KJ, Verity A, Clements PJ, Paulus HE. Association of L-Tryptophan and an illness resembling eosinophilic fasciitis: clinical and histpathologic findings in four patients with eosinophilia-myalgia syndrome. Arthritis Rheum. 1990; 33:918–929

117. Hertzman PA, Blevins WL, Mayer J, Greenfield B, Ting M, Gleich GJ. Association of the eosinophilia-myalgia syndrome with the ingestion of tryptophan. N Engl J Med. 1990; 322: 869–873

118. Silver RM, Heyes MP, Maize JC, Quearry B, Vionnet-Fausset M, Shernberg EM. Scleroderma, fasciitis and eosinophilia associated with the ingestion of tryptophan. N Engl J Med. 1990; 322:874–881

119. Shulman LE. The eosinophilia-myalgia syndrome associated with ingestion of L-tryptophan. Arthritis Rheum. 1990; 33:913–917

120. Shulman LE. Diffuse fasciitis with eosinophilia: a new syndrome? Trans Assoc Am Physicians. 1975; 88:70–86

121. Kilbourne EM, Swygert LA, Philen RM et al. Interim guidance on the eosinophilia-myalgia syndrome. Ann Intern Med. 1967; 112: 300–301

122. Wilson RH, McCormick WE, Tatum CF et al. Occupational acro-osteolysis – report of 31 cases. JAMA. 1967; 201:577–581

123. Dodson VN, Dinman BD, Whitehouse WM et al. Occupational acroosteolysis: III. A clinical study. Arch Environ Health. 1971; 22:83–91

124. Maricq HR, Johnson MN, Whetstone CL *et al.* Capillary abnormalities in polyvinyl chloride production workers. JAMA. 1976; 23:1368–1371

125. Gama C, Meria JBB. Occupational acro-osteolysis. J Bone Joint Surg. 1978; 60A: 86–90

126. Sluis-Cremer GK, Hessel PA, Nizodo EH et al. Silica, silicosis, and progressive systemic sclerosis. Br J Indust Med. 1985; 42: 838–843

127. Kumagai Y, Shiokawa Y, Medsger TA *et al.* Clinical spectrum of connective tissue disease after cosmetic surgery. Observations on eighteen patients and a review of the Japanese literature. Arthritis Rheum. 1984; 27:1–12

Smoking

128. Calabro JJ. Cancer and arthritis. Arthritis Rheum. 1967; 10:553–567

129. Graham GG, Haavisto IM, McNaught PJ, Browne CD, Champion GD. The effect of smoking on the distribution of gold in blood. J Rheumatol. 1982; 9:527–531

130. Larkin JG, Lowe GDO, Sturrock RD, Forbes CD. The relationship of plasma and serum viscosity to disease activity and smoking habit in rheumatoid arthritis. Br J Rheumatol. 1984; 23:15–19

131. Kelsey JL, Githens PB, O'Conner T, Weil U *et al.* Acute prolapsed intervertebral disc. An epidemiologic study with special reference to driving automobiles and cigarette smoking. Spine. 1984; 9:608–613

132. Typpo T. Osteoarthritis of the hip. Radiologic findings and etiology. Ann Chir Gynecol (Suppl.) 1985; 201:1–38

133. Biering-Srensen F, Thomsen C. Medical, social and occupational history as risk factors for low-back trouble in the general population. Spine. 1986; 11:720–725

134. Gilchrist C. Psychiatric and social factors related to low back pain in general practice. Rheumatol Rehab. 1976; 15:101–107

135. Daniell HW. Osteoporosis in the slender smoker. Vertebral compression fractures and loss of metacarpal cortex in relation to postmenopausal cigarette smoking and lack of obesity. Arch Intern Med. 1976; 136:298–304

136. McKinlay SM, Bifano NL, McKinlay JB. Smoking and age at menopause in women. Ann Intern Med. 1985; 103:350–356

137. Everson RB, Sandler DP, Wilcox AJ, Schreinemachers D, Shore DL. Weinberg effect of passive exposure to smoking on age at natural menopause. Br Med J. 1986; 1:792

138. Michnovicz JJ, Hershcopf RJ, Naganuma H *et al.* Increased 2-hydroxylation of oestradiol as a possible mechanism for the anti-oestrogenic effect of cigarette-smoking. N Engl J Med. 1986; 315:1305–1309

139. Daniell HW. Anti-oestrogenic effect of cigarette smoking. N Engl J Med. 1987; 316:1342

140. Schneider J, Bradlow HL, Strain G, Levin J, Anderson K, Fishman J. Effects of obesity on oestradiol metabolism: decreased formation of nonuterotropic metabolites. J Clin Endocrinol Metab. 1983; 56:973–978

141. Barbieri RL, Gochberg J, Ryan KJ. Nicotine, cotinine, and anabasin inhibit aromatase in human trophoblast in vitro. J Clin Invest. 1986; 77: 1727–1733

142. Jensen J, Christiansen L, Rodbro P. Cigarette smoking, serum estrogens, and bone loss during hormone-replacement therapy after early menopause. N Engl J Med. 1985; 313:973–975

143. Aloia JF, Vaswani AN, Yeh JK, Ross P, Ellis K, Cohn SH. Determinants of bone mass in post menopausal women. Arch Intern Med. 1983; 143:1700–1704

144. Rundgren A. The effect of tobacco smoking on the mineral content of the heel bone in 70, 75 and 79-year old men and women. In Christiansen C, Arnaud CD, Nordin BEC, Parfitt AM, Peck WA, Riggs BL, eds., Osteoporosis. Copenhagen, Aalborg Stiftsbogtrykkeri, 1984, pp. 377–379

145. Johnstone CC Jr, Norton J, Khairi MRA *et al.* Heterogeneity of fracture syndromes in postmenopausal women. J Endocrinol Metab. 1985; 61:551–556

146. McNair P, Christiansen MS, Madsbad S, Christiansen C, Binder C, Transbol I. Bone loss in patients with diabetes mellitus; effects of smoking. Mineral Electrolyte Metab. 1980; 3:94–97

147. Lindsay R. The influence of cigarette smoking on bone mass and bone loss. In DeLuca HF, Frost HM, Jee WSS, Johnston CC Jr, Parfitt AM, eds., Osteoporosis Recent Advances in Pathogenesis and Treatment. Baltimore, University Park Press, 1981, p. 481

148. Williams AR, Weiss NS, Ure CL *et al*. Effect of weight, smoking, and estrogen use on the risk of hip and forearm fractures in postmenopausal women. Obstet Gynecol. 1982; 60:695–699

149. Alarcon-Segovia D. Drug-induced systemic lupus erythematosus and related syndromes. Clin Rheum Dis. 1975; 1:573–582

150. Fakhro, AM, Ritchie, RF, Lowen B. Lupus-like syndrome induced by procainamide. Am J Cardiol. 1967; 20:367–373

151. Weinstein A. Lupus syndromes induced by drugs. In Schur PH, ed., Clinical Management of Systemic Lupus Erythematosus. Orlando, Grune and Stratton, 1983, pp. 221–231

152. Rothfield NF, Bierer WF, Garfield JW. The induction of antinuclear antibodies by isoniazid: a prospective study (Abstract). Arthritis Rheum. 1971; 14:182–183

153. Alarcon-Segovia D, Wakim KG, Worthington JW, Ward LE. Clinical and experimental studies on the hydralazine syndrome and its relationship to systemic lupus erythematosus. Medicine (Baltimore). 1967; 46:1–33

154. Quismorio FP, Bjarnasson DF, Dubois EL, Friou GJ. Chlorpromazine-induced antinuclear antibodies. Arthritis Rheum (Abstract). 1972;15:451

155. Alarcon-Segovia D, Fishbein E, Getina JA, Raya RJ, Barrera E. Antigenic specificity of chlorpromazine-induced antinuclear antibodies. Clin. Exp. Immunol. 1973; 15:543–548

156. Feltkamp TEW, Dorhoutmees EJ, Nieuwenhuis MG. Auto-antibodies related to treatment with chlorthalidone and α-methyldopa. Acta Med Scand. 1970; 187:219–223

157. Carstairs KC, Breckenridge A, Dollery CT, Worlledge SM. Incidence of a positive direct Coombs test in patients on α-methyldopa. Lancet. 1966; 2:133–135

158. Worlledge SM, Cairstairs KC, Dacie JV. Auto-immune haemolytic anaemia associated with α-methyldopa therapy. Lancet. 1966; 2:35–139

159. Jungers P, Dougados M, Pelissier C *et al*. Influence of oral contraceptive therapy on the activity of systemic lupus erythematosus. Arthritis Rheum. 1982; 25:618–623

160. Hess EV. Drug-related lupus: the same or different? In Lahita RG, ed., Systemic Lupus Erythematosus. New York, John Wiley, 1987

161. Reidenberg MM, Drayer MM. Genetic regulation of drug metabolism and systemic lupus erythematosus. In Lahita RG, ed., Systemic Lupus Erythematosus. New York. John Wiley and Sons, 1987

162. Harmon CE, Portanova JP. Drug-induced lupus. Clin Rheum Dis. 1982; 8:121–135

163. Alarcon-Segovia D. Drug-induced lupus syndromes. Mayo Clin Proc. 1969; 44:664–681

164. Blomgren SE, Condemi JJ, Vaughan JH. Procainamide induced lupus erythematosus: clinical and laboratory observations. Am J Med. 1972; 52:338–348

165. Hahn BJ, Sharp GC, Irvin WS, Kantor OS *et al*. Immune response to hydralazine and nuclear antigens in hydralazine induced lupus erythematosus. Ann Intern Med. 1970; 76:365–374

166. Dubois EL, Molina J, Bilitch M, Friou GJ. Procainamide-induced serologic changes in asymptomatic patients. Arthritis Rheum. 1911:477–478

167. Winfield JB, David JS IV. Anti-DNA antibody in procainamide-induced lupus erythematosus. Determinations using DNA fractionated by methylated albumin – Kieselguhr chromatography. Arthritis Rheum. 1974; 17:97–110

168. Hughes GRV, Rynes RI, Gharavi A, Ryan PFJ, Mansilla R. The heterogeneity of serologic findings and predisposing host factors in drug-induced lupus erythematosus. Arthritis Rheum. 1981; 24:1070

169. Batchelor JR, Welsh KI, Tinoco RM *et al*. Hydralazine-induced SLE: influence of HLA-DR and sex on susceptibility. Lancet. 1980; 1:1107–1109

170. Perry HM Jr, Tan EM, Carmody S, Sakamoto A. Relationship of acetyl transferase activity to antinuclear antibodies and toxic symptoms in hypertensive patients treated with hydralazine. J Lab Clin Med. 1970; 76:114–125

171. Alarcon-Segovia D, Fishbein E, Alcala H. Isoniazid acetylation rate and development of antinuclear antibodies upon isoniazid treatment. Arthritis Rheum. 1971; 14:748–752

172. Price Evans DA, Bullen MF, Houston J, Hopkins CA, Vetters JM. Antinuclear factors in rapid and slow acetylator patients treated with isoniazid. J Med Genet. 1972; 9:53–56

173. Reidenberg MM, Drayer DE, Levy M *et al*. Polymorphic acetylation of procainamide in man. Clin Pharmacol Ther. 1975; 17:722–730

174. Woosley RL, Drayer DE, Reidenberg MM *et al.* Effect of acetylator phenotype on the rate at which procainamide induces antinuclear antibodies and the lupus syndrome. N Engl J Med. 1978; 298:1157–1159

175. Reidenberg MM, Levy M, Drayer DE *et al.* Acetylator phenotype in idiopathic systemic lupus erythematosus. Arthritis Rheum. 1980; 23:569–573

176. Kluger J, Drayer DE, Reidenberg MM *et al.* Acetylprocainamide therapy in patients with previous procainamide-induced lupus syndrome. Ann Intern Med. 1981; 95: 18–23

Gout

177. Cannon PJ, Heinemann HO, Stacy WB, Laragh JH. Ethacrynic acid. Effectiveness and mode of diuretic action in man. Circulation. 1965; 31:5–18

178. DeMartini FE. Hyperuricemia induced by drugs. Arthritis Rheum. 1965; 8:823–829

179. Stason WB, Cannon PJ, Heinemann HO, Laragh JH. Furosemide. A clinical evaluation of its diuretic action. Circulation. 1966; 34:910–920

180. Steel TH. Diuretic-induced hyperuricemia. Clin Rheum. Dis. 1977; 3:37–50

181. Emmerson BT. Hyperuricemia and Gout in Clinical Practice. ADIS Health Science Press, 1983, p. 42

182. Manuel MA, Steele TH. Changes in renal urate handling after prolonged thiazide treatment. Am J Med. 1974; 57:741–746

183. Cannon PJ, Stason WB, DeMartini FE, Somners SC, Laragh JH. Hyperuricemia in primary and renal hypertension. N Engl J Med. 1966; 275:457–464

184. Breckenridge A. Hypertension and hyperuricaemia. Lancet. 1966; 1:15–18

185. Beevers DG, Hamilton M, Harpur JE. The long-term treatment of hypertension with thiazide diuretics. Postgrad Med J. 1971; 47:639–643

186. Steele TH. Evidence for altered renal urate reabsorption during changes in volume of extra-cellular fluid. J Lab Clin Med. 1969; 74:228

187. Steele TH, Oppenheimer S. Factors affecting urate excretion following diuretic administration in man. Am J Med. 1969; 47:564–574

188. Kelley WN. Hyperuricemia. In Kelley WN, Harris Jr ED, Ruddy S, Sledge CB, eds., Textbook of Rheumatology, 3rd edn, Philadelphia, WB Saunders, 1989, Chap 35, pp. 571–578

189. Ostberg Y. Renal urate deposits in chronic renal insufficiency. Acta Med Scan. 1968; 183: 197–201

190. Demartini FE *et al.* Effect of chlorthiazide on the renal excretion of uric acid. Am J Med. 1962; 32:572–577

191. Gutman AB, Yu TF, Berger L. Tubular secretion of urate in man. J Clin Invest. 1959; 38: 1778–1781

192. Weiner IM, Tinker JP. Pharmacology of pyrazinamide: metabolic and renal function studies related to the mechanism of drug-induced urate retention. J Pharmacol Exp Ther. 1972; 180:411–434

193. Pascale LR, Dubin A, Bronsky D, Hoffman WS. Inhibition of the uricosuric action of Benemid by salicylate. J Lab Clin Med. 1955; 45: 771–777

194. Yu TF, Dayton PF, Gutman AB. Mutual suppression of the uricosuric effects of sulfinpyrazone and salicylate. A study in interactions between drugs. J Clin Invest. 1963; 42:1330–1339

195. Brooks CD, Ulrich JE. Effect of ibuprofen or aspirin on probenecid induced uricosuria. J Int Med Res. 1980; 8:283–285

196. Nriagu JO. Occasional notes. Saturnine gout among Roman aristocrats. Did lead poisoning contribute to the fall of the empire? N Engl J Med. 1983; 308:660

197. Ball GV, Sorensen LB. Pathogenesis of hyperuricemia in saturnine gout. N Engl J Med. 1969; 280:1199

198. Emmerson BT, Knowles BR. Triglyceride concentrations in primary gout and out of chronic lead nephropathy. Metabolism. 1971; 20: 721–729

199. Rapado A. Gout and saturnism. N Engl J Med. 1969; 281:851

200. Halla JT, Ball GV. Saturnine gout: a review of 42 patients. Semin Arthritis Rheum. 1982; 11:307–314

201. Cullen MR, Robins JM, Eskenazi B. Adult inorganic lead intoxication: presentation of 31 new cases and a review of recent advances in the literature. Medicine. 1983; 62:221–247

202. Craswell PW, Price J, Boyle PD *et al.* Chronic renal failure with gout: a marker of chronic lead poisoning. Kidney Int. 1984; 26:319

203. Wright LF, Saylor RP, Cecere FA. Occult lead intoxication in patients with gout and kidney disease. J Rheumatol. 1984; 11:517–520

204. Behringer D, Craswell P, Mohl C, Stoeppler M, Ritz E. Urinary lead excretion in uremic patients. Nephron. 1986; 42:323

205. Colleoni N, Damico G. Chronic lead accumulation as a possible cause of renal failure in gouty patients. Nephron. 1986; 4:32

206. Campbell BC, Moore MR, Goldberg A *et al.* Subclinical lead exposure: a possible cause of gout. Br Med J. 1978; 2:1403

207. Graziano JH, Blum C. Lead exposure from lead crystal. Lancet. 1991; 337:141–142

208. Delbarre F, Auscher C, Brouilhet H, DeGery A. Action de l'ethanol dans la goutte et sur le metabolisme de l'acide urique. Semin Hop Paris. 1967; 43:659–664

209. Saker BM, Tofler OB, Burvill MJ, Reilly KA. Alcohol consumption and gout. Med J Aust. 1967; 1:1213–1216

210. Evans JG, Prior JAM, Harvey HPB. Relation of serum uric acid to body bulk, hemoglobin and alcohol intake in two South Pacific Polynesian populations. Ann Rheum Dis. 1968; 27:319–325

211. Lieber CS, Jones DP, Lasowsky MS, Davidson CS. Inter-relation of uric acid and ethanol metabolism in man. J Clin Invest. 1962; 41:1861

212. MacLachlan MJ, Rodnan GP. Effects of food, fast and alcohol on serum uric acid and acute attacks of gout. Am J Med. 1967; 42:38–57

213. Scott JT, McCallum FM, Holloway VP. Starvation, ketosis and uric acid excretion. Clin Sci. 1964; 27:209–221

214. Steenstrup OR. A note on hyperuricemia during labor. Scand. J Clin Lab Invest. 1960; 12:205

215. Handler JS. The role of lactic acid in the excretion of uric acid in toxemia of pregnancy. J Clin Invest. 1960; 39:1526

216. Kelley WM, Rosenbloom FM, Seegmiller JN, Howell RR. Excessive production of uric acid in type I glycogen storage disease. J Pediatr. 1968; 72:488–496

217. Kelley WN, Goldfinger SE, Hardy HL Hyperuricemia in chronic beryllium disease. Ann Intern Med. 1969; 70:977

218. Faller J, Fox IH. Ethanol-induced hyperuricaemia. Evidence for increased urate production by activation of adenine nucleotide turnover. N Engl J Med. 1982; 307:1598–1602

27. POSTINTERVENTIONAL RHEUMATIC PROBLEMS (CHEIROGENIC RHEUMATIC DISEASE)

Patrick J. Rooney and W. Watson Buchanan

In this chapter, rheumatic complaints following joint surgery and after arthrocentesis, renal transplantation, intestinal bypass surgery and silicone implantation will be discussed.

JOINT SURGERY

Over the past quarter of a century, surgical replacement of hips and knees have become the most common elective procedures in orthopedic practice, and it is estimated that nearly a million patients worldwide have had surgery to these regions and/or received one or more prosthetic joints[1]. One of the major problems of total joint replacement is infection, which occurs in 1–5% of patients[2]. Infection usually develops at the bone–cement interface and in 20–40% of patients is blood-borne[3,4]. Pyogenic skin infection can lead to staphylococcal and streptococcal infections; infection with gram-negative bacilli and anaerobic organisms may be due to genitourinary or gastrointestinal infections or procedures; dental treatment can also induce infection on a hematogenous basis[2]. Patients who appear to be at greatest risk for infection are the elderly, the malnourished, patients with rheumatoid arthritis, or those receiving corticosteroid therapy[2]. Prevention can be achieved by covering any dental, gastrointestinal and genitourinary procedures with antibiotic therapy, and treating skin sepsis or other infections with such therapy promptly and vigorously.

Joint infections that result from contaminated periarticular wounds, e.g. suture abscesses, hematomas, and ischemic necrosis[2] can be prevented by perioperative antibiotics[5], filtered laminar air flow systems in the operating room[6], and impregnation of the polymethylmethacrylate cement with antibiotics[7]. The last agent, however, carries the risk of systemic toxicity and protracted hypersensitivity reactions[2]. Prior to the revision of a prosthesis, it is prudent to carry out percutaneous aspiration, since many arthroplasties have been found to be infected, despite the lack of clinical suspicion[8]. Infection of an arthroplastic revision can be prevented by intensive antibiotic therapy prior to surgical revision of a joint[2].

ARTHROCENTESIS

Arthrocentesis of joints is rarely followed by joint injection. Hollander[9] reported an occurrence of only 0.005% of 400 000 injections. However, local infection of the skin or other periarticular joint structures are regarded as absolute contraindication to injection, and the presence of bacteremia is a relative contraindication, since trauma to the synovium caused by the injection may localize organisms to the joint. Prevention of joint infection as a result of joint injection can be further reduced by use of an aseptic 'no-touch' technique[10].

Earlier reports of cartilage damage secondary to corticosteroid injection have not been supported by subsequent experience[11]. A small number of all injectees report pain for 1–2 days following steroid injection, which may represent a gout-like reaction to crystalline material, or be caused by the preservative used in the formulation of the drug, which may respond to the simple expediency of changing the product being injected. The same may be true of the erythema which may follow injection[11].

RENAL DIALYSIS-RELATED ARTHROPATHY

Lucas[12] was the first to describe the connection between chronic renal failure and bone disease; this condition has been termed renal osteodystrophy for nearly half a century[13], and encompasses hyperparathyroidism, osteomalacia, osteoporosis, and soft tissue calcification[14]. With the advent of renal hemodialysis, it has become apparent that over time, patients successfully maintained on this therapy can develop a number of skeletal and articular abnormalities[15], which include erosions of the interphalangeal joints, as well as subperiosteal and intracortical osseous resorption in the shafts of the tubular bones in the hands[16,17], crystal-induced arthritis, avascular necrosis of bone, periarticular calcification, and recurrent hemarthrosis of the shoulders[15,18–22]. In addition, a clinical complex consisting of the carpal tunnel syndrome, chronic large joint destructive arthropathy, destructive spondylarthropathy, and bone cysts has been described in patients on long term dialysis treatment[20,23–35]. Spondylarthropathy may involve the entire spine, but the cervical segment appears to be most prominently affected[23,31,35]. Many of the lesions described are consistent with secondary hyperparathyroidism[23,31,35] and degenerative conditions may mimic several of these features[36].

The etiopathogenesis of dialysis-associated arthropathy remains unknown. A particular form of β_2-microglobulin amyloid has been found compressing the median nerves, and as a component of bone cysts and other affected tissues[26,27,33,37–45], although such deposits are usually asymptomatic[30,33,42,46]. Serum β_2-microglobulin concentration rises during dialysis[47,48], but no correlation has been found between the development of this clinical complex and β_2-microglobulin levels[46], and although Blumberg and Burgi[49] found a rise in serum β_2-microglobulin concentrations with increasing duration of dialysis, this was not confirmed by other workers[33,48]. Findings other than amyloid deposition have been reported in dialysis related arthropathy, including non-specific synovitis, synovial fibrosis, iron deposition, and crystals of calcium hydroxyapatite, calcium oxalate and calcium pyrophosphate[15,18,21,23,33,42,45,50]. Other factors that may contribute to the development of 'dialysis arthropathy' include the duration of dialysis, the patient's age, presence of hyperparathyroidism especially in the form of destructive spondylarthropathies, the actual type of dialysis membrane, and the action of acetate[23,33,45,50–56]. Aluminum is often increased in patients with chronic renal failure, as this metallic ion may be present in antacids and dialysate solutions; it may be toxic to various tissues[57], easily crosses the synovial membrane, and accumulates in synovial fluid[58]. Whether aluminium is toxic to joint tissues or whether it helps localize β_2-microglobulin in joint tissues is unknown[57]. In view of the increasing numbers of patients with renal failure now being successfully maintained by renal dialysis, an understanding of the etiopathogenesis of dialysis-associated arthropathy is urgently needed, as there is no known method of prevention.

ARTHRITIS AFTER INTESTINAL BYPASS SURGERY FOR MORBID OBESITY

Intestinal bypass surgery for marked obesity was introduced over three decades ago[59,60]. The original operation, a jejunocolic shunt[61] carried a high risk of life-threatening complications, and was replaced by the jejunoileal bypass procedure[62], which also leads to many complications[59,60] and has now been virtually abandoned[59,60,63]. The arthritis–dermatitis syndrome that resulted from this procedure has provided insights into the role played by intestinal bacteria and immune complexes in the pathogenesis of certain forms of arthritis. Inflammatory joint disease of both small and large joints, and occasionally the axial skeleton, has been reported in 6–52% of patients following jejunoileal bypass surgery[64–70]. The arthritis is more common in women, and usually develops within 3 years of operation[63,68], but has been reported by Stein and colleagues[71] as long as 9 years after surgery. Despite the intensity of synovial inflammation, joint erosions rarely occur[67,72]. Tests for rheumatoid and antinuclear antibodies are negative[63,71].

In addition to inflammatory polyarthritis, intestinal bypass surgery complications include tenosynovitis, carpal tunnel syndrome, polymyositis, pleurisy and pleural effusion, Raynaud's phenomenon, vasculitis and rashes[64,67,69,73–79]. The rashes usually appear either immediately before or accompanying the arthritis, and may be urticarial, maculopapular and papulovesicular lesions saffecting all parts of the body, as well as erythema nodosum-like lesions, nodular non-suppurative panniculitis, and necrobiosis lipoidica[64,67,69,71,73–78].

Synovial fluid analysis reveals leukocytosis, most commonly granulocytic, with counts as high as 50 000 cells/l[67,76]. Histological examination of the skin lesions often demonstrates some form of small vessel vasculitis[63,66,67,69,71,73,76,79–81]. It is of interest that cryoglobulinemia and cryoprotein complexes contain antibodies of different immunoglobulin classes directed against intestinal bacteria[71,73,82–85]. Inman[86] has proposed that the pathogenesis of bypass arthritis and the associated dermal lesions represent a response to an altered mucosal barrier in the non-functioning segment of small intestine, allowing increased absorption of bacteria and bacterial products leading to immune complex formation. In support of this hypothesis, immune complexes have been demonstrated both in the synovium of involved joints[67] and in the dermal lesions[75,84]. However, it is to be noted that immune complexes have also been described in patients who have not developed arthritis[67,69,76–78,87] and serum complement levels are normal[66,69]. Thus, other mechanisms may be responsible for the arthritis–dermatitis syndrome of intestinal bypass surgery.

SILICONE IMPLANTS

A foreign body type of arthritis may complicate the use of silicone joint implants in rheumatoid arthritis (*see* Chapter 22). As the benefit from this operation for deformed PIP joints is cosmetic rather than functional, the decision to use these prosthetic devices must be tempered by the possibility of a reaction to the material[88].

A generalized systemic disorder described as human adjuvant disease and resembling rheumatoid arthritis, systemic sclerosis or systemic lupus erythematosus may result from silicone implants for breast augmentation. This has been a particular problem in Japan[89]. Resolution after implant removal is usually incomplete, although one complete recovery is reported[90]. Clearly, this is a preventable disorder, and in future the risk of this procedure is unlikely to be considered justifiable for cosmetic operations[91].

REFERENCES
Joint surgery and injection
Joint infections following joint surgery and/or injections.
1. Harris WH, Sledge CB. Total hip and total knee replacement. N Engl J Med. 323:725–731, 323:801–807
2. Brause BD. Infections associated with prosthetic joints. Clin Rheum Dis. 1986; 12:523–536

3. Ahlberg A, Carlsson AS, Lindberg L. Hematogenous infection in total joint replacement. Clin Orthop Rel Res. 1978; 137:69–75

4. Lattimer GL, Keblish PA, Dickson TB, Vernbick CG, Finnegan WJ. Hematogenous infection in total joint replacement. JAMA. 1979; 242:2213–2214

5. Norden C. A critical review of antibiotic prophylaxis in orthopedic surgery. Rev Inf Dis. 1983; 5:928–932

6. Lidwell V, Lowbury E, Whyte E *et al.* Effect of ultraclean air in operating rooms on deep sepsis in the joint after total hip or knee replacement: a randomised study. Br Med J. 1982; 285:10–14

7. Wahlig H, Dingeldein E. Antibiotics and bone cements: experimental and clinical long-term observations. Acta Orthop Scand. 1980; 51:49–56

8. Gould ES, Potter HG, Rober SE. Role of routine percutaneous hip aspirations prior to prosthesis revision. Skel Radiol. 1990; 19:427–430

9. Hollander JL. Intrasynovial therapy. In McCarty DJ, ed., Arthritis and Allied Conditions: A Textbook of Rheumatology. 10th edn. Philadelphia, Lea and Febiger, 1985, p. 543

10. Dixon A St J, Graber J. Local Injection Therapy in Rheumatic Diseases. EULAR Monograph Series No. 4, Basel, EULAR, 1983

11. Owen DS. Aspiration and injection of joints and soft tissues. In Kelley WN *et al.*, eds., Textbook of Rheumatology. Philadelphia, WB Saunders, 1989

Renal dialysis-related arthropathy

12. Lucas RC. On a form of late rickets associated with albuminuria, rickets of adolescents. Lancet. 1983; 1:993–994

13. Liu SH, Chu HI. Studies of calcium and phosphorus metabolism with special reference to pathogenesis and effects of dihydrotachysterol (A.T.10) and iron. Medicine. 1946; 22:103–161

14. Sundaram M. Renal osteodystrophy. Skel Radiol. 1989; 18:415–426

15. Massry SG, Bluestone R, Klinenberg JR, Coburn JW. Abnormalities of the musculoskeletal system in hemodialysis patients. Semin Arthritis Rheum. 1975; 4:321–349

16. Meema HE, Rabinovich S, Meenas S, Lloyd GJ, Oreopoulos DG. Improved radiological diagnosis of systemic osteodystrophy. Radiology. 1972; 102:1–10

17. Duncan IJS, Hurst NP, Disney A, Sebben R, Milazzo SC. Is chronic renal failure a risk factor for the development of erosive osteoarthritis? Ann Rheum Dis. 1989; 48:183–187

18. Brown EA, Gower PE. Joint problems in maintenance hemodialysis. Clin Nephrol. 1982; 18:247–250

19. Rubenstein J, Campbell J, Saiphoo C. Erosive systemic osteoarthropathy. Arthritis Rheum. 1984; 27:1086–1094

20. Goldstein S, Winston E, Chung TJ, Chopra S, Priser K. Chronic arthropathy in long term hemodialysis. Am J Med. 1985; 78:82–86

21. Brown EA, Arnold IR, Gower PE. Dialysis arthropathy: complication of long-term treatment with hemodialysis. Br Med J. 1986; 292:163–166

22. Langevitz P, Buskila D, Stewart J, Sherrard DJ, Hercz G. Osteonecrosis in patients receiving dialysis: report of two cases and review of the literature. J Rheumatol. 1990; 17:402–406

23. Kuntz D, Naveau B, Bardin T, Drueke T *et al.*, Destructive spondyloarthropathy in hemodialyzed patients. Arthritis Rheum. 1984; 27:369–375

24. Schwarz A, Keller F, Seyfert S, Poll W *et al.*, Carpal tunnel syndrome: a major complication in long-term hemodialysis patients. Clin Nephrol. 1984; 22:133–137

25. Spertini F, Wauters JP, Poulenas I. Carpal tunnel syndrome: a frequent invaliding long-term complication of chronic hemodialysis. Clin Nephrol. 1984; 21:98–101

26. Munoz-Gomez J, Bergada-Barado E, Gomez-Perez R *et al.* Amyloid arthropathy in patients undergoing periodical hemodialysis for chronic renal failure: a new complication. Ann Rheum Dis. 1985; 44:729–733

27. Fenves AZ, Emmett M, White MG *et al.* Carpal tunnel syndrome with cystic bone lesions secondary to amyloidosis in chronic hemodialysis patients. Am J Kidney Dis. 1986; 7:130–134

28. McClure J, Bartley CJ, Ackrill P. Carpal tunnel syndrome caused by amyloid containing β_2-microglobulin: a new amyloid and a complication of long term hemodialysis. Ann Rheum Dis. 1986; 45:10007–1011

29. Bardin T, Kuntz D. The arthropathy of chronic hemodialysis. Clin Exp Rheumatol. 1987; 5: 379–386

30. Bardin T, Zingraff J, Shirahama T *et al.* Hemodialysis-associated amyloidosis and β_2-microglobulin; clinical and immunohistochemical study. Am J Med. 1987; 83:419–424

31. Kerr R, Bjorkengren A, Bielecki DK, Resnick D, Feinstein EI. Destructive spondyloarthropathy in hemodialysis patients. Report of four cases and prospective study. Skel Radiol. 1988; 17:176–180

32. Gerster JC, Carruzzo PA, Ginalski JM, Wauters JP. Cervico-occipital hinge changes during long-term dialysis. J Rheumatol. 1989; 16:146–1473

33. Hurst NP, van den Berg R, Disney A, Alcock M *et al.* Dialysis related arthropathy: a survey of 95 patients receiving chronic hemodialysis with special reference to β_2-microglobulin related amyloidosis. Ann Rheum Dis. 1989; 48:409–420

34. Kleinman KS, Coburn JW. Amyloid syndromes associated with hemodialysis. Kidney Int. 1989; 35:567–575

35. Orzincolo C, Bedani PL, Scutellari PN, Cardona P *et al.* Destructive spondyloarthropathy and radiographic follow-up in hemodialysis patients. Skel Radiol. 1990; 19:483–487

36. Farge D, Remy PL, Poignet JL, Menoyo V, Bariety J, de Vernejoul MC. Isolated bone end sclerosis simulating osteonecrosis after renal transplantation. Letter. Arthritis Rheum 1990; 33:1444–1445

37. Goldman AB, Pavlov H, Bullough P. Primary amyloidosis involving the skeletal system. Case report 137. Skel Radiol. 1981; 6:69

38. Charra B, Calemard E, Uzan M, Terrat JC *et al.* Carpal tunnel syndrome, shoulder pain and amyloid deposits in long term hemodialysis patients. Kidney Int. 1984; 26:549

39. Bardin T, Kuntz D, Zingraff J, Voisin M-C *et al.* Synovial amyloidosis in patients undergoing long term hemodialysis. Arthritis Rheum. 1985; 28:1052–1058

40. Geyjo F, Odani S, Yamada T *et al.* β_2-Microglobulin: a new form of amyloid protein associated with chronic hemodialysis. Kidney Int. 1986; 30:385–390

41. Huaux JP, Noel H, Malghem J, Maldague B *et al.* Erosive azotemic osteoarthropathy: possible role of amyloidosis. (Letter) Arthritis Rheum. 1985; 28:1075–1076

42. Cary NRB, Sethi D, Brown EA, Erhardt CC *et al.* Dialysis arthropathy: amyloid or iron? Br Med J. 1986; 293:1392–1394

43. Gorevic PD, Casey TT, Stone WJ, Di Raimondo CR *et al.* Beta-2-microglobulin is an amyloidogenic protein in man. J Clin Invest. 1985; 76: 2425–2429

44. Sebert JL, Fardellone P, Marie A *et al.* Destructive spondylo-arthropathy in hemodialyzed patients: possible role of amyloidosis. Arthritis Rheum. 1986; 29:301–302

45. Kaplan P, Resnick D, Murphey M. Destructive spondyloarthropathy in hemodialysis patients. Skel Radiol. 1987; 17:176–180

46. Zingraff J, Drueke T, Bardin T. Dialysis-related amyloidosis in the stenoclavicular joint. Nephron. 1989; 52:367

47. Karlsson FA, Wibell L, Eurin PE. Beta-2-microglobulin in clinical medicine. Scand J Clin Lab Invest. 1980; 40:27–37

48. Geyjo F, Homma N, Suzuki Y, Arakawa M. Serum levels of gamma β_2-microglobulin as a new form of amyloid protein in patients undergoing long term hemodialysis. N Engl J Med. 1986; 314:585–586

49. Blumberg A, Burgi W. Behavior of β_2-microglobulin in patients with chronic renal failure undergoing hemodialysis, hemodiafiltration and continuous ambulatory peritoneal dialysis (CAPD). Clin Nephrol. 1987; 27:245–249

50. Hardouin P, Lecomte-Houche M, Flipo RM *et al.* Current aspects of osteoarticular pathology in patients undergoing hemodialysis: study of 80 patients. Part 2. Laboratory and pathologic analysis: discussion of the pathogenetic mechanism. J Rheumatol. 1987; 14:784–787

51. Vanden Broucke JM, Jadoul M, Maldague B, Huaux JP *et al.* Possible role of dialysis membrane characteristics in beta amyloid osteoarthropathy. Lancet. 1986; 1:1210–1211

52. Bayer H, Lajons-Petter A, Debrand A, Herbst R. Investigations of Blood Diseases. Basel, EULAR Publishers, pp. 17–18

53. Bingel M, Lonneman G, Koch KM *et al.* Enhancement of in vitrium interleukin-1 by sodium acetate. Lancet. 1987; 1:14

54. Gaucher A, Kessler M, Netter P, Azoulay E *et al.* Dialysis arthropathy:the effect of age. J Rheumatol. 1988; 15:1880–1881

55. Netter P, Kessler M, Gaucher A et al. Aluminium and dialysis arthropathy. Lancet. 1988; 1: 886–887

56. Kleinman KS, Coburn A, Bannworth B. Amyloid syndromes associated with hemodialysis. Kidney Int. 1989; 35:567–575

57. Netter P, Kessler M, Bannworth B. Does aluminum have a pathogenic role in dialysis associated arthropathy. Ann Rheum Dis. 1990; 49:573–575

58. Netter P, Kessler M, Burnel D *et al.* Aluminum in the joint tissues of chronic renal failure patients treated with regular dialysis and aluminum compounds. J Rheumatol. 1984; 22:66–70

Jejunal surgery

59. Griffen WO Jr, Bivens BA, Bell RM. The decline and fall of the jejunoileal bypass. Surg Gynecol Obstet. 1983; 157:301–308

60. Ross CB, Scott HW, Pincus T. Jejunoileal bypass arthritis. Baillière's Clin Rheumatol. 1989; 3: 339–355

61. Payne JH, de Wind LT, Surgical treatment of obesity. Am J Surg. 1969; 118:141–147

62. Halverson JD, Wise L, Wazna MF, Ballinger WF. Jejunoileal bypass for morbid obesity. Am J Med. 1978; 64:461–475

63. Clarke J, Weiner SR, Bassett LW, Utsinger PD. Bypass disease. Clin Exp Rheumatol. 1987; 5:275–287

64. Shagrin JW, Frame B, Duncan H. Polyarthritis in obese patients with intestinal bypass. Ann Intern Med. 1971; 75:377–380

65. Fernandez-Herliky L. Arthritis after jejunoileostomy for intractable obesity. J Rheumatol. 1977; 4:135–138

66. Ginsberg MD, Quismoria FP, DeWind LT, Morgan ES. Musculoskeletal symptoms after jejunoileal shunt surgery for intractable obesity. Am J Med. 1979; 67:443–448

67. Zapanta M, Aldo-Genson MA, Biegel A, Madura J. Arthritis association with jejunoileal bypass: clinical and immunological evaluation. Arthritis Rheum. 1979; 22:711–717

68. Clegg DO, Samuelson CO Jr, Williams HJ, Ward JR. Articular complications of jejunoileal bypass surgery. J Rheumatol. 1980; 7:65–70

69. Leff RD, Towles W, Aldo-Benson, MA, Madura J, Biegel AA. A prospective analysis of the arthritis syndrome and immune function in jejunoileal bypass patients. J Rheumatol. 1983; 10:612–618

70. Bjorkengren AG, Resnick D, Sartoris DJ. Enteropathic arthropathies. Radiol Clin North Am. 1987; 25:189–198

71. Stein HB, Schlappner OLA, Boyko W, Gourley RH, Reeve CE. The intestinal bypass arthritis-dermatitis syndrome. Arthritis Rheum. 1981; 24:684–690

72. Leff RD, Aldo-Benso MA, Madura JA. The effect of revision of the intestinal bypass on post-intestinal bypass arthritis. Arthritis Rheum. 1983; 26:278–681

73. Drenick EJ, Razzaque A, Greenway MD, Olerud JE. Cutaneous lesions after intestinal bypass. Ann Intern Med. 1980; 93:557–559

74. Williams HJ, Samuelson CO, Zone JJ. Nodular nonsuppurative panniculitis associated with jejunoileal bypass surgery. Arch Dermatol. 1979; 115:1091–1093

75. Kennedy C. The spectrum of inflammatory skin disease following jejunoileal bypass for morbid obesity. Br J Dermatol. 1981; 105:425–435

76. Utsinger PD. Systemic immune complex disease following intestinal bypass surgery: bypass disease. J Am Acad Dermatol. 1980; 2:488–495

77. Heyn J, Hey H, Jans H. Episodic arthritis, skin manifestations and immune complexes following intestinal bypass operations for morbid obesity. Scand J Rheumatol. 1983; 12:257

78. Persellin ST, Griffing WL, Micket CJ Jr *et al.* Polymyositis associated with jejunoileal bypass. J Rheumatol. 1983; 10:637–639

79. Goldman JA, Casey HL, Davidsen ED *et al.* Vasculitis associated with intestinal bypass surgery. Arch Dermatol. 1979; 115:725–727

80. Jorrizo JL, Apisarnthanaraz P, Subrt P *et al.* Bowel-bypass syndrome without bowel bypass: bowel-associated dermatosis–arthritis syndrome. Arch Intern Med. 1983; 143:457–461

81. Dicken CH. Bowel-associated dermatosis-arthritis syndrome: bowel bypass syndrome without bowel bypass. Mayo Clinic Proc. 1984; 59:43–46

82. Wands JR, Lamond JT, Mann E, Isselbacher KJ. Arthritis associated with intestinal bypass procedure for morbid obesity. Complement activation

and characterization of circulating cryoproteins. N Engl J Med. 1967; 294:121–124

83. Rose E, Espinoza LR, Osterland CK. Intestinal bypass arthritis: association with circulating immune complexes and HLA B27. J Rheumatol. 1977; 4:129–134

84. Ely PH. The bowel-bypass syndrome; a response to bacterial peptidoglycans. J Am Acad Dermatol. 1980; 2:473–487

85. Clegg DO, Zone JJ, Samuelson CO Jr, Ward JR. Circulating immune complexes containing secretory IgA in jejunoileal bypass disease. Ann Rheum Dis. 1985; 44:239–244

86. Inman RD. Arthritis and enteritis – an interface of protein manifestations. Editorial. J Rheumatol. 1987; 14:406–410

87. Fagan EA, Elkon KB, Griffin GF *et al.* Systemic inflammatory complications following jejunoileal bypass. Q J Med. 1982; 51:445–460

Silicone implants

88. Christie AJ. Silicone synovitis. Semin Arthritis Rheum. 1989; 19:166–171

89. Kumagai Y, Shiokawa Y, Medsger T *et al.* Clinical spectrum of connective tissue disease after cosmetic surgery: observations on eighteen patients and a review of the Japanese literature. Arthritis Rheum. 1984; 27:1–12

90. Francisco J, Gutierez FJ, Espinoza LR. Progressive systemic sclerosis complicated by severe hypertension: reversal after implant removal. 1990; 89:390–392

91. Kaiser W, Zazgornik J. Late reactions following implantation of silicone prostheses. Urologie. 1991; 30:302–305

28. OCCUPATIONAL FACTORS

John A.D. Anderson

INTRODUCTION

Occupational physicians and their supporting staff, with their special skills in nursing and hygiene, are particularly concerned with prevention at the interface of the worker and his job; they attempt to maintain the best possible health by ensuring that hazards associated with the workplace are reduced to a minimum. The impact of heavy manual labor on the human condition is a problem recognized since biblical times[1], and was formally brought to the attention of physicians by Ramazzini who wrote nearly 300 years ago[2]:

> *The various and numerous train of diseases that accrues to artificers from the exercise of their respective trades, is in my opinion owing chiefly to two causes: namely, first the noxious quality of the matter that goes through their hands, which by breathing out nocive streams and thin particles offensive to human nature, gives rise to particular diseases; and in the next place, certain violent and disorderly motions and improper posture of the body by which the natural structure of the vital machine is so undermined as gradually to make way for grievous distempers.*

After the industrial revolution, the mechanical dangers of machinery to vulnerable groups were the first to receive attention. Legislation was passed to protect women, who, to the owners of factories, represented inexpensive labor, and children, who were cheaper and, being small, were able to squeeze into awkward places in a factory. After the gross hazards of unsafe machinery had received attention, the efforts of industrial physicians were directed toward reducing the effects of toxic chemical and materials used in manufacturing processes. These toxins, include volatile substances, fibers (prototypically, asbestos), allergenic plant and animal proteins and heavy metals which impact most prominently on the respiratory tract and skin, as well as the liver, kidneys, and bladder. Far less common, to the point of being anecdotal, are toxic substances that may damage the skeletal system, resulting in malalignment and secondary osteoarthritis. Nonetheless, the wonders of industrial modernization have resulted in limited epidemics of skeletal intoxications, to wit, radium intoxication, which induced malignancies in those who worked in a factory that manufactured clock faces in the USA in the 1920s, and the 'ouch-ouch' disease (itai-itai byo), which was related to cadmium intoxication in Japan in the 1960s, but these events are very rare (*see* Chapters 10 and 22).

Changes in morbidity patterns and acceptance of the need for preventive medicine and early identification of risk factors (a philosophy that is distinct from curative medicine for chronic locomotor diseases), has made the field of occu-

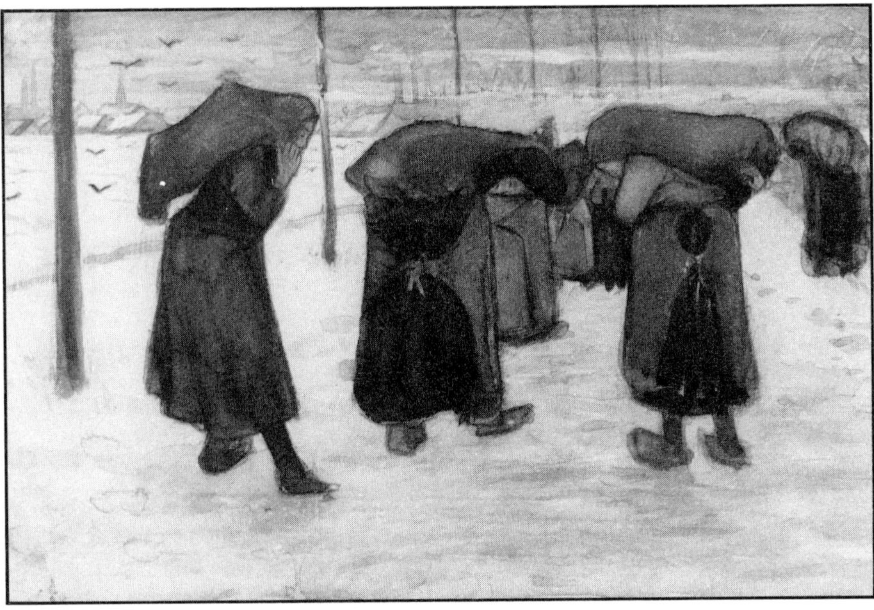

Figure 1 Van Gogh depicts the plight of nineteenth century women carrying coal, presaging back and neck pain, knee and first metatarsophalangeal joint osteoarthritis. (Reproduced with kind permission from Rijksmuseum, Knoller Muller, Otterloo, Holland)

pational medicine more relevant than it was a 100 years ago. This change in thinking has occurred throughout the developed world, and is epitomized by the shifts in policy and legislation in the United Kingdom during the past century. These policies resulted from the evolution of social welfare and social consciousness during the late nineteenth and early twentieth centuries, and were being implemented, albeit in a fragmented fashion, voluntarily or by statute in the age of Victorian and Edwardian prosperity. Other countries have evolved toward a similar attitude in relation to occupational medicine and prevention. Scandinavian countries are particularly advanced in this respect, but there are indications that even developing countries are striving to reach the goals of preventive medicine. These changes have culminated in the concept of 'Health for all by the year 2000'. Against this background, rheumatic complaints, which are often secondary to occupational insults, now ac-

count for annual losses of up to two thousand working days per thousand employees[3]. In the UK these concerns are formally addressed by the Occupational Health Services.

PREVENTING RHEUMATIC DISEASE

In terms of primary prevention, that is, the steps taken to avoid the onset of a disease process, there are four important conditions to be considered by the occupational health services relative to rheumatic complaints: back pain, osteoarthrosis, repetitive strain injury (overuse syndrome) and soft tissue rheumatism discussed in detail in Chapters 6 and 8.

Primary preventive measures for back pain have been discussed in Chapter 9 on both an environmental and individual basis. As far as osteoarthrosis is concerned, the heaviness of the loads being lifted or humped over prolonged periods of

326

work are also applicable[4], as depicted by Van Gogh over 100 years ago in Figure 1. However there is little evidence that posture is a risk factor for this condition, except for the knees in those who work in a kneeling position such as carpet layers[5].

Overuse syndrome, as its name implies, arises from repetitive use of muscles, tendons and ligaments, especially if the worker is unaccustomed to the task. Environmental prevention may thus be achieved by limiting overuse-type activities or even, if possible, changing from repetitive bench work to clerical work at intervals during the course of the day. Another environmental approach is the use of machines to do repetitive work, a measure which may offer economic payoffs to the employer, as well as health benefits to the workers. Also important in relation to overuse syndrome is the position required to perform a task, as is the height at which the arms are operating[6], as was discussed in relation to cervicoscapular back pain. Similarly, the need to reach or stretch to a point of discomfort may precipitate overuse symptoms. At the individual level, workers should be made aware of potential dangers or risk behaviors and encouraged to regulate their activities so that periods requiring repetitive movements are interspersed with periods of reduced repetition. It should be remembered that those suffering from overuse may also develop psychological problems and it is critical to ensure that workers have job satisfaction and morale is maintained through good staff relationships and a pleasant working environment.

It is often difficult to distinguish soft tissue rheumatism (also known as fibrositis) from overuse syndrome, particularly if the work being performed is of a repetitive nature. As with overuse syndrome, the height of the arms above the horizontal may contribute to fibromyalgia, as would undue reaching or stretching of either arms or legs. Inspection of the workplace usually enables a skilled observer to detect potential hazards or environmental factors, e.g. low temperatures and high humidity that may precipitate painful muscle spasms, and advise on evasive strategies. The simple expediency of protective clothing may solve the problem, if the work station itself cannot be appropriately modified, although it might be difficult to ensure that the workers will wear such clothing, especially if the protective clothing is cumbersome and makes it difficult to perform the tasks required. The psychological aspects of fibrositis are relevant to the acceptance or rejection of protective clothing as well as an understanding that stress, both at work and in the home, may be an aggravating factor in the onset and continuation of the symptoms.

IDENTIFICATION OF THOSE AT SPECIAL RISK

The unreliability and lack of specificity of presymptomatic screening for back pain by clinical examination, X-rays or ultrasound have been discussed in Chapter 9. Furthermore, there is little support for a relationship between recreational exercise and osteoarthrosis[7], although there is increasing evidence that occupational overuse does increase the risk of osteoarthrosis (*see* Chapter 10). It is generally accepted that meniscectomy predisposes to osteoarthrosis of the knees, and workers subjected to this type of knee surgery should, if possible, be advised against labors requiring repetitive knee flexion. Similar advice should also be given to those who have had an old fracture leading to malalignment of the articulation of an extremity.

As far as risk factors for other rheumatic complaints are concerned, opinions are guarded. Bjelle[6] has suggested that muscle strength tests may be helpful in identifying those at greatest risk for developing shoulder and arm problems arising from the joint capsules and tendons. Evidence that psychosocial stress predisposes to overuse syndrome and soft tissue rheumatism is largely anecdotal, and lacks the support of cohort studies. It is moreover difficult to correlate retrospectively vague etiological factors with painful conditions, especially when legal disputes arising therefrom may aggravate any dormant psychosocial component, and not be of themselves risk factors.

PREVENTION OF HANDICAP

Although prevention of disease, or the identification of those at special risk for a particular complaint are of critical importance. An important role played by the occupational physician and his team is in the prevention of permanent disability or handicap that might result from rheumatic diseases. An important point in understanding the prevention of handicap is an appreciation of the WHO's definitions of impairment, disability and handicap with the move towards a formal classification[8].

Prior to the publication of The International Classification of Impairments, Disabilities and Handicaps (ICIDH), there had been little formal attempt to standardize disability-related terminology – even among countries sharing a (supposedly) common language such as Australia, the UK and the USA. A brief summary of the relevant terms, their ICIDH-sanctioned (and WHO-blessed) definitions and their limitations, may help to put into perspective the concept of tertiary prevention of rheumatic disease through 'occupational health services'. It is being accepted increasingly that disease labels, as listed in the International Classification of Diseases[9], may be poorly applicable in the absence of well-defined boundaries among diseases. This means that for prevention, workers and occupational physicians should be more concerned with disablement than with precise diagnostic labels of the various rheumatic diseases.

The WHO term '*impairment*' includes both abnormalities (i.e., structural deviations from the norm, such as a cervical ribs) and malfunction (i.e. functional or locomotor abnormalities including the inability to move a joint or series of joints through the full range movement). Malfunctions also include those affecting intellect or emotion, which may have a bearing on the work capacity of someone developing a rheumatic disease. Thus, the recommended definition of impairment is '... any loss or abnormality of psychological, physiological or anatomical structure or function'; the explanatory notes accompanying this definition stress that an impairment is either present or absent and that the concept of a 'latent impairment' is unjustified – a comment that has some relevance to the concept of secondary prevention discussed above. Affected individuals may be unaware of impairments recognized by trained observers, e.g. doctors or nurses.

Where an *impairment* results in a limitation of normal activity for the affected individual, then the term *disability* is more appropriate, which the WHO would define as '... any restriction or lack (resulting from an impairment) of ability to perform an activity in a manner or within the range considered normal for a human being'. A person with a *disability* (e.g. stiffness or arthrodesis of a joint) cannot perform as well as his peers, for example, climb stairs or ladders, *and recognizes* his disability. However, such a loss of activity may cause little or no embarrassment to the individual; it is only when the limitation impinges directly on an activity which that individual wants to perform for maintenance or advancement of social, recreational or occupational status that it can be said to impose a *handicap*.

The suggested definition for *handicap* is '... a disadvantage for a given individual resulting from an impairment or a disability that limits or prevents the fulfilment of a role that is normal (depending upon age, sex and social or cultural factors) for that individual'. Thus, a handi-

328

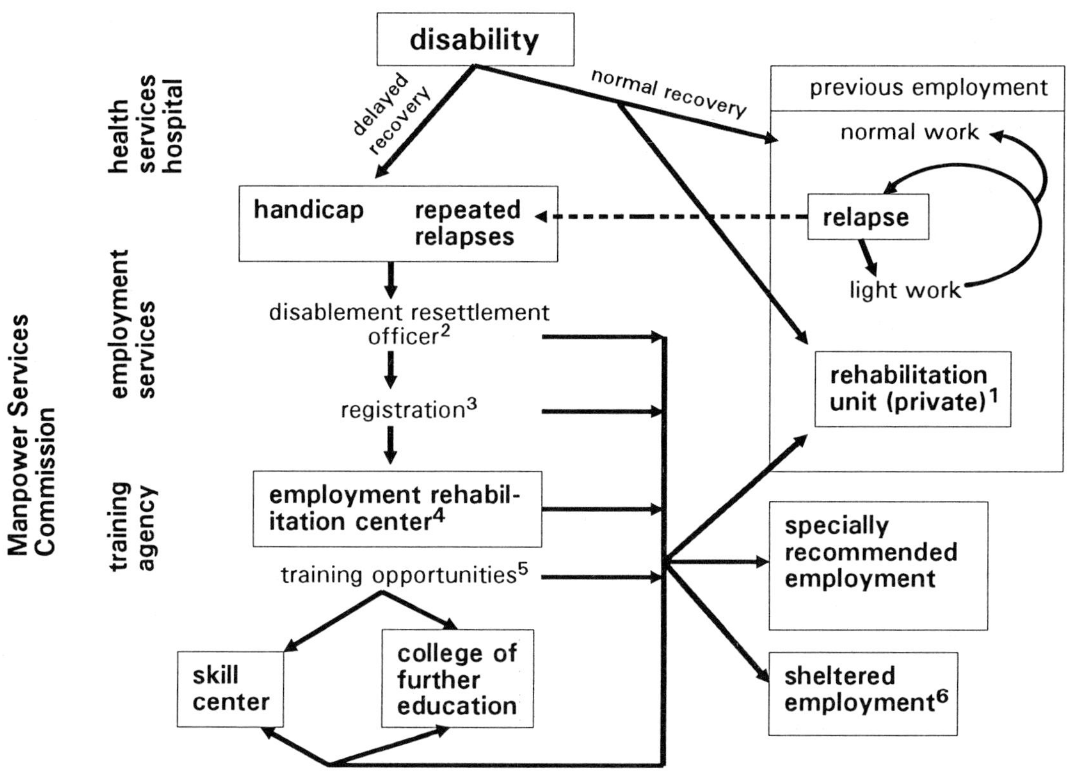

Figure 2 Diagram illustrating the help available to those with handicap in relation to work in UK. [1] Rehabilitation unit (private): administered by a firm for its own employees. A number of firms may share such a resource as part of a privately financed occupational health service; [2] Disablement resettlement officers are special officers of the employment service with local knowledge of the job opportunities for those with handicaps, and provide various services to employers prepared to accept handicapped staff; [3] Provides protection for those whose handicaps prevent them from performing certain tasks or who have prolonged and/or repeated periods of sick leave; [4] Employment rehabilitation center: assesses the potential of those requiring a job change, and has both clerical and industrial sections; these centers are also helpful in reacclimatizing those with erratic work attendance, with emphasis on rhythm in working routine by setting standards within functional capacity and insistence on compliance. A doctor and a gymnasium are available so that remedial programmes started elsewhere can be continued. NB: (1) Limited number of centers may pose traveling problems or necessitate temporary absence from home; (2) If the proportion of depressed patients among attending clientele is unduly high this may be detrimental to those with physical disabilities; [5] Training opportunities: courses arranged by the training agency or held at either a skill center or a college of further education, not exclusively for handicapped but for those officially recognized as being handicapped, stand a good chance of acceptance, particularly if previously assessed at an employment rehabilitation center; [6] Sheltered workshops: These are government maintained to provide employment for the severely handicapped, particularly those with below average production speeds. A limited number of able bodied supervisors may also carry out complicated and/or hazardous tasks

capped person is disadvantaged by the fact that he cannot achieve desired goals in terms of work performance, recreation or family activity; whereas impairments on their own or even disabilities if they are of no consequence to those affected, need not cause such disadvantage.

An 'occupational health service' is most concerned with preventing those handicaps that interfere with work performance and result in a reduction of the quality of life through pain (a common factor in any major rheumatic complaint) or through reduced earning capacity, either by lowering productivity or increasing sickness absence. In preventing handicap arising from rheumatic complaints, not only must potentially preventable disease processes be considered, as discussed earlier in this chapter, but also those diseases that cannot be prevented or cured, such as rheumatoid arthritis and ankylosing spondylitis. In these conditions, a worker may be chronically disabled, but still be able to work with suitable 'team' support: the late stages of these diseases may be incapacitating to the degree that work eventually becomes impossible. Prevention of occupational handicap requires evaluation by the occupational health team of the work station, the journey to and from the place of work and the route from the entrance to the work place to the work station itself. These efforts could contribute substantially to limiting handicap and keeping the individual in the work force. Prevention of occupational handicaps requires an adaptation of tasks and site where the work is performed to enable workers with a chronic rheumatic complaint, such as rheumatoid arthritis, osteoarthrosis or ankylosing spondylitis or back pain, to perform adequately.

The difficulty in assessing a disabled worker's ability to continue working is that a physician may certify a patient as: 'fit to return to work, but only for "light duties"'. This becomes problematic when the worker has no skills, e.g. clerical or academic, that can be translated into 'light duty'. Even so-called 'sedentary occupations' often require the employee to handle heavy ledgers or to reach and stoop to obtain material stored on high or low shelving; these are the very activities which a worker disabled by a rheumatic impairment may find difficult or even impossible, and therefore find himself at a disadvantage. Nonetheless, many of those with severe joint deformities, or limited back movement, may skilfully perform tasks at the workbench, which an ergonomist might classify as being at the heavy end of the spectrum. The difficulty in evaluating the extent of an individual rheumatic handicap is that these complaints fluctuate in intensity, during the day and from day to day.

A major obstacle observed in occupational medicine is that when a worker is 'on the job', the normal doctor–patient relationship seen in a therapeutic context, in which the patient believes the doctor to be 'on the patient's side', may not develop; the worker may distrust the occupational physician if redundancy or compensation are at issue. Distinction amongst the confounding factors of hysteria, anxiety or depression and their effects on symptoms and work performance on the one hand, and malingering on the other, may be a fine one. Furthermore the assistance of a psychiatrist or industrial psychologist, or even direct observation of work performance by an ergonomist may be rejected by a suspicious employee. This means that occupational physicians must understand and bear the brunt of the psycho-social evaluation and support in any given situation.

In view of the uncertainties of continued employment faced by someone with rheumatic complaints, it is advisable to ensure that he has the help of any statutory agencies designed to assist those with handicaps. In developing countries, resources are often limited to provision of only the most perfunctory of rehabilitation programs. Some countries, such as the oil-rich states of the Persian Gulf have a policy of importing inexpensive labor, and deporting those who develop chronic disease. This strategy absolves the host country from the need to provide rehabilitation services, while adding to the burden borne by poor countries. Most western countries have extensive rehabilitation services, which differ substantially in mode of operation and regulatory mechanisms.

In Britain, the Manpower Services Commission, established in 1974, was one such agency. Under the terms of the relevant legislation the Government accepted responsibility for job replacement and training, which includes special responsibility for those with handicap as a result of injury, chronic disease or congenital impairment from any cause. This was, in effect, a development of the postwar legislation which sought to give those disabled on active service, some protection in relation to obtaining jobs. Figure 2, together with the explanatory notes, gives an outline of the help available. A key person is the disablement resettlement officer and contact can be made through the nearest job center, though a few hospitals have such an officer seconded to work on the premises to ensure closer co-operation.

Some advantages arising from the British system include:

(1) Obligation by larger firms to include a percentage of those (registered) as disabled in their workforce;

(2) Insurance companies generally include (registered) persons in the employers' liability policy on the same terms as the able-bodied, since the inference is that account has been taken of the disability when allocating tasks;

(3) Help may be given with fares or transport to and from work to selected persons on the register;

(4) Special equipment to obtain or maintain employment may be provided (on loan); also structural adaptation of the workplace may be undertaken at public expense; and

(5) Registration tends to make it easier to obtain placement at an employment rehabilitation center, particularly for those in need of readjustment to the working situation following handicaps arising in later life or prolonged sickness absence. Such people are also more likely to obtain a place in the retraining scheme (e.g. at a skill center or college of further education).

Apart from the job itself, it is important to remember that transportation must be provided to and from the place of work for those with mobility handicaps. Individual invalid carriages or other conspicuous vehicles for the disabled are far less acceptable than adapted production models, not least because the latter can be used socially to transport other members of the family. Government funding is usually available for approved adaptations, and most local government authorities, which have responsibility for areas of high traffic congestion, give special dispensation to enable those with mobility handicap to park their vehicles.

Access to the factory is also the subject of legislation in Britain and ramps are becoming more commonplace in public and private buildings including factories. Where the factory has not got such special provision, the terms of legislation mentioned above allow for special adaptation at public expense to be made in very special circumstances.

SUMMARY

(1) Apart from very rare cases of malalignment of joints following fractures or chemical destruction of bone leading to joint deformity, primary prevention through weight limitation and hazard spotting with legally supported enforcement may be useful in relation to osteoarthrosis; however, evidence is less well documented than for back pain, where both absolute weight and its relative position to the body axis, as well as the posture adopted at work, are important (*see* Chapter 9).

(2) Screening by physical examination is unlikely to be helpful in deflecting workers from tasks that are potentially hazardous in terms of back pain, osteoarthrosis, repetitive strain syndrome and soft tissue rheumatism. However, a history suggestive of such problems, obtained through a self-completed questionnaire, may serve as a warning against allowing those affected be allocated to unsuitable tasks in terms of weight and posture.

(3) In practical terms, the greatest impact made by an occupational health service is by minimizing handicap among those with rheumatic problems, who are still able to work. Given that multiple factors are involved, individual detailed assessment of the physical, emotional, social and intellectual elements is required for each affected worker. It is also important to assess the tasks in the context of the working environment, which may require the involvement of psychologists and ergonomists with occupational physicians or nurses being required to sell such an idea to potentially handicapped workers.

(4) Statutory help with finding suitable jobs as well as (in rare cases) special equipment and help with transport to and from work are available in most western countries; the problems are to mobilize them to meet the identified needs of the affected workers and also to persuade those who may be depressed, anxious or paranoid as a complication of a chronic painful complaint to accept that such appraisals are in their best interests.

REFERENCES

1. Exodus, Chapter 6, v.v. 6–19
2. Ramazzini B. De Morbis Artificum Diatribe. Modena. 1700
3. Anderson JAD. Occupational aspects of low back pain. Clin Rheumatic Dis. 1980; 6:17–35
4. Lawrence JS. Rheumatism in Populations. London, Heinemann, 1977
5. Kivimaki J. Occupationally related ultrasonic findings in carpet and floor layers' knees. Scand J Work Environ Health. 1992; 18:400–402
6. Bjelle A. Scapulo humeral syndromes. Baillière's Clin Rheumatol. 1987; 1:547–559
7. Panush RS, Schmidt C, Caldwell J *et al.* Is running associated with degenerative joint disease. JAMA. 1986; 255:2252–2254
8. WHO International Classification of Impairments, Disabilities and Handicaps. Geneva, World Health Organization, 1980
9. WHO International Classification of Diseases. (9th revision). Geneva, World Health Organization, 1979

29. MEDICO-LEGAL ASPECTS OF PREVENTING WORK INCAPACITY FROM CHRONIC RHEUMATIC DISEASE

Nortin M. Hadler

INTRODUCTION

Much of this monograph attempts to identify environmental precipitants of rheumatic disease with a view toward primary prevention. However, avoiding all musculoskeletal symptomatology is an unrealistic goal. Regional musculoskeletal illnesses will afflict all of us, usually in an intermittent and remittent fashion, throughout our lives without overtly traumatic precipitants. Since musculoskeletal illness is predictably exacerbated by use of the afflicted body part, each episode places one's ability to maintain a prior level of physical functioning at some peril. The past century has witnessed attempts by every industrialized nation to provide recourse for individuals whose livelihood may be compromised by disease affecting this system. In this chapter I will provide an overview of such programs. I will also introduce a caveat that emerges from some of the sadder experiences with these exercises in ethical social legislation; for the unaware, ill-advised claimant there is potential for considerable iatrogenicity in what I have come to appreciate as a vortex of disability determination.

HISTORY OF REDRESS FOR WORK-RELATED INCAPACITY

Inability to support oneself or one's family is an age-old dread. Such individuals suffer the 'illness of work incapacity'. The equally age-old remedies of charity, altruism and philanthropy are as remarkable for their unevenness as for their magnanimity. In response to this dread, 'Poor Laws' were first codified in Elizabethan England[1]. These statutes required the nobility and landed gentry to identify the crippled and destitute on their lands and provide asylum care. Poor Laws represent the dawn of social legislation.

Just as they recognize a great human need, the Poor Laws also articulate a great western scruple; only the deserving are to be helped – the unworthy are to be ferreted out. This stipulation is the first of the two great western conundrums regarding redress for the illness of work incapacity. It survives today under the rubric of 'disability determination'. Well into the eighteenth century, the exercise of distinguishing the worthy from the unworthy poor was pursued with unconscionable zeal, indeed, corporal punishment was often specified for the malingerer. The zeal tempered, but the Poor Laws survived in Great Britain until they were finally condemned[2] and then superseded by the Social Insurance Acts of 1911 shepherded through the Edwardian Parliament by David Lloyd George.

The English Poor Laws were a watershed in social consciousness, but the ethic they served was distorted by the often arbitrary nature of the determination of worthiness and the stigmatizing nature of their largesse. Besides, they were no match for the social ramifications of the Industrial Revolution. No longer were your birthright and fate simply to work the land on which you were born; now you could or must seek employment. Furthermore, it was held that your employer discharged all his responsibilities to you by virtue of your salary; under common law the employer was not liable even should you be injured or incapacitated on the job by virtue of three tenets[3]:

(1) Employment is voluntary; in accepting employment, the employee accepts the risks inherent in such employment;

(2) If by his actions, the employee contributed in any way to his accident, the employer was exonerated of all liability; and

(3) In 1837 Abinger articulated the 'fellow servant' rule in the House of Lords which was imported into Boston in 1842 by Judge Shaw.

If a supervisor or other 'fellow servant' intervenes between the intent of the employer and the injury of the worker, the supervisor and not the employer bears any liability. This rule effectively blocked all redress for injured workers. In 1862 a journalist, Henry Mayhew, published a collection of his essays as *London Labour and the London Poor* which was recently republished by Dover Press[4]. He had set out 'to publish the history of a people, from the lips of the people themselves', the 'people' being those of the streets of London. He argued that the numbers of such people were greatly underestimated, that civil law treated them in a prejudicial fashion and that education was inaccessible to them. He urged compassion since it was the 'effects of uncertain labour (which) drive the labourers to improvidence, recklessness, and pauperism.' Mayhew was willing to champion, alike, 'those that will work, those that cannot work, and those that

will not work.' Mayhew stood alone. Society was still wedded to a need to exclude the unworthy poor, 'those that will not work', from compassion. And of those 'that cannot work', the human cost of industrialization was weighing heavy on the community conscience. The injured worker, deprived of redress by the Abinger rule, was a voice not long to be denied[5].

The social reform legislated in Germany in 1884 under Bismarck and imported into England in 1897 through Russell Cecil established two critical precedents: the continuing need for identifying the unworthy by means of 'disability determination', and the new need to single out those whose work incapacity is a consequence of accidental workplace injury for special treatment under Workers' Compensation programs. To this date in nearly all industrialized western countries, the latter category is maintained and the claimant so defined is provided with considerably more redress and recompense. However, defining both 'accident' and 'injury' is the second great western conundrum in providing redress for the illness of work incapacity.

THE SOCIOLOGY OF LOW BACK PAIN

In the discussion that follows, I will explain the fashion in which industrialized countries provide redress for individuals who suffer the illness of work incapacity in the context of low back pain. It will become clear that the very act of seeking redress confounds the experience of backache. Prerequisite to this insight is an appreciation of the sociology and medical anthropology of the experience. I will restrict my comments to individuals who are between the ages of 20 and 50 years, who suffer neither cauda equina symptoms nor severe leg weakness, whose backache was not precipitated by a discrete traumatic event involving external force, and who would be entirely well were it not for their backache. Such individuals suffer a regional backache; nearly

Table 1 The Health in Detroit survey. Incidence of musculoskeletal morbidity in 6 weeks. (Reproduced with kind permission from reference 6)

People experiencing musculo-skeletal symptoms	51%
Days with symptoms	11%
Average duration of symptoms	8 days

Table 2 The Health in Detroit survey. Characteristics of those with musculoskeletal morbidity. (Reproduced with kind permission from reference 6)

The majority were suffering from back or leg pain
  were otherwise asymptomatic
    thought they had 'arthritis'
    talked to their spouse
    consumed 'over the counter' remedies
    thought their symptoms were 'not very serious'
Less than 10%
  experienced neck or hand pain
  thought their symptoms were 'very serious'
    sought medical care (3%)
    received medical care (0.3%)

every single one of us will join their ranks in the very near future.

I base my auguring on several data sets. The 'Health in Detroit' study was a survey of one adult from each of a probability sample of 589 White households in the Detroit metropolitan area conducted in 1978 and published by Verbrugge and Ascione in 1987[6]. After an initial interview, participants maintained a daily diary for 6 weeks up to the closing interview. During the 6-week period the average adult had 16 symptomatic days; only 11% of men and 5% of women escaped symptom-free. Musculoskeletal morbidity (Table 1) ranked second only to respiratory symptomatology. Nearly half the people were experiencing musculoskeletal symptoms for 1 week out of 6! The quality of the experience

and the response to this unfortunate happenstance are highlighted in Table 2.

Clearly, episodes of backache color our lives for more than a few days each year. Some of the episodes are of such impact, even import, that well over 10% of us can recall prolonged episodes occurring in the past year[7,8]. Whenever we are faced with a backache, when we realise that the simplest of locomotor tasks can be confounded by increased pain, and we have a *predicament*[9,10]. There are three options available to us (Figure 1), and we have no choice but to consider these options, choose amongst them and act accordingly. This sequence I have termed 'processing the predicament'.

The vast majority of the people sampled in the Health in Detroit survey chose to cope with their regional backache by relying on their personal resources (Table 2). I have argued that this is advisable behavior[11] as the outcome with the other alternatives are far more problematic. After all, the majority of these predicaments remit spontaneously, albeit after challenging the sense of invincibility of more than one person so afflicted. Whether the average person can maintain sufficient self-confidence to cope within his personal sphere is itself problematic. Care, based usually on unproven remedies, is offered with conviction and a sense of urgency if not alarm by physicians and a myriad of alternative care givers. The sufferer is a market and the target of pervasive marketing in most countries.

One alternative is to cease to be a person with a predicament of backache and visit a physician. The moment one visits a physician, one is no longer a person with a predicament; one becomes a patient with the illness of backache. Although there are arguments questioning this approach[10,12], much of the interaction between the patient and physician relates to defining the cause of the backache in the hopes of effecting a cure.

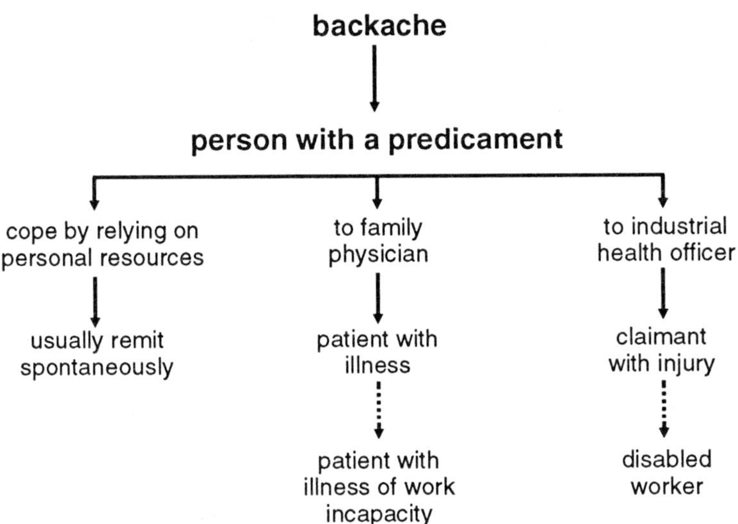

Figure 1 Most people will at one time or another (and often r peatedly) suffer from low back pain, and are confronted with a 'predicament' in each episode that requires that choices be made in this algorithm

Backache is one of the most frequently encountered illnesses in office practice[13]. The likelihood of a valid diagnosis of the underlying disease is exceedingly small; the likelihood of a diagnosis that leads to specific and reliably palliative intervention is vanishingly rare[10,14]. Nonetheless, contemporary medicine is wedded to this exercise for reasons that range from the self-serving to the service of the occasional patient who is benefited. Furthermore, since the traditional approach to diagnosis and therapy is seldom definitive but often sacrificing of time, money and healthfulness, the patient with the persistent incapacitating backache can well find himself afflicted with a confounding chronic illness, the illness of work incapacity. This fate, and the quest for a disability pension, will occupy our attention shortly.

There is a third option available to many with backache. If they perceive their backache to be a consequence of usage on the job, they can seek medical care as redress under Workers' Compensation statutes in all states in the USA and in most industrial countries. In so doing, they are no longer people with the predicament of regional backache; they transform into claimants with an injured back. Here the fate of a small percentage is also the chronic illness of work incapacity.

Between 1971 and 1975, the United States Health and Nutrition Examination Survey (HANES I) was carried out on a sample of non-institutionalized adults. One segment of the survey involved a detailed history and physical examination of 6913 adults aged 25 to 74 years. Table 3 presents

Table 3 Prevalence of backache and consequent incapacity in the HANES I survey. (Reproduced with kind permission from reference 8)

Total household sample	6 913
Recalled > 1 month of backache in past 2 years	1 189
Recalled incapacity from axial pain	389
with moderate/severe restrictions	69
causing job change	63
necessitating > 5 days off work	55

the prevalence of backache lasting at least 1 month and occurring within 2 years of the survey. Table 3 also yields some insights into the magnitude of the risk of the illness of work incapacity 25 years ago. It is clear from preceding chapters that the likelihood of choosing to be a claimant with a back injury and of suffering the illness of work incapacity has accelerated dramatically; it is equally clear that the likelihood of suffering the predicament or the illness of backache has not accelerated. After all, the predicament was already ubiquitous and the illness already overwhelmingly common in medical practice. Something has perturbed the processing and that 'something' is the quest of the remainder of this essay.

THE WORKERS' COMPENSATION PARADIGM

The turn of the century saw the rise of organized labor. Fueling the movement throughout the industrial world was the unconscionable lot of the average worker. Near the top of the list of grievances was the plight of workers who had been rendered 'worthy poor' as a consequence of injuries suffered on the job. The Prussian statutes established the precedent for offering special treatment to such individuals. All 58 American Workers' Compensation jurisdictions offer an exclusive, no-fault remedy to those who suffer a personal injury which arose 'out of and in the course of employment and occurred by accident'. Such individuals are afforded medical care, suffer little financial compromise while mending, and are compensated, in theory, for any permanent loss of wage earning capacity. The vast majority of claimants have suffered discrete traumatic events such as lacerations, amputations and the like. For these individuals, Workers' Compensation provides an efficient remedy which has provoked little controversy and relatively little consternation regarding the cost/benefit ratio of the program up to the present. The controversies relate to coverage for 'occupational diseases' and

for disorders where the precipitant is less discrete or less overtly work-related. The latter category includes such illnesses as 'stress on the job', 'cumulative trauma disorders'[15], and the like. So-called 'cumulative trauma disorders', 'repetitive strain injuries' and the like are covered in Chapters 7 and 8 of this monograph. It is my contention that these clinical labels are rubrics that obfuscate a heuristic concept[15] that is not only flawed but iatrogenic[16]. The near-epidemics of these illnesses in Japan and Australia have waned with lessons for us all that support my contention. However, the illness that continues to dominate in this regard is the regional backache. The compensable backache is a challenge for clinical medicine[17,18], econometrics[19] and labor relations[20]. The challenge relates to three pivotal determinations all of which masquerade as clinical constructs:

When is a regional backache an injury? Prior to World War II, regional backache was seldom conceptualized by the sufferer or by society as an 'injury'. Medicine provided an inventive differential diagnosis but trauma was felt to be improbable. In 1934, two surgeons, Mixter and Barr[21], first described the symptoms of discal herniation in a series of patients many of whom had cauda equina syndrome and several of whom improved following surgical intervention. They suggested that herniation was a common cause of regional backache, often amenable to surgical intervention; their hypothesis took hold rapidly in America and began to pervade the remainder of the industrial world. At least as dramatic was the implication of their label for the disease, 'rupture' of the disc. Everywhere, the judiciary held that if the clinical result was so violent as to be a 'rupture', the details of the causal event should not be determinative of the accidental nature of the illness. In this fashion regional backache became back injury, and backache occurring on the job and ascribed to discal herniation became compensable[22].

This line of reasoning dominates the administration of the American Workers' Compensation programs even today[17]; a regional backache diagnosed as a ruptured disc almost always elicits an award from Workers' Compensation. This is not the case in other countries[23,24]. Both New Zealand and Switzerland insure their entire adult populations separately for the clinical consequences of injury, regardless of work relatedness, with benefits that include medical care and compensation for lost wages. New Zealand provides ready, usually uncontested access to benefits; Switzerland offers a severe gauntlet to access in terms of the assertion of accidental cause of the backache, but once access is gained, benefits are more liberal. France demands sudden onset at work corroborated by a witness before providing liberal benefits. These programatic distinctions all reflect the need to come to grips with the issue of causality if one wishes to umbrella regional backache under a Workers' Compensation paradigm.

When is the worker with a back injury as healed as he is likely to get? All schemes for redress for the illness of work incapacity encourage, support, even nurture the possibilities of healing and of sufficient recovery to return to gainful employment. Many schemes, particularly Workers' Compensation schemes, will expend considerable sums on medical care and income substitution as long as steady progress is being made or likely to be made on the road to clinical recovery. The intent is noble. The pitfalls are obvious; therapeutic zeal is potentially unbridled and motivation toward rapid recovery tested. The point of maximum healing is termed 'fixed and stable' in America and often 'consolidation' elsewhere. Its definition can be quite contentious invoking the opinions of 'independent medical examiners' (IMEs) in America, the 'expert' in France, and sundry similar mechanisms in other jurisdictions[24]. The IME is an expensive solution sharing all the short-comings we shall discuss for con-

tracted examinations in disability insurance schemes. Its supporters argue that it is more humane than the fixed temporal cut-off employed by some countries.

DISABILITY INSURANCE SCHEMES

The distinction between a disabling backache and a disabling back injury is not trivial. In most countries, with notable exceptions such as Holland[24], disabling injuries that a rise out of and in the course of employment are traditionally afforded more generous and more comprehensive benefits than similarly disabling illnesses whose pathogenesis is unrelated to employment. The distinction was drawn from the outset of the social legislation and is nowhere more dramatic than in America where nearly half a century was to pass between writing Workers' Compensation statutes and national disability insurance.

In 1954, Social Security Disability Insurance (SSDI) was established. Wages were assessed, employers contributed, and the moneys accumulated in a separate fund that was restricted, until recently, to the payment of disability benefits. Requirements as to how long or how much one must contribute to the Disability Insurance Fund to be eligible for benefit in the event of disability have changed since 1954. Obviously workers may become disabled after contributing for brief periods and some individuals with work incapacity may never have contributed. Rather than totally liberalize SSDI, the Federal Government assumed administration of the Supplemental Security Income (SSI) program in 1973. This program insures those who are ineligible for SSDI because of inadequate contributions and draws on general tax revenues.

The intent of SSDI/SSI is quite different from Workers' Compensation insurance[18]; this program insures against poverty consequent to any illness while Workers' Compensation insurance is designed with income substitution as a goal. To

> C. Other vertebrogenic disorders (e.g. herniated nucleus pulposus, spinal stenosis) with the following persisting for at least 3 months despite prescribed therapy and expected to last 12 months. With both 1 and 2:
>   1. Pain, muscle spasm, and significant limitation of motion in the spine; **and**
>   2. Appropriate radicular distribution of significant motor loss with muscle weakness and sensory and reflex loss.

Figure 2 Section 1.05C of the Social Security Adminstration's Handbook for Physicians. This is the 'listing' for disabling regional backache

a large extent the SSDI/SSI program is modeled after the 'invalid pensions' of Europe that preceded it. To be eligible for SSDI/SSI one must be incapable of 'any substantial gainful activity by reason of any medically determinable physical or mental impairment or impairments which can be expected to result in death or which have lasted, or can be expected to last, for a continuous period of not less that 12 months' (20 Code of the US Federal Regulations 404.1591). Defining 'substantial gainful activity' is administratively straightforward; the current operational definition is US$ 300/month. In other words, you must be so ill that you cannot even earn US$ 300/month in any job anywhere within reason. As we discussed above, these programs are attempting to ferret out the 'unworthy', those who simply 'will not work' and therefore must establish some definition of the prerequisite illness. SSDI/SSI borrows from a tradition in workers' compensation that even Workers' Compensation administrations have largely abandoned – using impairment as the surrogate measure. Impairment 'results from anatomical, physiological or psychological abnormalities which are demonstrable by medically acceptable clinical and laboratory diagnostic techniques .. (symptoms) are, alone, insufficient .. ' (Code 20 of Federal Regulations 404.1501). SSDI/SSI is attempting to es-

tablish quantifiable criteria for pathoanatomical abnormalities that are assumed to be highly sensitive and specific for the most severe illness of work incapacity rendering one incapable for earning even US$ 300/month[25]. The criteria to be satisfied in order for a regional backache to qualify as disabling are given as Figure 2. If these criteria are met along with a determination that the claimant cannot maintain 'substantial gainful employment', an award will follow. This is seldom the case[26], the vast majority of claimants are denied and share the fate of many disabled under Workers' Compensation. These individuals enter the contest of disability determination wherein they have to prove they are dreadfully ill.

THE CONTEST OF DISABILITY DETERMINATION

Every disability program, whether a Workers' Compensation program or an invalid pension program such as SSDI/SSI, defines disability as free from volition. If one has the choice to return to work, one is ineligible for compensation and benefits. How does one prove to the administrators that the quest for a pension relates to forces outside one's control, and derive from the illness. In truth, impairment short of pathoanatomical catastrophe (such as coma) is seldom totally determinative of the incapacity. In fact, social exigencies in the workplace are major variables contributing to the processing of the predicament of backache as an injury claim, as schematically delineated in Figure 1. Disability determination is not a bureaucratic decree, it is a dynamic contest that places the claimant on the defensive. The claimant has to prove he is ill. Unsuspecting, under the mantle of social redress, with the encouragement of minions of bureaucrats, physicians and adjudicators, the claimant enters the contest that is itself iatrogenic. How can one possibly improve or heal if one has to prove one is ill (Figure 3). In SSDI/ SSI to the extreme[27], but in all schemes to some extent, physicians will be testing the veracity of the claimant against invalid, unreliable standards. The claimant under Workers' Compensation has the additional challenge of proving his regional backache is an injury in the face of assertions and contentions based on marginal ergonomic data. The entire unwieldy contest takes on a life of its own in which all parties seem to benefit except the claimant whose illness is so confounded that rehabilitation programs and pain clinics await him.

In SSDI/SSI, the claimant with a backache almost always loses the first round of the contest, played out before agency bureaucrats who review clinical records attempting to define impairment and apply the 'substantial gainful employment' rule. Often the agency will purchase objective clinical data, the so-called 'contracted examination', from a physician other than the claimant's physician. Over 250 000 contracted examinations are purchased each year. When analyzed as to their intellectual content, it is clear that contracted examinations for backache are not clinical exercises in that they give little if any weight to the claimant's symptoms in assessing his disability; physical signs and radiographic findings hold sway[27]. As reviewed elsewhere[28] and discussed below, tying disability determination to impairment criteria is invalid. Without acknowledging

this truth by programatic change, the SSDI/SSI has created a second level of the contest. Once denied by the agency (the fate of some 80% of claimants), there is ready recourse before an Administrative Law Judge in the Social Security Administration. Here the rules of the contest are expanded to permit the expression of symptoms, the corroboration of witnesses to the illness including the treating physicians, and the assistance of attorneys. Over 50% of contests are won before the Administrative Law Judge[26].

THE VORTEX OF DISABILITY DETERMINATION

Society is willing to go to great lengths to devise an objective measure of disability. The traditional approach is to invert the basic tenet of differential diagnoses. That tenet is that patients present with symptoms, their illness, and the physician is expected to deduce the underlying cause, the disease. For disability determinations, the converse asserts that if one knows and quantifies the disease, one can predict the illness. If there is sufficient disease, the illness should operate as the illness of work incapacity. This is the principle of 'impairment rating': seldom does it hold as much sway today as it does in America but it permeates thinking everywhere. I am convinced that the notion of impairment rating is fatally flawed and should be discarded. The illness of work incapacity is a necessary consequence only of global, catastrophic disease such as a massive stroke, terminal emphysema, end-stage heart disease, and the like. Short of these extremes, the illness of work incapacity is multivariate in precipitation and perpetuation. The work of Magora[29], Bigos and colleagues[30] and Deyo and Diehl[31] render this conclusion inescapable for low back pain; in fact, psychological and sociopolitical confounders overwhelm both disease and ergonomic measures in predicting the illness of work incapacity. Nonetheless, almost all systems persist in placing weight on impairments and seem fixated on finding objective measures in the face of the

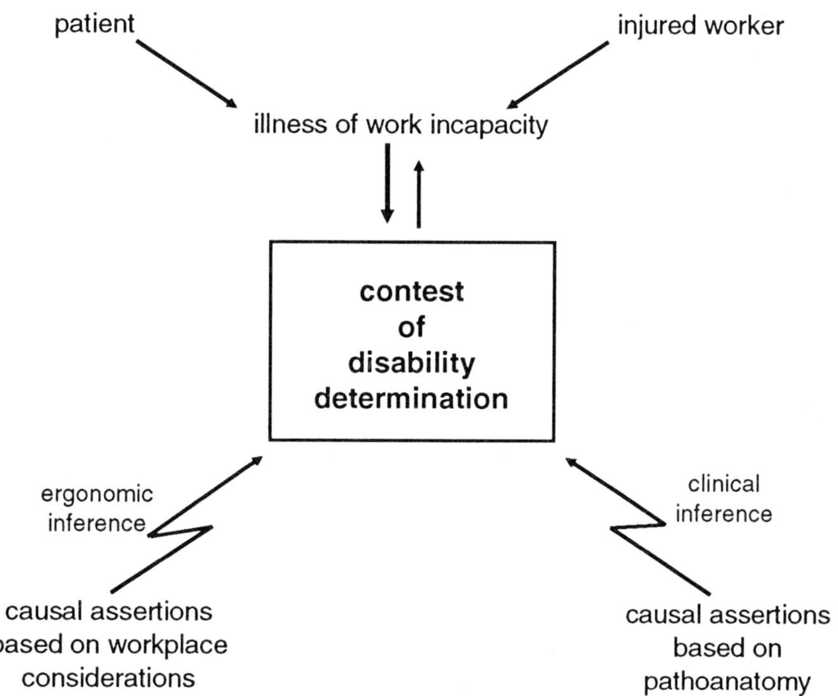

Figure 3 The contest of disability determination

daunting inadequacies of radiographic and electrodiagnostic criteria in this regard[32,33]. No wonder orthopedic surgeons seem to adopt their own idiosyncratic criteria for disability which they offer to the insurer under the guise of impairment rating[34]. In America, recourse is to the courtroom usually before an Administrative Law Judge within the system. Elsewhere, recourse is often before a panel of educated citizens, and more often impairment rating has been abandoned[24]. Disability insurance schemes are mandatory in an enlightened world. They must be made readily accessible and they must be salutary. We are now completing a century of experimentation and false starts. Let's hope the next generation of planners has learned the lessons.

REFERENCES

1. Hadler NM. Who should determine disability? Semin Arthritis Rheum. 1984; 14:45–51
2. Grigg J. Lloyd George: The People's Champion 1902–1911. London, Eyre Methuen, 1978
3. Larson A. The Law of Workmen's Compensation. New York, Matthew Bender, 1972, Section 4.30, pp. 25–32
4. Mayhew H. London Labour and the London Poor. London, Dover Press, 1983, vv. 1–4
5. Bohlen FH. A problem in the drafting of workmen's compensation acts. Harvard Law Review. 1912; 25:328–348
6. Verbrugge LM, Ascione FJ. Exploring the iceberg. Common symptoms and how people care for them. Medical Care. 1987; 25:539–569
7. Frymoyer JW, Pope MH, Costanza MC, Rosen JC et al. Epidemiologic studies of low-back pain. Spine. 1980; 5:419–422
8. Cunningham LS, Kelsey JL. Epidemiology of musculoskeletal impairments and associated disability. Am J Public Health. 1984; 74:574–579
9. Hadler NM. Medical Management of the Regional Musculoskeletal Diseases. Orlando, Grune and Stratton, 1984

10. Hadler NM. Clinical Concepts in Regional Musculoskeletal Illness. Orlando: Grune and Stratton, 1987

11. Hadler NM. The predicament of backache. J Occup Med. 1988; 30:449

12. Hadler NM. Regional back pain. N Engl J Med. 1986; 315:1090–1092

13. Cypress BM. Characteristics of physician visits for back symptoms. A national perspective. Am J Public Health. 1983; 73:389–395

14. Quebec Task Force on Spinal Disorders. Scientific approach to the assessment and management of activity-related disorders. Spine. 1987; 12 (Suppl. 1):S1–S59

15. Hadler NM. The roles of work and of working in disorders of the upper extremity. Baillière's Clin Rheumatol. 1989; 3:121–141

16. Hadler NM. Cumulative trauma disorders. J Occup Med. 1990; 32:38–41

17. Hadler NM. Legal ramifications of the medical definition of back disease. Ann Intern Med. 1978; 89:992–999

18. Hadler NM. Occupational illness. The issue of causality. J Occup Med. 1984; 26:587–593

19. Worrall JD, Appel D. The impact of Workers' Compensation benefits on low-back claims. In Hadler NM, ed., Clinical Concepts in Regional Musculoskeletal Illness. Orlando, Grune and Stratton, 1987, pp. 281–298.

20. Burton JF. Disability benefits for back disorders in workers' compensation In Hadler NM, Gillings DB, eds., Arthritis and Society. London, Butterworths, 1985, pp. 89–103

21. Mixter WJ, Barr JS. Rupture of the intervertebral disc with involvement of the spinal canal. N Engl J Med. 1934; 211:10–15

22. Hadler NM. Regional musculoskeletal diseases of the low back. Cumulative trauma versus single incident. Clin Orthop Rel Res. 1987; 221:33–41

23. Hadler NM. Industrial rheumatology. The Australian and New Zealand experiences with arm pain and backache in the workplace. Med J Aust. 1986; 144:191–195

24. Hadler NM. Disabling backache in France, Switzerland, and the Netherlands: contrasting sociopolitical constraints on clinical judgment. J Occup Med. 1989; 31:823–831.

25. Hadler NM. Medical ramifications of the federal regulation of the Social Security Disability Insurance program. Ann Intern Med. 1982; 96: 665–669.

26. Carey TS, Hadler NM. The role of the primary physician in disability determination for Social Security Insurance and Workers' Compensation. Ann Intern Med. 1986; 104:706–710

27. Carey TS, Hadler NM, Gillings D, Wallston T. Medial disability assessment of the back pain patient for the Social Security Administration: the weighting of presenting clinical features. J Clin Epidemiol. 1988; 41:691–697

28. Yelin E, Meenan R, Nevitt M, Epstein W. Work disability in rheumatoid arthritis: effects of disease, social, and work factors. Ann Intern Med. 1980; 93:551–556

29. Magora A. Investigation of the relation between low back pain and occupation. Psychological aspects. Scan J. Rehabil Med. 1973; 5:191–196

30. Bigos SJ, Spengler DM, Martin NA, Zeh J et al. Back injuries in industry: a retrospective study. III. Employee-related factors. Spine. 1986; 11:252–256

31. Deyo RA, Diehl AK. Psychosocial predictors of disability in patients with low back pain. J Rheum. 1988; 15:1557–64

32. Eisenberg RL, Hedgcock MW, Gooding GAW, DeMartini WJ, Akin JR, Ovenfors CO. Compensation examination of the cervical and lumbar spines: critical disagreement in radiographic interpretation. Am J Radiol. 1980; 134:519–522

33. Haldeman S, Shouka M, Robboy S. Computed tomography, electro-diagnostic and clinical findings in chronic Workers' Compensation patients with back and leg pain. Spine. 1988; 13:345–350

34. Brand RA, Lehmann TR. Low-back impairment rating practices of orthopaedic surgeons. Spine. 1983; 8:75–78

30. SPECIAL PROBLEMS IN DEVELOPING COUNTRIES

John Darmawan and Richard Wigley

INTRODUCTION

As noted in Chapter 3, population surveys have shown that rheumatic diseases are common in developing countries, and are frequently severe enough to lead to loss of work time. Low back pain, shoulder pain, and epicondylitis commonly occur in those with chronic rheumatic complaints, and are significant public health problems requiring preventive and therapeutic intervention.

Infectious diseases, in particular, those with diarrhea and/or association with malnutrition, have a very high priority for the limited budgetary resources available to the health care systems in developing nations. Infection control will, by extension have a beneficial impact on the joints and musculoskeletal system (*see* Chapters 12–18), when these are affected by such Third World diseases as arise from poor sanitation and malnourishment. Understandably and in general terms, other rheumatic diseases cannot be adequately prevented or treated by physicians and ancillary health care workers. With the taming of venereal, gastrointestinal and parasitic infections and improvement of nutritional status, the average age of these populations rises, as does the prevalence of rheumatic complaints, which begin to mimic the pattern seen in developed countries (Chapter 3).

Demographic problems
Of the 5.4 billion population of the world, 4.2 billion people live in developing countries, 80% of these live in the areas with inadequate housing, communications, sanitation, water and health care facilities.

Iatrogenic problems
The absence of government social security support and insurance coverage for most of those in developing nations means that only the wealthiest can afford western style health care. Moreover, the qualified rheumatologists are almost invariably located in major cities. For the rest of the population, less expensive western drugs, which might be regarded in advanced nations as being too toxic for certain rheumatic complaints, e.g. phenylbutazone, methampyrone, prednisone are available without prescription. The infirm, then often turn to traditional medicine including herbal remedies, which may be 'fortified' by cheap, but potent western drugs with major side effects, and potentially disastrous results[1]; minor self limiting complaints should not be treated with potentially dangerous drugs.

Regulation of these 'over the counter' concoctions is not effectively policed, as economic and commercial considerations do not allow viable alternatives. Salicylates, either alone or buffered with antacids, though cheap, are not well tolerated in developing countries where red peppers (jalapeña) containing capsainoids and tamarind which is also ulcerogenic, are routinely used in cooking. No formal studies have been done.

Smoking, alcohol and possibly strong coffee are additional factors predisposing to gastric intolerance and possibly ulceration. Paracetamol is tolerated well and is a cheap alternative but must be used with caution in those with liver disease, which is not uncommon in those nations that have a high prevalence of hepatitis.

Organization of services

In these countries, institutional care and physiotherapy are available only to urban wealthy. Those living in rural areas usually cannot afford to travel to one of the country's very few rheumatologists, and thus turn to the traditional masseurs who often have little or no formal training. It is heartening that in many developing countries, rheumatologists are forming associations affiliated to the international league, becoming more influential in medical and paramedical teaching and organizing national arthritis foundations to promote training and services. It is hoped that these will eventually have the resources to circulate educational material for the public and primary health workers.

Education

There is a need for general public education on the prevention of accidents, back injuries, and occupational problems. Infections, rheumatic fever, tropical, sexually transmitted diseases and dietary problems are covered to some extent by existing health programs. It is disturbing that in Indonesia's Central Java, where the thiamine deficiency disease beri-beri, was first shown to result from removal (polishing) of the husks of brown rice, thiamine deficiency continues to be the most common cause of limb discomfort, according to a COPCORD (Community Oriented Program for the Control of Rheumatic Disease) survey from 1983 to 1987[1], as thiamine-poor polished rice continues to be a staple food. A high prevalence of knee pain related to genu valgum in north China (Chapter 3) raises the possibility of vitamin D and/or calcium deficiency in a community where milk is rarely used and sunlight exposure is low. High sunlight in the south may

protect those on a low calcium diet from developing rickets.

The World Health Organization (WHO) is currently preparing a booklet on rheumatic conditions for use by primary health care workers[2]. In many countries, television is still not available widely enough for this purpose, and some villages have a single communal television. Written, audiotape, videotape and television educational material used in developed countries on the avoidance of back, neck and joint injury, overload and overuse cannot be used in a community without electricity, and whose communication with the outside world is via a portable radio. Pictomanuals to be published by WHO will be helpful in these communities[2], as are comic strip type pictographs[3], detailed below.

OCCUPATIONAL RHEUMATIC PROBLEMS

The primitive methods used in agriculture, e.g. use of a short hoe for ground crops as chronicled by Van Gogh, Figure 1, customs which continue to be used in developing nations. The COPCORD protocol could be extended to record occupational tasks such as the use of the short (65–81 cm) handled hoe for tilling the soil in certain Asian countries, e.g. in Indonesia[4], which weigh from 1 to 2 kg. In rice cultivation the irrigated soil is broken by men using these hoes and the clod is crushed at a second round. This is done in three minute cycles with 26 big strikes, 20 small strikes and seven crushings of clods with the foot interrupted by several seconds of spontaneous rest[4]. It is intriguing that this traditional pattern corresponds so closely to the frequent breaks now recommended for the overuse syndromes so prevalent in developed countries (Chapter 7). Conjunctivitis from splashing the eyes with infected water is a problem. Both this and presumably back pain would be reduced by the simple expediency of using a longer handle

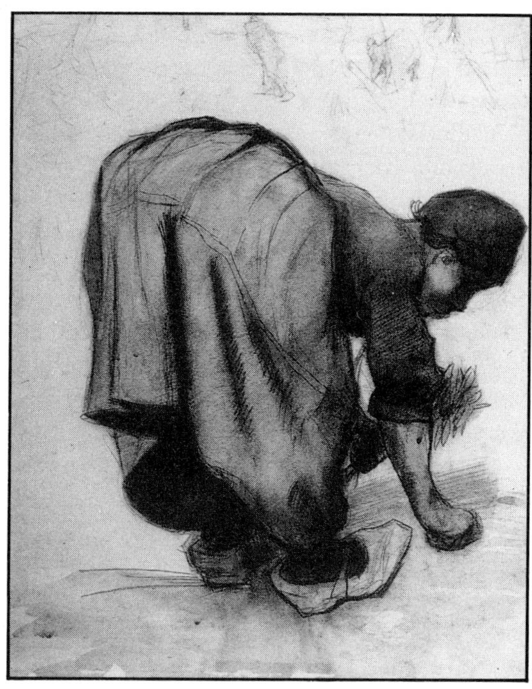

Figure 1 A drawing by Van Gogh depicting a woman harvesting a ground crop. (Reproduced with kind permission from Rijksmuseum, Knoller Muller, Otterloo, Holland)

for the same hoe, reducing the forward flexion required of the back, as has been recommended in the USA[5].

After levelling the paddies with an implement pulled by a boy-navigated buffalo, rice seedlings are planted by the women, who bend their backs from dawn to dusk once or twice a year during the planting seasons, potentially causing severe pain to the unaccustomed back. Harvesting the rice by cutting it close to the ground with a sickle also involves prolonged stooping; harvesting is less taxing to the back when a small finger knife is used to cut the rice stalk at the top while standing, and several breaks are taken during the day. Back pain though distressing during work, is relieved by a full night's rest. Unless these millennia-old methods for planting and harvest-

ing rice are proven scientifically invalid, they should not be tampered with. Further ergonomic research is needed, which addresses such issues as whether prolonged bending at the limit of flexion, allows muscle rest, since ligaments carry the static load (Figure 1). If not, the static load might produce an ischemic muscle repetitive strain syndrome type of pain.

Traditional carrying devices in the East may well minimize the risk of back strain, as for example, the flexible carrying pole, which allows lifting with the knees and a straight back. Carrying the load with a smooth ambling gait; the flexibility of the pole minimizes vertical shock loading; the balanced load eliminates lateral flexion stress, and there is no rotational stress, as all turning is from the feet. In the Indonesian COPCORD study, one retired man who had carried loads on such a pole to a city 30 miles away and returning the same day had thickened skin pads on the shoulders. These develop in some pole carriers[6], and can be painful. They presumably did not develop in the shaped shoulder yoke traditionally used for milk pails in Europe but these would be more rigid with more shock loading potential. Indonesian women use a sash of cloth to carry baskets, and may use two, with an infant in one and farm produce in the other, allowing heavy loads to be carried, at the considerable cost of back stress, incorrect posture while bending and torsion while lifting the load.

Head carrying by women of India and Africa, as well as the Philippines (Figure 2) might be expected to cause neck pain though the rhythmic swaying carriage would minimize strain. Lawrence[7] found increased severity of degenerative changes in the neck in head carrying Jamaican women but no proportionate increase in neck pain. Jamaicans had more severe cervical spine degeneration than African Blacks, who also carry loads on the head, a discrepancy that requires explanation. In Bali, women carry bricks lifted onto a board on

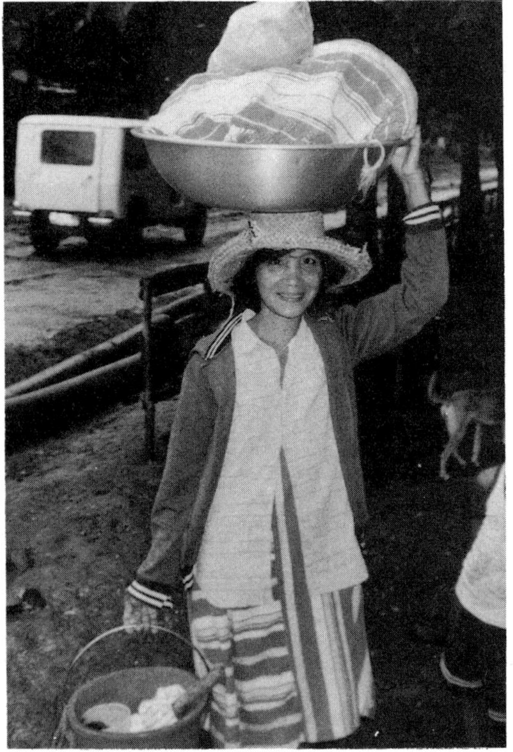

Figure 2 Woman carrying large weights on the head in the Philippines

their heads by another person but no studies of neck problems have been discovered.

In the COPCORD studies in Asia (Chapter 3), overuse or strain-type spinal pain is followed in frequency by shoulder and elbow pain. Other overuse syndromes have not been systematically studied, but typical repetitive syndrome was observed in basket weavers in the Philippines[8]. There is clearly a need for more ergonomic research in developing countries.

Gout

Gout is more common in Filipinos living in North America than in those living in the Philippines[9]. The prevalence of gout increased in the Tokelauans migrating to New Zealand where a west-ern diet and beer consumption result in a rise in weight and led to an increase in gout, implicating the western diet as a preventable risk factor[10]. Nonetheless, gout is relatively common in Indonesians[11] despite the marginal food supply, and being Muslim, they do not drink alcohol. This may be related to a genetic predisposition to gout.

Rheumatic fever

Rheumatic fever is a proportionally greater problem in developing countries, but is also prevalent in some ethnic groups in developed countries such as the Maori in New Zealand (*see* Chapter 11).

Rheumatoid arthritis

As in developed countries, prevention of rheumatoid arthritis (RA) is not feasible. Due to the direct access that the lay community has to potent therapeutic agents, and the ubiquity of gastrointestinal and respiratory infections, life expectancy may be shortened in RA in developing countries[12]. Misinformation may lead to untreated secondary drug-related disease and mortality. Though the Indonesian government, prompted by the findings of the COPCORD study, legislated against adding drugs such as prednisone and phenylbutazone to popular remedies, this is not well policed and the practice continues. Many will use western remedies as well as traditional methods which may not be harmless.

Osteoarthritis

Osteoarthritis of the knees is common in developing countries and carries a much greater handicap since squatting is a necessary part of daily living, in work and in defecation. Osteoarthritis may arise secondary to childhood rickets in association with genu varus, or occur in Kashin–Beck disease which causes secondary osteoarthritis particularly of the knees in endemic areas in northern China and parts of Siberia. Repeated overloading from the severe stresses generated in squatting and rising from the squat position may lead to premature cartilaginous degeneration[13]. This problem may resolve in newly industrialized countries when sitting at work, daily activities and at the toilet become the norm, although it may persist in those countries, e.g. Japan or segments of the population, e.g. certain religious orders, where tradition dictates kneeling and squatting on formal occasions.

Traditional medicine

Traditional medicine dispensed by herbalists, masseurs and shamanistic witch doctors continue to be used widely in developing countries. Since many rheumatic complaints remit spontaneously, often within short periods of time (and without treatment), it is unclear whether the beneficial effect (if any) of these medicines is due to the mere passage of time, a faith healing or placebo effect or a therapeutic effect greater than placebo[14]. It is also unknown whether these treatments by themselves are harmful (an issue the WHO is attempting to resolve[15]), although they are clearly pernicious if potentially toxic western drugs are added to a traditional formulation, delaying a more appropriate treatment. Nonetheless, if these regimens relieve anxiety, while nature effects spontaneous healing, then it can be argued that a valuable service has been rendered. In the West, alternative methods also abound, but are widely rejected by the medical establishment, and often frustrate any attempts by 'mainstream' physicians at preventive or therapeutic measures that are more effective than placebos.

Education

The leather puppet shadow play (wayang kulit) is a popular form of entertainment in rural and to a lesser extent, urban regions of certain parts of South East Asia, including Java and Madura, which have a population of more than one hundred million, and Malaysia. These puppets depict the Hindu epics of Mahabharata and Ramayana, and the puppeteer modifies his dialogue according to the needs of the audience.

In a pilot educational program by the WHO, the ability to modify the attitudes of a test population through the use of these puppets was studied. Those natives who had rheumatic pain within the last 2 weeks were subjected to a pictorial questionnaire on correct activities of daily living with respect to neck, back, and joint pain. Two primary health care workers (PHW) who understood the cultural characteristics, beliefs, values and local dialect of the people, obtained answers to a pictorial questionnaire on the correct way to perform some of the daily activities of living to minimize rheumatic problems from subjects and controls. A puppet shadow play incorporating an Arthritis Community Education (ACE) program was then shown to test subjects only[3]; in the play, the puppets subtly educated the audience with an improvised dialogue interwoven into a section of one of the most popular Hindu epics, using vocabulary and language understood by, and compatible with the traditional beliefs, customs, and ethics of a largely illiterate rural people.

The educational goals of this program did not include individual needs, or different stages of specific rheumatic disorders, but rather illustrated the correct and incorrect methods of carrying out daily living activities. The pictographs cover only the simple generalized teaching of proper posture, positioning, joint and back protection techniques, physical stress reduction and range retaining and strengthening exercises for the muscles of the involved joints. The program which focused on showing and doing, not reading and writing, emphasized behavioral and postural changes for improving performance. This had a definite, though short lived, effect of improved knowledge of appropriate daily living activity. At 1 and 6 months after the play, mean scores for the test group were 90% and 81% correct whereas the controls showed no change at 65% and 64%. Not surprisingly the better educated showed higher scores. The ACE program induced a significant improvement in knowledge of the correct activities of daily living in preventing or coping with musculoskeletal pains.

A number of important conclusions derive from this study. The vocabulary for community education must be within the range of the population (here a largely illiterate rural community), and must take into account their traditional beliefs, customs and ability to comprehend. In the absence of literacy and television, the shadow play is appropriate for mass education. Repetition is necessary as with the passage of time the learned responses decreased. The educator must also be sensitive to change as it appears that the younger generation appear to be losing interest in this type of folk art.

GENERAL COMMENTS

The rheumatic problems of developing countries are similar to those of industrialized countries, if one considers that the younger age of the population is offset by the increased incidence of complaints relating to physical labor, or that many tropical diseases (*see* Chapters 15–17) cause rheumatic symptoms. Clearly any intervention or educational effort must target the diseases peculiar to the region.

REFERENCES

1. Darmawan J, Valkenburg HA, Muirden KD, Wigley RD. Epidemiology of rheumatic complaints in rural and urban populations in Indonesia. A WHO–ILAR COPCORD study, Stage I, Phase II. Ann Rheum Dis. 1992; 51:525–528. SEAPAL Bull. 1986; 6–7
2. Bjelle A, Muirden KD. Handbook for Primary Health Care Workers. Geneva, World Health Organization (in press)
3. Darmawan J, Muirden KD, Wigley RD, Valkenburg HA. Arthritis community education by leather puppet (wayang kulit) show play in rural Indonesia (Java). Rheumatol Int. 1992; 12:97–101
4. Suzuki S. Conjunctivitis due to cultivation work observed among Indonesian peasants. Proceedings of the 10th Asian Conference on Occupational Health, Singapore, 1982; pp. 187–192
5. Dickerson OB. Practical ergonomics. In Zenz C, ed., Developments in Occupational Medicine. Chicago, Year Book Medical Publishers, 1980, pp. 159–167
6. Darmawan J, Valkenburg HA, Muirden KD, Wigley RD, Euldering F. Nodules of shouldergirdle in 2 Indonesian villages. Rheum Int. (in press)
7. Lawrence JS. Rheumatism in Populations. London, Heinemann, 1977, pp. 80–81
8. Wigley RD, Manahan L, Muirden KD, Caragay R, Pinfold B *et al.* Rheumatic disease in a Philippine village II: WHO-ILAR-APLAR COPCORD study, phases II and III. Rheum Int. 1991; 11:157–161
9. Dekker JL, Healey LA, Skeith MD. Ethnic variation in serum uric acid: Filipino hyperuricemia, the result of hereditary and environmental factors. Population studies in rheumatic diseases. Proc. 3rd International Symposium. 1959, p. 336
10. Wigley Rd, Prior IAM, Salmond C, Stanley D, Pinfold B. Rheumatic complaints in Tokelau. II. A comparison of migrants in New Zealand and non-migrants. The Tokelau migrant study. Rheumatol Int. 1987; 7:61–65
11. Darmawan J, Valkenburg HA, Muirden KD, Wigley RD. The epidemiology of gout and hyperuricaemia in a rural population of Java. J Rheumatol. 1992; 19:1595–1599
12. Darmawan J, Valkenburg HA, Muirden KD, Wigley RD. The epidemiology of rheumatoid arthritis in Indonesia. Br J Rheumatol. (in press)
13. Morimoto I. Attrition lesions of articular cartilage in Japanese knee joint due to formal sitting and squatting. J Anthrop Soc. Nippon. Suppl. 1982; 90:163–176
14. Wigley RD. Placebo and time therapy: Can they be used in rehabilitation research. Clin Rehabil. 1987; 1:47–52
15. Chronic disease control program. WHO, Regional office, Manila, 1990

31. EDUCATION IN DEVELOPED AND DEVELOPING NATIONS

Kenneth D. Muirden

GLOBAL PATTERNS

During the past century, there has been a dramatic decline in infant mortality and an improvement in the likelihood of reaching old age. In India, for example, life expectancy has risen from around 20 years to over 55 years[1]. As in Europe and other developed nations, this increase in life expectancy has been made possible by a decline in lethal infections, public health initiatives and improved nutritional status. An increased lifespan is also attributable, albeit in a less tangible fashion, to cultural and institutional changes and socioeconomic development, which results in less crowded housing, improved transportation and communication networks. Possibly more significant in this regard, has been an increase in literacy and education, in particular that of women who have enjoyed the benefits of increased autonomy. Indeed, low mortality rates are more related to a high level of literacy in women, as occurs in China, than to a high income or number of physicians per capita[1]. The schooling *per se* appears to be less important for the specific knowledge it imparts, than for reorienting a person from traditional to more cosmopolitan sources of knowledge. Education impacts not only on knowledge and skills, but more importantly, on attitudes[2] about, for example the potential controllability of disease(s), ultimately overriding a commonly held prejudice that little can be done to extend life span.

The decline in mortality from infections has been offset in many societies by a rise in the so-called 'diseases of affluence'. Whilst obesity is considered a risk factor for osteoarthritis of the knee joint[3], and gout can be associated with cultural changes including over-indulgence in food and alcohol[4], the label of 'affluence' is hardly appropriate for most rheumatic complaints. Moreover, it has been reported that hypertension and other cardiovascular diseases, diabetes mellitus and chronic lung conditions, back pain and several forms of arthritis, traditionally regarded as diseases of affluence, vary inversely with years of formal education in the USA[5]. The relative odds of developing any of these diseases range from 3:1 to 6:1 for individuals with less than 9 years versus those with more than 12 years of formal education, a finding not explained by differences in age, sex, race or smoking[5]. Lower levels of formal education have been associated with a poorer clinical status and a higher mortality from rheumatoid arthritis[6], and these findings are supported by surveys in Italy and Great Britain[7]. This linking of health status and formal education is probably multifactorial in nature, and reflect behavioral variables including diet, smoking, income, occupation, capacity to cope with physical and emotional stress, social isolation, and efficiency in use of medical services[7]. Low education status restricts employment possibilities to (heavy) manual work, or at least non-sedentary work, and the development of back pain or other forms of arthritis would be expected to take a greater toll on these workers, and enlarge welfare statistics for subjects with limited education. The cumulative effect of several behavioral risk factors, for which a low education level is an important marker, could lead to a disease or increase disease severity. It would seem appropriate therefore for health policy developers to study whether increased expenditure on childhood education might improve community health by a cost effective use of progressively limited resources.

Public education and the media

Although reduction in morbidity and mortality from non-communicable diseases in developed nations has been less impressive than from infections, a number of successes can be claimed. Public education efforts have been largely responsible for substantial reductions in tobacco use and tobacco-related disease, motor vehicle accidents, cardiovascular disease and substance abuses, both legal and illegal.

Unfortunately, prospects are more uncertain in the Third World. Many Departments of Health now have high profile preventative medicine policies being disseminated at great cost to the public purse warning the community about acquired immune deficiency syndrome (AIDS), smoking, alcohol and drugs. Tobacco advertizing, seemingly focused on young females in many western countries, has been banned in some enlightened societies but not without some bitterly fought campaigns where the wealth of the tobacco industry and its ability to influence politicians has often been more than evident. The tobacco debate has generated an important message for public education, to wit: *it is not sufficient in itself to prove that a particular habit is damaging to health for the problem to be solved.* An estimated 80–90% of smokers acknowledge that it is a damaging habit[8]. Factors sustaining a (bad) habit, such as smoking may include an erroneous perception of limited personal vulnerability (the so-called 'invincibility syndrome'), cultural or religious fatalism, peer pressure, lack of motivation, and an image generated by the advertizing industry that smokers are sophisticated, glamorous, and mature. Public health advertisements can present the other side of the picture and it is felt that their impact on consumers is high[9]. In some countries community service announcements on television receive government sponsorship, but television advertizing is expensive and its cost cannot be added to a purchase price, since public health is an intangible 'product'. Nonetheless, television has the advantage of reaching many socially and physically disadvantaged people, those isolated by distance and the illiterate. The *'Quit For Life'* antismoking campaign, and the *'Life Be In It'* advertizement to encourage an active exercise program have had some success[10]. In a similar vein, public education programs for other diseases, for example, weight control to prevent diabetes mellitus and hypertension may also benefit knee osteoarthritis, back pain and other rheumatic complaints. Formal evaluation of the effect of these measures are clearly needed.

Medical reporting in the popular press is often sensationalist, biased and inaccurate; moreover even when a medical authority provides balanced information, the details may be shortened and/or amended. The ensuing heated debate may provoke further publicity, which can be counter productive in achieving an accurate health message. Unlike the press release or media interview, the paid advertisement gives the advertiser near complete control over content. Few doctors are media specialists or qualified as public educators and they should be prepared to accept professional advice on how to present a clear and distinct message. Occasional media workshops for doctors and health educators are often inadequate in this regard. The use of well-known sports or entertainment figures suffering from a particular disease, often proves far more effective that a battalion of more eloquent experts, in presenting a health message. Commercial advertisers are well aware of the need for ancillary promotional support to add substance to an advertizing campaign. The same applies to preventative medicine, were mass media methods together with a community infrastructural support works better than the use of either alone[10]. Billboard advertizing is hard to evaluate and posters in doctors waiting rooms or in community health centers may be more effective as they do not have to compete for space as they do in the street. Media health campaigns have frequently been of an *ad hoc* basis without longitudinal support and follow-up. Lack of co-ordination and too little preliminary market and consumer research limits the effectiveness of programs. In the UK, the Health Education Council supervises and funds advertizing activities and similar bodies exist elsewhere; the Arthritis Foundations can play an important role in public education (*see* below).

PUBLIC EDUCATION IN DEVELOPING COUNTRIES

The wayang shadow play

It is not clear how effective 'media based interventions' are to less literate and poorer communities. Some parts of the world are spared the pervasive influence of television and here special initiatives for purveying health messages are required. An example of what is possible using imagination, enthusiasm and perseverance is an 'arthritis community education' program organized by Dr John Darmawan (Chapter 30) in a rural area in central Java, Indonesia[11,12] using the traditional leather puppet shadow play.

The role of arthritis foundations and patient support groups

Public perceptions about rheumatic problems are haphazard at best, especially when one considers the popularity and variety of folk remedies, manipulations and special diets that are used in both developed and developing regions for the treat-

ment of these complaints. 'Arthritis Foundations, now active in many parts of the world, are playing a growing role in combating misinformation and various forms of ignorance. These organizations may sponsor 'Arthritis Weeks' and may obtain media coverage through the use of sports personnel, whose role is to get across a simple health message to the effect of '. . . its your body: move it or lose it'. These foundations produce booklets on diet and exercise, and may support a 'phone in' service to answer in a timely and accurate fashion, public inquiries related to prevention of specific rheumatic diseases and/or their sequelae. Recently in Australia, several women's magazines ran articles on post menopausal osteoporosis and its prevention, provoking a flood of requests for information. The Arthritis Foundation of Australia responded by providing health professionals, with a seminar covering aspects of the cause, prevention and treatment of osteoporosis.

The International League against Rheumatism (ILAR) has expressed concern that there is little co-ordination among these foundations especially with regard to the preparation of educational material. Pamphlets, booklets, fact sheets, electronic media programs including films and video tapes developed at considerable time and cost could be applicable to other countries and save expensive duplication of efforts. Consequently a central ILAR database for public education, material and programs has been set up under the direction of Professor Rodney Grahame at Guy's Hospital, London.

These foundations may also adopt the role of a political lobby group, a logical step, since they represent both the needs of patients and their families, as well as professional groups, which translates into a sizeable political force. Health professionals attached to arthritis foundations can provide exercise classes including water exercises, which can have a preventive role by, for example, increasing the strength, bone density, ease of movement in the elderly, as well as improve their mental state and self esteem. Such programs are not necessarily confined to the elderly. Advice can also be given in the course of these programs on accident prevention and this includes warnings about home hazards such as loose mats or wires and slippery floors.

Self-help groups are popular and, if they have some professional supervision, are of value for the disabled and for those who feel physically isolated. Although support groups for certain conditions, e.g. back pain, play a role in prevention, in others, e.g. systemic lupus erythematosus and scleroderma, the support group provides emotional support in dealing with potential consequences of a disease with an inexorable course.

Undergraduate and postgraduate medical education

The importance to health of preventive measures as a principle has been slow to make an impact on medical undergraduate training in many universities. In one survey, 30% of family physicians felt their training was inadequate in teaching behavioral health risks[13]. It has further been suggested that the learning environment for clinical medicine in a teaching hospital ward with emphasis on the cure of disease may need alteration to better emphasize prevention, primary care, epidemiology and risk assessment[14]. Clinical training and the teaching on wards often concentrates on rare conditions that require elaborate diagnostic and therapeutic modalities, while neglecting the social and preventive aspects of more common conditions. In many centers, didactics in rheumatic diseases may be by non-rheumatologists who are reluctant to discuss epidemiology, posture and ergonomic principles; nonetheless, this deficiency does not exonerate rheumatologists. The better use of adequately resourced preventive and primary care units located within teaching hospitals or in suburban or rural health

centers would help redress this problem. Here undergraduate and postgraduate students could receive continued exposure to prevention-orientated general practice medicine. In this setting, there are two obvious difficulties: one is to amplify and reinforce the primary care physicians' knowledge about developments in preventative medicine; the second is that changing patient behaviors requires time. One study suggests that brief intervention is effective in behavioral change in the order of 5–10% of subjects taking part in the educational activity[15]. The use of ancillary staff, such as practice nurses, and in developing countries, community nurses and primary health workers becomes necessary. Unfortunately, in a busy general practice, time constraints (and governmental reimbursement plans) are financial disincentives that may tempt a physician to prescribe an anti-inflammatory drug for an overweight, osteoarthritic patient rather than encourage behavioral changes such as weight loss, dietary moderation, exercise and stress reduction.

Support groups such as 'Weight Watchers' and water exercise health clubs can help but do not replace the role of the doctor. Surveys continue to indicate that most patients perceive their doctor to be the most reputable and desired source of health information[16]. However, community, factory and medical group practice nurses, given appropriate training, can play an important role in emphasizing preventive strategies to the public.

Together with a more imaginative curriculum for undergraduate and postgraduate education, substantial expertise in public health is clearly required for an optimal understanding of preventative medicine and clinical epidemiology. Education, identification of disease risk factors, and appropriate preventive measures requires rheumatologists trained in epidemiological techniques for implementation. An epidemiology training course in rheumatic diseases in Moscow in 1989 is an example. The announcement in 1990 of an ILAR-COPCORD Epidemiology Fellowship is a direct response to the need for experts, and these are now available at McMaster University, Canada, Manchester, England and in Newcastle, Australia.

The Role of the World Health Organization (WHO) and ILAR

Both WHO and ILAR have a strong overall commitment to disease prevention and are co-operating in a number of areas where education strategies are important. The production of manuals such as *'Pain in the Joints: A Practical Guide'* directed at problems of primary health care and a manual on *'Standard Survey Methods'* will fill important gaps as they are focused specifically for developing countries. The COPCORD studies[12] have collected data on rheumatic complaints and disability in both developing and developed countries in the Asia/Pacific Area.

WHO has recognized the importance of health promotion in the workplace[17]. The advantages include accessibility of large groups of people who do not have regular contact with health care providers, easy follow up of workers and the opportunity for continued reinforcement and encouragement of workers involved in these programs. The advantages to an organization that implements such programs include better staff morale and lower staff turnover with a reduction in factory worker training costs. The implementation of preventive strategies will require careful evaluation, review mechanisms and field testing. Despite potential advantages, there has been little attempt to evaluate the cost-effectiveness of health promotion programs in industry. The same applies to community measures. Such a task is difficult but not impossible as has been shown with the Wayang shadow play (*see* Chapter 30).

REFERENCES

1. Powles J. Global patterns and disadvantaged populations. In McNeil JJ *et al.*, eds., A Textbook of Preventative Medicine. Melbourne, Edward Arnold, 1990, p. 238
2. Wright V, Harvey A. Rheumatology education in the late 20th century. Br J Rheumatol. 1989; 28:95–97
3. Hartz AJ, Fischer ME, Bril G *et al.* The association of obesity with joint pain and osteoarthritis in the HANES data. J Chronic Dis. 1986; 39:311–9
4. Stanhope JM, Prior IAM. The Tokelau Island migrant study. Alcohol consumption in two environments. N Z Med J. 1979; 19:419–421
5. Pincus T, Callahan LF, Burkhauser RV. Most chronic disease are reported more frequently by individuals with fewer than 12 years of formal education in the age 18–64, US population. J Chronic Dis. 1987; 40:865–874
6. Pincus TM, Callahan LF. Formal education as a marker for increased mortality and morbidity in rheumatoid arthritis. J Chronic Dis. 1987; 38:973–984
7. Pincus T. Editorial. Formal education level – a marker for the importance of behavioral variables in the pathogenesis, morbidity and mortality of most diseases. J Rheumatol. 1988; 15:1457–1460
8. Sanson-Fisher RW, Byles J. The role of health social science in preventative medicine. In McNeil JJ *et al.*, eds., A Textbook of Preventative Medicine. Melbourne, Edward Arnold, 1990, p. 284
9. Robinson P. The role of advertizing in preventative medicine. In In McNeil JJ *et al.*, eds., A Textbook of Preventative Medicine. Melbourne, Edward Arnold, 1990, pp. 304–315
10. Egger G, Fitzgerald W, Frape G *et al.* Results of large scale media anti-smoking campaign in Australia: North Coast 'Quit for Life' program. Br Med J. 1983; 287:125–1128
11. Darmawan J, Muirden KD, Wigley RD *et al.* Arthritis community education by puppet (wayang kulit) shadow play. Rheum Int. 1992; 12:97–101
12. Manahan L, Caragay R, Muirden KD, Wigley RD, Valkenburg H A. Rheumatic pain in a Philippine village; a WHO–ILAR COPCORD study. Rheumatol Int. 1985; 5:149–153

13. Orleans CT, George LK, Houpt JL, Brodie KH, Health promotion in primary care: a survey of US family practitioners. Prev Med. 1985; 14:636–47

14. Committee of Inquiry into Medical Education and Medical Workforce (the Doherty Committee). Australian Medical Education and Workforce into the 21st Century. AGPS, Canberra, 1988

15. Johns MB, Hovell MF, Ganiats T *et al*. Primary care and health promotion: a model for preventive medicine. Am J Prev Med. 1987; 3:346–355

16. Ford AS, Ford WS. Health education and the primary care physician: the practitioners perspective. Soc Sci Med. 1983; 17:1505–1512

17. WHO Health Promotion For Working Population. WHO Tech Rep Series No. 765, 1988

32. GENERAL CONCLUSIONS

Richard Wigley

This review has revealed many opportunities for the primary prevention of the ubiquitous rheumatic diseases which, broadly defined to include all musculoskeletal discomfort, afflict the majority of individuals in all communities at some time in their lives.

Medical knowledge has expanded with increasing rapidity this century so that it has become less practicable for those providing health services to be familiar with all the information required for every type of problem. In the Middle Ages, the barber surgeons were separated from the drug prescribing physicians. This division was perpetuated by Henry VIII in England in the sixteenth century with the formation of a Royal College of Surgeons and a separate Royal College of Physicians. General practitioners were expected to train in both fields. Variations on this theme apply in almost all countries but both groups have further subdivided either by different anatomical regions or, for ease of administration of institutions, by age groups, e.g. pediatrics and geriatrics.

Rheumatic diseases affecting the musculoskeletal system are of interest to rheumatologists, physical medicine specialists (psychiatrists, or physicians specialized in rehabilitation medicine) and orthopedic surgeons, and form a large part of the work of occupational physicians and general practitioners as well as physiotherapists occupational therapists, nurses psychologists, sociologists and other related professions. This division of interest has not helped in the presentation of a clear picture of the problem to the public and to legislators. Lay bodies such as the Arthritis and Rheumatism foundations have a valuable function in this respect.

As most rheumatic complaints are minor or transient, and relatively few are seriously disabling or potentially fatal, they are of more concern to primary care providers than to administrators and politicians. Diseases with a higher public profile related to the strong emotive effect of mortality attract more research, care, legislation and preventive efforts than the less dramatic but often more distressing rheumatic causes of prolonged suffering and disability. Because the interests of these planners of health care often lie in the concrete and tangible, such as mortality data and provision of hospital bed care, they tend to overlook the burgeoning need for relief of chronic pain and disability in the wider community. These chronic painful and disabling disorders not only impair the quality of life of the affected individual but place a heavy social and economic burden on family and friends. This may be intolerable leading to marital breakdown and loss of work with heavy costs to the social services and general economy. Traditionally then, less emphasis has been placed on research into causation (that would provide the information necessary for prevention), although public health specialists are now turning increasing attention to quality of life in allocating sparse resources to health care.

The economic cost of prevention and care is balanced against the probability of, and length of survival from a prevention program and the likelihood of enjoyment of life (versus suffering) during that period. On such a score, prevention of rheumatic fever would rate much higher than open heart surgery to repair rheumatic valve damage later in life. Likewise hip replacement would take priority over treatment of cancer in providing virtually certain improvement in quality of life over a longer period.

Pessimism among all professional groups towards the prospects of primary prevention and control of the rheumatic disorders has led to further inaction so that many of the lay public have lost faith in western medicine and resort to a vast array of 'alternative care providers', ranging from shamanistic African witch doctors to eastern herbalists, manipulators, purveyors of allegedly natural health foods and charlatans. The apparent success of these is guaranteed by the high rate of spontaneous recovery (regardless of treatment used), albeit often temporary, and the scientifically measurable faith healing effect in painful and/or emotionally disturbing complaints. This is further compounded by the fact that normal activity, especially when carried to extreme without training and preparation leads to musculoskeletal discomfort ('good' pain), which is nature's feedback control to prevent overuse, abuse or injury. These ubiquitous problems can obscure the more serious disorders in need of control. Debate has arisen concerning the need to compensate those so afflicted for loss of work capacity (*see* Chapters 7 and 30). It is notable that in developed countries, pain has not been considered a necessary and inevitable accompaniment of work for more than a century.

Narrow spectrum specialists or 'superspecialists' contribute most of the published literature, making it difficult to obtain a general view of the problems at hand. Psychiatrists, who are referred only cases with psychiatric symptoms, may extrapolate that all such symptoms are psychiatric in origin; neurologists may attribute disease to nerve entrapment or focal dystonia; orthopedists will lean to tenosynovitis and carpal tunnel syndrome; sociologists will impugn external social stresses; psychiatrists and manipulators will think that all arises in the neck; occupational physicians and ergonomists will look for mechanical causes in the work place and so on. Only the generalist and the epidemiologist take the broad view, considering appropriately all aspects of the problem.

Rhetorically, one might ask whether is it worse to die at 60 of cancer or to survive for 50 years in constant pain, dependent on others? Neither consideration is pleasant. Here we have presented in a single volume the currently known measures for preventing or ameliorating the effects of rheumatic diseases, with the hope that both health administrators and the public will apply these principles and to stimulate more research in this area.

GLOBAL CONTROL

Integration of preventive effort across artificial specialty barriers is clearly important (Tables 1 and 2). Human afflictions do not fit neatly into organ or age groups. Preventive measures appropriate for one health problem are often appropriate for others, and thus represent a cost-effective strategy. If a preventive measure such as weight control is a well established need for other reasons such as diabetes mellitus, then intervention is justified. Thus, while evidence that obesity predisposes to osteoarthritis of the knee is not strong, weight reduction is clearly advantageous for diabetes mellitus and coronary disease so

Table 1 This table summarizes the possibilities for control of infectious causes of rheumatic disease

Source	Causative agent	Disease	Control program
Water control			
	dysentery;	Reiter's disease	clean water
	salmonellae	typhoid; food poisoning	clean water
	enteroviruses	myalgia; paralysis	clean water
	cercaria	shistosomiasis	sewerage, water
	dracunculus	dracontiasis	control cyclops
	fluoride	fluorosis	water supply
Food control			
	shigellae	Reiter's disease	hot food
	salmonellae	food poisoning	tot food
	enteroviruses	poliomyelitis	vaccines
	hepatitis B	hepatitis	STD control
			vaccines
Air (droplet infection)			
	streptococci	rheumatic fever	housing, penicillin
	rubella virus	rubella arthritis	vaccine
	parvovirus	polyarthritis	nil
	meningococci	arthritis	isolation, penicillin
	pneumococci	pneumonia	antibiotic
	tuberculosis	TB joints	BCG; contact,
			milk pasteurization
Insect control			
mosquitoes	Ross River	endemic polyarthritis	tropical
	Chikungunya	endemic polyarthritis	tropical
	Onyongyong	endemic polyarthritis	tropical
	Mayaro	endemic polyarthritis	tropical
	Sindbis	endemic polyarthritis	tropical
	Dengue	acute myositis	tropical
	Filaria	elephantiasis	tropical
flies	Filaria	loiasis	clear bush
	Onchocerca volvulus	onchocerciasis	spray rivers
ticks	Spirillum	Lyme disease	ticks
	Rickettsia	tick typhus	vaccines
Reduviid bugs	trypanosomes	South American Chagas	local DDT
		disease	house spray
Animals			
goats	*Brucella melitensis*	brucellosis	testing and slaughter
cattle	*Brucella bovis*	brucellosis	testing and slaughter
cattle	mycobacterium TB	tuberculosis	testing and slaughter
possums	mycobacterium TB	tuberculosis	possum control
badgers	mycobacterium TB	tuberculosis	badger control
deer	*Borrelia burgdorferi*	Lyme disease	ticks; antibiotic
pigs	cestodes	onchocerciasis	cooking meat
	Trichinella spiralis	trichinosis	cooking pork
birds	fungal infections		
	psittacosis	myalgia	treat birds

Table 1 (continued)

Sexually transmitted disease			
	various	Reiter's disease	STD, food, water
	various	spondylarthropathy (SARA)	STD, food, water
	chlamydia	urethritis	STD
	chlamydia	lymphogranuloma I	STD
	Treponema pallidum	syphilis	STD
	HIV virus	AIDS	STD
Contact	*Treponema pertenue*	yaws	penicillin
	M. leprae	leprosy	contacts, treat
Skin	staphylococci	septic arthritis	skin hygiene
Needles (needle stick, transfusion, dialysis)			
	HIV	AIDS, addiction	sterility
	hepatitis B	hepatitis arthritis	sterility

general advice on weight control is recommended without need for complex evaluation. There are many other situations in which a number of objectives can be achieved by a single measure.

Integrated disease control

Weight control, is advantageous in preventing diabetes, atheroma, heart disease strokes, hypertension, as well as gout and probably osteoarthritis of the knees and trochanteric bursitis. The general control of bacterial, virus and parasitic diseases will reduce related rheumatism which is only one of the many manifestations of these infections. The provision of safe water and food supplies, the elimination of insect vectors and animal carriers and the avoidance of direct infection as with the sexually transmitted diseases universally demands high priority. The prevention of transmission by transfusion and needle stick injuries is important in control of HIV and hepatitis B infection and probably other diseases.

Work-induced symptoms due to overload of limbs and/or the back and neck, fractures and other injuries are preventable now. The prevention of accidents generally in the home, at work, in sport are preventable to a degree. Accidents on the roads can be controlled by controlling road traffic and alcohol abuse, reducing joint and back injuries leading to long term musculoskeletal disability. Alcohol control will also reduce accidental joint injury and reduce risk of gout, osteoporosis and liver disease. Although the hazard of smoke inhalation have long been recognized, it is only now that antismoking campaigns are beginning to have an impact. Those interested in reducing the morbidity of rheumatic diseases should not be frustrated if these programs do not take effect quickly. Tobacco control, in addition to reducing malignancies and respiratory diseases (and by extension, hypertrophic pulmonary osteoarthropathy), may also reduce back pain and probably osteoporosis. Although smoking is associated with lower weights, any possible advantage is far outweighed by the overt dangers of smoking with respect to cancer of the lung, mouth, larynx and bladder, bronchitis and emphysema and even sudden infant death syndrome (SIDS)[1]. Estrogens used post menopausally reduce the risk of both heart disease and osteoporosis. A low calcium intake in youth may

Table 2 This table summarizes control measures for dietary, chemical and physical causes of rheumatic problems including accidents and overuse syndromes

Source	Causative agent	Disease	Control program
Diet	urate	gout	diet
	calcium excess	calcinosis	excess vitamin D or calcium
	wheat fungus	Kashim–Beck disease	rice diet selenium
	food excess	obesity diabetes osteoarthritis	diet, exercise
	thiamine deficit	beriberi	unpolished rice
	urate, alcohol	gout	diet, drug control
	hypervitaminosis A	DISH	
	L-tryptophan	eosinophilia myalgia	remove drug
	maize oil	toxic oil syndrome	demarket oil
Surgery	adverse effects	i.e. spinal fusion	monitor outcome
	silicone breast implants	scleroderma	discontinue
	bowel shortening	polyarthritis	discontinue
Iatrogenic	diuretics	gout	monitor
	antiepileptics	SLE	monitor
	steroids	osteoporosis	monitor
Chemical	industrial chemicals	sclerodactyly	vinyl chloride
Accidents	joints	osteoarthritis	workplace design
	soft tissue	chronic pain	architecture
	back pain		ergonomics
Overuse	muscles	strains	repetition
	tendons	tenosynovitis	sustained load
	bursae	bursitis	overload
	diffuse	?muscle pain	ergonomics
Sport	fractures	joint injury	protective gear
	strains		rule changes
	overuse injuries		presport training
Legal measures	compensation	increases the sick role	feed-back prevention to compensation authority regulate load limits to anthropometry identify susceptibles

predispose to osteoporosis later in life in addition to causing rickets and bone and joint deformity. Various chemical and physical agents causing rheumatic problems may also affect other systems so must be included in any global prevention program.

It is increasingly accepted that social stresses and fatigue contribute to rheumatic symptoms as well as psychiatric problems and affect other systems such as the heart, blood pressure and gastrointestinal tract so a complete control plan would include education in stress management. Education on these global matters can be delivered in schools as well as to the general public. Technical education can be used to provide education on the prevention of work related overuse syndromes, i.e. in writing and keyboard technique and the use of tools.

Local control
Many rheumatic complaints occur in a particular locality or in a few susceptible individuals. For instance work related problems will depend on immediate circumstances in different factory settings so that effective control will depend on experts such as ergonomists and factory inspectors giving advice on the actual work site or factory. Exposure to chemicals from factory effluent, manufacturing processes, excess fluoride in a water supply and exposure to fungal toxin and/or giving selenium supplements in Kashin–Beck disease are examples of local or regional problems. In these educational effort will need to be locally directed.

There is a long list of rheumatic disorders that can result from prescribed drugs. These are all preventable though the frequency of such adverse effects is usually so low that a calculated risk may be considered to be justified by the benefit gained. This is important in medical education and in fully informing the public of the risks involved.

Multivariant causation
Many problems concern the individual and his total social and physical environment requiring a (w)holistic multifactorial approach to control. Obsession with single cause hypotheses can obscure the view of researchers to possible disease control by a multi-disciplinary approach. For instance, providing an expensive ergonomically ideal work station will not help if the many other factors involved are not attended to in occupational overuse syndrome.

DIRECTION OF FUTURE RESEARCH
Clearly, finely focused laboratory research to identify removable causes of disease must continue but such expensive research should be directed by population needs established by broadly based epidemiology. It is also the task of the epidemiologist with public health specialists and administrators to identify risk factors and to initiate intervention studies and to evaluate the effectiveness and economic feasibility of these and to consider possible educational, regulatory and legislational measures.

Legislation
There is scope for regulation i.e. mandatory reporting of disease to maintain case registers for disease control and weight lifting regulations but some legislation can impede primary and secondary prevention.

Workers compensation law for instance can, in some countries such as the USA, be such a slow process that people are encouraged to act out the sick role for prolonged periods so delaying rehabilitation while the expensive legal process consumes half of the benefit intended for the subject. Impairments, defined by the American Medical Association[2] as acceptable for compensation are limited to visible or measurable defects and limitation of range of motion of joints without distinction between limitation of active or passive motion of joints is regarded as significant in joint disability though loss of active movement and so function, is counted only in the neurological section. This gives rise to major anomalies since, as explained in Chapter 28, some visible impairments do not cause a handicap and many conditions causing disability and handicap do not have visible physical features. These would be included as disabled and/or handicapped using the more realistic WHO classification of impairments, disabilities and handicaps[3]. In the final assessment it is the handicap or limitation of work capacity which are most important for the individual[2].

The exaggerated sums claimed provide an incentive to maximize complaints. In the case of occupational overuse syndrome (RSI) in Australia the associated anxiety appears to have aggravated the symptoms making management and control much more difficult. A heavy handed government counter attack set a legal precedent making it difficult for the deserving to be compensated[4].

In the UK, the law has distorted reality by allowing some diagnoses to be acceptable for compensation whereas others only succeed at great expense since employer negligence has to be proved. For instance only one occupational overuse syndrome case has been compensated as employer negligence was established. Legal costs make this precedent unlikely to be successfully followed[5].

The New Zealand no fault system which depends on partial wage replacement rather than delayed large lump sum payments, favors early resumption of employment and prevention by minimizing media encouraged public anxiety. However, though lump sum payments, usually after two years are small they can encourage sick behavior.

The rules of law differ strikingly from those of clinical science in that far reaching conclusions are drawn, precedents are set, from single cases. Selection of the test case and the expertise of witnesses may be heavily biased[4]. The clinical researcher must select a representative sample of adequate number taking great pains to avoid bias if his findings are to be applied to other cases and his adversaries must take equal pains if they are to successfully challenge his conclusions.

Positive health

The concept of positive health being the ultimate goal as opposed to the idea that health is the absence of disease, is worth considering in the context of rheumatic problems. Most of the ingredients required for perfect health are needed in adequate but not excessive quantities. For instance dietary requirements all have minimum and maximum recommended levels. Increasing intake without limit as would seem to be advocated by some 'natural health food and vitamin' promoters either have no beneficial effect at high dosages or may have harmful effects, except on the purse of the purveyor. The current vogue for physical fitness does appear to lead to improved well being but again there is abundant evidence that, carried to excess, harmful effects arise such as amenorrhea and osteoporosis in young women athletes and the many sports induced overuse syndromes.

Accepting universal mortality as inevitable and that the remarkable human machine does not last for ever and that the final breaking down process is uncomfortable, especially in the joints, the concept of perfect positive health can only be real for a limited period. The WHO's goal of 'Health for All by the Year 2000' more realistically aims to achieve the maximum availability of health care to as many as possible by 2000 AD.

Finally, although prevention of some diseases such as rheumatoid arthritis is not currently possible and for others further research is needed to make prevention possible with available resources, primary prevention is feasible and affordable for many rheumatic complaints now and should be applied where possible in an integrated health program or otherwise tailored to affected countries, localities, work scenes, homes or individuals.

REFERENCES

1. Mitchell EA, Scragg R, Stewart AW *et al*. Results from the first year of the New Zealand cot death study. N Z Med J. 1991; 104:71–76
2. Guidelines to the Evaluation of Permanent Impairment. 3rd edn. Chicago, American Medical Association, 1990
3. WHO International Classification of Impairments, Disabilities and Handicaps. Geneva, World Health Organization, 1981
4. Reid J, Reynolds L. Requiem for RSI: the explanation and control of an occupational epidemic. Med Anthropol Q. 1990; 21:162–190
5. Willhoft T. Repetitive strain injury. Law Soc Gazette. 1991; 32–34

Index